CLINICAL NEUROPSYCHOLOGY AND COST OUTCOME RESEARCH
A beginning

Psychology Press
New York and Hove

CLINICAL NEUROPSYCHOLOGY AND COST OUTCOME RESEARCH: A Beginning

Edited by

George P. Prigatano

Neil H. Pliskin

Psychology Press
Taylor & Francis Group
LONDON AND NEW YORK

First published 2003 by Psychology Press, Inc.

Published 2014 by Psychology Press,

27 Church Road, Hove, East Sussex BN3 2FA, UK

711 Third Avenue, New York, NY 10017

First issued in paperback 2014

Psychology is an imprint of the Taylor & Francis Group, an informa business

Library of Congress Cataloging-in-Publication Data

Clinical neuropsychology and cost outcomes research : a beginning / [edited by] George P. Prigatano and Neil H. Pliskin

p. cm.

Includes bibliographical references and index.

ISBN 978-1-84169-025-4 (hbk)

ISBN 978-0-41576-357-8 (pbk)

1. Clinical neuropsychology. 2. Outcome assessment (Medical care)—Cost effectiveness. I. Prigatano, George P. II. Pliskin, Neil H.

[DNLM: 1. Neuropsychology—economics. 2.Cost and Cost Analysis—methods. 3. Nervous System Diseases—economics. 4. Nervous System Diseases—therapy. 5. Outcome Assessment (Health Care) WL 103. 5C6404 2002]

RC386.6.N48 C5273 2002

616.8—dc21 2002017806

Dedication

This book is dedicated to practicing clinical neuropsychologists, who are increasingly asked to justify the usefulness of their clinical work and to provide documentation regarding the cost effectiveness of their services and the impact those services have on health-care economics.

CONTENTS

PART II. CEREBRAL VASCULAR DISORDERS

PART III. NEOPLASMS

PART IV. DEMENTIA

PART V. EPILEPSY

PREFACE

There are three keys to the survivability and success of clinical neuropsychology as a profession in today's health-care environment. First, clinical neuropsychologists must continue to strive at integrating important insights from the neurosciences into their practice. Expanding the scientific basis of clinical neuropsychology is crucial for its contributions to the health-care system. Second, practicing clinical neuropsychologists must be constantly alert to factors that may improve services for the patients they serve. This includes being vigilant regarding how patients and families experience the services they receive and their degree of satisfaction with those services. A third, but frequently neglected area, focuses on the need of clinical neuropsychologists to demonstrate to health-care economists, government officials, and third-party payers the value of their services. As this book addresses, value has both subjective and objective markers. At times, value can be measured directly in terms of dollars saved, but most frequently it is measured by a health outcome that is not easily assessed by attaching a monetary figure. Nevertheless, clinical neuropsychologists must become acquainted with the broad area of cost outcome research in order to conduct studies that address this third dimension.

This book began with the intent of summarizing for clinical neuropsychologists and for those outside the field what, in fact, are the clinical utilities of various neuropsychological services. Second, we hoped to describe for clinical neuropsychologists concepts and methodologies that could be used when studying the economic and health-care benefits of their services. We realize this can be a daunting task, as most of us have only marginal training in economics, typically at the undergraduate level. We, therefore, consider this book a "beginning," not even an introduction to this rather complicated but important area of research.

Our hope is that clinical neuropsychologists, and particularly the membership of the National Academy of Neuropsychology (NAN), will benefit from reading this volume in numerous ways. We hope it will stimulate research projects that will aid neuropsychologists in demonstrating the utility of their work and the economic impact in our health-care environment. We also hope it will provide a resource neuropsychologists can turn to when explaining to others exactly what their work is about and how they are attempting to go about measuring its impact in our health-care environment. Finally, we hope it will consolidate useful clinical information for practicing clinical neuropsychologists.

When we began this project, we were fully aware that there were few empirical studies that dealt directly with such questions as the cost-effectiveness of the neuropsychological examination or neuropsychologically oriented rehabilitation. Nevertheless, we knew we had to begin somewhere. Initially, some potential publishers of this book declined to support the project for fear there was not enough empirical evidence to devote a book to this topic. We hope the readership will find those publishers wrong in their judgment. There is, in fact, a great deal of information available that indirectly bears on this important topic. It is true there are very few studies that directly measure the cost–outcome of our work, but the existing database provides a springboard for beginning research in this area. It is the intent of this book to provide such a beginning for clinical neuropsychologists.

As editors of this project, we wish to thank the 1998 and 1999 board of directors of NAN, who supported the idea of this book and authorized funds to help make it a reality. We also thank the Barrow Neurological Institute at St. Joseph's Hospital and Medical Center; Robert F. Spetzler, M.D., its director; Shelley A. Kick, Ph.D.; Eve DeShazer; and Judy Wilson for their economic, editorial, and secretarial help on this project. Special thanks also to Jerry Sweet, Ph.D., for his exceptionally helpful review of an earlier version of this manuscript.

The NAN membership will also note that this book carries with it an opportunity to obtain continuing educational credits (see the Appendix). We are hopeful that the book will provide valuable information and that clinical neuropsychologists can obtain continuing education credits in a cost-efficient manner.

Finally, we would like to express our special thanks to Alison Mudditt, of Psychology Press, for her support and belief in this project. Our organization should not forget the dedication of Psychology Press to this venture, as it indeed carries with it some risk, but we hope considerable benefit.

George P. Prigatano
Neil H. Pliskin
Phoenix, Arizona

CONTRIBUTORS

Editors/Authors

George P. Prigatano, Ph.D.
Barrow Neurological Institute
St. Joseph's Hospital and Medical Center
Phoenix, AZ

Neil H. Pliskin, Ph.D.
University of Illinois College of Medicine
Chicago, IL

Authors

Deborah Koltai Attix, Ph.D.
Duke University Medical Center
Durham, NC

Jeffrey Barth, Ph.D.
University of Virginia School of Medicine
Charlottesville, VA

Brian Bell, Ph.D.
University of Wisconsin
Madison, WI

Yehuda Ben-Yishay, Ph.D.
Rusk Institute
New York University Medical Center
New York, NY

Robert W. Butler, Ph.D.
Oregon Health Services Center
Portland, OR

Patricia S. Camplair, Ph.D.
Oregon Health Sciences University
Portland, OR

Scott B. Cantor, Ph.D.
University of Texas MD Anderson Cancer Center
Houston, TX

C. Munro Cullum, Ph.D.
University of Texas Southwestern Medical Center at Dallas
Dallas, TX

John DeLuca, Ph.D.
Kessler Medical Rehabilitation Research and Education Corporation
West Orange, NJ

Leonard Diller, Ph.D.
Rusk Institute
New York University Medical Center
New York, NY

Carl B. Dodrill, Ph.D.
University of Washington School of Medicine
Seattle, WA

Ruben J. Echemendia, Ph.D.
Pennsylvania State University
University Park, PA

Jonathan Evans, Ph.D.
Oliver Zangwill Centre for Neuropsychological Rehabilitation
Ely, UK

William D. Gouvier, Ph.D.
Louisiana State University
Baton Rouge, LA

Paul Lees-Haley, Ph.D.
Lees Haley Psychological Corporation
Woodland Hills, CA

Jill Hayes Hammer, Ph.D.
Louisiana State University School of Medicine
New Orleans, LA

Bruce Hermann, Ph.D.
University of Wisconsin
Madison, WI

Robert Heilbronner, Ph.D.
Independent Practice
Chicago, IL

Lorie A. Humphrey, Ph.D.
University of California at Los Angeles
Los Angeles, CA

T. Michael Kashner, Ph.D., JD, MPH
University of Texas Southwestern Medical Center at Dallas
Dallas, TX

Mark Lovell, Ph.D.
University of Pittsburgh Medical Center
Pittsburgh, PA

Muriel D. Lezak, Ph.D.
University of Oregon Health Science Center
Portland, OR

Roy Martin, Ph.D.
University of Alabama
Birmingham, AL

Douglas J. Mason, Ph.D.
Duke University Medical Center
Durham, NC

Stephen Mennemeyer, Ph.D.
University of Alabama
Birmingham, AL

Christina A. Meyers, Ph.D.
University of Texas MD Anderson Cancer Center
Houston, TX

Richard I. Naugle, Ph.D.
Cleveland Clinic Foundation
Cleveland, OH

Thomas A. Novack, Ph.D.
University of Alabama
Birmingham, AL

Mary Pepping, Ph.D.
University of Washington School of Medicine
Seattle, WA

Paul M. Richards, Ph.D.
Private Practice
Boulder, CO

Leslie D. Rosenstein, Ph.D.
Independent Practice
Austin, TX

Ronald M. Ruff, Ph.D.
University of California
San Francisco, CA

Paul Satz, Ph.D.
University of California at Los Angeles School of Medicine
Los Angeles, CA

Maria T. Schultheis, Ph.D.
New Jersey Medical School
Newark, NJ

Mark Sherer, Ph.D.
Methodist Rehabilitation Center
Jackson, MS

Lisa A. Sworowski, Ph.D.
University of Chicago Pritzker School of Medicine
Chicago, IL

Laetitia L. Thompson, Ph.D.
University of Colorado School of Medicine
Denver, CO

Kathleen A. Welsh-Bohmer, Ph.D.
Duke University Medical Center
Durham, NC

Barbara A. Wilson, Ph.D.
Medical Research Council
Cambridge, UK

Lanie Y. Zigler, Ph.D.
Private Practice
Phoenix, AZ

CHAPTER 1

George P. Prigatano

Health-Care Economics and Clinical Neuropsychology

Introduction

America's ideals and its economy are interrelated. The pursuit of life, liberty, and happiness implies the enjoyment of good health. Numerous studies have documented the obvious point that impaired health is readily associated with unhappiness (see Csikszentmihalyi, 1999). But what is the cost of "good health," and who is to pay for it? Kaplan (1999) noted that for the last 30 years economists have expressed concern about the rising costs associated with health care in America. He noted that almost 15% of the U.S. gross domestic product (GDP) is spent on health care, "while no other country in the world spends more than 10%" (p. 160). Moreover, economists question whether the rising health-care costs are actually associated with better health status (Gold, Siegel, Russell, & Weinstein, 1996).

Certain statistics raise the suspicion that the increased cost of medical care is, at least in part, related to poor business practices. For example, Stein and Foss (1995) compared the annual rate of change in "output, prices, and employment" between health-care delivery services and all private industry in the United States between 1977 and 1992. During that time the domestic output of all private industries grew at a rate of 2.6%, compared to 2.4% in the health industry. Yet prices for health industry services and products increased more than 8%, whereas "all domestic private industries grew at a 5% rate" (p. 236). Employment-compensation costs also increased dramatically compared to the private sector. Were Americans paying more but getting less compared to other services they were receiving?

Part of the problem in answering this question is that the health-care service arena had insufficient data to counter attacks on its business practices and to demonstrate that the health-care services provided to Americans were needed and valued by the public. The rapid changes in reimbursement schedules, difficulties encountered in receiving "good" hospital care, and restrictions on seeing doctors that patients knew and trusted have resulted in America's dissatisfaction with changes imposed by policy makers interested in lowering the costs of health care but not in understanding what health-care consumers actually experience as a result of those changes.

Although the percentage of "other professional services" (including psychological services) accounted for 10% to 12% of health expenditures in 1993 (Stein & Foss, 1995), psychologists are being asked to justify their services and their associated fees. This book is the first major effort by clinical neuropsychologists to state the utility of their clinical services and to provide consolidated information regarding studying cost outcomes. Like many areas within the health-care delivery system, few systematic data are available on this important topic. Consequently, this text attempts to help clinical neuropsychologists learn how to demonstrate the economic value of their work. The book was conceptualized as a first major effort to help clinical neuropsychologists meet the challenges imposed by contemporary health-care economic policies and procedures.

□ Economics and Health Care

Economics is "the science that deals with the production, distribution, and consumption of wealth" (*Webster's*, 1983, p. 574). It attempts to apply statistics, mathematical models, research designs, and, to the degree possible, controlled observations to understand how money is used and saved; how expenditures flow from certain principles of supply and demand; and how various business practices influence the distribution of wealth.

In their discussion of the American economy, Stein and Foss (1995) noted that the GDP for the United States has grown dramatically since the late 1890s. Consumer spending has fueled much of the growth. They compared the distribution of consumption expenditures during 1963 and 1993, noting that the proportion spent on food decreased dramatically during this period. Apparently, this is a well-recognized economic principle. The more wealthy a nation is, the less it spends proportionately on food. During the same time, however, a greater proportion of the GDP was spent on medical care and transportation. Regarding the increase in medical expenditures, they commented as follows: "The rising share of medical care reflects higher incomes, more new but costly medical procedures and drugs, an aging population, and the increasing prevalence of medical insurance that weakens patients' incentives to economize on medical care" (Stein & Foss, 1995, p. 22). The notion that the mere presence of health insurance may result in overutilization of a given health-care service is referred to as the "problem of demand response" (see Frank & McGuire, 1999).

In addition to a greater proportion of the GDP being spent on medical care, an equally large portion is now spent on transportation. Americans are more mobile and use their health-care system perhaps to a greater degree than in the past. Although efforts have been made to reduce the cost of air travel and health-care services, the public seems unhappy with the imposed changes. The news is frequently filled with discussions of the problem of crowded airplanes, delays, the failure to provide meals on long flights, and the failure of the airline industry to consider consumer complaints seriously. Yet the airline industry continued to flourish until the attack on America on September 11, 2001.

Likewise, concerns about health-care costs have resulted in briefer hospitalization stays, less nursing coverage, less and restricted access to physicians, and long delays in getting authorization to see physicians for services. Americans have become more vocal and contentious about their dissatisfaction with health maintenance organizations (HMOs). Lawsuits filed and won against HMOs seem to be on the increase. The liability suits often include emotional distress as well as failure to provide adequate physical care. In fact, a journal has appeared that provides attorneys with information dealing solely with lawsuits filed against managed care organizations (i.e., *Mealey's Managed Care Liability Report*).

Considerable inequity also is inherent in our present system. A case in point follows: The medical director of an HMO denied clinical neuropsychological evaluations for young adult traumatically brain-injured (TBI) patients covered under their organizational care. However, when that medical director suffered a mild head injury, he arranged for his corporation to authorize a clinical neuropsychological examination by a clinical neuropsychologist who was out of the network. These arrangements reflected his perception that a clinical neuropsychologist would provide the most expert evaluation of his cognitive difficulties.

Despite the absence of statistics justifying the service for a large number of enrollees under their insurance policy, the medical director's "subjective" or personal perception revealed that, in fact, he considered the service important enough to get it for himself. This "subjective" side of health-care expenditures should also be monitored and not forgotten when the utility of our services, their costs, and the perceived and actual benefits of such services are studied. A growing literature has emerged around the topic of the impact managed care has had on the utilization of psychological testing in general and neuropsychological testing in particular. The reader is referred to several recent publications focusing on this topic including Groth-Marnat (1999); Kubiszyn, Finn, Kay, Dies, Meyer, Eyde, Moreland, and Eisman (2000); Maruish (2001); Norcross, Karg, and Prochaska (1997); Piotrowski (1999); Piotrowski, Belter, and Keller (1998); Stout (1997); Stout and Cook (1999); and Sweet, Moberg, and Suchy (2000).

□ Productivity and Standard of Living

Many practicing clinical psychologists and clinical neuropsychologists report that they must work several more hours each week than they once did to maintain their present income. As managed care policies have resulted in less financial reimbursement for health-care services in the United States, physicians report the same phenomenon. Managed care often is a misnomer for managed costs. How the quality and quantity of health-care services are related to their cost is the true question. Answering this question requires not only accounting and statistical skills but innovative ways of measuring the direct and indirect benefits (and costs) of neuropsychological services.

In the broad economic picture, of which health-care costs are only a portion, some basic economic ideas need to be considered. In a free enterprise economic system, three basic points are often made. First, "production is important because it determines income, and income determines consumption" (Junior Achievement, 1996, p. 82). Second, standard of living is measured in part by "the amount of goods and services available to citizens" (Junior Achievement, 1996, p. 82). Third, the average citizen's "piece" of the GDP is an index of the funds available within a country to purchase goods and services to increase or maintain the standard of living.

In the present health-care environment, clinical neuropsychologists must be very productive to generate an adequate income to keep themselves and their profession alive and healthy. These services must provide a higher standard of living for the people whom they serve without substantially increasing that proportion of the GDP devoted to health-care costs in this country. Squarely stated, these are the hard facts confronting our profession.

In the early 1990s, the apparent perception of many business and government leaders was that the U.S. economy needed to reduce health care costs to remain competitive in various international markets. Thus, managed care began to influence health care delivery services in the early and mid-1990s.

Our institution (St. Joseph's Hospital and Medical Center) was greatly affected by reimbursement patterns superimposed by managed care. By mid-1995, the Department of Clinical Neuropsychology within Barrow Neurological Institute (BNI), St. Joseph's Hospital and Medical Center, faced a major dilemma. Its billed services covered the overall cost of the department, but the percentage of revenue actually collected seriously jeopardized the survivability of the department. An accountant-oriented administrator simply asked the question: Could the revenues collected justify the maintenance of the Department of Clinical Neuropsychology? When the answer appeared to be no, that administrator took steps to eliminate all salaried positions for clinical neuropsychologists in that department.

The department, however, had been in existence for almost 10 years and had been productive from research, clinical, and teaching perspectives. Its services had been appreciated by the patients, families, and physicians who had requested those services. The director of the BNI (a physician) convinced hospital administrators that the Department of Clinical Neuropsychology should be maintained because the services these psychologists provided were important for the continuum of quality care for neurological patients. With this level of support, the department survived the economic crisis of the mid-1990s precipitated by managed care and its associated reduction in reimbursement. The department is now economically solvent in terms of productivity, and percentages of collections are improving. Barriers to collecting fees for services that were once approved by insurance companies have been identified progressively and handled in a businesslike manner. Consequently, salaried psychology positions have remained. Clinical neuropsychologists continue to provide services to patients and families and are encouraged to engage in research and educational activities.

From my perspective, the message of this story is that the "bean counter" mentality of given administrators can greatly damage a department of clinical neuropsychology. However, if that department has demonstrated its true utility from both scientific and clinical perspectives, then visionaries will support its maintenance during difficult times. In the long run, clinical neuropsychologists will be able to maintain their positions if they can demonstrate the value of their services unequivocally. This value often is a subjective perception on the part of the individuals receiving services, but it can have certain "objective" markers. It results from psychologists taking seriously the need to care for patients, to study the efficacy of their work, and to publish both positive and negative findings associated with their clinical and research efforts (Prigatano, 1999; 2000). With this approach, clinical neuropsychologists can and will survive the crisis imposed by the "managed care-managed cost" movement in the health-service industry in America.

In the present health-care environment, clinical neuropsychologists must continue to articulate the value and usefulness of their clinical services. They must measure that value from the consumer's perspective as well as from that of the physicians who refer those patients. They must further demonstrate that in some instances clinical neuropsychological services reduce other related health-care costs (thus reducing the percentage of the GDP devoted to health care).

These tasks require clinical neuropsychologists to become acquainted with a new vocabulary; new journals; new sources of information; and new research questions, methodologies, and measurements.

☐ A New Vocabulary for Clinical Neuropsychologists

Hargreaves, Shumway, Hu, and Cuffel (1998) have written a useful text that describes methods for assessing cost–outcomes in the field of mental health. The terminology they described is important for clinical neuropsychologists. From an economic perspective, they described four models for studying cost–outcomes associated with mental health care. Although clinical neuropsychology partially relates to mental health services, it also partially relates to general health services. Thus, their methodology and terminology have to be understood in terms of our own specialty.

Perhaps the first form of study that is driven from economic theory could be described as the study of *cost-efficiency*. In this case, the major goal is to minimize the cost of a given outcome. In business, many examples reflect this type of study. For example, suppose you are a builder and you want to construct a series of homes for $125,000 or less in a metropolitan area. Those homes would then be sold for $250,000. The question is how to keep the cost at $125,000 or less. An analyses of the cost of labor, materials, land, and so on would be necessary to determine how to produce a home for that amount of money. The economics are straightforward. The skill is in defining where costs can be cut to achieve a certain financial goal.

Applied to health care, the question can be reframed as follows. If the goal is to spend no more than $50,000 a year to rehabilitate a brain-dysfunctional patient to the point that he or she can return to work, what is the most cost-efficient manner of achieving this goal? Should money be spent for a day-treatment program, outpatient therapies, or a job coach? To answer this question, one must clearly understand the services one is buying and also the nature of the patient's needs to determine whether a certain form of therapy is appropriate for the patient. In this case, the choice of therapy may initially appear cost-efficient, but it may not necessarily prove to be cost-efficient in the long run. Demonstrating cost-efficiency is important for clinical neuropsychologists.

As Hargreaves et al. (1998) noted, "cost efficiency studies are usually not practical (in health care) because there is rarely sufficient evidence to demonstrate that treatment alternatives have equal treatment outcomes" (pp. 40–41). The advent of the case manager model attempted to apply a cost-efficiency mentality to the management of brain-dysfunctional patients. In this instance, however, it should be noted that the outcome is determined by many "patient variables" as well as by many "therapist variables." Consequently, cost-efficiency studies of the health care of patients who are typically seen by neuropsychologists are quite difficult to accomplish. However, there may be instances when this type of study is possible.

A second form of economic analysis has been referred to as *cost–benefit studies.* In this approach, cost and outcome are expressed in economic terms. For example, in nonhealth-care economics, one could study the cost of building a database for a retail merchandise company and calculate the dollars one would expect to save using a computer system rather than a manual monitoring system. One could show that activities such as inventory monitoring and producing payroll will result in substantially fewer errors and less cost to the employers if they purchase such a database system with appropriate computer software and hardware. Simple rules of accounting demonstrate the cost–benefit of such an approach, and many accounting firms flourish because of it.

Can this type of approach also be applied to health care? Hargreaves et al. (1998) noted that outcomes in the health-care area can seldom be examined only in terms of dollars because the services involve health, and health represents both physical and psychological well-being. Therefore, it can be extremely difficult to use a purely financial measure to evaluate outcomes. Consequently, strict cost–benefit studies can be especially difficult in the health-care arena.

A third type of economic analysis, which has gathered considerable promise in health care, is that of *cost-effectiveness.* Hargreaves et al. (1998) pointed out that "cost-effectiveness analysis, unlike cost benefit analysis, is used when both outcomes and costs are expected to differ. In cost-effective analysis, however, outcomes, or effectiveness, are measured in units that seem more natural than dollars" (p. 41). A perfect example of this statement, as applied to health care, is measurement of the cost-effectiveness of psychotherapy.

Miller and Magruder (1999) edited a text entitled *Cost-Effectiveness of Psychotherapy: A Guide for Practitioners, Researchers, and Policymakers.* In that text, Howard, Lueger, Martinovich, and Lutz (1999) made some important distinctions relevant to the practice of clinical neuropsychology. In our traditional, Western empirical approach to science, randomized controlled studies are the gold standard for determining if a treatment has an effect. We can refer to such studies as *efficacy studies.* Another type of question centers around the effectiveness of a given treatment when delivered by clinicians in the field, not necessarily by researchers conducting a controlled scientific investigation. Studies in health-care economics involve cost-effectiveness rather than efficacy. These studies focus on whether a given intervention provided by a typical clinician results in some measurable benefit to the patient or person who is being served.

Different models can be used when conducting such cost-effectiveness studies. In an informative example, Howard et al. (1999) reanalyzed Hans Eysenck's data, which previously criticized the value or the efficacy of psychotherapy. They noted the following:

> For example, a reanalysis of Eysenck's data (McNeilly & Howard, 1991) has qualified Eysenck's (1952) conclusion that spontaneous remission is as effective as psychotherapy. Indeed, it is, if a 2-year end point analysis is made of the Eysenck's data. As Figure 4.2 shows, psychotherapy accomplishes in 16 sessions what spontaneous remission does in 2 years. Half of psychotherapy patients are improved with 8 sessions, whereas the comparable rate of improvement under spontaneous remission conditions takes approximately 1 year. (p. 44)

This interesting analysis makes a poignant statement about careful assessment of what could be described as patient "improvement" and how it varies as a function of the number of psychotherapy sessions. It reveals important data that can escape scientific analysis but are extremely relevant when attempting to establish the clinical usefulness of a service in terms of affecting a person's standard of living. Throughout this text, examples are given of how cost–outcome analyses can be applied to problems that clinical neuropsychologists confront.

A fourth model for assessing the economic cost of clinical outcomes has been referred to as *cost–utility* studies. Hargreaves et al. (1998) noted the following:

> Cost utility analysis extends cost-effectiveness analysis by incorporating measures of the relevant importance of the multiple outcome domains. A variety of methods have been developed for quantifying preferences for, or "the utility" of different health outcomes. These methods yield numerical weights that can be combined with the original outcome measures to compute a single comprehensive outcome indicator. (p. 42)

The work of Kaplan (1999) has provided examples of how cost–utility studies can be used in health-care research and has considerable relevance for clinical neuropsychologists. Kaplan described various methods for measuring the quality of life, and one scale—referred to the "quality of well-being scale"—seems to hold considerable promise. It attempts to measure the relative value that persons served apply to different types of symptom reduction or different levels of both physical and psychological health. The methodology for establishing such psychometric instruments is complex. Considerable research is being performed to provide such metrics, which ultimately will have to be incorporated in clinical neuropsychological research.

A summary of the four major economic analyses used in assessing cost outcomes in a health-care environment is given in Table 1.1. Additional theoretical (and real) neuropsychological examples are presented. The four major analyses listed were discussed further by Drummond, O'Brien, Stoddart, and Torrance (1998).

Further Analysis of Cost-Effectiveness in Clinical Neuropsychology

Clinical neuropsychologists must understand the rationale behind cost-effectiveness analysis and how it is used by policy makers. Russell, Siegel, Daniels, Gold, Luce, and Mandelblatt (1996) noted that cost-effectiveness analysis is not a simple, straightforward procedure. The concept behind it is relatively simple; the actual methodology used can be debated (see "Introduction," Gold et al., 1996).

In its simplest form, cost-effectiveness analysis attempts to establish a ratio between the costs of a service divided by its outcome (the *cost-effectiveness analysis ratio*). How one calculates costs and how one calculates outcome can be narrow or broad. It can reflect the interest of a particular group or society as a whole. For example, the cost of a medical or health service can be measured purely in Medicare dollars spent for the services (reflecting the government's most immediate cost), or it can reflect supplementary insurance expenditures. It also can include costs associated with transportation to obtain the services as well as costs associated with lost income from being out of work to obtain the services. Obviously, the list can be extended.

Outcome can likewise be measured in many ways. Outcome measures can reflect medical outcomes such as the reduction of neural tube defects in a given population over time, the increase in life expectancy after cancer treatment, or the avoidance of predictable dementia after placement of a shunt for low-pressure hydrocephalus. It

TABLE 1.1. A Summary of Four Basic Cost Outcome Analyses That Could Be Used in Clinical Neuropsychology

Type of Cost Analysis	Design	Possible Clinical Examples: Outcome Desired	Cost of Services	Considerations
Efficiency (or minimization)	Costs of a service to produce an expected outcome	Identification of cognitive deficits indicative of early dementia	Neuropsych assessment: Option 1: (2 hrs., $300) Option 2: (4 hrs., $600) Option 3: (two separate testing sessions, 4 hrs. each; $1,200)	Odds of achieving desired outcome: Option 1, 70% Option 2, 90%† Option 3, 99%
Benefit	Cost of service in dollars compared to costs saved in dollars by providing the service	Reduce health-care costs following severe TBI	Holistic neuropsychological rehabilitation of TBI patients conducted in Denmark, 162,000 DKK/yr.	Public savings over 3.5 yrs. after rehabilitation, 190,400 DKK. Cost of program vs. savings, 28,200 DKK.††
Effectiveness	Cost of two or more treatments to produce similar clinical outcomes	Reduce irritability and enhance social integration after TBI	Service #1: 1–yr. psychotherapy, $7,000 Service #2: antidepressant medications alone for 1–yr., $2,000	Changes in ratings on the Katz Adjustment Scale for Irritability and Belligerence are compared to the cost of treatments. Number of friends counted before and after each treatment. The two treatments and the two outcomes are then compared on these relative measures and associated costs.

Utility	Cost and outcome of different services to impact some health-care problems	Improve quality of life of TBI patients. Reduce depression in family members of TBI patients Return TBI patients to gainful employment	1-yr. holistic neuro-psychologically oriented rehabilitation, $60,000 U.S.* versus cost of just paying disability benefits over 3 yrs.	Base outcomes on improved quality of life for TBI patients (Outcome Measurement Questionnaire). Reduced signs of depression in family members (Beck Depression Index). Maintenance of gainful employment 3 to 5 yrs. after treatment.‡

TBI = traumatic brain injury. * = estimated cost. †Most patients would be identified by Option 2; therefore, it provides the most cost-efficient outcome given the probability of success. ††Over 3.5 yrs this rehabilitation program demonstrated cost benefits. ‡This outcome measure could be measured in various subcomponents such as job satisfaction, reduction of psychiatric disability, dollars the patient paid in taxes, and reduction of disability benefits by workmen's compensation insurance.

also can reflect quality of life variables such as a decrease in depression and the enhancement of memory function. It can further include broader psychosocial variables such as the number of days the individual has been able to maintain work after rehabilitation (or surgery). And it can measure any reduction in disability payments following a certain form of medical or health intervention. Each investigator must struggle with which variables will be placed in the denominator and which will be placed in the numerator of this ratio. How each variable will be measured and weighted in the final analysis requires considerable skill and sophistication. Clearly, this can be a daunting task; nevertheless, some approach is needed to answer various policy maker's questions regarding what clinical neuropsychologists do and how it affects health outcomes and associated costs.

It should be kept in mind that in true cost-effectiveness analysis one is always comparing the cost–outcome of a certain form of care with the cost outcome of another form of care. That is, in strict cost-effective analysis one is comparing different types of outcomes with different associated costs. To understand how cost-effectiveness analysis is used in decision making, it is also important to keep in mind that at least two other issues are relevant to policy makers beyond this analysis. Policy makers ask questions such as these: *How serious is the health problem that is being addressed* (e.g., the management of a tension headache versus surgical resection to cure epilepsy)? *How effective is a given intervention in reducing the problem* (Russell et al., 1996, p. 7)?

These serious questions often have been answered by physicians and the public at large. However, political forces influence expenditures because vested interest groups can emphasize the importance of a certain health problem for a section of the American public (for example, the human immunodeficiency virus problem). The effectiveness of treatment is supposed to be determined by scientific investigations, which has driven the so-called *evidence-based medicine* movement into health-care practice. Here is where clinical neuropsychologists must become articulate when they perform studies. Besides carrying out methodologically sound studies of cost-effectiveness, they must articulate (and demonstrate) the seriousness of the problem they are evaluating as well as the effectiveness of an intervention that would modify or reduce the problem. To do so, clinical neuropsychologists must see the "big picture" of their work and be innovative about evaluating which variables should be in the denominator and which in the numerator of their cost-effectiveness analysis ratio. To do such research, however, clinical neuropsychologists must expose themselves to new journals and books outside the field of clinical neuropsychology, and develop new ways of thinking about how to measure the impact of their clinical and scientific work in health economic terms.

☐ New Journals for Clinical Neuropsychologists

The data collected relevant to cost outcome studies in health care can be found in a large array of journals. In the fields of neurology, psychiatry, clinical psychology, and clinical neuropsychology, a number of studies are being published relevant to cost–outcomes research in such journals as the *Archives of General Psychiatry, American Journal of Psychiatry, Acta Psychiatrica (Scandinavia), The New England Journal of Medicine, Neurology, Annals of Internal Medicine, Epilepsy, Journal of the American Geriatric Society, Dementia and Geriatric Cognitive Disorders, Journal of Geriatric Psychiatry, British Journal of Psychiatry, Journal of Clinical Psychology, Journal of Consulting and Clinical Psychology, Clinical Neuropsychologist, Professional Psychology: Research and Practice,* and the *Journal of the American Medical Association (JAMA).*

However, numerous papers in other journals that we seldom read ultimately bear on our work as well. These are the journals commonly read by health economists and policy makers. A perusal of the references listed in Hargreaves et al. (1998), Miller and Magruder (1999), and Gold et al. (1996) suggests that the following journals should become more common reading for neuropsychologists interested in cost–outcome studies: *American Journal of Managed Care; Health Economics; Health Policy; International Journal of Technology Assessment in Health Care; Human Resources; Journal of Health Politics, Policy and Law; Controlled Clinical Trials, Milbank Quarterly; Medical Decision-Making; Quality of Life Research; Medical Care; Health Services Research; Health Care Demand and Disease Management;* and *Health Affairs.* Other important journals in this area include *Health Care Finance Review, Journal of Health Care Finance,* and *Behavioral Health Care Tomorrow.*

By reading journals focused on health-care economics and policies, we will become more familiar with studies that affect the delivery of our services and familiarize ourselves with how to address questions commonly asked by health economists.

☐ New Sources of Information: Two Examples

To highlight how reading health-care economic journals opens new vistas for clinical neuropsychologists, a recent study is described. Rizzo et al. (1998) studied the costs of falls in the Medicare population. As people age, falls become quite common. In their data analysis, Rizzo et al. (1998) noted:

> the probability of incurring hospital costs increased monotonically with fall severity and that subjects that incurred one or more injurious falls were more than three times as likely to receive hospital care as were nonfallers and were more than 16 times as likely to receive nursing home care." (p. 1179)

Their estimate for just hospital costs for one injurious fall was almost $14,000. For an individual who had one noninjurious fall, the cost was less than $7,000. What differentiated an injurious from a noninjurious fall? Their data analysis clearly showed that the presence of mental impairment, as measured by a mental status examination, was related to whether individuals suffered injurious falls. The implication is that special management of elderly patients with cognitive impairments might result in fewer injurious falls which, in turn, would result in a substantial economic savings. Neuropsychologists must be aware of such data and design studies to demonstrate that both brief assessment and appropriate behavioral management in terms of cognitive assessment result in a substantial economic savings for Medicare patients—and therefore for the government.

Nowack (1997) also presented provocative data for clinical neuropsychologists interested in cost-effectiveness issues. Nowack discussed the costs associated with misdiagnosis of epilepsy. Substantial expenditures are associated with individuals with nonepileptic seizures who are diagnosed as having epilepsy. Nowack estimated that the cost of such misdiagnosis was somewhere between $650 million and $4 billion. Whether these figures are accurate is difficult to determine. They are, however, staggering. They suggest that if clinical neuropsychologists can help differentiate patients who have nonepileptic seizurelike events from those with true epilepsy, they may well save the health-care system millions of dollars. The chapter by Martin, Bell, Hermann, and Mennemeyer in this text partially addresses this important question.

By being aware of such studies, neuropsychologists can construct scientifically sound studies that demonstrate the potential financial impact of effective clinical neuropsychological work. The remainder of this book describes clinically useful aspects of our services and clarifies which existing data are relevant to the cost-effectiveness of our work. Equally important, each chapter suggests research ideas that may be helpful in conducting cost outcome research pertinent to the practice of neuropsychology.

Plan of Text

The following chapters discuss a select but representative sample of the types of services provided by clinical neuropsychologists to the various patient populations they serve. Each chapter has the following goals:

- Review relevant research concerning the state of knowledge related to a given problem area.
- Describe the utility of the neuropsychological services provided for different patient populations.
- Summarize studies that have been done or could be done to address how neuropsychological services can be studied within the context of cost outcomes research.

References

Csikszentmihalyi, M. (1999). If we are so rich, why aren't we happy? *American Psychologist, 54*(10), 821–827.

Drummond, M. F., O'Brien, B. J., Stoddart, G. L., & Torrance, G. W. (1998). *Methods for the economic evaluation of health care programmes.* New York: Oxford University.

Eysenck, H. J. (1952). The effects of psychotherapy: An evaluation. *Journal of Consulting Psychology, 16,* 319–324.

Frank, R. G., & McGuire, T. G. (1999). Pricing psychotherapy: Lessons from health care reform. In N. E. Miller & K. M. Magruder (Eds.), *Cost-effectiveness of psychotherapy: A guide for practitioners, researchers, and policymakers* (pp. 134–152). New York: Oxford University.

Gold, M. R., Siegel, J. E., Russell, L. B., & Weinstein, M. C. (1996). *Cost-effectiveness in health and medicine.* New York: Oxford University.

Groth-Marnat, G. (1999). Financial efficacy of clinical assessment: Rational guidelines and issues for future reference. *Journal of Clinical Psychology, 55,* 813–824.

Hargreaves, W. A., Shumway, M., Hu, T.-W., & Cuffel, B. (1998). *Cost-outcome methods for mental health.* San Diego: Academic Press.

Howard, K. I., Lueger, R. J., Martinovich, Z., & Lutz, W. (1999). The cost-effectiveness of psychotherapy: Dose-response and phase models. In N. E. Miller & K. M. Magruder (Eds.), *Cost-effectiveness of psychotherapy: A guide for practitioners, researchers, and policymakers* (pp. 143–152). New York: Oxford University.

Junior Achievement. (1996). *Economics™ Student Text.* Colorado Springs: Author.

Kaplan, R. M. (1999). Health-related quality of life in mental health services evaluation. In N. E. Miller & K. M. Magruder (Eds.), *Cost-effectiveness of psychotherapy: A guide for practitioners, researchers, and policymakers* (pp. 160–173). New York: Oxford University.

Kubiszyn, T., Finn, S., Kay, G., Dies, R., Meyer, G., Eyde, L., Moreland, K., & Eisman, E. (2000). Empirical support for psychological assessment in clinical health care settings. *Professional Psychology: Research and Practice, 31,* 119–130.

Maruish, M. (2001). *Psychological testing in the age of managed care.* Mahwah, NJ: Erlbaum.

McNeilly, C., & Howard, K. I. (1991). The effects of psychotherapy: A reevaluation based on dosage. *Psychotherapy Research, 1,* 74–78.

Mealey's Managed Care Liability Report. (2000). Box 62090, King of Prussia, PA 19406-0230.

Miller, N. E., & Magruder, K. M. (1999). *Cost-effectiveness of psychotherapy: A guide for practitioners, researchers, and policymakers.* New York: Oxford University.

Norcross, J., Karg, R., & Prochaska, J. (1997). Clinical psychologists and managed care: Some data from the Division 12 membership. *The Clinical Psychologist, 50,* 4–8.

Nowack, W. J. (1997). Epilepsy: A costly misdiagnosis. *Clinical Electroencephalography, 28*(4), 225–228.

Piotrowski, C. (1999). Assessment practices in the era of managed care: Current status and future directions. *Journal of Clinical Psychology, 55,* 787–796.

Piotrowski, C., Belter, R., & Keller, J. (1998). The impact of managed care on the practice of psychological testing: Preliminary findings. *Journal of Personality Assessment, 70,* 441–447.

Prigatano, G. P. (2000). Neuropsychology, the patient's experience, and the political forces within our field. *Archives of Clinical Neuropsychology, 15*(1), 71–82.

Prigatano, G. P. (1999). *Principles of neuropsychological rehabilitation.* New York: Oxford University.

Phelps, R. Eisman, E., & Kohout, J. (1998). Psychological practice and managed care: Results of the CAPP practitioner survey. *Professional Psychology: Research and Practice, 29,* 31–36.

Rizzo, J. A., Friedkin, R., Williams, C. S., Nabors, J., Acampora, D., & Tinetti, M. E. (1998). Health care utilization and costs in a Medicare population by fall status. *Medical Care, 36*(8),1174–1188.

Russell, L. B., Seigel, J. E., Daniels, N., Gold, M. R., Luce, B. R., & Mandelblate, J. S. (1996). Cost-effective analysis as a guide to resource allocation in health: Roles and limitations. In M. R. Gold, J. E. Siegel, L. B. Russell, & M. C. Weinstein (Eds.), *Cost-effectiveness in health and medicine* (pp. 3–24). New York: Oxford University.

Stein, H., & Foss, M. (1995). *The new illustrated guide to the American economy.* Washington, DC: AEI Press.

Stout, C. (1997). *Psychological assessment in managed care.* New York: Wiley.

Stout, J., & Cook, L. (1999). New areas for psychological assessment in general health care settings: What to do today to prepare for tomorrow. *Journal of Clinical Psychology, 55,* 797–812.

Sweet, J., Moberg, P., & Suchy, Y. (2000). Ten-year follow-up survey of clinical neuropsychologists: Part II. Private Practice and Economics. *The Clinical Neuropsychologist, 14,* 479–495.

Webster's new universal unabridged dictionary. (1983). Cleveland: New World Dictionaries/Simon & Schuster.

2

CHAPTER

George P. Prigatano
Lanie Y. Zigler
Leslie D. Rosenstein

The Clinical Neuropsychological Examination: Scope, Cost, and Health-Care Value

☐ Introduction

Meyer et al. (2001) recently provided a systematic summary of the utility of psychological assessment methods, with reference to certain neuropsychological measures. Among their conclusions are that "psychological test validity is strong and compelling" and "psychological test validity is comparable to medical test validity" (p. 128). They also specifically mentioned the utility of judgments made by clinical neuropsychologists. These findings and conclusions clearly support the work of clinical neuropsychologists.

In this chapter, the focus will be on defining the scope of the clinical neuropsychological examination and its clinical utility. It is emphasized that there are both subjective and objective markers of value of such a service that need to be considered when conducting cost outcome research studies. In this regard, economic variables important for such analyses will be discussed.

Generally speaking, the clinical utility of a neuropsychological examination is threefold. It can answer three interrelated questions:

1. Is there objective evidence of disturbed higher cerebral (or integrated) brain functions?
2. Do the pattern and level of the clinical neuropsychological test findings suggest a diffuse, lateralized, or regionalized cerebral dysfunction?
3. Are the pattern and level of disturbed functions compatible with a known or suspected brain disorder in a given patient?

The answers to these questions can be used in a variety of ways. Prigatano and Redner (1993) identified seven uses of neuropsychological testing in behavioral neurology (Table 2.1).

TABLE 2.1. Seven Uses of Neuropsychological Testing

1. To describe disturbances in higher cerebral dysfunction in patients with known or suspected brain disorder quantitatively and qualitatively
2. To monitor changes in higher cerebral functioning over time with and without treatment
3. To help diagnose and identify clinically relevant syndromes
4. To describe neuropsychological processes that affect a patient's ability to be independent at home or to return to work
5. To develop an outline of the nature of disturbed higher cerebral dysfunctions and how they might be managed within the context of rehabilitation
6. To provide a database with which to counsel patients and families concerning life decisions given existing higher cerebral dysfunctions (Does the patient appear cognitively capable of living alone? Of being unsupervised? Of returning to work?)
7. To motivate further research in brain–behavioral relationships

Adapted from Prigatano and Redner (1993). With permission from W.B. Saunders.

As other chapters in this text highlight, this information can be used to counsel patients and their family members, to help physicians make medical and surgical decisions, to aid rehabilitationists, and to expand educational and research endeavors.

Determining the cost of a clinical neuropsychological examination requires an assessment of the professionals' and paraprofessionals' time spent in providing the service, the materials involved in the examination process, the clarity of information provided by the findings, and how the information is used by a variety of people (i.e., the referring neurosurgeon, neurologist, psychiatrist, patient, patient's family, school teachers, disability claims specialists, attorneys, and so on).

☐ The Scope of the Clinical Neuropsychological Examination

Reitan (1986) pointed out that "insufficient information is presently available to develop a battery of tests that would reflect the full range of behavioral correlates of brain functions" (p. 3). Yet, each day clinical neuropsychologists are faced with the practical questions of how best to examine a given patient's higher cerebral functions and which tests and measurements will produce the most scientifically valid and clinically useful information.

In her description of several important issues related to interviewing and examining patients from a neuropsychological perspective, Lezak (1995) discussed several broad categories of behavior that must be considered. She refrained, however, from listing a specific set of functions that should be evaluated or tests that should be administered. The patient's clinical presentation, the diagnostic or rehabilitation questions raised, and the skill of the neuropsychological examiner determine how functions are sampled and what tests are administered.

In broad terms, some researchers have attempted to outline what dimensions should be considered when conducting a neuropsychological evaluation. Twenty-five years ago, Benton (1975) listed 10 major cognitive skills that should be assessed by neuropsychological tests: visual perception, auditory perception, tactile perception, constructional praxis, "body schema" functions, abstract reasoning, retention and memory, sensorimotor performance, language functions, and aphasia.

Elsewhere, Prigatano (1999) emphasized that the nature of higher cerebral or integrative brain functions is not purely cognitive. They seem to reflect an integration of thinking and feeling functions that is crucial for problem solving and that allow social (and physical) adaptation. These functions have "convergent" and "emergent" properties (p. 43). Based on this formulation, Table 2.2 lists 10 dimensions that are considered relevant to a clinical neuropsychological examination. Again, the time spent and the tests administered to assess these dimensions are determined by several factors. When examining a patient with a known or suspected brain disorder, a clinical neuropsychologist typically keeps these dimensions in mind. Certainly, each dimension has several subcomponents that may require greater delineation depending on the patient's symptom picture, the diagnostic problem, or the specific referral questions asked of the practicing clinical neuropsychologist.

The reader is referred to other volumes that summarize the studies documenting the validity, reliability, and normative data for several neuropsychological tests (Lezak, 1995; Mitrushina, Boone, & D'Elia, 1999; Spreen & Strauss, 1998). Questions about the clinical utility of the neuropsychological examination for different patient populations are considered throughout this book. This section considers what is involved in conducting a clinical neuropsychological examination and provides some examples of what constitutes normal performance.

Steps in Conducting a Clinical Neuropsychological Examination

The first step is to obtain adequate information to plan the examination. The information needed includes demographic characteristics (age, education, gender, and so on) as well as the pertinent medical and psychosocial history that seem to have prompted the referral. This record review can be brief or lengthy, depending on the clinical situation. The time and cost spent in obtaining this background information must be added to the overall cost of conducting a neuropsychological examination.

After the relevant information is reviewed, the second step is to interview the patient (and sometimes family members) to help clarify the patient's clinical condition and how the patient (and family) describes his or her functioning. Depending on the questions being posed, this step also can be relatively brief or time consuming. How patients actually describe their condition, however, was recognized by Luria years ago to be an important part of a clinical neuropsychological examination (Christensen, 1979).

After historical information has been obtained and the patient and family members have been interviewed, the patient is in a position to undergo the actual examination. The patient's level and pattern of performance on various standardized (and in some instances nonstandardized) tests provide the systematic observations on which the clinical neuropsychologist makes statements concerning the nature of the patient's higher cerebral or integrative functions.

Issues in Conducting a Neuropsychological Examination

Depending on the patient's clinical condition and referral questions, each of the 10 dimensions listed in Table 2.2 can be assessed briefly or extensively. It is the profes-

TABLE 2.2. Ten Dimensions of a Clinical Neuropsychological Examination

1. Speech and language functions
2. Perceptual skills (auditory, visual, and tactual)
3. Attention and concentration skills
4. Learning capacity
5. Memory
6. Intellectual level and executive function
7. Speed of new learning
8. Speed and coordination of simple motor responses
9. Emotional and motivational characteristics
10. Self-awareness of level of functioning and judgments regarding psychosocial implications

sional and ethical responsibility of the clinical neuropsychologist to determine what is necessary for individual cases. This individualized approach, however, makes it difficult to apply a specific cost to conducting a neuropsychological examination. Typically, the charges (not the costs) of conducting a neuropsychological examination are based on the time spent in reviewing records, interviewing, testing, scoring the tests, interpreting tests results, and dictating the report. Lundin and DeFilippis (1999) provided specific information about the time it takes to administer, score, interpret, and report results for commonly used neuropsychological tests. Based on their findings, a "brief" examination can easily take 2 hours, with extensive testing requiring 8 to 10 hours.

Before clinical neuropsychologists can determine whether various aspects of higher cerebral functioning are impaired, they must understand what constitutes a normal performance on neuropsychological tests for different individuals of different ages and educational and cultural backgrounds. Acquiring this expertise requires lengthy training, and the cost of providing services must consider the cost of training someone to perform these services. As an example of how clinical neuropsychologists must have a broad background to conduct a comprehensive and competent examination, consider the important role of statistics and normative data in determining whether a patient has a brain dysfunction.

Clinical neuropsychologists rely heavily on well-standardized neuropsychological tests. These tests are empirically derived and include normative data used to determine whether a performance is "average" or "below average." Soundly derived psychometric norms are of great value to clinical neuropsychologists, but in certain instances they can be misleading. There is always a range of scores in any normal distribution (Keppel & Zedick, 1989). The mean (average) score of a normative sample may or may not be "normal" for a given individual. Thus, the clinical neuropsychologist must estimate the patient's premorbid cognitive status to determine whether a level of test performance actually indicates a brain disorder.

These and other observations led Reitan (1986) to postulate that level of performance is only one indication of brain function or dysfunction. The pattern of test findings, in addition to the presence of certain "pathognomonic" signs, also is important when evaluating neuropsychological test findings. Building on these observations, other researchers and clinicians have noted that certain "demographic" variables may greatly influence level of performance on standard neuropsychological tests. Age and education are two such variables (Prigatano, 1999; Prigatano, Amin, & Rosenstein, 1995; Prigatano & Parsons, 1976; Vega & Parsons, 1967). Therefore, the interpretation of test findings often requires appropriate norms for age and, at times, for education and gender (Heaton, Grant, & Matthews, 1991). Level of motivation to perform also is recognized as a potential influence on a patient's performance on psychological tests (Reitan, 1956). Research on suspected malingerers has documented this same point (Prigatano & Amin, 1993; Prigatano, Smason, Lamb, & Bortz, 1997).

Against this background, "normal" performance on the 10 dimensions included in a neuropsychological examination is described. For simplicity, we focus on what is normal for young to middle-aged adults with a high-school education examined in the United States.

□ Markers of Normal Neuropsychological Status

Language function provides the first neuropsychological window of observation of brain function. The person being examined must understand what is being asked of him or her and have sufficient speech and language skills to respond. Students of aphasia have suggested that there are "markers" of normal language function (Goodglass & Kaplan, 1983). Speech production must be fluent; that is, the number of words uttered per unit of time must flow at a rate that is normal for a given culture and age. The utterances must be free of paraphasic errors (except an occasional error), and there should be no dysarthria during speech production. Although psychometric measures of fluency and dysarthria are difficult to construct, clinicians reliably judge the normality of these functions (Goodglass & Kaplan, 1983).

In the standardization of the BNI Screen for Higher Cerebral Functions (BNIS), 200 normal individuals between the ages of 15 and 84 years had no difficulties in these areas. Moreover, a simple verbal command (i.e., touch the small red circle and the large white square) was easily understood aurally and executed by more than 95% of the normal subjects the first time they heard the verbal command. Failures often were attributed to problems of attention, and individuals easily passed the task given a second request (Prigatano, Amin, & Rosenstein, 1995).

Likewise, young adults (15 to 39 years old) were able to name common objects and to repeat a six-word sentence 100% of the time. The older population made only minor errors (Prigatano, Amin, & Rosenstein, 1995). Thus, most normal adults are able to speak in a fluent manner; to demonstrate no paraphasic errors in free speech; to demonstrate no dysarthria; and to demonstrate basic auditory comprehension, naming, and sentence repetition skills. Errors in any of these dimensions raise the possibility of a subtle speech and language impairment that could reflect brain dysfunction.

The second dimension of a clinical neuropsychological examination is the assessment of perceptual skills. Are the patient's auditory, visual, and tactile perceptions adequate for further examination? Disturbances in any of these perceptual realms can influence performance on neuropsychological tests and help to determine whether a patient's higher cerebral functions are impaired. For example, the presence of left homonymous hemianopsia documents a visual disturbance related to brain dysfunction. Several screening tests, including the sensory-perceptual examination, incorporate a basic assessment of these perceptual skills. Assuming that the clinical examiner judges that a patient's perceptual skills are adequate, attention, concentration, and "working memory" skills are evaluated next.

Assessing the capacity to attend to various forms of sensory stimulation and to show adequate concentration (working memory) is an important part of the neuropsychological examination. Hyperactive children, emotionally distressed patients, and persons with various somatic difficulties (e.g., intense headache or severe lower back pain) may perform below average on tests of attention and concentration. Lesions of the brain stem and parietal and frontal lobes also can influence these functions negatively. Therefore, the examination must include an assessment of these interrelated but complex functions. Certain clues can help clinicians with this differential diagnosis. For example, McDowell, Whyte, and D'Esposito (1997) showed that normal individuals demonstrate a mild decline when doing two cognitive tasks at once (i.e., a visual reaction time task while repeating digits). Patients with traumatic brain injury (TBI), however, show proportionally more difficulty performing these two tasks simultaneously. The relative amount of difficulty patients exhibit can help clinicians to determine the presence or absence of brain dysfunction.

A fourth dimension of the clinical neuropsychological examination focuses on the learning capacity of the individual. During the last 50 years, a number of psychologists have emphasized the importance of rote verbal learning (Zangwill, 1947). The basic question is whether individuals can learn a "normal amount" of information with repetition and whether they show a normal "learning curve." Geffen, Moar, O'Hanlon, Clark, and Geffen (1990) amply demonstrated the learning curve associated with adolescents and young to middle-aged adults attempting to learn a series of words read to them over repeated trials. Normal aging may influence the amount of information learned with practice, but it does not seem to influence the learning curve per se. In normal individuals, all age groups exhibit a serial position effect: Words at the beginning and end of a list tend to be learned better than words in the middle. In the elderly, failure to show the primacy effect may be related to early dementia (Bayley et al., 2000). This type of information, in addition to level of performance, can help clinical neuropsychologists involved in the differential diagnosis of brain dysfunction.

Next, neuropsychologists assess the fifth dimension of a neuropsychological examination—namely, memory function. After a patient has learned verbal information, he or she is distracted briefly and then asked to recall the learned information. Frequently, a 20- or 30-minute delay follows and the same information is again requested. Typically, healthy young adults can recall 75% to 80% of what they learned with practice and repetition, especially when rote verbal learning tests are involved. This finding reflects the normal amount of forgetting (or, conversely, memory capacity) that one would expect individuals to exhibit on tasks such as the Rey Auditory Verbal Learning Test (RAVLT; Geffen et al., 1990).

This information is useful when attempting to document whether higher brain functions are normal or abnormal. In fact, memory impairment is the most prominent of the earliest symptoms of a number of neurological conditions, including but not limited to anoxic encephalopathy (Caine & Watson, 2000; Cummings, Tomiyasu, Read, & Benson, 1984), multiple sclerosis (Rao, Leo, & St. Aubin-Faubert, 1989), dementia of the Alzheimer's type (Bayley et al., 2000), and temporal lobectomy (Milner, 1958).

The sixth dimension of the clinical neuropsychological examination is the assessment of intellectual level. This task can be difficult because it is greatly influenced by educational background and cultural factors. Nevertheless, a comprehensive neuropsychological examination should attempt to assess intelligence. In the United States, the typical measure used for adults is the Wechsler Adult Intelligence Scale, which is in its third edition (WAIS-III, Wechsler, 1997). We agree with Gardner (1983) that multiple forms of intelligence exist and that standardized intelligence tests sample just a few of them. For clinical purposes, however, the WAIS-III is presently the single best measure of intellectual performance. By obtaining a WAIS-III Full-Scale Intelligence Quotient (IQ), Verbal IQ, and Performance IQ, the clinical examiner is in a good position to judge a patient's level of intellectual functioning and whether the pattern of functioning is compatible with the individual's history (both educational and occupational). Sometimes, differences between these scores can help determine the presence of a lateralized higher brain dysfunction (Anderson, Damasio, & Tranel, 1990).

Related to intelligence is the construct of "executive function" (Lezak, 1995). The early work of Hebb (1939; 1941) showed that the performance of patients on standard IQ tests who had undergone a frontal lobectomy did not necessarily decline. In fact, on some tests they actually showed a practice effect; that is, their performance improved. Later work documented that many patients who showed no changes on standard IQ tests did exhibit difficulties on tasks that sampled abstract reasoning and planning skills. Milner (1963) demonstrated that such patients may show impairment on abstract reasoning tasks not sampled by standard IQ tests. Thus, practicing clinical neuropsychologists distinguish between intellectual performance and executive functioning. There are various tests of executive function, but the Halstead Category Test, the Wisconsin Card-Sorting Test, the Stroop Test, and the Trail-Making Tests Parts A and B are often used to assess these functions.

The seventh dimension of a clinical neuropsychological examination focuses on the speed at which information is learned. Developmentally, the speed at which information is learned is a marker of cognitive growth or development (Case, 1985; Kail, 1991). Several markers can be used to assess the speed of information processing. A simple marker is the level of performance on the Digit Symbol-Coding Subtest of the WAIS-III. This particular test is highly sensitive to brain dysfunction and even to the estimated size of a brain lesion (Chapman & Wolff, 1959; Johnson, Bigler, Burr, & Blatter, 1994; Reitan, 1955, 1986).

The eighth dimension of a neuropsychological examination deals with the speed and coordination of simple motor responses. Costa, Vaughan, Levitan, & Farber (1963) noted that performance on the Purdue Groove Pegboard Test was a reliable predictor of brain dysfunction. Moreover, recent literature has documented that speed of motor performance is negatively influenced by severity of TBI (Dikmen, Machamer, Winn, & Temkin, 1995). Speed of finger movement can be affected by mild to moderate injuries and often recovers less than grip strength after such injuries (Haaland, Temkin, Randall, & Dikman, 1994). Assessing the speed of finger tapping over time and considering the differences between the right and left hands can provide useful information about a patient's neuropsychological status. The ability to sustain fast finger movements when fatigued may involve multiple anterior brain regions (Johnson & Prigatano, 2000). It may underlie the correlation of speed of finger tapping to the achievement of inpatient rehabilitation goals after acute brain injury (Prigatano & Wong, 1997).

The ninth dimension focuses on an individual's emotional and motivational characteristics. This component of the neuropsychological examination is challenging and has been neglected by many test batteries. Yet, patients' capacity to generate affect in their tone of voice, to perceive facial affect, and to show spontaneous affect is unequivocally related to brain injury and rehabilitation outcomes (Borgaro & Prigatano, in press; Prigatano & Wong, 1999). Evaluating these three simple functions is a place to begin assessing patients' emotional and motivational characteristics. Much more work, however, is needed in this area.

The last and perhaps the most difficult of all areas to assess in a neuropsychological examination is the degree to which patients are aware of their disturbances in higher brain function. The problem of impaired self-awareness and issues involved in its assessment and rehabilitation have been discussed elsewhere (Prigatano, 1999). There are, however, markers of impaired awareness. By asking patients to rate certain capacities (on a scale from 0 to 10, 0 meaning no difficulty and 10 meaning a severe problem), clinicians can form an idea of whether individuals appear to make judgments compatible with their performance on the neuropsychological examination. Comparing patients' ratings of their abilities to relatives' ratings provides another index of potentially impaired awareness (Prigatano, 1999). Cross-cultural studies have repeatedly shown that brain-dysfunctional patients' ratings of their behavioral competence tend to correlate poorly with their test performance on neuropsychological measures. In contrast, relatives' ratings of patients' neuropsychological abilities correlate well with patients' neuropsychological test performance (Table 12.2; Chapter 12; Prigatano, 1999). Recent work on assessing patients with dementia highlights this point and shows the importance of disturbances of awareness (or insight) to the differential diagnosis (Kertesz, Nadkarnin, Davidson, & Thomas, 2000).

Clinical neuropsychologists should have freedom on how they assess each of these dimensions. By their training, they are bound by both professional and ethical standards for how much time should be spent in evaluating a given patient and what tests are appropriate to administer. Selected studies (Table 2.3) have documented the usefulness of neuropsychological tests for assessing normal and abnormal higher cerebral functions. The present health-care market, however, also demands that clinical neuropsychologists address the costs of performing these services.

TABLE 2.3. Selected Studies that Document the Utility of Neuropsychological Test Performance to Distinguish Normal and Abnormal Higher Cerebral Functions

Dimensions	Selected Studies
Speech and language function	Goodglass and Kaplan (1983)
Perceptual skills	Robertson and Halligan (1999)
Attention/concentration skills (and working memory)	McDowell, Whyte, and D'Esposito (1997) De Renzi and Vignolo (1962)
Learning	Rosenstein, Prigatano, and Nayak (1997)
Memory	Goldstein and Levin (1995) Crosson et al. (1993)
Intellectual level and executive functioning	Johnson et al. (1994) Levin et al. (1994)
Speed of new learning	Johnston et al. (1994)
Speed and coordination of simple motor responses	Dikmen et al. (1995)
Emotional and motivational characteristics	Kertesz et al. (2000) Prigatano and Wong (1999)
Self-awareness	Prigatano (1991; 1999)

Costs, Charges, Fees, and the Value of the Clinical Neuropsychological Examination

The costs of conducting a clinical neuropsychological examination can be defined as the amount of dollar resources *needed* to provide the services. Charges refer to the amount of dollars *billed* for the services. Fees refer to the amount of dollars actually *paid* for the services. Value refers to the *benefit* someone experiences as a result of undergoing a neuropsychological examination. This benefit can be measured "objectively" or "subjectively." Both objective and subjective markers of value are needed when studying the cost outcome of a clinical neuropsychological examination. Finally, comparing costs with fees collected provides information about profit and loss for an individual, a hospital, or a corporation that provides this neuropsychological service.

Costs

The costs of providing neuropsychological services, and particularly clinical neuropsychological examination services, can be viewed from the perspective of individual practitioners or groups (corporations). In both cases, direct and indirect costs must be considered. The costs of not providing the service from the corporation's perspective must also be considered (i.e., failure to provide the services might affect other clinical services negatively). The cost of *not* providing this service also must be estimated from the perspective of society.

The direct dollar resources needed to establish and maintain a small department of clinical neuropsychology in a nonprofit hospital or medical center may well reach \$500,000 to \$600,000 per year (this sum covers the salaries of three to four clinical neuropsychologists, secretarial support, and neuropsychology residents). Salaries account for 80% to 90% of these costs.

Assuming that an additional 20% of indirect costs are absorbed by the corporation in the form of various benefits (e.g., medical insurance and retirement plans), the total dollar costs for the corporation may range from \$600,000 to \$720,000 per year. What does the corporation receive for this expenditure?

Charges

Theoretically, clinical neuropsychologists spend 25 to 30 hours per week providing neuropsychological services. In reality, however, this is probably an underestimate. Many of these services include time devoted to the clinical evaluation of patients. Typically, hours of service are billed at a rate considered professionally responsible for a given geographical location and for the type of service provided. In many places in the United States, fees range from \$140 to \$200 per hour, although this is not a strict range of costs for services. Assuming that the average clinical neuropsychologist bills 25 hours of work per week for 48 weeks (factoring in 4 weeks of vacation and time for continuing medical education credits), the charges would be about 1,200 hours × \$140 = \$168,000 per year. Three psychologists would bill \$504,000 per year; four psychologists would bill \$672,000 per year. If these fees were collected, the hospital would "break even" (in the spirit of a nonprofit organization). Since the advent of the managed care movement, however, charges never reflect the actual fees received.

Fees

In almost all aspects of medicine and health care today (in the United States), the actual dollars paid for services are considerably lower than the charges. A recent Blue Cross and Blue Shield (BCBS) of Arizona provider prevailing fee report (dated 7/1/00) for mental and behavioral health highlighted this reality.

Psychotherapies are reimbursed at the rate of $100 per hour (per 40- to 50-minute hour) and neuropsychological testing at $80 per hour. The amount of reimbursement from any health-care provider, however, varies in different parts of the country. The same is true for Medicare reimbursements. Presently in Arizona, Medicare reimburses neuropsychologists for approximately $71 per unit (hour) of psychometric testing.

If a clinical neuropsychologist bills 1,000 hours per year in neuropsychological testing (1,000 × 80 or 1,000 × 71), the revenue received would be between $80,000 and $71,000 per year. If 250 additional hours per year are spent providing psychotherapy services for brain-dysfunctional patients, the revenue for that year would be $25,000 (250 × 100). So, in reality, the revenue produced by a given clinical neuropsychologist would be between $105,000 and $96,000 per year. If four psychologists generated revenue at this rate, the hospital would collect between $420,000 and $384,000 per year. Under such circumstances, the dollar *loss* for the hospital would be between $105,000 and $288,000 per year. No wonder many salaried psychology positions have disappeared in university hospitals and private hospital medical settings throughout the United States.

As a result, many clinical neuropsychologists have gone into private practice. Some report working fewer hours and experiencing much less stress by dealing with insurance carriers and the Medicare system directly. Such a setting often imposes no other administrative responsibilities. Their incomes vary, but an informal survey of private practice psychologists suggests that their reimbursement and salary levels match if not exceed those of psychologists who work for an organization. Private practice, however, deprives neuropsychologists of the opportunity to do research and to train fellow psychologists, two activities important to many practitioners. For departments of clinical neuropsychology to survive these realities, others sources of revenue must be obtained.

Additional Sources of Revenue (and Hidden Other Costs)

Like some private practitioners, salaried hospital clinical neuropsychologists may see patients for medicolegal purposes. Again, fees vary. If, however, one or two experienced neuropsychologists evaluate one medicolegal case every 10 days, revenue would be boosted by about $3,000 per case (say, 30 cases per year × $3,000 = $90,000). Such evaluations could greatly offset the negative profit–loss statement described above.

In an active clinical neuropsychology department, clinical neuropsychologists often are engaged in clinical research. Research raises the opportunity to offset the remaining dollar losses with grant support. This strategy, however, requires extra effort on the part of the clinical neuropsychologists to obtain grant funds, to publish their research findings, and to present those findings at scientific meetings.

To perform these extra activities, clinical neuropsychologists working in nonprofit settings need to spend more than 40 hours a week in discharging their duties. When involved in clinical and research activities, clinical neuropsychologists in such settings often work 50 to 60 hours per week. Such a workload can take a toll on morale and health, not to mention personal and family relationships. No one has studied the spiraling economic costs to society as adults spend more and more of their "leisure time" pursuing revenue-generating activities.

Objective Markers of Value

Value refers to the "worth" of a service (or commodity; *Webster's*, 1983, p. 2018). In purely economic terms, value refers to the dollar (or money) equivalent of the service (or commodity) received. Economists and stockbrokers, for example, refer to a stock as being a "good value" when the amount paid for it is less than the actual (or potential) worth (in dollars). This type of definition also can be applied to health care. The value of a neurosurgical procedure can be measured by comparing the costs of the neurosurgical procedure to the actual dollars saved by avoiding other health-care costs as well as the dollars saved by returning an individual to work. The value of a neuropsychological rehabilitation program after TBI (as illustrated in Chapter 1) can be measured by the dollars a government agency saves by providing this health-care service to individuals after brain injury (Mehlbye & Larsen, 1994). Value also can be measured in nondollar, but still objective, terms. In health care, the efficacy of a medical intervention often is assessed in terms of quality of life variables (see Chapter 1). Five to six objective markers can be used to measure the potential value of a clinical neuropsychological examination (Table 2.4).

One objective marker of value is the cost–benefit ratio calculated as a result of objectively describing a patient's higher cerebral functioning and the medicolegal implications of the description. For example, assume that a young male in the beginning years of his productivity suffers a TBI. Documentation of the extent and nature of his neuropsychological impairments can demonstrate that his capacity to maintain the line of

TABLE 2.4. Suggested Objective and Subjective Markers of Value of a Clinical Neuropsychological Examination

Objective Markers

- Reduce costs and liabilities by describing disturbances of higher cerebral functioning.
- Improve quality of life by describing disturbances in higher cerebral functioning.
- Assess the effectiveness of treatment by assessing disturbances in higher cerebral functioning.
- Direct treatment procedures by assessing disturbances in higher cerebral functioning.
- Provide a continuum of care and help maintain accreditation standards.
- Improve physician education and decision making.

Subjective Markers

- Reduce patients' sense of psychological aloneness with daily problems.
- Reduce patients' confusion and frustration about the nature of their higher cerebral disturbances.
- Help family members feel less guilty in making decisions regarding brain-dysfunctional adults and children by describing their disturbances in higher cerebral functioning objectively.
- Compare whether individuals value the service for themselves or for others when they need a neuropsychological examination.

work for which he was preparing is now reduced. This information can translate into hundreds of thousands of lost dollars as a result of the brain injury. Much of this lost potential income can be captured via litigation. The cost of conducting such an examination and providing testimony may vary, but even if the attorney or patient pays as much as $5,000 for such a comprehensive service, the benefits greatly offset the costs.

Perhaps less dramatic, but no less important, are the savings associated with differential diagnoses. Many individuals in their early 60s complain of memory disorder, and some individuals show mild cognitive impairments associated with early Alzheimer's disease (Bayley et al., 2000). Depending on the amount of time spent and the geographical location in which the patient is seen, a neuropsychological examination in a setting like ours (the BNI) for such individuals costs about $840.[1] If a neuropsychological examination reveals that the patient most likely suffers from depression, psychiatric treatment may help the individual to regain a productive lifestyle. If the findings are indicative of early dementia of the Alzheimer's type, further medical expenditures (e.g., brain imaging studies or APOE genotype testing) may follow. In the long run, however, the diagnostic information can help the patient and family plan for the patient's early and significant decline in cognitive and behavioral functioning.

Objectively describing disturbances in higher cerebral functioning after TBI also can help families make decisions about the need for supervision after brain injury. For example, a 16-year-old girl suffered a severe TBI while driving a car under the influence of alcohol. Within 2 weeks of her injury, she exhibited no obvious neurologic impairments. Her mother noted, however, that her daughter's thinking seemed less clear and that she showed unexpected memory difficulties. The family debated whether this girl could return to school and live independently. A neuropsychological examination documented unequivocal memory disturbances as well as reduced awareness of her limitations. With this information, the disagreement in the family about what needed to be done was reduced. This young woman received supervision and consequently avoided the potential risks had she engaged in harmful behavior while unsupervised. Again, the examination cost about $840: It could well have cost the family literally thousands of dollars, not to mention a potentially substantial decrease in the girl's quality of life, if her parents had allowed her to function independently.

Another example highlights the cost of failing to request a neuropsychological examination. A 55-year-old businessman underwent surgical resection of an arteriovenous malformation (AVM) in the left temporal lobe. His neurological recovery was substantial, and his attending neurosurgeon identified no cognitive or linguistic disturbances. The patient pressed his neurosurgeon to allow him to return to work as soon as possible. The neurosurgeon, pleased with the outcome of his surgical interventions, agreed to do so. Within 3 months, this individual lost more than $100,000 in poor investments for his company. He was fired and was not placed on medical disability. He was referred for a neuropsychological examination that documented unequivocal impairments of his higher-order language and memory functions that contributed to his errors in judgment. Eventually, the individual was helped to obtain a level of employment lower than his previous level of functioning. He might well have been spared the loss of resources and the emotional trauma if he had undergone a neuropsychological examination before returning to work.

---

[1]This is an estimated cost in our setting. The actual cost vary within our setting as well as across settings. It should not be taken as an absolute value of the charges common for neuropsychological testing, but is used only for illustrative purposes.

A third objective marker of the value of the clinical neuropsychological examination is its capacity to determine the effectiveness of various treatments. Throughout the United States, drug companies are trying to identify medications that will retard the effects of Alzheimer's disease. As a part of these scientific investigations, neuropsychological tests are often administered to participants to assess whether their memory function has improved. These neuropsychological measures can help determine whether a drug is affecting higher cerebral functioning and whether the treatment is efficacious. Neuropsychological test findings also can help determine the benefit of medical or surgical interventions, as various chapters throughout this text highlight.

A fourth objective measure of a clinical neuropsychological examination is its ability to guide treatment successfully. Two brief examples are offered. Whether a patient undergoes surgical intervention for epilepsy depends partially on the pattern of neuropsychological test findings obtained when there is evidence of gliosis in the mesial temporal lobe (see Chapter 11). Neurologists and neurosurgeons need to know whether a patient may be further harmed, from a neuropsychological perspective, by undergoing such surgery.

In the future, combining a neuropsychological assessment with neuroimaging may help guide neurosurgical interventions. Recently, for example, an 8-year-old child was evaluated at the BNI for resection of a tumor in the left frontal lobe. Selected language functions were assessed while the child underwent functional magnetic resonance (MR) imaging (personal communication, Sterling Johnson, 2000). Because naming and word-generation skills were embedded in a certain region surrounding the tumor, the surgeon decided to alter his surgical approach for removing a portion of the malignant neoplasm.

The fifth objective marker of the value of the clinical neuropsychological examination is its capacity to provide a true continuum of care for patients and the effect it may have on institutional care. For example, the Department of Clinical Neuropsychology at the BNI provides neuropsychological consultations to inpatients on the neurorehabilitation unit. Studies have documented that brief but focused neuropsychological findings can predict outcomes from inpatient neurorehabilitation (Prigatano & Wong, 1997, 1999). This brief but focused approach to neuropsychological assessment for patients on a brain-injury rehabilitation unit has been well recognized as a valuable service. The unit's continuing accreditation by the Commission on Accreditation of Rehabilitation Facilities (CARF) partially reflected the availability of these neuropsychological services. Neuropsychologists also consult with family members about the nature of a patient's higher cerebral deficits. The consultation provides the family with information that helps prepare them to deal with the intermediate and long-term cognitive and behavioral deficits exhibited by many brain-dysfunctional patients (see Chapter 5).

A final but related source of value of the clinical neuropsychological examination is related to the continuing education of physicians. Physicians as well as psychologists need to better understand how various brain disturbances actually affect higher cerebral functions. Without that information, physicians can make poor decisions, such as returning patients to work prematurely, as noted earlier. Such decisions can cause considerable pain and suffering for patients and families and have catastrophic economic and personal consequences. Research on clinical decision making by physicians who use and do not use neuropsychological test findings to manage brain-dysfunctional patients would be a fruitful area of investigation.

Subjective Markers of Value

Table 2.4 also illustrates four subjective markers of value of the clinical neuropsychological examination. Many brain-dysfunctional patients experience disturbances in higher cerebral functioning that they feel others do not understand. For example, a patient was referred for a neuropsychological evaluation because she exhibited memory and speech difficulties associated with extreme fatigue. She was tested when she was "tired" and when she was "not tired." Her speed of information processing and concentration were better when she was not fatigued, but she showed unequivocal signs of subtle but real problems with verbal learning and speed of finger movement. These findings suggested that her subjective complaints had "objective" correlates. Unfortunately, the findings were compatible with the clinical hypothesis that she might be in the early stages of multiple sclerosis. The patient, however, voiced considerable relief in knowing that her problems were real instead of imagined. Many patients express this sentiment when they have deficits their family physicians had assumed were psychological.

In other instances, the patient and family clearly understand that disturbances in higher cerebral functions are present but may not understand the implications of those impairments. Both patients and families can be confused about what patients need given their memory or judgment disturbances. For example, a 56-year-old man had problems with language function, and a clinical neuropsychological examination was requested. His previous neurological evaluation had been negative for Alzheimer's disease. His neuropsychological test findings suggested a pattern indicative of primary progressive aphasia, documenting objective signs of dementia, but not of the Alzheimer's type. This information helped reduce the patient's confusion and frustration over what he was experiencing. Although saddened by the findings, both he and his wife were relieved to know what was "wrong."

A third subjective marker of the value of the clinical neuropsychological examination can be obtained by asking families to identify the benefits of having objective information concerning a brain-injured loved one. Many family members struggle with the issue of placing a patient with dementia in a residential setting and feel guilty about doing so. A neuropsychological examination that documents dementia and the patient's risk for hurting him- or herself or others provides the family a rationale for making this difficult decision. Many family members have expressed relief when the clinical neuropsychologist clarifies what is wrong with a parent with dementia.

A related example involves family members who are exhausted by their attempts to manage the behavior of a brain-injured child. The family often worries that they have done something to produce the problem. When they understand that the problem is not caused by psychodynamic problems or faulty childrearing experiences, but is the result of brain dysfunction, the family often reports considerable relief. To date, no one has had the courage to ask families the value of gaining that relief and reducing their confusion. This line of research is against the grain of traditional health care, which is reluctant to assign a dollar value to helping patients with their psychological suffering. Yet, future studies may need to ask such difficult questions to demonstrate to third-party payers that neuropsychological examinations provide value.

The fourth and final subjective marker of the neuropsychological examination was mentioned in Chapter 1. Recall the administrator of a managed care organization who repeatedly refused to authorize neuropsychological examinations for young adults under his care who had suffered a TBI. When he suffered a concussion, however, he became anxious about his condition. He knew that a neuropsychological examination might help clarify what was wrong and guide him in managing the effects of his concussion. He was able to convince his organization to pay for a neuropsychological assessment, even though he had denied this service to many others. As discouraging as this scenario is, it is a powerful example of how individuals can value a service even though they are unwilling to pay for the service for others. This "hidden" and subjective marker of value should be included when trying to demonstrate the utility and cost-effectiveness of the neuropsychological examination.

☐ Methods for Assessing Cost–Outcomes of a Clinical Neuropsychological Examination

Drummond, O'Brien, Stoddart, and Torrance (1997) described quantitative methods for evaluating the economic impact of health-care services. They note that the "real cost" of a service is not the number of dollars "budgeted by an institution to provide these services, but rather the impact of placing those dollars in one clinical arena versus another" (p. 8). From the perspective of this chapter, the "costs" of a clinical neuropsychological examination ultimately must be based on what resources are used to provide the services and what the economic benefit or losses to a health-care system would be if those dollar resources were allocated to another clinical service. Such an economic analysis can be quite complex, but clinical neuropsychologists need to "start somewhere" to demonstrate the utility and cost-effectiveness of a clinical neuropsychological examination.

Drummond et al. (1997) provided a useful model for conceptualizing how to compare the costs of health-care services with outcomes or consequences (see their Figure 2.2, p. 99). By substituting the term "clinical neuropsychological assessment" for "healthcare programs" in their model, one can follow the pathways for assessing the impact on the health of an individual and the value and types of resources that could potentially be saved. Their model also includes the concept of "willingness to pay" as an important variable when conducting cost–benefit analysis. Simple formulae (Table 2.5) can be used to evaluate the economics of a health-care service (Drummond et al., 1997). These formulae are applied to a few examples to highlight how cost–benefit, cost–utility, and cost-effectiveness of a clinical neuropsychological examination can be calculated. Drummond et al. (1997) used the following equation to analyze costs–benefits:

$$[(W + V + S_1, + S_2, + S_3) - (C_1, + C_2, + C_3)],$$

where W = willingness to pay, V = value measured in dollars, S_1 = health-care savings, S_2 = savings in patient/family resources, S_3 = savings in "other resources," C_1 = health-care costs, C_2 = patient/family resources used (costs), and C_3 = costs in other "sectors."

As noted, the 55-year-old man who returned to work prematurely after an AVM was resected lost $100,000 for his company and was terminated from his position. After surgery, he had seen no need for a clinical neuropsychological examination and, therefore, W would equal 0. The value, as measured in dollars of the examination at the time, could not be estimated. Consequently, a 0 value was put in its place. At the time, the patient was temporarily medically disabled and the savings involved in him being

TABLE 2.5. Possible Formulations of Economic Evaluation

Cost-minimization analysis
$(C_1 - S_1)$
$(C_1 + C_2 + C_3) - (S_1 + S_2 + S_3)$
Cost-effectiveness analysis
$(C_1 - S_1) / E$
$[(C_1 + C_2 + C_3) - (S_1 + S_2 + S_3)] / E$
Cost–utility analysis
$(C_1 - S_1) / U$
$[(C_1 + C_2 + C_3) - (S_1 + S_2 + S_3)] / U$
Cost-benefit analysis†
$(W') - (C_1 + C_2 + C_3)$
$[(W + V + S_1 + S_2 + S_3) - (C_1 + C_2 + C_3)]$

E and U represent *changes* in effectiveness or health status, compared to an alternative. †CBA results can also be expressed as ratios, although this model is not recommended. Adapted from Drummond et al. (1997).

evaluated also was 0. The savings that would have been incurred by the family if he had stayed on medical disability for 6 months would have been about 50% of his regular salary (i.e., $5,000 × 6 = $30,000); the savings to the company (the other sector savings) would have been $100,000. The cost of the examination and consultation for the health-care system was $1,120 (a 7-hour examination at $140 per hour and a 1-hour consultation at $140). The resources used by the family would have been about $30 for transportation to attend the examination. No productivity time would have been lost if the patient had been examined, because he was on medical disability. The cost–benefit was therefore calculated as follows: (0 + 0 + 0 + $30,000 + $100,000) – ($1,120 + $30 + 0) = $128,850. Not a bad deal.

Drummond et al. (1997) used the following equation for a cost-utility analysis:

$$(C_1+C_2+C_3) - (S_1+S_2+S_3)] \div U,$$

where C_1, C_2, C_3, S_1, S_2, S_3 are defined above, and U refers to some nondollar but objective measure of health-care benefit. In many medical analyses, U refers to the quality-adjusted life years (or QALYs).

This measure of U may or may not be appropriate for assessing the cost–utility of a clinical neuropsychological examination. For the moment, let us apply it to a college athlete who has sustained a concussion. Assume that the athlete sustained multiple concussions (three before the examination) and that the last one occurred about 1 month before the neuropsychological examination. The patient had difficulties with headaches and dizziness and also reported problems with decreased memory and concentration skills. He did not know if he should end his college athletic career because of his concussions. How to manage his symptoms and whether it would be advisable for him to avoid further concussions by dropping his athletic pursuits were the basic referral questions.

In this case, C_1 = $540 for the first examination and $140 for the follow-up examination, for a total C of $680. C_2 = 1 hour of lost time to interview the father, estimated at a cost of $100 to the father. The patient was not working at the time and therefore incurred no cost to be examined. Travel costs were estimated at $30. In this case C_3 = essentially 0. S_1 is difficult to estimate. Without the examination, however, the athlete might have been placed on medications for headache (estimated cost = $120). If he continued to play and had sustained a fourth concussion, the estimated health cost could have been substantial. It certainly would have included neuroimaging studies such as MR imaging, which would have cost $1,500 at minimum. S_2, the estimated savings to the family, also is difficult to determine. Conceivably, it could have been several hundreds of dollars because they would have had to care for him while he was unable to attend school. S_3 also is difficult to estimate. In this case U = one-half of a quality-adjusted life years, or 6 months. That is, 6 months of the student's life would have been disrupted if he had not been evaluated properly and given appropriate recommendations. This analysis leads to the following equation: ($680 + $100 + 0) – ($120 + $1,500) = – $840, a "savings," for an estimated one-half of QALY.

Drummond et al. (1997) used the following equation for assessing the cost-effectiveness of a clinical service:

$$[(C_1 + C_2 + C_3) - (S_1 + S_2 + S_3)] \div E,$$

where the C and S values are the same as noted above, and E refers to the effect obtained in the health-care status of an individual or group as a result of the service. In a strict cost-effective analysis, "E and U represent changes in effectiveness of a health state, compared to an alternative" (Drummond et al., 1997, p. 21). This distinction is extremely important. Health-care economics do not just consider the cost of a service for a specific outcome but ask that question in relationship to an alternative treatment. Thus, for clinical neuropsychologists to study the cost-effectiveness of a clinical neuropsychological examination, they must compare the cost of the service to obtain the outcome to some other service that would attempt to achieve the same or another health-care outcome. This issue is important to consider when attempting to do innovative research on the cost-effectiveness of a clinical neuropsychological examination.

Assume for a moment that the decision about whether the athlete should continue playing football was based on the Mini-Mental Status Examination (a 15-minute examination) or on 3 hours of extensive neuropsychological testing. The cost of the Mini-Mental Status Examination may be less than $30, compared to $680 for the neuropsychological examination. But is the outcome the same? We would argue that the outcome is not the same. The Mini-Mental Status Examination misses many neuropsychological deficits that are covered by the more extensive neuropsychological examination. In fact, this difference is the reason individuals are referred for a neuropsychological examination. A brief neurological assessment examination is inadequate. Studies need to be conducted to document what clinicians seem to recognize in their daily work.

Determining What Patients and Their Families Experience After a Neuropsychological Consultation: A Research Example

This chapter outlines a number of points that define a neuropsychological examination and measure its cost outcome. However, it is important to provide practical examples about how practicing clinical neuropsychologists can translate this information into simple but useful research projects.

A simple approach is to ask patients about their degree of satisfaction after consulting with a clinical neuropsychologist. Figure 2.1 shows a letter sent to individuals who have received a neuropsychological examination consultation from the Department of Clinical Neuropsychology at the BNI. It is replicated here to illustrate how patient and family can be questioned about simple information after they are seen for a consulta-

Dear Patient:

You recently were seen for a neuropsychological examination/consultation in the Department of Clinical Neuropsychology at St. Joseph's Hospital and Medical Center. We would appreciate hearing from you regarding your experience and its relative value for you. If you would please take a few minutes to answer the following questions and return this survey to our department in the postage-paid envelope, I would greatly appreciate it.

Sincerely,

George P. Prigatano, Ph.D.

Item		
1. The office/clerical staff was helpful and courteous.	Yes_____ No_____	
2. The neuropsychologist who saw me was helpful and courteous.	Yes_____ No_____	
3. The results of the examination were clearly explained to me.	Yes_____ No_____	
4. My physician received the neuropsychological report in a timely fashion.	Yes_____ No_____	Don't know____
5. I feel the time spent in the examination provided useful information to me, my family, and/or my doctor.	Yes_____ No_____	Don't know____
6. If I had to pay for this consultation/examination out of my own pocket, I would be willing to do so.	Yes_____ No_____	Don't know____
7. My bill was clear and understandable, and I thought the cost reasonable.	Yes_____ No_____	Don't know____
8. My experience with the billing department was	Positive____ Negative___	Neutral____

Thank you for your feedback.

Patient's name (optional)________________________________

My neuropsychologist was (please check):

Dr. Prigatano____ Dr. Zigler____ Dr. Hahn_____

Dr. Baxter______ Dr. Johnson____

FIGURE 2.1. Patient satisfaction survey. Department of Clinical Neuropsychology, Barrow Neurological Institute, St. Joseph's Hospital and Medical Center, Phoenix, Arizona. With permission from Barrow Neurological Institute.

tion. The questions focus not only on how well the clients were treated but on whether they felt the time spent was useful. The question of whether they would be willing to pay for the consultation themselves is key to this chapter.

As Sweet (personal communication) noted, patients who experience the two ends of the spectrum of patient satisfaction (i.e., very happy, very unhappy) appear to many surveyors to be the most motivated to respond. Yet, this type of information is important in our clinical practice. Neuropsychologists need to ask such questions in a scientific, reliable, and professionally responsible manner to determine the value of their work from the perspective of patients and families they serve. Questionnaires are difficult to construct and response rate is often low, but work in this area is very much needed. Armed with this information, neuropsychologists can make better business decisions and deal with the administrators to whom they report.

Summary and Conclusions

This chapter described the components of a neuropsychological examination, what it attempts to measure, and the kinds of questions it can answer. Depending on the context, the answers to these questions can have different values that can be measured both objectively and subjectively.

This chapter also described methods of studying the cost outcomes of a clinical neuropsychological examination. Economic formulae presented by Drummond et al. (1997) were reviewed and applied to the neuropsychological examination. A brief patient satisfaction survey derived from the considerations discussed in this chapter was provided as an example of how practicing clinical neuropsychologists can measure the value of their work as experienced by the patients and families who see them.

The remaining chapters of this book further clarify these basic ideas and how they can be applied to different patient populations and clinical settings.

References

Anderson, S. W., Damasio, H., & Tranel, D. (1990). Neuropsychological impairments associated with lesions caused by tumor or stroke. *Archives of Neurology, 47,* 397–405.

Bayley, P. J., Salmon, D. P., Bondi, M. W., Bui, B. K., Olichney, J., Delis, D. C., Thomas, R. G., & Thal, L. J. (2000). Comparison of the serial position effect in very mild Alzheimer's disease and amnesia associated with electroconvulsive therapy. *Journal of the International Neuropsychology Society, 6*(23), 290–298.

Benton, A. (1975). Neuropsychological assessment. In D. B. Tower (Ed.), *The nervous system, Vol 2: The clinical neurosciences,* (pp. 67–74). New York: Raven.

Borgaro, S., & Prigatano, G. P. (in press). Early cognitive and affective sequelae of traumatic brain injury. *The Journal of Head Trauma Rehabilitation.*

Caine, D., & Watson, J. D. G. (2000). Neuropsychological and neuropathological sequelae of cerebral anoxia: A critical review. *The Journal of International Neuropsychology Society, 6,* 86–89.

Case, R. (1985). *Intellectual development. Birth to adulthood.* San Diego, CA: Academic Press.

Chapman, L. F., & Wolff, H. G. (1959). The cerebral hemispheres and the highest integrative functions of man. *Archives of Neurology, 1,* 357–424.

Christensen, A. L. (1979). *Luria's neuropsychological investigation text* (2nd ed.). Denmark: Munksgaard.

Costa, L. D., Vaughan, H. G., Levita, E., & Farber, N. (1963). Purdue Pegboard as a predictor of the presence and laterality of cerebral lesions. *Journal of Consulting Psychology, 27,* 133–137.

Crosson, B., Sartor, K. J., Jenny, A. F., Nabors, N. A., & Moberg, P. J. (1993). Increased intrusions during verbal recall in traumatic and nontraumatic lesions of the temporal lobe. *Neuropsychology, 7,* 193–208.

Cummings, J. L., Tomiyasu, U., Read, S., & Benson, D. F. (1984). Amnesia with hippocampal lesions after cardiopulmonary arrest. *Neurology, 34,* 679–681.

De Renzi, E., & Vignolo, L. A. (1962). The token test: A sensitive test to detect disturbances in aphasics. *Brain, 85,* 667–678.

Dikmen, S. S., Machamer, J. E., Winn, H. R., & Temkin, N. R. (1995). Neuropsychological outcome at 1-year post head injury. *Neuropsychology, 9*(1), 80–90.

Drummond, M. F., O'Brien, B. J., Stoddart, G. L., & Torrance, G. W. (1997). *Methods for the economic evaluation of health care programmes* (2nd ed.). Oxford: Oxford University.

Gardner, H. (1983). *Frames of mind.* New York: Basic Books.

Geffen, G., Moar, K. J., O'Hanlon, A. P., Clark, C. R., & Geffen, L. B. (1990). Performance measures of 16- to 86-year-old males and females on the Auditory Verbal Learning Test. *The Clinical Neuropsychologist, 4*(1), 45–63.

Goldstein, F. C., & Levin, H. S. (1995). Post-traumatic and anterograde amnesia following closed head injury. In A. D. Baddeley, B. A. Wilson, & F. N. Watts (Eds.), *Handbook of memory disorders* (pp. 187–209). West Sussex, UK: John Wiley & Sons.

Goodglass, H., & Kaplan, E. (1983). *The assessment of aphasia and related disorders.* Philadelphia, Lea & Febiger.

Haaland, K. Y., Temkin, N., Randahl, G., & Dikmen, S. (1994). Recovery of simple motor skills after head injury. *Journal of Clinical and Experimental Neuropsychology, 16*(3), 448–456.

Heaton, R. K., Grant, I., & Matthews, C. G. (1991). *Comprehensive norms for an expanded Halstead-Reitan battery.* Odessa, FL: Psychological Assessment Resources.

Hebb, D. O. (1941). Human intelligence after removal of cerebral tissue from the right frontal lobe. *Journal of General Psychology, 25,* 257–265.

Hebb, D. O. (1939). Intelligence in man after large removals of cerebral tissue: Report of four left frontal lobe cases. *Journal of General Psychology, 21,* 73–87.

Johnson, S. C., Bigler, E. D., Burr, R. B., & Blatter, D. D. (1994). White matter atrophy, ventricular dilation, and intellectual functioning following traumatic brain injury. *Neuropsychology, 8*(3), 307–315.

Johnson, S. C., & Prigatano, G. P. (2000). Functional MR imaging during finger tapping. *BNI Quarterly, 16*(3), 37–41.

Kail, R. (1991). Developmental change in speed of processing during childhood and adolescence. *Psychological Bulletin, 109*(3), 490–501.

Keppel, G., & Zedick, S. (1989). *Data analysis for research design.* New York: W.H. Freeman.

Kertesz, A., Nadkarni, N., Davidson, W., & Thomas, A. W. (2000). The frontal behavioral inventory in the differential diagnosis of frontotemporal dementia. *The Journal of the International Neuropsychology Society, 6,* 460–468.

Levin, H. S., Mendelsohn, D., Lilly, M. A., Fletcher, J. M., Culhane, K. A., Chapman, S. B., Harward, H., Kusnerik, L., Bruce, D., & Eisenberg, H. M. (1994). Tower of London performance in relation to magnetic resonance imaging following closed head injury in children. *Neuropsychology, 8*(2), 171–179.

Lezak, M. D. (1995). *Neuropsychological assessment.* New York: Oxford University.

Lundin, K. A., & DeFilippis, N. A. (1999). Proposed schedule of usual and customary test administration times. *The Clinical Neuropsychologist, 13*(4), 433–436.

McDowell, S., Whyte, J., & D'Esposito, M. (1997). Working memory impairments in traumatic brain injury: Evidence from a dual-task paradigm. *Neuropsychologia, 35*(10), 1341–1353.

Mehlbye, J., & Larsen, A. (1994). Social and economic consequences of brain damage in Denmark: A case study. In A. L. Christensen & B. P. Uzzell (Eds.), *Brain injury and neuropsycho-*

logical rehabilitation: International perspectives (pp. 257–267). Hillsdale, NJ: Lawrence Erlbaum.

Meyer, G., Finn, S., Eyde, L., Kay, G., Moreland, K., Dies, R., Eisman, E., Kubiszyn, T., & Reed, G. (2001). Psychological testing and psychological assessment: A review of evidence and issues. *American Psychologist, 56,* 128-165.

Milner, B. (1963). Effects of different brain lesions on card sorting. *Archives of Neurology, 9,* 90–100.

Milner, B. (1958). Psychological deficits in temporal lobe excision. *Research Publication of the Association for Research of Nervous and Mental Disorders, 36,* 244–257.

Mitrushina, M. N., Boone, K. B., & D'Elia, L. F. (1999). *Handbook of normative data for neuropsychological assessment.* New York: Oxford University.

Prigatano, G. P. (1999). *Principles of neuropsychological rehabilitation.* New York: Oxford University.

Prigatano, G. P. (1991). Disturbances of self-awareness of deficit after traumatic brain injury. In G. P. Prigatano & D. L. Schacter (Eds.), *Awareness of deficit after brain injury: Theoretical and clinical issues* (pp. 111–126). New York: Oxford University.

Prigatano, G. P., & Amin, K. (1993). Digit Memory Test: Unequivocal cerebral dysfunction and suspected malingering. *Journal of Clinical Experimental Neuropsychology, 15*(4), 537–546.

Prigatano, G. P., Amin, K., & Rosenstein, L. D. (1995). *Administration and scoring manual for the BNI screen for higher cerebral functions.* Phoenix, AZ: Barrow Neurological Institute.

Prigatano, G. P., & Parsons, O. A. (1976). The relationship of age and education to Halstead test performance in different patient populations. *Journal of Consulting Clinical Psychology, 44,* 527–533.

Prigatano, G. P., & Redner, J. R. (1993). The uses and abuses of neuropsychological testing in behavioral neurology. *Neurological Clinics, 11*(1), 219–231.

Prigatano, G. P., Smason, I., Lamb, D., & Bortz, J. (1997). Suspected malingering and the Digit Memory Test: A replication and extension. *Archives of Clinical Neuropsychology, 12*(7), 609–619.

Prigatano, G. P., & Wong, J. L. (1999). Cognitive and affective improvement in brain dysfunctional patients who achieve inpatient rehabilitation goals. *Archives of Physical Medicine and Rehabilitation, 80,* 77–84.

Prigatano, G. P., & Wong, J. L. (1997). Speed of finger tapping and goal attainment following unilateral CVA. *Archives of Physical Medicine and Rehabilitation, 78,* 847–852.

Rao, S. M., Leo, G. J., & St. Aubin-Faubert, P. (1989). On the nature of memory disturbance in multiple sclerosis. *Journal of Clinical Experimental Neuropsychology, 11*(5), 699–712.

Reitan, R. M. (1995). *Manual for administration of neuropsychological test batteries for adults and children.* Tucson, AZ: Reitan Neuropsychology Laboratories.

Reitan, R. M. (1986). Theoretical and methodological bases of the Halstead-Reitan Neuropsychological Test Battery. In I. Grant & K. M. Adams (Eds.), *Neuropsychological assessment of neuropsychiatric disorders* (pp. 3–30). New York: Oxford University.

Reitan, R. M. (1956). Investigation of relationships between "psychometric" intelligence and "biological" intelligence. *Journal of Nervous Mental Disorders, 123,* 536–541.

Robertson, I. H., & Halligan, P. W. (1999). *Spatial neglect: A clinical handbook for diagnosis and treatment.* East Sussex, UK: Psychology Press.

Rosenstein, L. D., Prigatano, G. P., & Nayak, M. (1997). Differentiating patients with higher cerebral dysfunction from patients with psychiatric or acute medical illness with the BNI Screen for Higher Cerebral Functions. *Neuropsychiatry, Neuropsychology and Behavioral Neurology, 10*(2), 113–119.

Spreen, O., & Strauss, E. (1998). *A compendium of neuropsychological tests: Administration, norms, and commentary.* New York: Oxford University.

van Zomeren, A. H. (1981). *Reaction time and attention after closed head injury.* Lisse, The Netherlands: Swets & Zeitlinger B.V.

Vega, A., Jr., & Parsons, O. A. (1967). Cross-validation of the Halstead-Reitan tests for brain damage. *Journal of Consulting Psychology, 31,* 619–625.

Webster's new universal unabridged dictionary. (1983). Cleveland: New World Dictionaries, Simon & Schuster.

Wechsler, D. (1997). *Wechsler adult intelligence scale–revised.* San Antonio, TX: The Psychological Corporation.

Zangwill, O. L. (1947). Psychological aspects of rehabilitation in cases of brain injury. *British Journal of Psychology, 37,* 60–69.

PART

I

TRAUMATIC BRAIN INJURY

3

CHAPTER

Mark Sherer
Thomas A. Novack

Neuropsychological Assessment After Traumatic Brain Injury in Adults

Introduction[1]

Chapter 2 outlined the scope, cost, and health-care value of clinical neuropsychological examinations. This chapter considers in greater detail the value of neuropsychological assessment for monitoring the recovery of adults after significant traumatic brain injury (TBI) and for making treatment recommendations.

TBI can produce a wide range of physical, cognitive, behavioral, and emotional impairments. Initially, physical impairments may be prominent, especially after a severe TBI. Cognitive, behavioral, and emotional impairments, however, have the greatest impact on long-term outcomes (Brooks, Mckinlay, Symington, Beattie, & Campsie, 1987; Corrigan, Smith-Knapp, & Granger, 1998). Therefore, neuropsychological assessments include (a) review of preinjury functioning; (b) review of medical data regarding the nature and severity of the brain injury; (c) measurement of neuropsychological functions (as outlined in Chapter 2); and (d) assessment of behavioral and emotional characteristics through an interview with the patient and, when possible, with family and significant others. Patients with a TBI also should be observed directly.

In clinical practice, neuropsychological assessments for adults with a TBI are useful for describing disturbances in higher cerebral functioning, for monitoring changes that occur with time, treatment, or both, and for helping patients make practical decisions about their care and capacity to function independently and return to work (as outlined in Table 2.1). This chapter focuses on the need to document neuropsychological

[1]Preparation of this chapter was partially supported by the National Institute on Disability and Rehabilitation Research TBI Model Systems grants H133A980035–the TBI Model System of Mississippi and H133A980010–the University of Alabama/Birmingham Traumatic Brain Injury Care System. Editor G. P. Prigatano helped prepare the section on cost outcomes.

disturbances in this group of patients and on how that information is used to determine patients' capacity to make decisions, to live safely and independently, and to resume driving and work. The epidemiology of TBI, the typical neuropsychological impairments associated with TBI, the timing of evaluations, and expected outcomes in the course of recovery are reviewed. Finally, the use of cost–outcome methods to study the impact of neuropsychological assessment after TBI on health-care economics is considered.

☐ Epidemiology of TBI

Several different methods have been used to classify the severity of TBI. The most widely used method relies on the Glasgow Coma Scale (GCS; Teasdale & Jennett, 1974). Severe, moderate, and mild injuries are designated by scores between 3 and 8, 9 and 12, and 13 and 15, respectively (Hannay & Sherer, 1996; Levin & Eisenberg, 1991). A low GCS score associated with a space-occupying lesion suggests severe injury, especially in children (Levin, 1998).

Based on their review of previously published studies, Kraus, McArthur, Silverman, and Jayaraman (1996) estimated that the overall incidence of TBI in the United States is 200 per 100,000 population each year. Kraus and colleagues (1996) estimated that approximately 80% of patients admitted to hospitals after TBI have suffered mild injuries, 10% have moderate injuries, and 10% have severe injuries. A more recent study conducted by the Centers for Disease Control and Prevention (Thurman & Guerrero, 1999) indicated that hospitalization rates for TBI have decreased to 98 per 100,000 population per year. However, the incidence of moderate and severe TBI requiring hospitalization reported by Thurman and Guerrero (1999) is essentially the same as that estimated by Kraus and colleagues (1996). The decrease in the rate of hospitalization appears to reflect a tendency to hospitalize fewer individuals with mild TBI. This decrease likely does not reflect a true decrease in the incidence of mild TBI; rather, it probably reflects managed care practices in the United States.

☐ Neuropsychological Impairments Caused by TBI

People who experience blunt head trauma from motor vehicle collisions, falls, sport accidents, or other causes exhibit a characteristic pattern of impairment and recovery that has important implications for neuropsychological assessment. Typically, a period of posttraumatic amnesia (PTA; Levin, 1993) follows TBI. PTA is characterized by confusion and an inability to form new memories (Stuss et al., 1999). After the PTA has resolved, patients with a moderate or severe TBI usually still have some degree of physical, cognitive, or behavioral impairment. The prognosis for recovery of physical function after a blunt head injury is good, although some patients have persistent spasticity, dysphagia (impaired swallowing), dysarthria, balance disturbances, or other impairments (Horn & Sherer, 1999). Patients with focal injuries such as a large intracerebral hemorrhage or TBI from a gunshot wound may have residual hemiparesis, visual field deficits, or both. In a small percentage of patients, recovery is diminished by late complications such as posttraumatic epilepsy (Yablon, 1996) or posttraumatic hydrocephalus (Yu, Yablon, Ivanhoe, & Boake, 1995). The duration of PTA is related to later memory complaints (van Zomeren & van Den Burg, 1985).

Cognitive and neurobehavioral deficits are the most common residual impairments in the postacute period, and most contribute to long-term difficulties (Brooks, Campsie, Symington, Beattie, & McKinlay, 1986; Jennett, Snoek, Bond, & Brooks, 1981). Diffuse brain injury caused by blunt head trauma results in a typical pattern of cognitive deficits that includes slowed fine motor movements, decreased attention, slowed cognitive speed, memory impairment, impaired complex language skills and discourse, and impaired executive functions (Levin, 1993). Executive functions include working memory, problem solving, monitoring performance, allocating resources, and organizing behavior (Levin, 1998). Deficits in executive functions may be related to impaired self-awareness of deficits. Both are hypothesized to be caused by a prefrontal injury. Impaired self-awareness is common after moderate and severe TBI and contributes to poor functional outcomes (Sherer, Bergloff, Levin, High, Oden, & Nick, 1998). Severe persistent aphasia or visual perceptual impairment is uncommon after diffuse injury but may occur in patients with focal injuries (Levin, 1993).

After a moderate or severe TBI, cognitive impairment mostly recovers in the first 6 months but continues for 18 months or longer (Levin, 1993; Tabbador, Mattis, & Zazula, 1984). The risk for persistent cognitive impairment is related to the initial severity of injury but is difficult to predict. Existing data indicate that almost all, if not all, patients with a moderate or severe TBI have detectable cognitive impairments 1 month after injury (Dikmen, McLean, Temkin, & Wyler, 1986). One year after a severe injury (time to follow commands ≥ 14 days), patients continue to exhibit cognitive impairment. More than half of patients who are able to follow commands between 1 hour and 13 days after injury have residual deficits (Dikmen, Machamer, Winn, & Temkin, 1995). Although function is expected to recover until a plateau is reached, limited evidence suggests that a subgroup of persons with TBI may show a late decline (12 to 18 months after injury) in cognitive function (Ruff et al., 1991).

Overall, cognitive recovery after mild TBI is expected to be excellent. Typically, initial impairments of memory, speed of processing, and attention recover to baseline within 3 months of injury (Dacey, Vollmer, & Dikmen, 1993; Levin, et al., 1987). Nonetheless, some persons with a mild TBI remain impaired in the postacute period (see Chapter 4).

Common neurobehavioral problems reported by persons with TBI include increased irritability, headache, anxiety, difficulty concentrating, fatigue, restlessness, and depression (Oddy, Humphrey, & Uttley, 1978a; Satz et al., 1998). Neurobehavioral impairments are inherently more subjective and therefore more difficult to assess than physical or cognitive impairments. Several studies, however, indicate that neurobehavioral impairments may be even more common than cognitive or physical impairments in the postacute period and also may influence long-term functional outcomes more (Brooks, McKinlay, Symington, Beattie, & Campsie, 1987). Contrary to the course of recovery associated with physical and cognitive deficits, neurobehavioral impairments, as judged by a relative's report, may become more common and disruptive in the postacute period (Brooks et al., 1986). Relatives report that TBI patients exhibit slowness, irritability, fatigue, depression, rapid mood changes, and anxiety, among other symptoms. Family members often report more behavioral problems than patients do, and the difference likely reflects patients' impaired self-awareness (Sherer, Boake, Levin, Silver, Ringholz, & High, 1998).

Global Outcomes After TBI

The interpretation of TBI outcome studies is complicated by the different criteria used to establish severity of injury (e.g., GCS criteria vs. duration of coma), different study populations (e.g., consecutive admissions to a trauma center vs. admissions to inpatient rehabilitation), and different standards of care likely provided at different times and locations. The most commonly used global outcome measure is the Glasgow Outcome Scale (GOS; Jennett & Bond, 1975). The GOS outcome categories are:

1. death,
2. vegetative state (i.e., unable to follow commands or communicate),
3. severe disability (i.e., conscious but requiring assistance to meet basic physical and cognitive needs such as feeding, toileting, grooming, or personal safety),
4. moderate disability (i.e., able to meet basic physical and cognitive needs, to use public transportation, and to work in a sheltered workshop, but unable to return to nonsheltered work or to resume other major social roles), and
5. good recovery (i.e., able to return to nonsheltered work, although perhaps in a decreased capacity, and to resume social roles, although some neurological or psychological impairments may remain).

Unfortunately, the capacity of the GOS to meaningfully describe outcome after TBI is limited by the small number of outcome categories and the frequent observation that even people designated as having a "good recovery" may still experience significant problems. Such patients are often referred for neuropsychological rehabilitation programs or need some form of cognitive rehabilitation (see Chapters 14 and 16).

Mortality rates for patients hospitalized after severe TBI range from mid-30% to 50% (Levin & Eisenberg, 1991; Marion, 1996; Murray et al., 1999). Vegetative state is a rare outcome after severe TBI. Three months after injury, the incidence is less than 10% (Choi & Barnes, 1996), and it decreases to 4% at 6 months (Murray et al., 1999) and to 2% or 3% at 12 months. About 50% of patients who are vegetative at 3 months improve to severe or moderate disability 1 year after injury, 25% die, and 25% remain in a vegetative state (Choi & Barnes, 1996).

Within 3 months of injury, about 32% of persons with severe TBI recover to severe disability, as defined by the GOS, (Choi & Barnes, 1996), and 16% recover to severe disability within 6 months of injury (Murray et al., 1999). About 10% of all cases or about 20% of surviving cases remain at that level 1 year after injury (Choi & Barnes, 1996; Jennett & Teasdale, 1981; Levin et al., 1990). More than 65% of those with a severe disability at 3 months recover to moderate disability or make a good recovery 1 year after injury. Three to 6 months after injury, approximately 20% of all patients with severe TBI have recovered to moderate disability; 10% to 17% of all patients or 20% to 34% of surviving patients remain moderately disabled at 1 year (Choi & Barnes, 1996; Jennett & Teasdale, 1981; Levin et al., 1990; Murray et al., 1999). Choi and Barnes (1996) reported that 74% of patients with moderate disability 3 months after injury improved to a good recovery 1 year after injury, and no patient declined to a lower GOS category. Good recovery, as defined by the GOS, is experienced by approximately 15% of all patients with severe TBI 3 months after injury. More than 20% of all patients and more than 40% of surviving patients improve to good recovery within 6 months to 1 year of injury (Choi & Barnes, 1996; Jennett & Teasdale, 1981; Murray et al., 1999;

Williams, Levin, & Eisenberg, 1990). Good recovery is the most common outcome for patients who survive a severe TBI.

The death rates associated with moderate TBI range from 7% to 9% (Levin & Eisenberg, 1991; Murray et al., 1999). The incidence of vegetative state after moderate TBI is trivial or nonexistent (Murray et al., 1999). Severe disability after moderate TBI is rare. Murray and colleagues (1999) found that 14% of persons with moderate TBI were severely disabled 6 months after injury; others (Jennett et al., 1981; Levin et al., 1990; Williams et al., 1990) have found no patients who initially had a moderate TBI to be severely disabled 6 to 12 months after injury.

Based on the GOS, about 25% of patients with a moderate TBI have moderate disability at 6 months (Murray et al., 1999; Williams et al., 1990). Within 6 months of injury, 53% to 73% of patients with a moderate TBI improve to a good recovery (Murray et al., 1999; Williams et al., 1990). Functional outcomes for persons with a complicated mild TBI (initial GCS = 13 to 15 with positive initial findings on computed tomography) are similar to those experienced by patients with a moderate TBI (Williams et al., 1990).

Data on the outcome of mild TBIs are incomplete because many persons with a mild TBI may never reach the attention of medical professionals. Uncomplicated mild TBI is associated with favorable outcomes for most patients. Death, vegetative state, and severe disability have not been reported for these patients (van der Naalt, van Zomeren, Sluiter, & Minderhoud, 1999; Williams et al., 1990). Van der Naalt and colleagues (1999) found that 82% of patients with initial GCS scores of 13 and 14 attained good recovery within 1 month of injury, whereas 18% remained moderately disabled. Williams and colleagues (1990) found that 97.1% of patients with an uncomplicated mild TBI attained a good recovery within 6 months of injury, and only 2.9% remained moderately disabled. The economic and personal costs of these various levels of disability have not been calculated.

☐ Functional Outcomes After TBI

Classification of moderate disability or good recovery based on the GOS is based on the clinician's rating of the patient's ability to live or work independently rather than on the patient's actual functional status (Jennett & Bond, 1975). Such ratings avoid the potential bias of motivational factors, economic conditions, and availability (or lack of availability) of environmental supports or accommodations. These may be valid concerns, but it is also interesting to determine the actual employment and independent living outcomes of persons with TBI. Employment outcomes have been investigated extensively. Independent living as an outcome is less well studied, possibly because of methodological difficulties (Sherer, Madison, & Hannay, 2000).

Rates of return to work after TBI vary from 22% to 66% (Sander, Kreutzer, Rosenthal, Delmonico, & Young, 1996). Differences among studies reflect methods of classifying injury, time to follow-up, patient population, and definition of employment. Studies of consecutive admissions of TBI patients to trauma centers provide the most useful data. Groups of patients studied after admission to rehabilitation facilities may be biased by socioeconomic factors that determine which patients receive inpatient rehabilitation services. In one series of trauma center admissions, Brooks, McKinlay, and colleagues (1987) found a 29% rate of return to work for survivors of severe TBI assessed 2 to 7 years after injury. Dikmen and colleagues (1994) found that the rate of return to work was 37% for survivors of severe TBI and 64% for survivors of moderate TBI 2 years after injury. In long-term follow-up studies of patients with mild TBI, the rate of return to work has ranged between 83% and 87.5% (Dikmen et al., 1994; Stambrook, Moore, Peters, Deviaene, & Hawryluk, 1990).

Typical studies of independent living have been restricted to patients followed after inpatient rehabilitation and thus may not reflect all TBI survivors. In an investigation of 114 persons with severe and moderate TBIs evaluated from 3.5 months to 13.3 years after injury, Boake (1996) found that 14% were fully independent, 11% received overnight supervision, 49% received part-time supervision, 15% received full-time indirect supervision, and 11% received full-time direct supervision. This study may have overestimated the need for supervision because some patients were assessed before they had recovered maximally. Of 95 patients discharged from inpatient rehabilitation and followed for 5 years, Corrigan and colleagues (1998) found that the need for assistance or supervision decreased as time elapsed after injury. Although more than 60% of patients received assistance or supervision 6 to 12 months after discharge from rehabilitation, only 25% received assistance or supervision 4 to 5 years after discharge. Severity of injury was not reported but can be inferred to be severe or moderate, because patients with uncomplicated mild TBI rarely require inpatient rehabilitation.

□ The Utility of Neuropsychological Assessment for Persons with TBI

The neuropsychological assessment is unique in terms of the breadth of information obtained about the integrity of higher brain functions. A comprehensive neuropsychological evaluation of TBI patients assesses motor and sensory functioning, multiple areas of cognitive function, and behavior, and also considers emotional and psychiatric issues. The broad and objective assessment of skills is important. Information obtained from such evaluation can be used in a number of ways (see Table 3.1).

Feedback to Family Members

Family members' need for feedback about their patient's cognitive and behavioral problems caused by TBI is best understood in the context of the stresses placed on the

TABLE 3.1. Utility of Neuropsychological Assessment in Adults with TBI

Documentation of cognitive, behavioral, and emotional status
Feedback to family members
Feedback to improve patient awareness
Guiding treatment efforts
Assessing effectiveness of drug trials
Determination of ability to function independently
Decision-making capacity
Capacity for safe and independent functions
Driving capacity
Timeliness of return to work

TBI = traumatic brain injury

family. As described by Camplair, Butler, and Lezak (Chapter 5), the injured person's behavioral difficulties, emotional status, and (to a lesser extent) cognitive limitations after TBI are strongly associated with the perceived burden of the primary caregiver and surpass the contribution of severity of injury or physical limitations (Groom, Shaw, O'Connor, Howard, & Pickens, 1998; Wallace et al., 1998). Problems such as forgetfulness, disorientation, disorganized communication, impatience, diminished insight, poor decision-making capacity, increased sensitivity, and irritability have been identified consistently as major concerns of family caregivers and as sources of stress (Marsh, Kersel, Havill, & Sleigh, 1998; Oddy, Humphrey, & Uttley, 1978b). Such stress has been associated with an increased use of medications, diminished employment, and poor financial status among family members of patients with TBI (Hall, Karzmark, Stevens, Englander, O'Hare, & Wright, 1994). In contrast, age, education, length of coma, duration of PTA, and degree of physical disability are not consistent predictors of the caregiver's burden, even years after injury (Brooks, Campsie, Symington, Beattie, & McKinlay, 1987; Allen, Linn, Gutierrez, & Willer, 1994).

Although a caregiver's stress is multidimensional and partly determined by the caregiver's coping style (Sander, High, Hannay, & Sherer, 1997), the effect of cognitive and behavioral difficulties on the caregiver's level of stress warrants providing caregivers with objective information about those difficulties. This issue has not been explored empirically, but providing such information may have an innoculatory effect on caregivers coping with injured relatives. In several studies, families reported a lack of information from treatment staff as a significant frustration that added to their perceived burden.

Feedback to Increase Patient Awareness

Lack of awareness of capabilities, particularly of deficits, is a major issue in recovery from TBI, because limited awareness can result in poor judgment and an inability to focus on restorative therapies. Objective evaluation of awareness of deficits suggests that persons with severe TBI overestimate their abilities compared to family members' perceptions (Burgess, Alderman, Evans, Emslie, & Wilson, 1998; Sherer, Boake, et al., 1998) and relative to their actual test performance (Boake, Freeland, Ringholz, Nance, & Edwards, 1995). Awareness of deficit is a unique ability that is not easily explained by cognitive status in other areas, such as memory, attention, or language skills (Prigatano & Altman, 1990). Examining patients a mean of 7 years after injury, Trudel, Tryon and Purdum (1998) found that diminished awareness was associated with a lower vocational and residential status and the presence of maladaptive behavior. In contrast to Prigatano and Altman (1990), diminished awareness was associated with injury severity (as indicated by PTA duration), memory deficit, and global impairment. Prigatano and colleagues (1998) later also found a relationship between the degree of impaired self-awareness and severity of TBI as indicated by admitting GCS score in a study of Spanish TBI patients.

By providing objective information about cognitive abilities, the neuropsychological evaluation provides a rationale for family members and rehabilitation therapists who must point out to brain-injured patients that their functional ability may be less than their subjective experience of their ability. The results of clinical studies (Rebmann & Hannon, 1995; Youngjohn & Altman, 1989) indicate that providing feedback to TBI patients about the discrepancy between their expectations and their actual performance on cognitive tests can improve the accuracy of the patients' expectations about the performance on specific tasks.

Guiding Treatment Efforts

Neuropsychological services are an accepted component of acute and postacute rehabilitation services for individuals with TBI. The role of the neuropsychologist on the rehabilitation team, particularly in acute treatment settings, is still evolving. Early in acute rehabilitation, patients with severe injuries often are unable to participate in lengthy testing procedures, because basic cognitive systems such as arousal, attention, and communication are too disrupted. This situation led to the development of brief screening procedures that enable clinicians to estimate cognitive skills.

Prigatano and Wong (1999) described a screening procedure that requires 10 to 25 minutes and can be administered at the patient's bedside to assess orientation, memory, language, attention, and visuospatial skills. Items also focus on awareness and affect. In a preliminary study of 95 individuals (24% with TBI), the total score of the screening scale on admission significantly differentiated those who met rehabilitation goals from those who did not. The relationship, however, between goal attainment and performance on the scale was much stronger at discharge. Affective improvement also was strongly associated with goal attainment. Prigatano and Wong (1999) also provided an excellent example of how cognitive test results and knowledge of brain–behavior relationships can guide interventions to improve cognition during rehabilitation.

Cognitive remediation represents a special instance in which neuropsychological evaluation is essential. Before any cognitive remediation program is initiated, cognitive abilities must be evaluated to provide a baseline for comparison. Posttreatment evaluation also is a standard procedure, even when the evaluation of community activities is emphasized in addition to cognitive abilities. Cognitive remediation studies have provided ample evidence of the use of neuropsychological assessment (Ben-Yishay, Silver, Piasetsky, & Rattok, 1987; Harrington & Levandowski, 1987; Ruff & Baser, 1990). Reviews of cognitive remediation techniques have underscored the importance of assessment of skills (Sohlberg & Mateer, 1989; Wilson, 1991), and the Guidelines for Cognitive Rehabilitation established by the Head Injury Interdisciplinary Special Interest Group of the American Congress of Rehabilitation Medicine (1992) have indicated the need for intake and discharge evaluations.

Assessing Effectiveness of Drug Trials

The necessary low tolerance for cognitive side effects associated with pharmaceutical interventions after TBI has led to a strong reliance on neuropsychological evaluation in drug trials. This reliance is particularly evident in the development of anticonvulsants, where newer medications often are claimed to have fewer cognitive side effects than established interventions (Gillham et al., 1988; Meador et al., 1991; Meador, Loring, Huh, Gallagher, & King, 1990). The potential for negative cognitive side effects has almost led to neuroleptics being abandoned in cases of TBI, particularly early in recovery (Stanislav, 1997).

Neuropsychological assessment also has played an essential role in assessing the effectiveness of medications intended to benefit cognition. Several studies, for instance, have explored the use of methylphenidate after TBI (Kaelin, Cifu, & Matthies, 1996;

Plenger et al., 1996; Whyte et al., 1997). Although results have been mixed, neuropsychological assessment was central to the design of the studies and to their conclusions. The development of pharmaceutical interventions for memory disorders also has relied heavily on neuropsychological assessment as a standard to determine efficacy. Although much of this work has focused on patients with degenerative disorders, studies focusing on these medications have begun to surface in the TBI literature (Bohnen, Twijnastra, & Jolles, 1993; Taverni, Seliger, & Lichtman, 1998).

Determination of Ability to Function Independently

Information obtained through neuropsychological assessment must be useful in practical ways. It is not enough to document the presence of neuropsychological deficits without providing some impression about how those deficits are translated into daily living. Providing information about the capacity to perform daily activities may be useful, but the accuracy of such feedback is difficult to evaluate empirically. The ecological validity of traditional neuropsychological tests has been questioned, despite evidence that functional skills and cognitive abilities are related in some populations. In the case of chronic obstructive pulmonary disease, measures of motor speed and visuomotor processing were predictive of functioning in a number of areas, including basic activities of daily living and hobbies (McSweeny, Grant, Heaton, Prigatano, & Adams, 1985). Many neuropsychological tests in use today, however, were developed to localize cerebral lesions and may not translate well to predicting daily functioning, thereby necessitating the development of new approaches (Hart & Hayden, 1986; Wilson, 1993). Many factors can influence a person's ability to perform daily activities, and it would be unrealistic to expect cognitive deficits to be the only, or even the primary, predictor of the capacity to perform such activities. To the extent that neuropsychological test results—whether derived from traditional assessment approaches or from new techniques—can contribute to such prediction, collecting the information is justified.

Capacity to Make Decisions

Evaluating patients' capacity to make decisions about their medical treatment, finances, and living independently represents a major challenge for clinicians who provide TBI rehabilitation. In many cases, rehabilitation, including the introduction of pharmacological agents, must be pursued at a time when severely injured persons are incapable of giving consent but have not been adjudicated as incapable of making such decisions. This situation raises legal and ethical issues (Banja, 1999). Consent to medical treatment requires that individuals have the capacity to understand the issues involved and to respond appropriately. This capacity depends on many cognitive abilities, including language skills, orientation, and awareness (Alexander, 1988). Guidelines for evaluating the capacity to provide consent to medical treatment after TBI have been generated (Haffey, 1989) but are not yet used consistently.

Few studies have focused specifically on the decision-making capacity of those with a TBI. Callahan and Hagglund (1995) described a quadriparetic person with a brain injury from a gunshot wound who refused nonemergent care. The neuropsychological data were helpful in determining the patient's capacity to refuse such care. Auerbach and Banja (1996) found that professional raters who viewed videotaped structured interviews were consistent in rating the subjects' capacity to make decisions about medical treatment. The group studied was predominantly composed of individuals with TBI, and raters were provided background information, including medical history and the results of a mental status screening. Interestingly, the ratings of professionals—including physicians, neuropsychologists, and attorneys—differed significantly from the ratings of the team treating the patients. The latter were more likely to perceive the subject as being incapacitated. This discrepancy underscores the need to establish greater objectivity and clarity in this area.

The capacity to make decisions receives considerable attention in persons experiencing degenerative disorders, such as Alzheimer's disease. In the process of developing instruments to assess decision making specifically, Marson, Chatterjee, Ingram, and Harrell (1996) found that the capacity of Alzheimer's patients to make medical decisions is predicted by their performance on neuropsychological tests. Instruments focusing on the capacity to consent to treatment originally developed for use with psychiatric patients (Grisso, Applebaum, & Hill-Fotouhi, 1997) also may have an application for persons with TBI. Neuropsychological evaluation may be very informative in this area, particularly as tests specific to competency issues are developed.

Capacity to Function Safely and Independently

This area focuses directly on the relationship between neuropsychological evaluation and the daily activities involved in independent functioning. The issues of safety and independence in activities of daily living have been addressed by neuropsychologists working with patients who have experienced a cerebrovascular accident (CVA; particularly with respect to the impact of sensory neglect) to a greater extent than by those working with TBI patients. Nonetheless, several studies have established a relationship between objective assessment and daily functioning in people with TBI.

Malec, Zweber, and DePompolo (1990) found that memory functioning and attentional skill accounted for 36% of the variance in scores on a measure of psychosocial functioning. The authors, however, stressed that the limited correlations between neurocognitive measures favor a broad assessment rather than measures of memory and attentional skill alone. Klonoff, Costa, and Snow (1986) obtained similar results from a sample composed mostly of persons with mild injuries. Memory abilities, constructional skills, and fine motor skills predicted psychosocial outcomes, including the performance of daily activities such as social interaction, ambulation, and eating. The severity of injury and the presence of structural lesions in the frontal area also played important roles.

Leahy and Lam (1998) examined 58 individuals 6 to 12 months after they sustained a severe head injury and found that intellectual ability and concentration, but not memory capacity, were significantly diminished in those who required assistance with daily activities. The authors speculated that memory functioning may not have been essential to daily tasks that were overlearned and that the emphasis on compensatory strategies during the rehabilitation program may have diminished the impact of the memory disorder. In 90 individuals (half of whom had a TBI), a significant relationship existed between falls during inpatient rehabilitation and executive and visuospatial functioning, but not with memory abilities, attentional skills, or verbal skills (Rapport, Hanks, Millis, & Deshpande, 1998). In addition, executive and visuospatial functioning contributed to the ability to predict falls beyond those predicted by demographic information and a measure of functional status on admission to rehabilitation. Neistadt (1993) examined 54 subjects a mean of 7 years after TBIs of variable severity. Spatial and motor tasks were used to predict the capacity to make a simple meal of a cold sandwich and hot beverage. All of the spatial motor tasks correlated significantly with success at meal preparation, even after motor abilities and sensory neglect were considered.

Wang and Ennis (1986) developed new measures of cognitive skills to increase the ecological validity of assessments. Tasks included demonstrating the sequence of daily activities using cards, recalling a grocery list and prices, sorting mail, summing money, and answering questions about safety, among others. The scale was used to differentiate 10 people living independently from 8 people who required at least partial assistance on a daily basis. Why the latter group needed assistance was not specified, but the case examples suggested a range of neurological disorders. With the exception of items that assess personal information, all components of the scale differentiated the two groups. The finding suggests the impact of cognitive limitations on independent living. Alone, this study is insufficient to recommend the scale strongly, and its use has not yet been reported again in the literature. However, this work provides an idea of how a scale can be developed and applied based on knowledge of cognitive abilities.

The studies reviewed suggest that neuropsychological evaluation is generally predictive of personal safety and the ability to live independently. Making specific predictions for individual patients is more difficult. In some situations, their incapacity is clear (e.g., severe and broad deficits are present). The challenge arises with individuals with milder problems, particularly when issues such as judgment and impulsivity must be addressed. This area appears to be fruitful for research in neuropsychology, which is positioned better than other specialties to deal with such issues.

Capacity to Drive

For many patients, driving is an important activity, and it can be related to the ability to achieve employment and live independently. To the extent that cognitive deficits predict the capacity to drive, performance on neuropsychological tests provides important information. Most studies in this area have involved small sample sizes and have often combined people with different diagnoses, particularly those with TBI and CVA. Based on a small sample (Katz et al., 1990), there is no indication that people with a severe TBI are more likely than matched controls to be involved in crashes or to receive moving violations. Individuals in this study, however, underwent a driving assessment that included a neuropsychological evaluation before they were permitted to drive again. Thus, it is possible that positive neuropsychological results, along with other factors in the driving assessment, were predictive of good driving outcomes.

Multiple studies indicate that TBI is associated with disruption of driving skills and that cognitive deficits are at the core of that disruption. For instance, van Zomeren, Brouwer, Rothengatter, and Snoek (1988) evaluated driving objectively (e.g., lateral positioning within the lane) and found that persons with TBI were impaired compared to controls. Poor results from tests of visual memory, speed of visual processing, and digital manipulation significantly correlated with poor driving performance.

Studies examining the correlation of cognitive tests with on-the-road performance have demonstrated that poor performance on measures of perceptual speed, accuracy of visual perception, and visual problem solving is associated with driving difficulties

(Mazer, Korner-Bitensky, & Sofer, 1998). In a study of persons with TBI tested at least a year after injury, measures of perceptual speed and reaction time, when combined with duration of coma and driving experience, accounted for 35% of the variance in open-road driving capability (Korteling & Kaptein, 1996). The results did not warrant substituting a cognitive evaluation for on-the-road testing but indicated that cognitive evaluation may serve as a screening tool before a driving evaluation.

Processing speed also is a major factor in predicting driving performance among subjects with TBI (Gouvier et al., 1989). Sivak and colleagues (1984) trained eight people with mixed neurological problems who exhibited cognitive problems and poor performance on open-road driving. Training, which lasted 8 to 10 hours, focused on visual scanning, spatial perception, figure-ground differentiation, attentional capacity, and problem solving. Evaluations during the course of training revealed that improved performance on visual perceptual cognitive tests corresponded with an improvement in driving performance. The results of these studies indicate that neuropsychological test results have predictive value for driving ability and may serve as a screening tool before individuals undergo on-the-road evaluation of their driving ability.

Timing of Return to Work

Returning persons with TBI to productive activity is a major goal of rehabilitation. Neuropsychological evaluation is an accepted means of identifying individuals who might be ready to participate in a vocational rehabilitation program or who might be able to return directly to productive activity. Ability to participate in vocational evaluation was examined in a sample of 80 individuals with TBI of unspecified severity (Ryan, Sautter, Capps, Meneese, & Barth, 1992). A discriminant function analysis revealed a 78% correct rate of classification based on cognitive tests, including reading comprehension, memory functioning, language skills, and depression. Ruff and colleagues (1993) examined 93 individuals with severe TBI 6 months after their injury; 55 subjects returned to work 1 year after injury. Return to work was best predicted by measures of selective attention, expressive vocabulary, and age. In 94 individuals with severe TBI examined at least 1 year after injury (Fabiano & Crewe, 1995), measures of intellectual capacity were found to be the predominant contributors in a discriminant function analysis. Those who were able to return to work after their injury were identified with an accuracy of 62%. In contrast, the injured person's education, age, and occupational history were not predictive of return to work. Memory functioning also differentiates employed from unemployed individuals after TBI (Cifu et al., 1997).

Awareness of deficits may surpass other cognitive variables in predicting a return to work. Sherer, Bergloff, and colleagues (1998) found clinician-rated awareness as well as the difference between client and family ratings of awareness to be predictive of employment. These variables exceeded the contribution of injury severity, chronicity, employment status before injury, history of substance abuse, and general rating of cognitive functioning on admission to rehabilitation. With the inclusion of the awareness information, 82% of the subjects were correctly classified in terms of their employment status. Although it is disconcerting that consistency is not greater in the areas identified, these studies indicate that a number of cognitive abilities influence return to employment.

Neuropsychological test results definitely contribute to the prediction of return to productive activity, but they are not the only variables that do so. For instance, Gollaher and colleagues (1998) examined 99 individuals with severe TBI and found that age, education, preinjury level of productivity, GCS score, and Disability Rating Scale score on admission to rehabilitation correctly discriminated 75% of those who returned to employment within 3 years of injury from those who did not. Similar results were obtained by Ponsford, Olver, Curran and Ng (1995). Dikmen and colleagues (1994) have explored return to work in great depth and found that the significant relationship between return to work and a global measure of neuropsychological impairment obtained 1 month after injury was enhanced by measures of injury severity and preinjury job stability. As in other areas of outcome, it would be inappropriate to consider cognitive abilities as the sole predictors of return to work. Nonetheless, evidence indicates that level of cognitive abilities contributes to prediction of return to productivity.

Assessment of cognitive abilities may predict not just a return to productive activity but the types of activity and whether accommodations may be necessary. For instance, Ezrachi, Ben-Yishay, Kay, Diller, and Rattok (1991) found that verbal aptitude (a composite of several intelligence scale subtests) was the most consistent significant predictor of the return to productive activity, including participation in a sheltered workshop and return to work with accommodations 6 months after completion of a day program. According to Kibby, Schmitter-Edgecombe, and Long (1998), measures of memory and executive functioning were not predictive when return to work was measured dichotomously. Memory functioning, however, was significant in hierarchical regression analyses focusing on a scale measuring the supervision and accommodations required on the job, even after accounting for physical disability, emotional distress, and the use of memory-compensation strategies. In contrast, executive functioning was significantly related to occupational status, suggesting that the impact of deficits of executive functions may be greater in more demanding occupations.

The studies reviewed indicate that those who are able to participate in vocational programs and who return to productive activity perform better on neuropsychological testing than those who do not engage in such activities. This outcome is not equivalent to being able to predict unerringly who will return to work. However, when combined with other information, neuropsychological evaluation has a role in ascertaining readiness for employment. A promising area that needs to be explored further is the need for accommodations at the work site and differentiating those able to return to previous jobs from those who will need less demanding positions.

Timing of Evaluations

There is consensus that most cognitive recovery occurs in the first 6 to 12 months after a severe TBI (Levin, 1993; Stuss & Buckle, 1992) and over a shorter period for less severe injuries. Consistent with this observation, Clifton, Hayes, Levin, Michel, and Choi (1992) recommended baseline evaluations of persons with TBI at resolution of PTA, follow-up evaluations for persons with severe TBI 6 and 12 months after injury, and follow-up evaluations for persons with moderate TBI 3 and 6 months after injury for purposes of research.

Cognitive abilities may continue to improve 2 to 3 years after severe TBI (Mandleburg & Brooks, 1975; van Zomeren & Deelman, 1978). These findings indicate that neuropsychological assessment in the postacute period of recovery from TBI may continue to detect meaningful changes in cognitive status. A schedule of assessments for persons with mild, moderate, and severe TBI has been recommended based on review of empirical findings, published recommendations, and a survey of 41 neuropsychologists regarding timing of neuropsychological evaluation after TBI (Table 3.2). Survey participants were selected based on board certification, published research on TBI, and current participation in research on outcomes of TBI. Of those surveyed, 33 responded, including 23 with board certification. Respondents reported a median of 20 years of clinical experience in examining patients with TBI (range = 7 to 35 years). The recommended times for evaluation are general suggestions. Determining the appropriate times to assess a specific patient is a clinical decision based on the evaluation of factors unique to that patient.

☐ Research on Cost Outcomes and Neuropsychological Assessment After TBI

Costs for neuropsychological services after severe TBI represent a small proportion of the entire cost of care. Billing records of 40 consecutive TBI admissions at the University of Alabama at Birmingham revealed that charges of neuropsychological assessment accounted for 1.2% of the rehabilitation charges and 0.2% of the total hospital charges, including all therapy services but excluding physician billing. Even if interventions for cognitive remediation and postacute rehabilitation are added to this picture, clinical neuropsychological services are not a major contributor to the cost of treatment. Nonetheless, insurance carriers want objective information regarding the costs–benefits of neuropsychological assessment.

Despite the important role of a neuropsychological examination in evaluating TBI patients, woefully few, if any, data are available on the health-care value and economic impact of such services. Research in this area, however, is eminently possible. Information obtained from a neuropsychological examination (Table 3.1) can help families understand the extent and nature of disturbed higher cerebral functions in an injured loved one. This information can provide a subjective sense of relief as family members better understand what is wrong with the patient and may also help reduce their burden of care.

The reduction of burden and its economic worth can and should be calculated. Suppose family members are asked to rate on a scale from 0 to 100 the degree to which they experience "burden" in the daily care of a brain-injured relative. Assume 0 equals no burden and 100 the maximum they could tolerate. Given Family 1's economic re-

TABLE 3.2. Suggested Schedules for Neuropsychological Evaluations After TBI

Time of Evaluation	Severe TBI	Moderate TBI	Mild TBI
At resolution of PTA	X	X	X
1 week to 1 month after injury			X
3 months after injury	X	X	X
6 months after injury	X	X	
1 year after injury	X	X	X
2 years after injury	X	X	

TBI = traumatic brain injury; PTA = posttraumatic amnesia

sources, what would they be willing to pay to reduce the burden by 10 points for 1 year? Assume that Family 1 reports that they are willing to pay $5,000 if such relief can be obtained. Family 2, with fewer financial resources, may also experience considerable burden, but could pay only $1,000 to reduce their burden by 10 points.

Using the method suggested by Drummond, O'Brien, Stoddart, & Torrance (1998; and described in Chapter 2), the following cost–benefit analysis could be calculated:

$$(W') - (C_1+C_2+C_3)$$

Assume Family 1 reports a 20-point drop in burden over 1 year (that would be worth $10,000 to them). The cost of two examinations for 1 year and providing information to the family is estimated at $1,700 ($C_1$). The total cost of travel (C_2) and time needed (C_3) to obtain this information for this family is $500. The following equation results:

$$(\$10{,}000) - (\$1{,}700 + \$500) = \$7{,}800$$

For Family 1, the neuropsychological evaluation and the information it provided were worthwhile. The value was good for the dollars spent.

Assume Family 2 reports only a 5-point drop in burden over 1 year as a result of receiving neuropsychological information. Assume it costs them $100 to take time off from work and to travel to obtain this information. In their case, the cost–benefit analysis is not beneficial.

$$(\$500 - \$1{,}700 + \$100 = -\$1{,}300)$$

Individual cost–benefit analysis, using a willingness-to-pay model, may be a fruitful way to assess both subjectively and objectively the value of such information for different families.

Another area of potential useful analysis focuses on the cost savings associated with providing appropriate supervision. Specific cost-minimization can be calculated. Assume that with proper supervision, the tendency to fall substantially decreases after brain injury. Falls that occur during inpatient rehabilitation have been related to impairments in executive and visuospatial functions (Rapport et al., 1998). This information may predict falls beyond that obtained from demographic information or measured functional status at admission obtained by rehabilitation specialists.

With this observation in mind, the following cost-effectiveness outcome could be calculated (medical costs of a fall with hip fracture are estimated at $21,000: $14,000 for hospital costs and $7,000 for physician's costs). The cost of a functional assessment is estimated at $160. The cost of a neuropsychological examination is estimated at $280 (for a 2-hour examination at $140 per hour). A neuropsychological examination is assumed to identify 14 of 20 fall victims, and the functional assessment would identify 6 of 20.

The cost of 20 falls with hip fractures would be $21,000 × 20 = $420,000. The cost of 20 neuropsychological examinations would be $280 × 20 = $5,600. The cost of 20 functional assessments would be $160 × 20 = $3,200. Identifying 14 of 20 potential hip fractures would save $294,000 ($S_1$). Identifying 6 of 20 hip fractures would save $126,000 ($S_2$). Thus, the expenditure of an extra $2,400 would produce considerable dollars savings ($294,000 – $126,000 = $168,000). This type of research could easily be conducted if accurate economic information from various medical sources were available.

The third example relates to an objective marker of value of neuropsychological testing when determining if a TBI patient can return to work. Although no such database exists, it would be an ideal area to assess the cost-effectiveness of neuropsychological examinations and to compare them with the clinical judgment of rehabilitation physicians and rehabilitation therapists.

Assume that in 100 consecutive admissions to an inpatient neurorehabilitation unit, 50 patients have TBI. Further assume that of these 50 patients, there is a serious question about whether 40 can return to work. Thus, the physician requests a neuropsychological examination for each of these 40 patients. The initial examination occurs within the hospital environment and typically takes about 2 hours, with an estimated charge of $280 in our setting. A second examination requested after discharge is 4 hours long with a 1-hour consultation, for a total of 5 hours (estimated cost = $700). Thus, the two examinations with consultation have an estimated cost of $980.

In this model, each of the 40 patients would be tested, so the total cost for such a consultation would be $39,200. Assume, for simplicity, that 20 patients would have been released by their physician and rehabilitation therapist too soon for work. The costs associated with these patients returning to work would then be calculated. These costs could include lost revenue from the employer, salary spent for ineffective work, the cost of correcting errors made by the TBI patient, the cost of poor customer satisfaction, and, finally, the cost associated with having to terminate the employee. In addition, the patient and family would experience costs. There would be costs associated with losing a job and the time and effort involved in finding a new one. The more difficult costs to calculate deal with the emotional distress of being fired. Finally, the family would bear costs by likely having to stay home to help the patient find a new position. Calculating all these costs determines the degree to which the expenditure of $39,200 would save in other costs incurred for society. Again, no such databases exist, but this analysis could be calculated.

Both individual cost–benefits and a group analysis on cost-effectiveness could be analyzed to justify reasonable assessments and to provide managed care interests with an explanation of how neuropsychological assessment can be cost-effective and cost-beneficial in different settings and for different families.

Conclusions

Evaluation of cognitive–behavorial and emotional disturbances via neuropsychological assessment is an essential component of a comprehensive evaluation and treatment plan for persons with TBI. The prevalence and persistence of neuropsychological deficits after TBI underscore the importance of such evaluations, particularly given the relationship between cognitive disabilities and outcome. The neuropsychological evaluation can contribute to decisions about independent living, effectiveness of treatment, and prognosis. Such information is valuable to those who have sustained injury, their families, and those providing treatment to persons with TBI.

Further research is needed to examine the usefulness of neuropsychological evaluations. For instance, it would be helpful if specific protocols could be established for people with injuries of various severity to be administered at intervals after the onset of injury. Such protocols would allow comparisons across samples and assess the rate of recovery of a particular person. Neuropsychologists also need to augment the use of general measures of outcome, such as the GOS, with more specific measures that focus on functional activities important to independent living. Predicting outcome in these areas will increase the utility of the neuropsychological evaluation. For example, prediction of return to work is an important goal of neuropsychological assessment, but specific predictions regarding the type of work and needed accommodations would be more useful. This type of prediction will require the development of new assessment strategies tailored to specific questions, as is occurring already in the area of managing finances. Finally, it is important to measure the impact of feedback provided to patients and family members about cognitive deficits after TBI. Such feedback should leave those involved, including the neuropsychologist, with a sense of direction and purpose.

References

Alexander, M. P. (1988). Clinical determination of mental competence: A theory and a retrospective study. *Archives of Neurology, 45,* 23–26.

Allen, K., Linn, R. T., Gutierrez, H., & Willer, B. S. (1994). Family burden following traumatic brain injury. *Rehabilitation Psychology, 39,* 29–48.

Auerbach, V. S., & Banja, J. D. (1996). Assessing client competence to participate in rehabilitation decision making. *Neurorehabilitation, 6,* 123–132.

Banja, J. D. (1999). Ethical dimensions of severe traumatic brain injury. In M. Rosenthal, E. R. Griffith, J. S. Kreutzer, & B. Penthland (Eds.), *Rehabilitation of the adult and child with traumatic brain injury* (3rd ed., pp. 413–434). Philadelphia: Davis.

Ben-Yishay, Y., Silver, S. M., Piasetsky, E., & Rattok, J. (1987). Relationship between employability and vocational outcome after intensive holistic cognitive rehabilitation. *Journal of Head Trauma Rehabilitation, 2*(1), 35–48.

Boake, C. (1996). Supervision Rating Scale: A measure of functional outcome from brain injury. *Archives of Physical Medicine and Rehabilitation, 77,* 765–772.

Boake, C., Freeland, J. C., Ringholz, G. M., Nance, M. L., & Edwards, K. E. (1995). Awareness of memory loss after severe closed-head injury. *Brain Injury, 9,* 273–283.

Bohnen, N. I., Twijnastra, A. T., & Jolles, J. (1993). A controlled trial with vasopressin analogue (DGAVP) on cognitive recovery immediately after head trauma. *Neurology, 43,* 103–106.

Brooks, N., Campsie, L., Symington, C., Beattie, A., & McKinlay, W. (1987). The effects of severe head injury on patient and relative within seven years of injury. *Journal of Head Trauma Rehabilitation, 2*(3), 1–13.

Brooks, N., Campsie, L., Symington, C., Beattie, A., & McKinlay, W. (1986). The five year outcome of severe blunt head injury: A relative's view. *Journal of Neurology, Neurosurgery, and Psychiatry, 49,* 764–770.

Brooks, N., McKinlay, W., Symington, C., Beattie, A., & Campsie, L. (1987). Return to work within the first seven years of severe head injury. *Brain Injury, 1,* 5–19.

Burgess, P. W., Alderman, N., Evans, J., Emslie, H., & Wilson, B. A. (1998). The ecological validity of tests of execution function. *Journal of International Neuropsychology Society, 4,* 547–558.

Callahan, C. D., & Hagglund, K. J. (1995). Comparing neuropsychological and psychiatric evaluation of competency in rehabilitation: A case example. *Archives of Physical Medicine and Rehabilitation, 76,* 909–912.

Choi, S. C., & Barnes, T. Y. (1996). Predicting outcome in the head-injured patient. In R. K. Narayan, J. E. Wilberger, & J. T. Povlishock (Eds.), *Neurotrauma* (pp. 779–792). New York: McGraw-Hill.

Cifu, D. X., Keyser-Marcus, L., Lopez, E., Wehman, P., Kreutzer, J. S., Englander, J., & High, W. (1997). Acute predictors of successful return to work 1 year after traumatic brain injury: A multicenter analysis. *Archives of Physical Medicine and Rehabilitation, 78,* 125–131.

Clifton, G. L., Hayes, R. L., Levin, H. S., Michel, M. E., & Choi, S. C. (1992). Outcomes measures for clinical trials involving traumatically brain-injured patients: Report of a conference. *Neurosurgery, 31,* 975–978.

Corrigan, J. D., Smith-Knapp, K., & Granger, C. V. (1998). Outcomes in the first 5 years after traumatic brain injury. *Archives of Physical Medicine and Rehabilitation, 79,* 298–305.

Dacey, R. G., Jr., Vollmer, D., & Dikmen, S. S. (1993). Mild head injury. In P. R. Cooper (Ed.), *Head injury* (pp. 159–182). Baltimore: Williams & Wilkins.

Dikmen, S. S., Machamer, J. E., Winn, H. R., & Temkin, N. R. (1995). Neuropsychological outcome at 1 year post head injury. *Neuropsychology, 9,* 1–11.

Dikmen, S., McLean, A., Temkin, N. R., & Wyler, A. R. (1986). Neuropsychologic outcome at one-month postinjury. *Archives of Physical Medicine and Rehabilitation, 67,* 507–513.

Dikmen, S. S., Temkin, N. R., Machamer, J. E., Holubkov, A. L., Fraser, R. T., & Winn, R. (1994). Employment following traumatic head injuries. *Archives of Neurology, 51,* 177–186.

Drummond, M. F., O'Brien, B. J., Stoddart, G. L., & Torrance, G. W. (1998). *Methods for the economic evaluation of health care programmes.* New York: Oxford University.

Ezrachi, O., Ben-Yishay, Y., Kay, T., Diller, L., & Rattok, J. (1991). Predicting employment in traumatic brain injury following neuropsychological rehabilitation. *Journal of Head Trauma Rehabilitation, 6*(3), 71–84.

Fabiano, R. J., & Crewe, N. (1995). Variables associated with employment following severe traumatic brain injury. *Rehabilitation Psychology, 40,* 223–231.

Gillham, R. A., Williams, N., Wiedmann, K., Butler, E., Larkin, J. G., & Brodie, M. J. (1988). Concentration-effect relationships with carbamazepine and its epoxide on psychomotor and cognitive function in epileptic patients. *Journal Neurology, Neurosurgery, and Psychiatry, 51,* 929–933.

Gollaher, K., High, W., Sherer, M., Bergloff, P., Boake, C., Young, M. E., & Ivanhoe, C. (1998). Prediction of employment outcome one to three years following traumatic brain injury (TBI). *Brain Injury, 12,* 255–263.

Gouvier, W. D., Maxfield, M. W., Schweitzer, J. R., Horton, C. R., Shipp, M., Neilson, K., & Hale, P. N. (1989). Psychometric prediction of driving performance among the disabled. *Archives of Physical Medicine and Rehabilitation, 70,* 745–750.

Grisso, T., Appelbaum, P. S., & Hill-Fotouhi, C. (1997). The MacCAT-T: A clinical tool to assess patients' capacities to make treatment decisions. *Psychiatric Services, 48,* 1415–1419.

Groom, K. N., Shaw, T. G., O'Connor, M. E., Howard, N. I., & Pickens, A. (1998). Neurobehavioral symptoms and family functioning in traumatically brain-injured adults. *Archives of Clinical Neuropsychology, 13,* 695–711.

Haffey, W. J. (1989). The assessment of clinical competency to consent to medical rehabilitative interventions. *Journal of Head Trauma Rehabilitation, 4*(1), 43–56

Hall, K., Karzmark, P., Stevens, M., Englander, J., O'Hare, P., & Wright, J. (1994). Family stressors in traumatic brain injury: A two-year follow up. *Archives of Physical Medicine and Rehabilitation, 75,* 876–885.

Hannay, H. J., & Sherer, M. (1996). Assessment of outcome from head injury. In R. K. Narayan, J. E. Wilberger, & J. T. Povlishock (Eds.), *Neurotrauma* (pp 723–747). New York: McGraw-Hill.

Harrington, D. E., & Levandowski, D. H. (1987). Efficacy of an educationally-based cognitive retraining program for traumatically head-injured as measured by LNNB pre- and post-test scores. *Brain Injury, 1,* 65–72.

Hart, T. & Hayden, M. E. (1986). The ecological validity of neuropsychological assessment and remediation. In B. P. Uzzell & Y. Gross (Eds.), *Clinical neuropsychology of intervention* (pp. 21–50). Boston: Martinas Nijhoff.

Head Injury Interdisciplinary Special Interest Group of the American Congress of Rehabilitation Medicine. (1992). Guidelines for cognitive rehabilitation. *Neurorehabilitation, 2,* 62–67.

Horn, L. J., & Sherer, M. (1999). Rehabilitation of traumatic brain injury. In M. Grabois S. J. Garrison, K. A. Hart, & L. D. Lehmkuhl (Eds.), *Physical medicine and rehabilitation the complete approach* (pp. 1281–1304). Cambridge, MA: Blackwell Science.

Jennett, B., & Bond, M. (1975). Assessment of outcome after severe brain damage. *Lancet, 1,* 480–484.

Jennett, B., Snoek, E. J., Bond, M. R., & Brooks, N. (1981). Disability after severe head injury:

Observations on the use of the Glasgow Outcome Scale. *Journal of Neurology, Neurosurgery, and Psychiatry, 44,* 285–293.

Jennett, B., & Teasdale, G. (1981). *Management of head injuries*. Philadelphia: F.A. Davis.

Kaelin, D. L., Cifu, D. X., & Matthies, B. (1996). Methylphenidate effect on attention deficit in the acutely brain-injured adult. *Archives of Physical Medicine and Rehabilitation, 77,* 6-9.

Katz, R. T., Golden, R. S., Butter, J., Tepper, D., Rothke, S., Holmes, J., & Sahgal, V. (1990). Driving safety after brain damage: Follow-up of twenty-two patients with matched controls. *Archives of Physical Medicine and Rehabilitation, 71,* 133–137.

Kibby, M. Y., Schmitter-Edgecombe, M., & Long, C. J. (1998). Ecological validity of neuropsychological tests: Focus on the California Verbal Learning Test and the Wisconsin Card Sorting Test. *Archives of Clinical Neuropsychology, 13,* 523–534.

Klonoff, P. S., Costa, L. D., & Snow, W. G. (1986). Predictors and indicators of quality of life in patients with closed-head injury. *Journal of Clinical and Experimental Neuropsychology, 8,* 469–485.

Korteling, J. E., & Kaptein, N. A. (1996). Neuropsychological driving fitness tests for brain-damaged subjects. *Archives of Physical Medicine and Rehabilitation, 77,* 138–146.

Kraus, J. F., McArthur, D. L., Silverman, T. A., & Jayaraman, M. (1996). Epidemiology of brain injury. In R. K. Narayan, J. E. Wilberger, & J. T. Povlishock (Eds.), *Neurotrauma* (pp. 13–30). New York: McGraw-Hill.

Leahy, B. J., & Lam, C. S. (1998). Neuropsychological testing and functional outcome for individuals with traumatic brain injury. *Brain Injury, 12,* 1025–1035.

Levin, H. S. (1998). Cognitive function outcomes after traumatic brain injury. *Current Opinions in Neurology, 11,* 643–646.

Levin, H. S. (1993). Neurobehavioral sequelae of closed head injury. In P. R. Cooper (Ed.), *Head injury* (pp. 525–551). Baltimore: Williams & Wilkins.

Levin, H. S., & Eisenberg, H. M. (1991). Neurobehavioral outcome. *Neurosurgery Clinic of North America, 2,* 457–472.

Levin, H. S., Gary, H. E., Eisenberg, H. M., Ruff, R. M., Barth, J. T., Kreutzer, J. S., High, W. M., Portman, S., Foulkes, M. A., Jane, J. A., Marmarou, A., & Marshall, L. F. (1990). Neurobehavioral outcome 1 year after severe head injury: Experience of the Traumatic Coma Data Bank. *Journal of Neurosurgery, 73,* 699–709.

Levin, H. S., Mattis, S., Ruff, R. M., Eisenberg, H. M., Marshall, L. F., Tabaddor, K., High, W. M., Jr., & Frankowski, R. F. (1987). Neurobehavioral outcome following minor head injury: A three center study. *Journal of Neurosurgery, 66,* 234–243.

Malec, J., Zweber, B., & DePompolo, R. (1990). The Rivermead Behavioral Memory Test, laboratory neurocognitive measures, and everyday functioning. *Journal of Head Trauma Rehabilitation, 5*(3), 60–68.

Mandleberg, I. A., & Brooks, D. N. (1975). Cognitive recovery after severe head injury. 1. Serial testing on the Wechsler Adult Intelligence Scale. *Journal of Neurology, Neurosurgery, and Psychiatry, 38,* 1121–1126.

Marion, D. W. (1996). Outcome from severe head injury. In R. K. Narayan, J. E. Wilberger, & J. T. Povlishock (Eds.), *Neurotrauma* (pp. 767–777). New York: McGraw-Hill.

Marsh, N. V., Kersel, D. A., Havill, J. H., & Sleigh, J. W. (1998). Caregiver burden at 1 year following severe traumatic brain injury. *Brain Injury, 12,* 1045–1059.

Marson, D. C., Chatterjee, A., Ingram, K. K., & Harrell, L. E. (1996). Toward a neurologic model of competency: Cognitive predictors of capacity to consent in Alzheimer's disease using three different legal standards. *Neurology, 46,* 666–672.

Mazer, B. L., Korner-Bitensky, N. A., & Sofer, S. (1998). Predicting ability to drive after stroke. *Archives of Physical Medicine and Rehabilitation, 79,* 743–749.

McSweeny, A. J., Grant, I., Heaton, R. K., Prigatano, G. P., & Adams, K. M. (1985). Relationship of neuropsychological status to everyday functioning in healthy and chronically ill persons. *Journal of Clinical and Experimental Neuropsychology, 7,* 281–291.

Meador, K. J., Loring, D. W., Allen, M. E., Zamrini, E. Y., Moore, E. E., Abney, O. L., & King,

D. W. (1991). Comparative cognitive effects of carbamazepine and phenytoin in healthy adults. *Neurology, 41,* 1537–1540.

Meador, K. J., Loring, D. W., Huh, K., Gallagher, B. B., & King, D. W. (1990). Comparative cognitive effects of anticonvulsants. *Neurology, 40,* 391–394.

Murray, G. D., Teasdale, G. M., Braakman, R., Cohadon, F., Dearden, M., Iannotti, F., Karimi, A., Lapierre, F., Maas, A., Ohman, J., Persson, L., Servadei, F., Stocchetti, N., Trojanowski, T., & Unterberg, A. (1999). The European Brain Injury Consortium survey of head injuries. *Acta Neurochir (Wien), 141,* 223–236.

Neistadt, M. E. (1993). The relationship between constructional and meal preparation skills. *Archives of Physical Medicine and Rehabilitation, 74,* 144–148.

Oddy, M., Humphrey, M., & Uttley, D. (1978a). Subjective impairment and social recovery after closed head injury. *Journal of Neurology, Neurosurgery, and Psychiatry, 41,* 611–616.

Oddy, M., Humphrey, M., & Uttley, D. (1978b). Stresses upon the relatives of head-injured patients. *British Journal of Psychiatry, 133,* 507–513.

Plenger, P. M., Dixon, C. E., Castillo, R. M., Frankowski, R. F., Yablon, S. A., & Levin, H. S. (1996). Subacute methylphenidate treatment for moderate to moderately severe traumatic brain injury: A preliminary double-blind placebo-controlled study. *Archives of Physical Medicine and Rehabilitation, 77,* 536–540.

Ponsford, J. L., Olver, J. H., Curran, C., & Ng, K. (1995). Prediction of employment status 2 years after traumatic brain injury. *Brain Injury, 9,* 11–20.

Prigatano, G. P., & Altman, I. M. (1990). Impaired awareness of behavioral limitations after traumatic brain injury. *Archives of Physical Medicine and Rehabilitation,* 71, 1058–1064.

Prigatano, G. P., Bruna, O., Mataro, M., Munoz, J. M., Fernandez, S., & Junque, C. (1998). Initial disturbances of consciousness and resultant impaired awareness in Spanish traumatic brain injured patients. *Journal of Head Trauma Rehabilitation, 13*(5), 29–38.

Prigatano, G. P., & Wong, J. L. (1999). Cognitive and affective improvement in brain dysfunctional patients who achieve inpatient rehabilitation goals. *Archives of Physical Medicine and Rehabilitation, 80,* 77–84.

Rapport, L. J., Hanks, R. A., Millis, S. R., & Deshpande, S. A. (1998). Executive functioning and predictors of falls in the rehabilitation setting. *Archives of Physical Medicine and Rehabilitation, 79,* 629–633.

Rebmann, M. J., & Hannon, R. (1995). Treatment of unawareness of memory deficits in adults with brain injury: Three case studies. *Rehabilitation Psychology, 40,* 279–287.

Ruff, R. M., & Baser, C. A. (1990). An experimental comparison of neuropsychological rehabilitation. In J. S. Kruetzer & P. Wehman (Eds.), *Community integration following traumatic brain injury* (pp. 85–102). Baltimore: Brooks.

Ruff, R. M., Marshall, L. F., Crouch, J., Klauber, M. R., Levin, H. S., Barth, J., Kreutzer, J., Blunt, B. A., Foulkes, M. A., Eisenberg, H. M., Jane, J. A., & Marmarou, A. (1993). Predictors of outcome following severe head trauma: Follow-up data from the Traumatic Coma Data Bank. *Brain Injury, 7,* 101–111.

Ruff, R. M., Young, D., Gautille, T., Marshall, L. F., Barth, J., Jane, J. A., Kreutzer, J., Marmarou, A., Levin, H. S., Eisenberg, H. M., & Foulkes, M. A. (1991). Verbal learning deficits following severe head injury: Heterogeneity in recovery over 1 year. *Journal of Neurosurgery, 75,* S50–S58.

Ryan, T. V., Sautter, S. W., Capps, C. F., Meneese, W., & Barth, J. T. (1992). Utilizing neuropsychological measures to predict vocational outcome in a head trauma population. *Brain Injury, 6,* 175–182.

Sander, A. M., High, W. M., Jr., Hannay, H. J., & Sherer, M. (1997). Predictors of psychological health in care givers of patients with closed head injury. *Brain Injury, 11,* 235–249.

Sander, A. M., Kreutzer, J. S., Rosenthal, M., Delmonico, R., & Young, M. E. (1996). A multicenter longitudinal investigation of return to work and community integration following traumatic brain injury. *Journal of Head Trauma Rehabilitation, 11*(5),70–84.

Satz, P., Zaucha, K., Forney, D. L., McCleary, C., Asarnow, R. F., Light, R., Levin, H., Kelly, D.,

Bergsneider, M., Hovda, D., Martin, N., Caron, M. J., Namerow, N., & Becker, D. (1998). Neuropsychological, psychosocial, and vocational correlates of the Glasgow Outcome Scale at 6 months post-injury: A study of moderate to severe traumatic brain injury patients. *Brain Injury, 12,* 555–567.

Sherer, M., Bergloff, P., Levin, E., High, W. M., Jr., Oden, K. E., & Nick, T. G. (1998). Impaired awareness and employment outcome after traumatic brain injury. *Journal of Head Trauma Rehabilitation, 13*(5), 52–61.

Sherer, M., Boake, C., Levin, E., Silver, B. V., Ringholz, G., & High, W. M., Jr. (1998). Characteristics of impaired awareness after traumatic brain injury. *Journal of the International Neuropsychological Society, 4,* 380–387.

Sherer, M., Madison, C. F., & Hannay, H. J. (2000). Outcome after moderate and severe closed head injury: Implications for life care planning. *Journal of Head Trauma Rehabilitation, 15,* 767-782.

Sivak, M., Hill, C. S., Henson, D. L., Butler, B. P., Silber, S. M., & Olson, P. L. (1984). Improved driving performance following perceptual training in persons with brain damage. *Archives of Physical Medicine and Rehabilitation, 65,* 163–167.

Sohlberg, M. M., & Mateer, C. A. (1989). *Introduction to cognitive rehabilitation theory and practice.* New York: Guilford.

Stambrook, M., Moore, A. D., Peters, L. C., Deviaene, C., & Hawryluk, G. A. (1990). Effects of mild, moderate and severe closed head injury on long-term vocational status. *Brain Injury, 4,* 183–190.

Stanislav, S. W. (1997). Cognitive effects of antipsychotic agents in persons with traumatic brain injury. *Brain Injury, 11,* 335–341.

Stuss, D. T., Binns, M. A., Carruth, F. G., Levine, B., Brandys, C. E., Moulton, R. J., Snow, W. G., & Schwartz, M. L. (1999). The acute period of recovery from traumatic brain injury: Posttraumatic amnesia or posttraumatic confusional state? *Journal of Neurosurgery, 90,* 635–643.

Stuss, D. T., & Buckle, L. (1992). Traumatic brain injury: Neuropsychological deficits and evaluations at different stages of recovery and in different pathologic subtypes. *Journal of Head Trauma Rehabilitation, 7*(2), 40-49.

Tabbador, K., Mattis, S., & Zazula, T. (1984). Cognitive sequelae and recovery course after moderate and severe head injury. *Neurosurgery, 14,* 701–708.

Taverni, J. P., Seliger, G., & Lichtman, S. W. (1998). Donepezil mediated memory improvement in traumatic brain injury during post acute rehabilitation. *Brain Injury, 12,* 77–80.

Teasdale, G., & Jennett, B. (1974). Assessment of coma and impaired consciousness: A practical scale. *Lancet, 2,* 81–84.

Thurman, D., & Guerrero, J. (1999). Trends in hospitalization associated with traumatic brain injury. *Journal of the American Medical Association, 282,* 954–957.

Trudel, T. M., Tryon, W. W., & Purdum, C. M. (1998). Awareness of disability and long-term outcome after traumatic brain injury. *Rehabilitation Psychology, 43,* 267–281.

van der Naalt, J., van Zomeren, A. H., Sluiter, W. J., & Minderhoud, J. M. (1999). One year outcome in mild to moderate head injury: The predictive value of acute injury characteristics related to complaints and return to work. *Journal of Neurology, Neurosurgery, and Psychiatry, 66,* 207–213.

van Zomeren, A. H., & van Den Burg, W. (1985). Residual complaints of patients two years after severe head injury. *Journal of Neurology, Neurosurgery, and Psychiatry, 48,* 21–28.

van Zomeren, A. H., Brouwer, W. H., Rothengatter, J. A., & Snoek, J. W. (1988). Fitness to drive a car after recovery from severe head injury. *Archives of Physical and Medical Rehabilitation, 69,* 90–96.

van Zomeren, A. H., & Deelman, B. G. (1978). Long-term recovery of visual reaction time after closed head injury. *Journal of Neurology, Neurosurgery, and Psychiatry,* 41, 452–457.

Wallace, C. A., Bogner, J., Corrigan, J. D., Clinchot, D., Mysiw, W. J., & Fugate, L. P. (1998). Primary caregivers of persons with brain injury: Life change 1 year after injury. *Brain Injury, 12,* 483–493.

Wang, P. L., & Ennis, K. E. (1986). Competency assessment in clinical populations: An introduction to the cognitive competency test. In B. P. Uzzell & Y. Gross (Eds.), *Clinical neuropsychology of intervention* (pp. 119–133). Boston: Martinus Nijhoff.

Whyte, J., Hart, T., Schuster, K., Fleming, M., Polansky, M., & Coslett, B. (1997). Effects of methylphenidate on attentional function after traumatic brain injury. *American Journal of Physical Medicine and Rehabilitation, 76,* 440–450.

Williams, D. H., Levin, H. S., & Eisenberg, H. M. (1990). Mild head injury classification. *Neurosurgery, 27,* 422-428.

Wilson, B. (1993). Ecological validity of neuropsychological assessment: Do neuropsychological indexes predict performance in everyday activities? *Applied and Preventive Psychology, 2,* 209–215.

Wilson, B. (1991). Theory, assessment, and treatment in neuropsychological rehabilitation. *Neuropsychology, 5,* 281–291.

Yablon, S. A. (1996). Posttraumatic seizures. In L. J. Horn & N. D. Zasler (Eds.), *Medical rehabilitation of traumatic brain injury* (pp. 363–394). Philadelphia: Hanley & Belfus.

Youngjohn, J. R., & Altman, I. M. (1989). A performance-based group approach to the treatment of anosognosia and denial. *Rehabilitation Psychology, 34,* 217–222.

Yu, E. J., Yablon, S. A., Ivanhoe, C. H., & Boake, C. (1995). Posttraumatic hydrocephalus: Incidence and outcome following screening of consecutive admissions [Abstract]. *Archives of Physical Medicine and Rehabilitation, 76,* 1041.

4

CHAPTER

Ronald M. Ruff
Paul M. Richards

Neuropsychological Assessment and Management of Patients with Persistent Postconcussional Disorders

Introduction

As noted in Chapter 3, approximately 80% of all patients with traumatic brain injury (TBI) who were admitted to hospitals are considered to have suffered a "mild" brain injury. Although mild does not mean insignificant, many of these individuals show a remarkable recovery within the first 30 to 90 days postinjury. However, as will be discussed, a small proportion of these patients do report persistent symptoms. Clinical neuropsychologists often are asked to examine these individuals and render an opinion as to whether their complaints are compatible with a brain injury versus a psychiatric disturbance, or a combination of both. This is one of the most challenging areas for practicing clinical neuropsychologists and has serious economic implications for the patient's health care.

Epidemiological and Economic Considerations

It is estimated that 1.3 million individuals sustain a mild traumatic brain injury (MTBI) each year in the United States (Kay, Newman, Cavallo, Czrachi, & Resnick, 1992). Approximately 10% to 20% of these individuals present with chronic difficulties (Alexander, 1995; Binder, 1997; McLean, Temkin, Dikmen, & Wyler, 1983; Rimel, Giordany, Barth, Boll, & Jane, 1981; Rutherford, Merrett, & McDonald, 1978). Although multiple factors can play a major role, such as premorbid vulnerabilities (Ruff, Mueller, & Jurica, 1996), from an economic standpoint this translates to a significant loss. The annual cost for all

TBI patients in the United States (severe, moderate, and mild) is approximately $4 billion (Max, McKenzie, & Rice, 1991). With a conservative estimate of 10%, or 130,000 MTBI patients, experiencing chronic difficulties for which they receive $10,000 worth of services, the cost would be $1.3 billion annually in terms of health-care expenses alone, without considering loss of wages.

Several factors compound the economic loss. The majority of MTBI patients fall between the ages of 15 and 35 (Kraus & Nourjah, 1989) and thus have 30 or more years of vocational productivity at stake if the postconcussive disorder reduces their overall work efficiency. In addition, brain injury occurs most often among three subgroups: teens and young adults, males, and persons with low income who live alone (Sosin, Sniezek, & Thurman, 1996). Because many of these individuals do not have medical insurance, the total costs for taxpayers are in the hundreds of millions of dollars each year.

MTBI symptoms include physical, emotional, and cognitive disturbances. Thus, MTBI patients do not fit within the expertise of any single discipline (Ruff, 1999). Even if evaluations by multiple health-care professionals (i.e., neurology, psychiatry, and neuropsychology) are paid for, the benefits for patients typically fall short due to a lack of explicit integration and coordination among the disciplines. An incomplete diagnosis of the postconcussional residua can lead to years of costly treatments that, in the long term, may only offer limited effectiveness.

Given the Zeitgeist of our current managed care system, there exists an attitude that a neuropsychological examination following MTBI may not be necessary, and that the cost may not justify the benefits. In this chapter, we will attempt to demonstrate the utility of neuropsychological services for MTBI patients and the barriers to providing cost-effective services.

In order to diagnose a postconcussional disorder (PCD), it is essential to develop a clear definition of cerebral concussion (Ruff, 1999). We will use the term concussion synonymously with MTBI. In the first part of this chapter, definitions for both MTBI and PCD are presented. Issues in the assessment and management of cognitive disorders associated with MTBI will then be considered. The neuropsychologist plays a special role in assessing the cognitive and the emotional sequelae associated with PCD. Thus, issues in the assessment of the emotional sequelae also will be presented. Future research directions for studying the cost–outcomes associated with neuropsychological services for this population will then be outlined.

□ Reasonable Definitions: Defining MTBI and PCD

The Glasgow Coma Scale (GCS) is internationally accepted as a measure for rating severe, moderate, and mild TBI (Teasdale & Jennett, 1974). Typically administered upon admission to the emergency room, the trauma physicians and neurosurgeons rate severity along the three dimensions of eye opening, verbal response, and motor response. Prior to admission, paramedics also may administer GCS measurements. A GCS score between 3 and 8 is classified as a severe TBI, a score between 9 and 12 as moderate, and (as noted in Chapter 3) scores of 13, 14, or 15 denote MTBI.

There are two principal shortcomings of relying exclusively on GCS for defining MTBI. First, the GCS captures only current status and, in the case of MTBI, frequently there is only a brief loss of consciousness (LOC) or posttraumatic amnesia (PTA). Thus, if the health-care professionals arrive at the scene after the patient has regained consciousness and continuous memory, the GCS will not reflect the occurrence of these states. Thus, the GCS is not designed to retrospectively evaluate LOC and PTA. Instead, the GCS is administered at relatively arbitrary time points that depend on when, for example, the paramedics arrive or at what time after the accident the individual is admitted to a medical center. Second, Kay and colleagues (1992) estimated that a majority of individuals who sustain a concussion either see their treating physicians only days postaccident or never seek medical care at all. Thus, the GCS is most appropriate for decision making by the trauma physicians. However, for health-care professionals who evaluate the patient hours, days, or even months after the accident, a retrospective diagnostic measure for MTBI is needed.

Definition by the American Congress of Rehabilitation Medicine

The American Congress of Rehabilitation Medicine (ACRM, 1993) published an MTBI classification system that can be used retrospectively (see Table 4.1). Note that no specific procedures were provided to capture the parameters, but many neuropsychologists use the Galveston Orientation and Amnesia Test (Levin, Eisenberg, & Benton, 1989; Levin, O'Donnell, & Grossman, 1979) to assess transient LOC and PTA. However, clinical inference is essential for the retrospective diagnosis of MTBI.

One of the criteria of the ACRM definition is an alteration of mental state at the time of accident (which can include being dazed, disoriented, or confused). The experienced clinician realizes that asking patients retrospectively to recall specific events before and after the accident can be challenging. On one hand, there are individuals who describe in great detail a definite gap during which no information is retained, and this gap typically is consistent with PTA. On the other hand, difficulties arise for patients who are, for example, emotionally traumatized to the degree that their recall is affected. Being emotionally upset or in shock is not sufficient for diagnosing MTBI, and a differential diagnosis for these latter individuals can be challenging.

Because PTA exceeds LOC, it is impossible for patients to recall whether during PTA they were initially unconscious. Thus, the reliance should be on PTA rather than LOC, especially if the diagnosis is rendered retrospectively.

Table 4.1. ACRM Definition for MTBI

Inclusion Criteria—One or more must be manifested

- Any period of loss of consciousness
- Any loss of memory for events immediately before and after the accident
- Any alteration of mental state at the time of accident (e.g., feeling dazed, disoriented, or confused)
- Focal neurological deficit(s) that may or may not be transient

Exclusion Criteria—One or more must be manifested

- Loss of consciousness exceeding approximately 30 minutes
- After 30 minutes, the GCS falling below 13
- Posttraumatic amnesia (PTA) persisting longer than 24 hours

DSM-IV: Is a Five-Minute Loss of Consciousness a Reasonable Cutoff?

The fourth edition of the *Diagnostic and Statistical Manual of Mental Disorders* (*DMS-IV*; American Psychiatric Association, 1994) for the first time included an experimental definition for PCD. A PCD is diagnosed 3 months following a concussion and is composed of persistent physical, emotional, and cognitive sequelae. *DSM-IV* also suggests a 5-minute LOC as a criterion for this diagnosis. On one hand, it is reasonable to set cutoffs. On other hand, in a three-center study (Levin, Mattis, Ruff, et al., 1987), we were able to determine the length of LOC in only half of our patients. Even for individuals who at one point in time were observed to be unconscious, the duration could not be reliably estimated. Moreover, as stated earlier, for patients with a PTA the duration of LOC is not obtainable. Thus, a 5-minute cutoff is overly restrictive for the diagnosis of MTBI. (For a more detailed discussion of the pros and cons of the *DSM-IV* definition, see Ruff & Grant, 1999.) As an alternative, the following gradation for MTBI is offered.

A Diagnostic Framework for MTBI

In order to bridge the ACRM and *DSM-IV* definitions, Ruff (1999) and Ruff and Jurica (1999) have proposed a subdivision of MTBI, in which Type I matches the ACRM definition, Type III matches the *DSM-IV* definition, and Type II bridges the two (see Table 4.2).

Neuropsychological testing is *not* essential for diagnosing an MTBI. A concussion occurs when the brain is sufficiently impacted to cause LOC, PTA, or neurological symptoms such as anosmia, vertigo, and posttraumatic headaches (Alexander, 1995).

Levin, Williams, Eisenberg, High, and Guinto (1992) have proposed the following subdivisions: uncomplicated MTBI for those individuals with no positive neuroimaging and complicated MTBI for those with positive computed tomography (CT) or magnetic resonance (MR) images. It is generally accepted that static neuroimaging with CT and MR imaging is not conclusive for diagnosing MTBI (Alexander, 1995; Levin, Amparo, et al., 1987; Levin et al., 1992). However, in most cases where positive neuroimaging is associated with the brain trauma, a concussion can be conclusively diagnosed.

For the so-called uncomplicated patients, the confidence of the MTBI diagnosis is based on the reliability of the quantification of the LOC or PTA. If a qualified healthcare professional gives a GCS score of 13 or 14 in the field or upon admission, then an

TABLE 4.2. Classifications for MTBI

	Type I	Type II	Type III
LOC	altered state or transient loss	definite loss with time unknown or < 5 minutes	loss of 5–30 minutes
PTA	1–60 seconds	60 seconds–12 hours	>12–24 hours
Neurological symptoms	one or more	one or more	one or more

Reproduced from Ruff (1999, p. 107).

MTBI can be diagnosed with a high degree of confidence. In those cases where PTA and LOC are examined retrospectively without available medical records, the diagnosis depends, in part, on the clinician's experience and interpretation. One of the pitfalls to avoid is rendering an opinion that there was no concussion, based on the absence of the individual being seen in an emergency room or having a physician administer a GCS. Moreover, it also has become unacceptable to only diagnose an MTBI if the patient was unconscious. At this point in time, it is reasonable to render a diagnosis of MTBI after clinically delineating a transient alteration of consciousness (ACRM, 1993). However, if the diagnosis is uncertain, this needs to be stated. Finally, if the patient has full recall of the impact and events during the accident, and then, a few minutes after, feels dizzy or does not remember information, an MTBI is unlikely. An MTBI is a neurological event and, as a rule, results in LOC and PTA as a consequence of the impact (i.e., without any time delays).

Diagnosing a PCD

The diagnostic criteria established by the *DSM-IV* (APA, 1994) for PCD provides a useful form of departure. Criteria include "documented cognitive deficit in either attention (concentration, shifting focus of attention, performing simultaneous cognitive tasks) or memory (learning or recalling information)" (p. 704). These cognitive disturbances must be assessed carefully with neuropsychological testing. Other cognitive disturbances also can be part of the picture, such as slowed motor movement, problems with executive functioning, or word-finding difficulties. The *DSM-IV* also recognizes that the PCD should not be diagnosed if there are only cognitive disturbances. There must also be

> three (or more) symptoms that are present at least three months following the closed head injury. These include becoming easily fatigued; disordered sleep; headache; vertigo or dizziness; irritability or aggression on little or no provocation; anxiety, depression, or affective lability; apathy or lack of spontaneity; or other changes in personality (e.g. social or sexual appropriateness). (APA, 1994, p. 704)

This definition emphasizes that a PCD is composed of cognitive, physical, and emotional sequelae.

The Importance of Assessing Persistent Cognitive Deficits

The cognitive difficulties that are typically experienced after an MTBI are well documented (e.g., Levin et al., 1989; Varney & Roberts, 1999), and as such are not controversial. As stated earlier, the principle areas that are affected are attention, memory, and learning. Other deficits include word finding (Jay, Goka, & Arakaki, 1995) and slowed speed of information processing (Gronwall & Wrightson, 1974; Wrightson. & Gronwall, 1999). Although problems in speed of processing, multitasking, working memory, and learning typically occur immediately following an MTBI, there is strong evidence that these difficulties improve significantly within 1 to 3 months postinjury. In the three-center study, Ruff, Levin, et al. (1989) found that patients underwent significant memory gains from baseline testing (at 1 week) to 1 month postinjury followed by more gradual recovery from 1 to 3 months. Dikmen, Temkin, and Armsden

(1989) documented that a single uncomplicated minor head injury generally results in near normal neuropsychological functioning within 1 to 3 months. Hence, MTBI clearly results in early cognitive difficulties, but a recovery takes place for the great majority of people who sustain no permanent cognitive deficits. Nevertheless, a minority of individuals (estimated between 10% and 20%) present with chronic cognitive deficits and, therefore, are the focus of neuropsychologists. That this so-called miserable minority (Ruff, Camenzuli, & Mueller, 1996) exists is not debated as hotly as whether persistent cognitive difficulties are organic or psychological in nature, or some combination thereof.

Are the Cognitive Deficits Psychogenic or Neurogenic?

The psychogenic vs. neurogenic controversy is still evolving, with a strong need for continued research. The studies to date have provided some support for each side of the argument in addition to suggesting a combination of both explanations as the most likely etiology for continued symptoms in the minority of individuals who do not improve within the expected timeline. The following review is not exhaustive, but represents a sampling of the recent literature on this controversy.

In a pilot study, selective MTBI patients who presented with neurocognitive deficits following months or years postaccident were studied (Ruff et al., 1994). Nine individuals with little or no evidence of brain damage upon nonfunctional neuroimaging (such as MR imaging and CT) but who evidenced positive neuropsychological test findings also were examined with positron emission tomography (PET). Four of the patients suffered PTA with no loss of consciousness, but the remaining five had an LOC that ranged from less than 1 minute to a maximum of 20 minutes; all met the ACRM diagnostic criteria (see Table 4.1). There was a "corroboration" between the positive neuropsychological findings and PET results with all nine MTBI patients. Documented changes on PET included hypometabolism in the prefrontal and anterior temporofrontal regions.

Varney et al. (1995) conducted a similar study using single photon emission computed tomography (SPECT) to study MTBI patients with positive neuropsychological findings. Their data demonstrated a similar corroboration, with frontotemporal changes occurring most frequently. Also, Kant, Smith-Seemiller, Isaac, and Duffy (1997), used SPECT and found that this technique was more sensitive to changes following MTBI, compared to structural neuroimaging techniques such as MR imaging and CT.

Binder, Rohling, and Larrabee (1997) conducted a meta-analytic review of neuropsychological studies of MTBI with the following inclusion criteria: (a) Patients were studied at least three months after MTBI, (b) selection was based on a history of MTBI rather than because they were symptomatic, and (c) within the samples studied the attrition rate was less than 50% for follow-up. Studies of children were not considered. The authors concluded:

> The meta analysis provides some support for the hypothesis that there is an association between MHT (mild head trauma) and cognitive deficits in a small percentage of MHT patients, or that there is a small reduction in cognitive functioning in a larger percentage of patients. However, we suggest that the small effect sizes should force a clinician to exercise considerable caution before diagnosing brain injury after MHT. (p. 430)

In a follow-up, Binder (1997) suggested that for most MTBI patients with chronic complaints, an alternate explanation should be used for the differential diagnosis. He pointed to a medical or psychiatric explanation, as the neurological basis for sustaining neuropsychological problems most often can be dismissed.

Miller and Mittenberg (1998) reviewed the literature regarding treatment and prevention of persisting PCD, focusing on studies in both adults and children. They suggested that, although PCD initially may have a neurological basis, the syndrome likely perpetuates because of psychological factors. These authors recommended relatively brief psychological treatment, which they suggested may significantly reduce the severity and duration of such symptoms. The dangers of misattributing persistent symptoms to organic factors were discussed as "iatrogenic."

Paniak, Toller-Lobe, Durand, and Nagy (1998) compared the following treatment modes in 111 adults with MTBI: Those randomly assigned to the first treatment received an education-oriented single session that provided information on what to expect and how to cope with common problems. The patients were assured that a good outcome was likely. The second group received treatment as needed, which commenced with neuropsychological and personality assessment followed by access to a multidisciplinary outpatient treatment program. Both groups improved at a similar rate after a period of 3 to 4 months, and the authors suggested that a single education-oriented session appears adequate for most MTBI survivors. The same cohort was reexamined at 1 year postinjury and the initial gains made at 3 to 4 months were maintained at follow-up (Paniak, Toller-Lobe, Reynolds, Melnyk, & Nagy, 2000). Indeed, the recovery rate between 3 to 4 months and 12 months was negligible, and again no differences emerged between the two groups. The authors therefore propose, similarly to Miller and Mittenberg (1998), a brief psychological and educational intervention.

Forces sufficient to produce brain damage might not result in just a neurological event. Miller (1998) discussed the "motor vehicle accident triple threat" in terms of postconcussion syndrome, whiplash injury, and posttraumatic stress disorder (PTSD), along with the implications toward diagnosis, treatment, and litigation. Miller opined that it is rare to find an accident case that comes to clinical and forensic attention that does not present at least two of these syndromes.

Weight (1998) reviewed the relevant literature showing that the anticipated resolution of MTBI symptoms occurs within 3 months. Also discussed were noncognitive, psychosocial, and motivational issues as well as symptom invalidity and premorbid emotional factors. It was postulated that such factors may serve as explanations of instances when a positive recovery or outcome is not obtained. Persistent symptoms that are primarily subjective in nature were discussed in terms of their inability to be differentiated from base rates of the normal, noninjured population.

Machulda, Bergquist, Ito, and Chew (1998) conducted two investigations studying the relationship between severity of PCD's impact of daily stress, and level of perceived stress over the past month in a group of young adults (aged 18 to 22 years). Several significant relationships were found, and the investigators suggested that persistent symptoms in some individuals with PCD are due, at least in part, to individual differences in the perceived stress of incurring an MTBI.

Bryant and Harvey (1999) studied postconcussive symptoms, postulating that they may be exacerbated by anxiety associated with PTSD. Postconcussive symptoms were significantly correlated with PTSD symptoms, leading the authors to conclude that PCD may be mediated by an interaction of neurological and psychological factors.

This conclusion stands in contrast to earlier studies that reported no evidence of PTSD following MTBI (Mayou, Bryant, & Duthie, 1993). Sbordone and Liter (1995) argued that, to some extent, the distinction between PTSD and MTBI is mutually exclusive, as a loss of memory surrounding the impact (i.e., LOC or PTA) would alleviate the traumatic reaction, which is the hallmark feature of PTSD.

Reitan and Wolfson (1999) performed an interesting study in which they evaluated three different groups of MTBI patients along with a control group. The control group (Group 1) consisted of patients with no history of brain damage but who did have psychiatric (excluding psychosis) and physical conditions, such as spinal cord injury. Groups 2 and 3 were composed of individuals with MTBI; however, the groups differed by the presence of "structural tissue damage" with focal neurologic signs and deficits vs. MTBI without such. All patients in Groups 2 and 3 were members of an ongoing research study who clearly met criteria for MTBI but who were not necessarily complaining of symptoms at the time of evaluation. A majority had a positive LOC and a period of PTA. Group 4 participants consisted of "relatively mild" MTBI patients who were not part of research but who had been referred for neuropsychological evaluation because of ongoing clinical complaints. The General Neuropsychological Deficit Scale (GNDS) was found to be quite sensitive in differentiating the four groups with only "a 10% overlap between the group with definite brain damage and the controls" (p. 199). More importantly, however, was the fact that Group 4 participants with ongoing clinical complaints were significantly more impaired than the MTBI research groups who were routinely tested irrespective of whether they had symptoms. Several important conclusions about research design and procedures were raised by the authors. First, conceptualizing MTBI as a homogenous category is not appropriate. Second, the subgroup of MTBI patients that the researcher uses, will likely lead to different results and conclusions about the neuropsychological consequences of MTBI.

Etiologies of Persistent Cognitive Disturbances

Agreement exists that there are patients who sustain an MTBI with a clear neurologic component that accounts for persistent neuropsychological deficits. Moreover, when untreated problems from a clear brain-related etiology are superimposed over preexisting psychological difficulties, significantly impaired cognitive and emotional functioning often are intermixed. An example of this type of poor outcome is exemplified by the case of a 40-year-old male who underwent neuropsychological assessment 2 years after sustaining an MTBI secondary to a fall from approximately 25 feet. He experienced an LOC that was witnessed by coworkers and estimated to be 3 to 4 minutes in duration. In addition, the PTA exceeded 12 hours, but the retrograde amnesia was minimal (i.e., a few seconds). In the 2 years between the accident and the testing, he experienced consistent organizational and attentional problems as well as severe temper outbursts and depression. Despite good effort and cooperation on most of the testing, a self-critical attitude, low frustration tolerance, and tendencies to give up easily adversely affected his performance, particularly during memory testing and on a sustained attention test (i.e., PASAT). Despite the confounding influence of his psychological reaction on selected neurocognitive tests, the examiner concluded that there were valid declines in immediate visual attention (i.e., block span was mildly to moderately impaired) and in the ability to shift cognitive set (i.e., WCST was borderline impaired), and there was a cluster of verbal deficits (including reduced verbal fluency) as well as difficulties in the area of reading comprehension. The remaining scores were average (or higher) and consistent with what would be expected in comparison to his male peers of comparable age and education.

Given that his MTBI was clearly diagnosed and he demonstrated cognitive deficits, this patient's poor outcome also was understood within the context of his preexisting problems with depression and anger. Based on clinical interviews, these difficulties were thought to have been exacerbated by the fall. Thus, even a patient with premorbid psychological problems can evidence neurocognitive deficits as a result of an MTBI. One important contribution to the assessment of patients is a neuropsychological evaluation that considers how both premorbid factors as well as factors associated with brain injury may contribute to the symptom picture. In this regard, it is extremely important to attend to the patient's premorbid personality characteristics as a part of a neuropsychological assessment.

☐ Persistent Emotional Disorders

When adults sustain brain trauma, they have not been living their lives in a vacuum. That is, problems stemming from MTBI are superimposed over normal life problems. Might the ways a person has previously coped with significant life stressors—such as loss, illness, disease, or bankruptcy—therefore predict how stress is handled following an MTBI? This brings up the well-known consideration that it is not only how the brain was damaged that's important, but what kind of brain was damaged. Historically speaking, neuropsychologists have emphasized the cognitive testing and typically added a personality questionnaire such as the Minnesota Multiphasic Personality Inventory (MMPI) or Millon Clinical Multiaxal Inventory (MCMI). However, particularly for MTBI patients, a more thorough evaluation of premorbid and postmorbid emotional variables are need. The focus of the following section is primarily on identifying premorbid personality factors that may render an individual more vulnerable to the effects of MTBI.

Personality "Disorders"

Millon (1981; 1983; 1985; 1986a; 1986b) has written extensively on personality disorders, conceptualizing such conditions as chronic, maladaptive ways of thinking, feeling, and perceiving which interfere with social and occupational functioning. Personality disorders are further conceptualized as "ego-syntonic"—that is, not necessarily distressing or apparent to the patient—in contrast to "ego-dystonic" conditions such as anxiety or depression, which produce great anguish and motivation for treatment. Millon has further integrated an understanding of personality disorders into the multiaxial *DSM* framework in terms of Axis II or long-standing characterological conditions. Accordingly, three different clusters of personality disorders, totaling 10 unique conditions and 1 "not otherwise specified" condition, are routinely diagnosed and treated by clinicians. Although it is not within the scope of this chapter to review such work, the point is that personality disorders and brain injury are not mutually exclusive, and when both are present there is an interactive effect. Personality disorders, by definition, imply premorbid (long-term) dysfunctioning and therefore contribute to the tremendous variance in recovery after MTBI that is both seen in clinical practice and described in the neuropsychological literature. However, a paucity of literature exists regarding the evaluation of Axis II diagnoses in MTBI patients (Ruff, Mueller, & Jurica, 1996). Nonetheless, we have found it very helpful to also evaluate long-term personality functioning via the Millon Clinical Multiaxial Inventory–III (Millon, 1994) as a routine part of a comprehensive neuropsychological evaluation. Although less aligned with *DSM-IV*, the MMPI can capture preexisting personality disorders (Cripe, 1999). Similarly, in the experienced clinician's hands, the Thematic Apperception Test and Rorschach also can be used effectively. For all of these tests, corrections are needed to consider the direct MTBI residua of the accident, such as pain, headache, fatigue, frustration, and irritability, so as not to falsely attribute these to preexisting psychological disturbances such as a somatoform disorder.

"Personality Styles"

There are other, less pathological approaches to understanding personality functioning. Shapiro (1965) proposed the obsessive-compulsive, paranoid, hysterical, and impulsive ("neurotic") personality styles. Rather than suggesting a personality disorder or other *DSM* condition, he conceptualized these four types as a "form or mode of functioning . . . ways of thinking and perceiving, ways of experiencing emotion" (p. 1) that do not necessarily interfere with social or occupational functioning. Might a chronically obsessive person coping via attention to detail, rigidity, and focus on intellect be exacerbated by the changes brought on by MTBI? Would an MTBI survivor's long-term hypervigilance and suspicion of others turn into distrust of health-care providers and insurance representatives that could interfere with getting the needed treatments?

"Vulnerable" Personalities

In line with the notion of examining personality styles (as opposed to a more pathological personality disorder), Ruff, Mueller, and Jurica (1996) described a number of premorbid psychological traits that result in likely postmorbid reactions to the effects of TBI. Such coping styles are theorized to color or complicate recovery. For instance, the "overachiever" derives self-esteem from accomplishments that are often accompanied by obsessive, Type–A characteristics. The likely postmorbid reaction to TBI for such a personality would be a "catastrophic" reaction if a drop in performance was perceived. Additional postmorbid reactions from these so-called vulnerabilities are described in Table 4.3.

The Psychogenic Profile: Know When the Pieces Do Not Fit

In clinical practice, neuropsychologists evaluate patients whose subjective complaints and overall level of disability are grossly in excess of what would be expected following an MTBI. Moreover, there are patients with prolonged needs for treatment or whose symptoms progressively worsen for months postinjury. Establishing an accurate diagnosis is not only important to effectively treat these patients, but within a medicolegal context, it is essential to determine permanence of injury, causation, and need for future treatment in order to determine damages. When such inconsistencies exist, one must search for and rule out alternative explanations for a person's deficits. Issues surrounding the so-called psychogenic profile might best be illustrated via the following case study.

TABLE 4.3. Vulnerable Preinjury Personality Styles

Style	Premorbid Psychological Traits	Postmorbid Reactions
Overachiever	Sense of self derived from driven accomplishments, which is frequently accompanied by obsessive-compulsive traits	Catastrophic reaction if drop in performance is perceived
Dependency	Excessive need to be taken care of, frequently leading to submissive behavior and fear of separation	Paralyzed by symptoms if a critical erosion of independence occurs
Borderline Personality Characteristics (not disorder)	Pattern of instability in interpersonal relationships and self-image, with fear of rejection or abandonment	Exacerbation of personality disorganization, including despair, panic, impulsivity, instability, and self-destructive acts
Insecurity	Weak sense of self, which can include shame, guilt, and dependency needs	Magnification of symptoms
Grandiosity	Overestimation of abilities and inflating accomplishments; can include need for admiration and lack of empathy	Minimization or denial of symptoms; if failure results, crash of self-esteem can result in catastrophic reaction
Antisocial Behavior	Tendency to be manipulative or deceitful, temperamental, impulsive, and irresponsible; lacks sensitivity to others	Possible exaggeration or malingering; increased risk taking, irritability; takes little responsibility for recovery
Hyperactivity	Restless, unfocused, and at times disorganized	Attentional difficulties and impulsivity may be compounded; possible oppositional behavior
Depression	Mood fluctuations dominated by negative affect	Increase of depressive symptoms, despondency
Histrionic Style	Emotionality and attention-seeking behavior	Dramatic flavor to symptom presentation, blaming behavior
Somatic Orientation	Preoccupation with physical well-being, reluctance to accept psychological conflicts	Endorsement of multiple premorbid physical symptoms intermixed with new or changing TBI residua
Posttraumatic Stress Disorder	Prior stressors produced an emotional reaction of fear and helplessness	Decreased coping ability, cumulative effect of traumas with exaggerated reaction to current crisis

Reproduced from Ruff and Richardson (1999, p. 326).

A 29-year-old, single, white female presented at an outpatient rehabilitation clinic for comprehensive neuropsychological assessment with a medical history of two different work-related injuries, the first of which occurred approximately 4 months prior to initially being seen at the clinic. At that time, she ran up a curving slide and accidentally ran into a metal crossbar on the top of the slide, striking the top of her head. There was no loss of consciousness and no retrograde or posttraumatic amnesia; in fact, the patient denied being stunned, with no nausea, dizziness, or blurred vision. Apparently she did not think she was injured, and the incident was never reported to her employer. Approximately 2 months later, a second injury occurred while outdoors when she reportedly "forgot to duck" and hit the top part of her head on a branch of a tree. Again, there was no loss of consciousness and no indication whatsoever of retrograde or posttraumatic amnesia. In fact, medical attention was not immediately sought as the patient did not think she was that injured; nevertheless, she did call her physician the following day because of her concern about her ability to function safely as a child-care worker. Photographs of the tree branch revealed it to be a relatively small branch, which almost certainly would have given way or bent, had anyone run into it. Although this patient was not at all symptomatic after the first incident, she declined quickly after the second insult to her head, developing severe physical, cognitive, and emotional symptoms, and did not return to work. She moved in with her sister, who basically took over almost all of the patient's responsibilities. Despite her numerous self-reported impairments, the patient's presentation was marked by an unusual focus on detail (often to the point of challenging conclusions in reports and editing the grammar of health-care providers she had consulted) and repeated requests for clarification and additional diagnostics.

Validity testing and other motivational checks revealed excellent effort throughout a battery of approximately 25 neuropsychological tests. There were no neuropsychological deficits identified, with all of her performances falling at least in the average range when she was compared to her female peers with comparable education and in the same age group. Moreover, several of her performances were well above average, placing her in the superior range of functioning. Personality testing with the MMPI-2 revealed significant emotional distress, characterized not only by a high number of somatic complaints but by marked tendencies on the patient's behalf to dwell, brood, and ruminate about her physical functioning. The MMPI-2 suggested an individual who characteristically used the defenses of repression, denial, and somatization. Additional testing with the MCMI-III revealed a probable Axis II diagnosis of obsessive personality disorder.

This case not only highlights the need for personality testing but points to the importance of conducting a thorough interview/psychosocial history. Specifically, this patient reported a quite extensive history of sexual abuse that resulted in a lengthy inpatient psychiatric hospitalization approximately 3.5 years before the alleged brain injuries. Additionally, she apparently had received consultation from a physician prior to neuropsychological testing and was advised that she had "probably sustained a mild traumatic brain injury." Needless to say, the patient was quite adamant and thorough in searching for a medical explanation for her difficulties, and she continued to fear, despite reassurance to the contrary, that she did have an MTBI. Her insistence and fear that she had sustained an MTBI (in the absence of positive LOC, PTA, or radiological findings) was discussed in terms of her past history of sexual abuse and preexisting personality disorder. The likelihood that physical symptoms had stirred up unresolved abuse issues thereby complicating this patient's recovery also resulted in an Axis I diagnosis of a somatoform disorder.

A Summary of the Clinical Utility of a Neuropsychological Examination for Patients with Persistent Cognitive and Emotional Disturbances

A neuropsychological examination includes more than psychometric testing. It incorporates a careful history taking, in which the clinician asks the patients to describe a number of events surrounding the presumed brain injury as well as assessing the cognitive sequelae following this assumed or known injury. Thus, an important part of a clinical neuropsychological examination is taking a careful history by an experienced clinician.

The neuropsychological examination should not only yield a description of cognitive impairment, as predictable cognitive disorders are associated with MTBI. Thus, the clinical neuropsychological examination allows for (a) an assessment of cognitive deficits known to be associated with MTBI and (b) cognitive assessment of functions believed not to be influenced by MTBI. Thus, the neuropsychological examination can provide a twofold assessment to determine whether the strengths and weaknesses within the profile are compatible with a history of MTBI.

Finally, the clinical neuropsychologist is clearly aware that the emotional disorders associated with MTBI may interact in complicated ways with the patients' premorbid personality characteristics. Thus, the clinical neuropsychologist should determine whether or not preexisting personality disorders or styles interact with the presentation of cognitive and medical symptoms. It is the appreciation of the interactions of the cognitive physical and emotional disturbances that is at the heart of a careful and clinically useful neuropsychological examination. Table 4.4 summarizes the clinical utility of a neuropsychological assessment for patients who demonstrate persistent postconcussional disorders.

☐ Management of Patients with PCD

Ruff, Camenzuli, and Mueller (1996) have proposed a model that views stressors as cumulative; the miserable minority represents a population that suffers from a combination of pre-, co-, and postmorbid stressors. If the accumulation exceeds an individual's

TABLE 4.4. Utility of a Neuropsychological Assessment for Patients with Persistent Postconcussional Disorders

1. Careful history-taking to determine if a period of posttraumatic amnesia existed
2. Psychometric assessment of cognitive functioning and possible impairments
3. Clinical assessment of emotional disorders in light of premorbid personality characteristics
4. Sophisticated appreciation of the interactions between cognitive, physical, and emotional disturbances in arriving at a statement of whether or not a mild brain injury has most likely occurred

maximal capacity to handle stress, the patient "loses it." This phenomenon can be experienced in forms of anger outbursts, panic attacks, or even a catastrophic reaction. If the patient remains at elevated stress levels, then productivity is affected and the individual is more vulnerable to future overloads. Thus, individuals are less productive when stress levels exceed their coping skills. (see Figure 4.1).

The stressors that make up our lives do not originate from just the physical, cognitive, and emotional domains; in addition to this intrapersonal dynamic, there are extrapersonal sources that result in daily stressors. These external sources include school or vocation, finances, social life, recreational activities, and the overall direction and meaning in life (for some, also known as spirituality; Ruff, 1999).

The first point that needs to be made is that individuals who do not have an MTBI can have moderate to high stress levels based on the demands placed on their lives. The second point is that when an individual sustains an MTBI, these premorbid stressors do not evaporate–instead, the new stressors of the MTBI accumulate on top. Therefore most MTBI patients have relatively high stress levels. Some patients suffer a drop in job or school performances that is stressful. Others sustain financial setbacks from taking off work or incurring new medical bills. For others, social life is affected because they are more fatigued or irritable. In addition, recreational activities, such as their favorite sports, are not tolerated due to pain or headaches. Thus, they are prevented from having their key stress release in place. These examples show that most MTBI patients are placed under higher levels of stress, which, by itself, can reduce their overall productivity and well-being.

The management of these patients should focus on early intervention (1 to 3 months postinjury) by a neuropsychologist with the provision of regular support and educa-

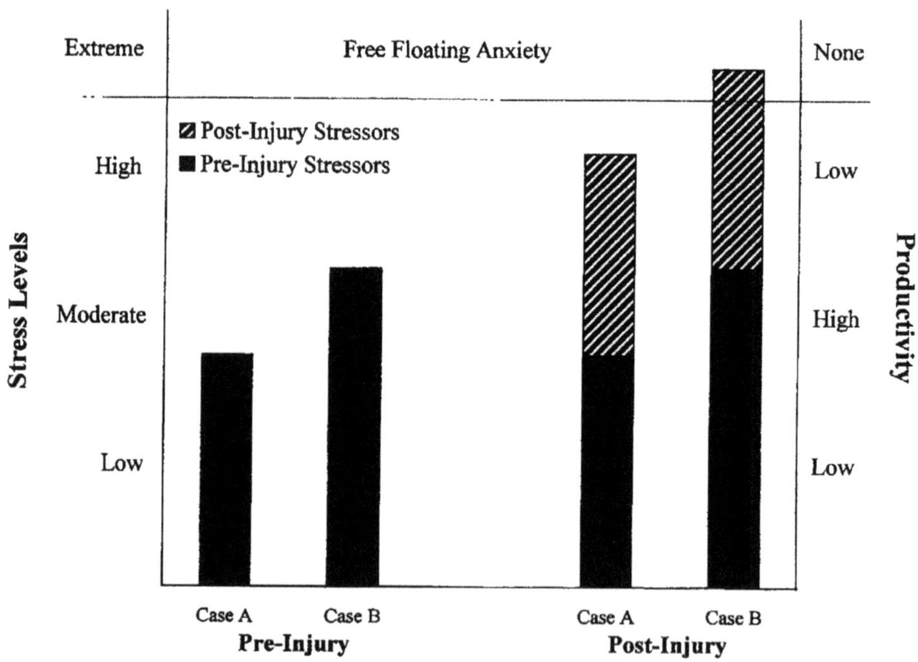

FIGURE 4.1. The effects of pre- vs. postinjury stressors on patient's perceived stress levels and productivity. Reproduced from Ruff, Camenzuli, and Mueller (1996, p. 559).

tion as well as assessment at appropriate intervals, such as that suggested in Chapters 2 and 3. Patients need to know early in their recovery from MTBI that cognitive and emotional symptoms are "normal" and should resolve with time and treatment. Most MTBI patients are unfamiliar with what to expect, and this uncertainty adds stress. Thus early educational interventions should become the standard of care. Alves, Macciocchi, and Barth (1993) reported that, in addition to education, MTBI patients should receive reassurance of a good outcome. In their study comparing two types of treatments, the MTBI patients receiving educational information and reassurance were at a lower risk for persistent postconcussional symptoms than those who received the same education without reassurance. Paniak and colleagues (1998) also included in their educational interventions the assurance of a good outcome. They provided suggestions about how to cope with the symptoms, especially encouraging their patients to rest and return to work and other activities at a gradual pace.

If cognitive difficulties persist following 3 months postinjury, then referrals to further treatments are warranted. Particularly a referral to a cognitive/speech therapist should be considered. Effective compensatory strategies typically can be learned in 6 to 12 1-hour sessions. Further treatments are warranted if specific cognitive limitations surface at work, school, and so on. Misattribution of common neuropsychological base rate symptoms (Lees-Haley & Brown, 1993; Raskin & Mateer, 2000) to organic factors also must be addressed directly. Persistent emotional problems need to be carefully managed by the neuropsychologist with targeted cognitive–behavioral therapies as well as referral to a physician for management of factors such as sleep problems, vestibular dysfunction, headaches, and psychiatric medication. If recovery exceeds the expected timelines, the neuropsychologist must carefully rule out alternate explanations and determine which symptoms (if any) represent an exacerbation of a premorbid condition or vulnerable personality style, and apportion causative factors and treatment accordingly.

The challenge to our field is to continue evaluating the efficacy of key treatments such as cognitive remediation. Although support exists for more formalized remediation of attention, memory, problem solving, and spatial deficits in various brain-injured populations (Ben-Yishay & Prigatano 1990; Niemann, Ruff, & Baser, 1990; Ruff, Baser et al., 1989; Ryan & Ruff, 1988), others (Levin, 1990) have referred to cognitive rehabilitation as "unproved but promising." In short, there is a need for better designed clinical trials to corroborate the efficacy of neurorehabilitation. The recent work of Diller (2000), Raskin and Mateer (2000), and Wood, McCrea, Wood, and Merriman (1999) is a step in this direction and exemplifies the cost-effectiveness of providing cognitive rehabilitation with good outcomes.

☐ Future Research

In the future, it is imperative that the trauma physicians and neuropsychologists develop methods by which they can separate those individuals who will (a) most likely have a positive recovery from those who will (b) potentially have a poor recovery. Treatment, then, should be tailored primarily to the latter group, whereas the first group should receive educational information and reassurance that a good outcome is likely. As mentioned earlier, it is a mistake to think of the patients within the miserable minority as a homogenous group of individuals with either only psychogenic or neurogenic problems. Instead, the miserable minority is composed of a very heterogeneous population with different premorbid risk factors and variable co- and postmorbid presentations. An early identification of the miserable minority would be most cost-effective.

Alves et al. (1993), Miller and Mittenberg (1998), and Paniak et al. (2000) have demonstrated that a relatively brief educational intervention is as effective as more intense interventions, and such findings no doubt could influence reimbursement practices. However, such a conclusion is not only premature but also likely flawed. Because the majority of MTBI patients recover by 3 months, the most relevant question is whether such interventions are applicable for the miserable minority? Note that none of these studies attempted such a separation, and thus we do not know if their samples included patients from the miserable minority. If, for example, 100 MTBI patients are randomly assigned to two treatments, then one should expect that 80% to 90% would have a favorable outcome by 3 months even without any treatments. Thus, treatments that benefit the 10% to 20% with persistent problems could be falsely rejected as not being efficacious. This is a serious limitation of the treatment research conducted so far. Consider the following analogy: If 80% to 90% of all breast tumors were nonmalignant, who would compare treatments for cancer in a sample that combines women with and without malignancy? In short, future research must evaluate various treatment modes that are tailored to the heterogeneous needs of the miserable minority.

For those individuals with MTBIs who are involved in litigation, a further compounding factor enters the picture. There has been an explosion of tests to capture "malingering." Indeed, it is a mistake to classify as malingerers those patients who fall in the miserable minority without the brain damage being the primary cause. It is beyond the scope of this chapter to deal with malingering and forensic issues. However, this is where neuropsychologists have placed great efforts. In comparison, little attention is paid that fewer neurologists, neurosurgeons, and trauma physicians are referring MTBI patients for neuropsychological testing, as managed care has started to dominate health care. Instead, it is becoming more common that attorneys are referring MTBI patients to neuropsychologists.

Cost Outcome Research as It Relates to the Problems of MTBI and PCD

Many of the points made in Chapters 2 and 3 regarding cost outcomes research apply to those with MTBI or PCD as well as TBI. However, because the confident diagnosis of MTBI can be problematic at times, the clinical neuropsychologist needs to spend extra time in the thorough review of an individual's history prior to the accident. This entails not only detailed analyses of medical records but also corroboration of the history from significant others, including the use of a standardized "significant-other" questionnaire such as the Cognitive Behavioral Rating Scale (Williams, 1987). Perhaps the most helpful tool is that of a detailed clinical interview with both the patient and significant others (Sbordone, Seyranian, & Ruff, 1998). The patient's pre-, peri-, and postnatal complications must be investigated. Determining whether developmental milestones were achieved on time and if learning disabilities existed, and obtaining documentation of such (if any) is imperative. A thorough medical, family, vocational, and psychosocial history can be obtained not only from a clinical interview but also from questionnaires such as SYNAPSIS (Mueller, 1996). This time-saving instrument can be completed prior to the neuropsychological evaluation and offers increased reliability to the person providing the information in that the person providing that information must sign the questionnaire attesting to its accuracy.

The point of this is that it takes extra time to determine whether additional information is necessary to consider when the syndromes are associated with PCD. It is beyond the scope of this chapter to delineate all of the steps a clinician might wish to consider in evaluating a given patient. However, one of the most cost-effective contributions of the clinical neuropsychological examination is the skill of an experienced clinician in bringing together multiple sources of information to arrive at a diagnosis and, at times, a treatment plan. To our knowledge, no study has yet appeared to evaluate the cost-effectiveness of this approach. It would seem, however, eminently practical. One could assess the economic impact of an experienced clinical neuropsychologist evaluating all of the information associated with a potential MTBI and compare that to the cost-effectiveness of having specific medical disciplines carry out such an evaluation. The end points could potentially be many, including whether the individual ultimately goes back to work, whether specific symptoms are reduced with the passage of time or therapy, and the capacity of this information to ultimately determine the outcome of litigation. Although this type of research again is not common for clinical neuropsychologists, any serious effort at assessing the cost–outcomes of a thorough clinical neuropsychological examination for this patient population should consider these dimensions.

In Chapter 1, the financial consequences of misdiagnosing epilepsy (vs. pseudoseizures) were discussed. In a similar vein, false positives and false negatives of the MTBI diagnosis carry significant ramifications not only in a financial sense but with respect to human consequences as well. Failing to correctly identify an MTBI, and instead dismissing it as a psychiatric or general medical condition (or no condition at all), can result in endless doctor shopping, lost wages, and frustration. In turn, both authors have seen instances of individuals who do not meet the diagnostic criteria for MTBI and were inappropriately treated as though they had this condition. If one considers the provision of weekly psychotherapy and cognitive remediation, multiple neuropsychological evaluations, and referral to other experts, the costs to these patients (or their payer of service) are high. Also to be considered are larger costs to society in terms of private or Social Security Disability benefits, workers' compensation, and strains on the health-care and legal systems. One year of such a scenario could easily result in $10,000 to $20,000 of unnecessary treatment and perhaps $30,000 in lost wages for a typical blue-collar worker. The latter figure might have to be doubled or tripled in instances of more highly trained professional employees. In both situations, the anxiety associated with not having an accurate diagnosis, diminished quality of life, and reduced productivity are immeasurable. Suffice it to say that an accurate and early diagnosis might be the best way to control costs and expedite return to previous levels of productivity.

Also in line with Chapter 2, the subjective value of a neuropsychological consultation and evaluation following MTBI should not be ignored. Many patients find a sense of relief in understanding the nature of their symptoms and finding a method to at least begin to coping with them. Again, to our knowledge, no one has studied the subjective value of a neuropsychological consultation examination for these patients. A study that could be conducted is comparing what patients would be willing to pay for such a neuropsychological evaluation versus what they would be willing to pay for a psychiatric consultation, a neurological evaluation, and so on.

The fact that attorneys appear to be sending many such patients for neuropsychological evaluation provides a powerful testimony that such evaluations, in fact, may have special relevance in cases of litigation. It is important that neuropsychologists take seriously the need to further study the impact of concussion on neuropsychological functioning and how various factors may influence the symptom picture. As Chapter 17 documents, the study of professional athletes may be especially helpful in this regard. We will end this section by emphasizing one point: Clinical neuropsychologists can assess the cost–outcome of their work with this patient population by asking the basic question, who benefits from the neuropsychological assessment and management of these individuals? Certainly, the medical health-care environment could benefit tremendously, because many of these individuals use large numbers of resources because of persistent complaints, even though no one has adequately studied this problem. Second, attorneys clearly benefit from this type of assessment, if the information is helpful in documenting that a true injury to the brain has occurred and that compensation can therefore follow. Perhaps, however, the third and most important benchmark of information is whether or not the patients themselves actually benefit in symptom reduction by such an evaluation. The early work of Mittenberg and Paniak provided a potentially useful model for assessing the cost–outcome of such interventions. Their work argued that if patients with MTBI are given appropriate early education and assurance, many of the symptoms do not develop. However, as mentioned earlier, the efficacy of treatments should focus on the miserable minority. At this point, it seems reasonable to conclude that postdischarge all MTBI patients should receive educational information and assurance. If in addition a measurement could be identified to identify early on those individuals who fall in the miserable minority, this could potentially lead to a significant cost savings.

Summary and Conclusions

This chapter has outlined some of the relevant issues in the neuropsychological assessment and management of patients with MTBI who also present with postconcussional symptoms. This patient population presents formidable diagnostic challenges to the clinical neuropsychologist. The clinical neuropsychologist, however, is in a unique position to synthesize multiple bits of information to arrive at a diagnosis and begin to explore how various treatment programs could provide the greatest assistance. Studying the cost outcomes of interventions with this population is, indeed, a timely venture.

References

Alexander, M. P. (1995). Mild traumatic brain injury: Pathophysiology, natural history and clinical management. *Neurology, 45,* 1253–1260.

Alves, W., Macciocchi, S., & Barth, J. (1993). Postconcussive symptoms after uncomplicated mild head injury. *Journal of Head Trauma Rehabilitation, 8,* 48–59.

American Congress of Rehabilitation Medicine. (1993). Definition of mild traumatic brain injury. *Journal of Head Trauma Rehabilitation, 8*(3), 86–87.

American Psychiatric Association (1994). *Diagnostic and statistical manual of mental disorders* (4th ed.). Washington, DC: Author.

Ben-Yishay, Y., & Prigatano, G. P. (1990). Cognitive remediation. In M. Rosenthal & M. R. Bond (Eds.), *Rehabilitation of the adult and child with traumatic brain injury* (2nd ed., pp. 393–409). Philadelphia: Davis.

Binder, L. M. (1997). A review of mild head trauma: Part II: Clinical implications. *Journal of Clinical and Experimental Neuropsychology, 19,* 432–457.

Binder, L. M., Rohling, M. L., & Larrabee, G. J. (1997). A review of mild head trauma. Meta-analytic review of neuropsychological studies. *Journal of Clinical and Experimental Neuropsychology, 19*(3), 421–431.

Bryant, R. A., & Harvey, A. G. (1999). Postconcussive symptoms and posttraumatic stress disorder after mild traumatic brain injury. *Journal of Nervous Mental Disorders, 187*(5), 302–305.

Cripe, L. I. (1999). The use of the MMPI with mild closed head injury. In N. R. Varney & R. J. Roberts (Eds.), *The evaluation and treatment of mild traumatic brain injury* (pp. 291–314). New York: Erlbaum.

Dikmen, S. S., Temkin, N., & Armsden, G. (1989). Neuropsychological recovery: Relationship to psychosocial functioning and postconcussional complaints. In H. S. Levin, H. M. Eisenberg, & A. L. Benton (Eds.), *Mild head injury* (pp. 229–241). New York: Oxford University Press.

Diller, L. (2000). Cognitive rehabilitation during the industrialization of rehabilitation. In *Critical issues in neuropsychology* (pp. 315–325). New York: Kluwer Academic Plenum Publishers.

Gronwall, D., & Wrightson, P. (1974). Delayed recovery of intellectual function after minor head injury. *Lancet, 2,* 605–609.

Head Injury Interdisciplinary Special Interest Group: American Congress of Rehabilitation Medicine. (1993). Definition of mild traumatic brain injury. *Journal of Head Trauma Rehabilitation, 8*(3), 86–87.

Jay, G., Goka, R., & Arakaki, A. (1995). Minor traumatic brain injury: Review of clinical data and appropriate evaluation and treatment. *Minor Traumatic Brain Injury, 27*(4), 262–282.

Kant, R., Smith-Seemiller, L., Isaac, G., & Duffy, J. (1997). Tc-HMPAO SPECT in persistent post-concussion syndrome after mild head injury. Comparison with MRI/CT. *Brain Injury, 11,* 115–124.

Kay, T., Newman, B., Cavallo, M., Ezrachi, O., & Resnick, M. (1992). Toward a neuropsychological model of functional disability after mild traumatic brain injury. *Neuropsychology, 6,* 371–384.

Kraus, J. F., & Nourjah, P. (1989). The epidemiology of mild head injury. In H. S. Levin, H. M. Eisenberg & A. L. Benton (Eds.), *Mild head injury* (pp. 8–22). New York: Oxford University Press.

Lees-Haley, P., & Brown, R. S. (1993). Neuropsychological complaint base rates. *Archives of Clinical Neuropsychology, 8*(3), 203–210.

Levin, H. S. (1990). Cognitive rehabilitation: Unproved but promising. *Archives of Neurology, 47*(2), 223–224.

Levin, H. S., Amparo, E., Eisenberg, H. M., Williams, D. H., High, W. M. Jr., McArdle, C. B., & Winer, R. L. (1987). Magnetic resonance imaging and computerized tomography in relation to the neurobehavioral sequelae of mild and moderate head injuries. *Journal of Neurosurgery, 66,* 706–713.

Levin, H. S., Eisenberg, H. M., & Benton, A. L. (1989). *Mild head injury*. New York: Oxford University Press.

Levin, H. S., Mattis, S., Ruff, R. M., Eisenberg, H. M., Marshall, L. F., Tabaddor, K., High ,W. M., Jr., & Frankowski, R. F. (1987). Neurobehavioral outcome following minor head injury: A three-center study. *Journal of Neurosurgery, 66,* 234–243.

Levin, H. S., O'Donnell, V. M., & Grossman, R. G. (1979). The Galveston Orientation and Amnesia Test: A practical scale to assess cognition after head injury. *Journal of Nervous and Mental Disorders, 167,* 675–684.

Levin, H. S., Williams, D. H., Eisenberg, H. M., High, W. M., & Guinto, F. C. (1992). Serial MRI and neurobehavioral findings after mild to moderate closed head injury. *Journal of Neurology, Neurosurgery, and Psychiatry, 55,* 255–262.

Machulda, M. M., Bergquist, T. F., Ito, V., & Chew, S. (1998). Relationship between stress, coping, and post-concussion symptoms in a healthy adult population. *Archives of Clinical Neuropsychology, 13*(5), 415–424.

Mayou, R., Bryant, B., & Duthie, R. (1993). Psychiatric consequences of road accidents. *British Medical Journal, 307,* 647–651.

Max, W., MacKenzie, E. J., & Rice, D. P. (1991). Head injuries: cost and consequences. *Journal of Head Trauma Rehabilitation, 6,* 76–91.

McLean, A., Temkin, N. R., Dikmen, S., & Wyler, A. R. (1983). The behavioral sequelae of head injury. *Journal of Clinical Neuropsychology, 5,* 361–376.

Miller, L. J., & Mittenberg, W. (1998). Brief cognitive behavioral interventions in mild traumatic brain injury. *Applied Neuropsychology, 5*(4), 172–183.

Miller, L. (1998). Motor vehicle accidents: Clinical, neuropsychological, and forensic considerations. *Journal of Cognitive Rehabilitation, 16*(4), 10–23.

Millon, T. (1994). *Millon Clinical Multiaxial Inventory (manual).* Minneapolis: National Computer Systems.

Millon, T. (1986a). A theoretical derivation of pathological personalities. In T. Millon & G. L. Klerman (Eds.), *Contemporary directions in psychopathology: Toward the DSM-IV* (pp. 639–679). New York: Guilford.

Millon, T. (1986b). Personality prototypes and their diagnostic criteria. In T. Millon & G. L. Klerman (Eds.), *Contemporary directions in psychopathology: Toward the DSM-IV* (pp. 671–672). New York: Guilford.

Millon, T. (1985). The MCMI provides a good assessment of DSM-III disorders: The MCMI-II will prove even better. *Journal of Personality Assessment, 49,* 379–391.

Millon, T. (1983). *Millon Clinical Multiaxial Inventory manual,* (3rd ed.). Minneapolis: National Computer Systems.

Millon, T. (1981) *Disorders of personality. DSM-III, Axis II.* New York: Wiley.

Mueller, J. (1996). *SYNAPSIS: A medical profile questionnaire.* Odessa, FL: Psychological Assessment Resources.

Niemann, H., Ruff, R. M., & Baser, C. A. (1990). Computer-assisted attention retraining in head injured individuals: A controlled efficacy study of an outpatient program. *Journal of Consulting and Clinical Psychology, 58,* 811–817.

Paniak, C., Toller-Lobe, G., Durand, A., & Nagy, J. (1998). A randomized trial of two treatments for mild traumatic brain injury. *Brain Injury, 12,* 1011–1023.

Paniak, C., Toller-Lobe, G., Reynolds, S., Melnyk, A., & Nagy, J. (2000). A randomized trial of two treatments for mild traumatic brain injury: 1 year follow-up. *Brain Injury, 14,* 219–226.

Raskin, S. A., & Mateer, C. A. (2000). *Neuropsychological management of mild traumatic brain injury.* New York: Oxford University Press.

Reitan, R. M., & Wolfson, D. (1999). The two faces of mild head injury. *Archives of Clinical Neuropsychology, 14*(2), 191–202.

Rimel, R. W., Giordani, B., Barth, J. T., Boll, T. J., & Jane, J. A. (1981). Disability caused by minor head injury. *Neurosurgery, 9,* 221–228.

Ruff, R. M. (1999). Discipline-specific approach vs. individual care. In N. R. Varney & R. J. Roberts (Eds.), *Mild head injury: Causes, evaluation and treatment* (pp. 99-113). Mahwah, NJ: Erlbaum.

Ruff, R. M., Baser, C. A., Johnston, J. W., Marshall, L. F., Klauber, S. K., Klauber, M. R., & Minteer, M. (1989). Neuropsychological rehabilitation: An experimental study with head injured patients. *Journal of Head Trauma Rehabilitation, 4*(3), 20–36

Ruff, R. M., Camenzuli, L. F., & Mueller, J. (1996). Miserable minority: Emotional risk factors that influence the outcome of a mild traumatic brain injury. *Brain Injury, 10,* 551–565.

Ruff, R. M., Crouch, J. A., Troster, A. I., Marshall, L. F., Buchsbaum, M. S., Lottenberg, S., & Somers, L. M. (1994). Selected cases of poor outcome following a minor brain injury: Comparing neuropsychological and positron emission tomography assessment. *Brain Injury, 8*(4), 297–308.

Ruff, R. M. & Grant, I. (1999). Postconcussional disorder: Background to DSM-IV and future considerations. In N. R. Varney & R. J. Roberts (Eds.), *Mild head injury: Causes, evaluation and treatment* (pp. 315-325). Mahwah, NJ: Erlbaum.

Ruff, R. M. & Jurica, P. (1999). In search of a unified definition for mild traumatic brain injury. *Brain Injury, 13,* 943–952.

Ruff, R. M., Levin, H. S., Mattis, S., High, W. M., Marshall, L. F., Eisenberg, H. M., & Tabaddor, K. (1989). Recovery of memory after mild head injury: A three center study. In H. S. Levin, H. M. Eisenberg, & A. L. Benton (Eds.), *Mild head injury* (pp. 176–188). New York: Oxford University Press.

Ruff, R. M., Mueller, J., & Jurica, P. J. (1996). Estimating premorbid functioning levels after traumatic brain injury. *Neurorehabilitation, 7,* 39–53.

Ruff, R. M. & Richardson, A. M. (1999). Mild traumatic brain injury. In J. Sweet (Ed.), *Forensic neuropsychology: Fundamentals and practice* (pp. 315–338). Exton, PA: Swet and Zeitlinger.

Rutherford, W. H., Merret, J. D., & McDonald, J. R. (1978). Symptoms at one year following concussion from minor head injuries. *Injury, 10,* 225–230.

Ryan, T. V., & Ruff, R. M. (1988). The efficacy of structured memory retraining in a group comparison of head trauma patients. *Archives of Clinical Neuropsychology, 3*(2),165–179.

Sbordone, R. J. & Liter, J. C. (1995). Mild traumatic brain injury does not produce posttraumatic stress disorder. *Brain Injury 9,* 405–412.

Sbordone, R. J., Seyranian, G. D., & Ruff, R. M. (1998). Are the subjective complaints of traumatically brain-injured patients reliable? *Brain Injury, 12,* 505–515.

Shapiro, D. (1965). *Neurotic styles*. New York: Basic Books.

Sosin, D. M., Sniezek, J. E., & Thurman, D. J. (1996). Incidence of mild and moderate brain injury in the United States, 1991. *Brain Injury, 10*(1), 47–54.

Teasdale, G., & Jennett, B. (1974). Assessment of coma and impaired consciousness: A practical scale. *Lancet, 2,* 81–84.

Varney, N. R., Bushnell, D. L., Nathan, M., Kah, D., Roberts, R., Rezai, K., Walker, W., & Kirchner, P. (1995). NeuroSPECT correlates of disabling mild head injury: Preliminary findings. *Journal of Head Trauma Rehabilitation, 10,* 18–28.

Varney, N. R. & Roberts, R. J. (1999). *The evaluation and treatment of mild traumatic brain injury*. Mahwah, NJ: Erlbaum.

Weight, D. G. (1998). Minor head trauma. *Psychiatric Clinics of North America, 21*(3), 609–624.

Williams, J. M. (1987). *Cognitive behavioral rating scale: Psychological assessment resources*. Odessa, FL: Psychological Assessment Resource.

Wood, R. L., McCrea, J. D., Wood, L. M., & Merriman, R. N. (1999). Clinical and cost-effectiveness of post-acute neurobehavioral rehabilitation. *Brain Injury, 13*(2), 69–88.

Wrightson, P., & Gronwall, D. (1999). *Mild head injury: A guide to management*. New York: Oxford University Press.

5 CHAPTER

Patricia S. Camplair
Robert W. Bulter
Muriel D. Lezak

Providing Psychological Services to Families of Brain-Injured Adults and Children in the Present Health-Care Environment

□ Introduction

Besides physicians and other health-care providers needing objective information about the effects of traumatic brain injury (TBI) on neuropsychological functioning, families often need and deserve such information. It has long been recognized that the family plays a pivotal role in supporting their injured relative and contribute to the patient's rehabilitation outcome (Livingston, 1985; Romano, 1974). Equally striking have been the stressors and suffering that family members endure, particularly when a relative has sustained a severe, character-altering TBI (Lezak, 1978).

Family members' reactions and needs differ from family to family and may change over the course of early hospitalization and later rehabilitation phases (Lezak, 1986). These varied and fluctuating family reactions and needs reflect (a) the extent of behavioral and other injury-related disorders; (b) the nature and quality of premorbid family relationships; (c) preexisting resources and characteristics of caregivers and families; and (d) a host of external factors, such as the availability and quality of social, community, and professional support. Increasing attention to milder brain injuries, which may result in subtle and perplexing symptoms, also has illuminated the need to provide consultation to relatives, even when such problems are transient (Casey, Ludwig, & McCormick, 1987; Kibby & Long, 1997; Lezak, 1988b).

Clinicians' observations have been crucial in bringing typical family reactions to light and in portraying the burdens so often shouldered by the family. In fact, a considerable literature provides clinically and theoretically derived guidelines for working with TBI families. To date, most empirical studies have examined the impact of brain injury on relatives, usually primary caregivers, and in some cases on the family unit. Factors associated with relatives' reactions also have been widely investigated. Studies examining the efficacy of treatment with TBI families or caregivers have just begun to emerge in the literature. Empirical study specifically addressing the cost-effectiveness of providing services to TBI families is lacking, although findings regarding family reactions and needs underscore the importance of family support and intervention.

Services provided by neuropsychologists to family members cover a wide range of activities, including education, counseling, psychotherapy, family/marital therapy, training or mentoring, and social/community support interventions. Some of these activities may be covered by rehabilitation or mental health insurance benefits (e.g., provision of neuropsychological test results, conjoint treatment), whereas others fall beyond the scope of patient-related benefits (e.g., therapy for family members' problems, facilitating family support groups). Whether covered or not, most brain injury programs provide services to families because the importance of working with the survivor's support system is so clearly necessary (see Chapter 14).

This chapter presents an updated summary of the literature addressing the most common reactions, problems, and needs of families of TBI adults and children. It emphasizes postacute to chronic phases of rehabilitation and moderate to severe injury and considers findings pertinent to mild brain injury as well. An overview of family services also is provided, with an emphasis on recent research findings and innovative treatment approaches. Finally, working with families in the current environment of managed care and cost–outcome concepts as applied to family services are explored.

Family Reactions and the Family's Importance in Rehabilitation

Beginning with the postacute stage in the course of moderate and severe TBI, issues of uncertain survival and medical stabilization are no longer at the forefront, and the often dramatic early improvements in survivor functioning have occurred. At this point, patients with better outcomes may be discharged to home and more impaired patients may enter postacute rehabilitation programs or other structured environments (e.g., skilled nursing facilities or foster care). Families to whom the injured person is returned face different issues than families whose injured relative receives ongoing inpatient or residential rehabilitation or care. This chapter focuses on families who assume primary care of their injured relative.

Not all families possess the needed resources for outpatient or community-based rehabilitation. In the absence of adequate preparation, relatives may be left with overwhelming responsibilities for their injured relative (e.g., for supervision, continuing rehabilitation interventions, and advocating for activities and services). In addition, relatives often are faced with an increasing awareness that the patients' cognitive, behavioral, and emotional problems are not resolving as they had hoped or expected (Lezak, 1996). Understandably, relatives may experience strong emotional reactions, including anxiety, anger, and despair. Consider also that brain-injured persons may have little awareness of their condition (i.e., anosognosia; Prigatano et al., 1986) and may be experiencing intense emotional reactions themselves, and one can readily begin to appreciate the enormous challenges confronting these families.

Brain Injury in Adults

Early published descriptions of frequently encountered family reactions first drew attention to the plight of these families. Panting and Merry (1972) described the great strain placed on relatives of severely brain-injured persons. Romano (1974) described a phenomenon of denial among family members of severely injured persons, particularly during the acute phases of recovery. For example, relatives made statements that the injured person had not changed, despite the presence of obvious deficits. This difficulty in appreciating the survivor's actual condition hindered the relative's ability to assist the survivor's rehabilitation. Lezak (1978) observed that the characterological alterations associated with severe brain injury—such as dependent, childlike, ill-mannered, or aggressive traits—were particularly burdensome for families. In later reports (Lezak, 1986; 1988a), the adaptation of family members to the consequences of severe TBI were depicted as a phasic process (see Table 5.1).

Formalized surveys and investigational research also have improved our understanding of what TBI patients' families experience. In addition to challenges presented by altered behavior and decreased functioning of the TBI patient, several other significant sources of strain can affect the family. Medical and rehabilitation costs and loss of income for adult survivors and family caregivers can create severe financial burdens (Mazzucchi, Cattelani, Gugliotta, Brianti, & Janelli, 2000). Family members may sacrifice jobs or careers to devote much of their time to the needs of the injured person (Jacobs, 1988). TBI survivors tend to become dependent on family members for social and recreational needs, which can result in social isolation for the entire family (Finset, Dyrnes, Krogstad, & Berstad, 1995). Quality of life for both survivors and family members is curtailed when survivors have difficulty keeping themselves occupied (Tennant, MacDermott, & Neary, 1995).

Caregiver Burden and Affective Disturbance. TBI family members often experience significant distress and affective disturbance. High levels of distress have been reported as early as 1 month after injury and may continue unabated for years (e.g., Brooks, Campsie, Symington, Beattie, & McKinlay, 1986; Oddy, Humphrey, & Uttley, 1978; Thomsen, 1984). In England, Brooks and colleagues (1986), for example, found that 90% of relatives reported a sense of severe burden 5 years after injury. Researchers in the United States have found that 40% to 50% of caregivers report significant levels of emotional disturbance months to years after their relative's injury (Kreutzer, Gervasio, & Camplair, 1994a). High prevalence rates of a significant sense of burden, along with anxiety, depression, decreased social adjustment, psychosomatic disorders, and associated use of tranquilizing medication or alcohol, have been found among these relatives (Camplair, Kreutzer, & Doherty, 1990; Kreutzer, Marwitz, & Kepler, 1992).

Ratings of burden, as well as caregiver affective disturbance, have consistently been associated with emotional and behavioral (i.e., personality) changes in the injured person (for reviews, see Camplair et al., 1990; Florian, Katz, & Lahav, 1989; Kreutzer et al., 1992). Thus, empirical study strongly confirms earlier clinical observations. Cognitive/communicative deficits have been associated with adverse caregiver reactions to a lesser extent. Time since injury, medical measures of injury severity, and residual physical limitations have *not* been consistently related to caregivers' distress.

Other factors of potential importance to caregivers' functioning include preexisting risk factors (e.g., caregiver vulnerability to depression), extent and nature of coping

TABLE 5.1. Stages in the Evolution of Family Reactions to a Brain-Damaged Member*

Stage	Time Since Hospitalization (months)	Perception of Patient	Expectation	Family Reaction
I	0–1 to 3	A little difficult because of fatigue, inactivity, weakness	Full recovery by 1 year	Happy
II	1–3 to 6–9	Not cooperating, not motivated, self-centered	Full recovery if patient tries harder	Bewildered, anxious
III	6–9 to 9–24; can continue indefinitely	Irresponsible, self-centered, irritable, lazy	Independence if knew how to help	Discouraged, guilty, depressed, going crazy
IV	9 or more; can continue indefinitely	A different, difficult, childlike person	Little or no change	Depressed, despairing, "trapped"
V	15 or more; usually time-limited	A different, difficult, childlike person	Little or no change	Mourning
VI	18–24 or more	A different, difficult, childlike person	Little or no change	Reorganizing—emotionally if not physically disengaged

Source: Lezak (1986).

*These common responses, expectations, and concerns do not necessarily evolve as a progression, as suggested by this table. Some family members skip a stage, some get stuck in a stage, and many experience periods in which hope or fears or bewilderment or resignation predominate, fluctuating back and forth with changing circumstances, both external and internal.

strategies used by caregivers, and the perceived adequacy of social support (Gillen, Tennen, Affleck, & Steinpreis, 1998; Sander, High, Hannay, & Sherer, 1997). For example, Sander et al. (1997) found that the use of emotion-focused coping strategies (e.g., denial and wishful thinking) predicted greater levels of distress in caregivers. These authors described methods to enhance appropriate problem-focused strategies that are likely to reduce caregivers' reliance on the less effective emotion-focused strategies. The extent to which coping strategies and perceptions of social support affect the adaptation of caregivers or families is of interest given the need to prioritize family services. However, it also is important to emphasize strategies that can reduce the stressors faced by families, such as helping families gain access to adequate services for the TBI patient.

Impact on Marital Relationships. Marital relationships are particularly vulnerable to the impact of TBI. Unlike parents, who may have the aid of a partner, spouses typically are left to shoulder caregiving burdens alone. Changes in role and conflicts may arise when a spouse has been severely injured and rendered more-or-less dependent on the intact partner (Cavatorta et al., 2000; Lezak, 1988a). Higher levels of burden and emotional distress often are reported for spouses when compared to parents (Gillen et al., 1998; Kreutzer et al., 1994a), although there have been exceptions to this finding (e.g., Brooks et al., 1987).

One indicator of relationship strain is the extent to which these marriages fail. Separation and divorce rates within the TBI population are higher than the national average in the United States (Jacobs, 1988). For example, Wood and Yurdakul (1997) found that between 58% and 89% of those married at the time of injury later separated or divorced. Percentages varied with injury severity, and relationships most frequently dissolved 5 to 6 years after injury. Longevity in a marriage also corresponded to how long a couple had been married before the injury occurred. Some spouses stayed with their partner in the role of caregiver only, and some separated partners were willing to provide support to their injured spouse but did not wish to live with him or her.

A number of studies have evaluated couples who remain together after TBI. Rosenbaum and Najenson's (1976) early Israeli study found higher levels of depression in wives of brain-injured veterans than in wives of spinal cord-injured and noninjured veterans. A more recent study of married couples one year or more after TBI documented high levels of depression and anxiety among both injured partners and their spouses (Linn, Allen, & Willer, 1994). Not surprisingly, marital adjustment diminishes as the severity of the injury increases and is more strongly and positively related to the injured person's level of functioning than to the spouse's personality or coping style (Peters, Stambrook, Moore, & Esses, 1990).

Impact of Parental TBI. Investigators have begun to address altered parental behavior and its effects on children within TBI families. Negative behavioral changes in children are associated with severity of the TBI and with parenting difficulties for both injured and intact parents (Pessar, Coad, Linn, & Willer, 1993). TBI parents tend to show less interest in their children, are more apt to be impatient or angry with them, and assume less responsibility for them. A decrease in positive parental behaviors, such as praising children or having fun with them, also is reported. Other research indicates that both parents and children in TBI families are prone to depression (Uysal, Hibbard, Robillard, Pappadopulos, & Jaffe, 1998).

Impact of TBI on the Family Unit. Investigating the implications of a family member's TBI for the family system as a whole has been a more difficult undertaking. Validated measures of family functioning have only recently been developed and assessed for use with TBI populations (see DePompei & Zarski, 1991, for discussion). Earlier research indicated that TBI tends to have a more dramatic impact on the family than other types of disability (Rosenbaum & Najenson, 1976). Later research has incorporated standardized measures to study the effects of TBI on family functioning. For example, Kreutzer et al. (1994a) used the Family Assessment Device (FAD; Epstein, Baldwin, & Bishop, 1983) with families whose members had sustained moderate to severe injuries (a minority had mild injures). General family functioning was rated as *unhealthy* by more than 50% of primary caregivers, with poor communication and diminished interest in family activities rated as the most disruptive family problems. Greater dysfunction was reported when TBI families were compared to medical and nonpatient families, but they suffered less dysfunction than families with a psychiatric patient (based on FAD norms). Healthier family functioning was positively correlated with time since injury (Kreutzer, Gervasio, & Camplair, 1994b), providing evidence that these families can adjust satisfactorily, at least in some respects. Unhealthy family functioning was associated with more behavioral problems demonstrated by the TBI family member, but injury severity and independence in activities of daily living were unrelated to family functioning.

An Australian study of TBI adults and their primary caregivers found that open communication and freedom from conflict, aspects of family functioning assessed via the Family Environment Scales (FES; Moos & Moos, 1994), were associated with multiple factors (Douglas & Spellacy, 1996). Higher levels of caregiver depression and unfavorable perceptions of patient competency were related to poorer family functioning, whereas caregivers' use of coping strategies and satisfaction with social supports predicted better family communication and interactions. Lending further support to a common finding, a patient's poor neurobehavioral status, as assessed in an interview-based measure, also was associated with poorer family functioning. This association between a patient's neurobehavioral status and family functioning was documented again in 1998 (Groom, Shaw, O'Connor, Howard, & Pickens, 1998).

Families report ongoing needs for a variety of services for their brain-injured member and for training to deal more effectively with the injured person (McCaffrey, Pollock, & Burns, 1987). In fact, 70% to 80% of Brain Injury Association members living in Iowa, whose survivors averaged 7 years since injury, reported low satisfaction with assistance in obtaining information about brain injury, about resources for survivors and relatives, and about long-term consequences of TBI (McMordie, Rogers, & Barker, 1991). Serio, Kreutzer, and Gervasio, (1995) reported that just over half the relatives of 180 TBI patients rated various needs as being met. The greatest unmet needs were for emotional and professional support. Similar to research on correlates of caregivers' distress and family functioning, reported needs of family members tend to correspond to the extent of the TBI survivor's neurobehavioral problems.

The Family's Influence on Outcome. In accord with the dynamic, interactional nature of family functioning, one study evaluated the extent to which aspects of family functioning were predictive of depression among TBI adults (Leach, Frank, Bouman, & Farmer, 1994). Using an interview-based family assessment measure (F-Copes; McCubbin, Larsen, & Olson, 1985), Leach and associates found that a family's effective problem solving and behavioral coping were associated with less severe depression for TBI patients. The influence that family variables may exert on the survivor's functioning has been considered in more detail in pediatric populations (see "Brain Injury in Children," below).

Clinicians working with adults also have commented on the importance of the family in facilitating a positive rehabilitation outcome (Cohadon, Castel, Richer, Mdazaux, & Loiseau, 1998; Prigatano et al., 1994). In fact, Prigatano and colleagues studied the importance of a working alliance between families and rehabilitation staff in connection with their neuropsychologically oriented milieu rehabilitation program for adolescents and adults with acquired brain injuries (Klonoff, Lamb, Henderson, & Shepherd, 1998; Prigatano et al., 1994). Families were provided with information and support during individual family meetings, relatives' groups, and observation of rehabilitation therapies. The strength of the alliance with families, as assessed at the time of the patient's discharge from the program, predicted productivity levels for the person with brain injury.

Brain Injury in Children

Only in the past several years has attention been directed toward family influences and effects associated with brain injury in a child. This delayed interest may partially reflect the fact that changes in dependency roles after a child's brain injury are more subtle than those associated with brain injury in adulthood. Although some regression clearly can occur after a child's brain injury, additional dependency needs likely place less dramatically altered demands on the parents than, for example, the disruption that results when a spouse must care for the basic needs of a marital partner. Some may have assumed that family factors were less important in child brain injury, but recent research is demonstrating that family variables can have a significant impact on the child's rehabilitation process.

Head injury is one of the most common neurological complications of childhood (Kraus, 1995). Thus, most research on family factors and their impact on psychological adjustment and neurobehavioral outcome has focused on pediatric TBI. As with adults, mild head injury, commonly defined as no or brief loss of consciousness (less than 15 minutes) and little change in sensorium, also is most prevalent in children (Annegers, 1983). Mild head injury in children and adolescents usually is not associated with significant lasting neurocognitive, behavioral, or academic changes (Light et al., 1998; Satz et al., 1997), although careful follow-up study may uncover persistent cognitive deficits in some children (Wrightson, McGinn, & Gronwall, 1995). In contrast, moderate to severe head injury in children clearly causes neuropsychological impairment (Anderson, Morse, & Klug, 1997; Broman & Michel, 1995; Max et al., 1999).

Severity of trauma is positively associated with the number of stress-related family changes that follow brain injury (Rivara et al., 1996). Lower levels of family-based control and increased familial communication and expressiveness correlated with better outcomes after severe trauma as much as 3 years after injury. Families that were rated as more intact on a number of dimensions before the head injury also tended to have children who experienced less severe neurobehavioral consequences.

Another group of researchers followed a cohort of families with a brain-injured child and a control group of families with children with orthopedic injuries (Taylor et al., 1999; Wade, Taylor, Drotar, Stancin, & Yeates, 1998; Yeates et al., 1997). Families of children with severe TBI consistently experienced significant levels of distress, burden, and psychological disturbance.

Pediatric malignancies produce another population of children who have incurred insults to the brain. The two most common cancers of childhood, the leukemias and brain tumors, are both associated with neuropsychological impairment from the disease itself, from treatments, or from both. Several studies of this population have identified familial factors that appear to moderate how much a child improves and long-term outcome. Single-parent families and a younger mother appear to be predictive of behavioral problems in children diagnosed with a brain tumor (Mulhern, Carpentieri, Shema, Stone, & Fairclough, 1993). Measures of maternal adjustment over the course of treatment for leukemia have predicted the child's psychological adjustment 2 years after diagnosis (Sawyer, Streiner, Antoniou, Toogood, & Rice, 1998). Within the leukemia population, there also is evidence that the child's disease, its treatment, and the late effects of treatment may result in enduring psychological changes in the parents, including increased anxiety and other stress-related symptoms (Kazak et al., 1998).

Little research has been directed toward the adjustment of siblings after pediatric TBI. One study suggests that such siblings have an increased risk for adjustment disturbances and psychological distress (Orsillo, McCaffrey, & Fisher, 1993). Based on clinical observation, factors thought to contribute to this increased risk have included jealousy of the increased attention allotted to the brain-injured sibling, guilt about resenting the injured sibling, and feeling less important to the parents (Conoley & Sheridan, 1996). Another research group focusing on the pediatric cancer population reported a significant increase in behavioral problems among siblings after cancer was diagnosed (Sahler et al., 1994).

Clearly, evaluations of a brain-injured child should now include an assessment of the parent's psychological adjustment, the marital relationship, and familial stability. Table 5.2 provides a list of nine published objective psychological measures for these three

TABLE 5.2. Assessment Measures for Parent and Child Adjustment, Marital Adjustment, and Familial Integrity

Measure	Respondent(s)	Subject Age
Parent/Child Adjustment		
Parenting Alliance Measure[1]	Parent	1–19 years
Parenting Stress Index[2]	Parent	1 mo–12 years
Stress Index for Parents of Adolescents[3]	Parent	13–19 years
Marital Adjustment		
Marital Satisfaction Inventory-Revised[4]	Self	Adult
Taylor-Johnson Temperament Analysis[5]	Self/Other	Adult
Social Skills Inventory[6]	Self	14 years and older
Family Integrity		
Family Environment Scale[7]	Self	Adolescent through adult
Family Environment Scale–Children's Version[8]	Self	5–12 years
McMaster Family Assessment Device[9]	Self	Adolescent through adult

[1]Abidin and Konold (1999);[2] Abidin (1995);[3] Sheras, Abdin and Konold (1998);[4] Snyder (1997);[5] Taylor and Morrison (1996);[6] Riggio (1989);[7] Moos and Moos (1994);[8] Pino, Simons, and Slawinowski (1995); and [9]Epstein, Baldwin, and Bishop (1983).

areas. This list is not exhaustive but, rather, represents measures found to be useful in the second author's pediatric neuropsychology clinic. These measures all have acceptable reliability and validity, and most have an extensive research database.

Psychological Services for Families

Approaches to helping families vary widely, depending on the rehabilitation setting, the extent of neurobehavioral problems presented by the injured family member, and the needs of individual families. Treatment modalities include education, counseling, psychotherapy, family or marital therapy, training or mentoring of family members, and social or community network interventions. These modalities have many overlapping features and are variously defined in the literature. Methods for working with families are organized here to highlight key features and to present information concerning efficacy when available.

Education

Given the array of possible difficulties that can arise after brain injury; the complicated blend among neurologically produced, reactive, and preinjury personality traits (Prigatano et al., 1986); and the lack of information among the general public regarding brain injuries, it is not surprising that relatives report needs for information during all phases of rehabilitation. Soon after the patient has been injured, families need information about the early and late effects of brain injury provided in a manner that they can assimilate (Lezak, 1996). Repetition is required, given the complexity of the information as well as the emotional reactions that can prevent family members from absorbing information. Information can be conveyed by books and pamphlets, videotapes, explanations from clinical or rehabilitation staff, presentations, and referral to libraries or to sound information on the Internet.

The following goals should be considered when educational resources are developed: (a) to provide a variety of modalities, as preferences vary widely among individuals; (b) to maintain a range of materials with respect to literacy level and use of technical terms; (c) to provide materials in languages suited to local cultural groups; (d) to tailor information to phase of rehabilitation/course to avoid overwhelming relatives; and (d) to make local resource and referral information available.

Holland and Shigaki (1998) offered an example of a resource bibliography organized by phase of rehabilitation. These writers proposed a model of *guided study* as a cost-effective supplement–not a replacement–for more patient-specific education and counseling needed during rehabilitation. Guided study implies that clinicians will be assessing family members' understanding of information reviewed. The National Brain Injury Association is an excellent resource for educational materials (see Internet site www.biausa.org, or call 1-800-321-7037 for help with reference materials and local services).

Unfortunately, some attempts to evaluate the success of educational programs have been disappointing (Acorn, 1995; Reeber, 1992). These studies failed to find evidence that education, with or without additional support, improved family members' coping skills, self-esteem, well-being, or family functioning, although Acorn did report high levels of participant satisfaction. Rather than focusing on relatives' coping skills or family functioning, however, a brief and circumscribed education program would be evaluated more appropriately by assessing knowledge gained, along with participant satisfaction.

Counseling

Typically, family counseling is intended to help families understand and cope with their injured relative's residual deficits and distress as well as with their own emotional reactions to the patient's altered abilities or behavior. For example, feedback given during the course of neuropsychological assessment can help relatives understand the nature of the patient's problems. During family conferences or counseling sessions, the clinician also may advise relatives on how to minimize difficulties related to the patient's cognitive, emotional, and behavioral problems. For example, the spouse of a patient struggling with a mildly inefficient information-processing capacity can be encouraged to slow down and pause when speaking or to avoid interrupting the injured person when he or she is focused on a task. Relatives also may require counseling without the survivor present so that they can express feelings of grief, despair, uncertainty, or frustration. Counseling can assist relatives by helping them acknowledge the loss of their family member as he or she was before the injury and to gradually accept the person he or she has become (refer to Table 5.1). Counseling and psychotherapy are important in helping relatives acknowledge and attempt to meet their own needs, in addition to those of the patient (Prigatano, 1999).

Families of persons with *mild brain injury* also require information and guidance to support these patients appropriately and to prevent the development of adjustment difficulties for the patient and the family (Casey et al., 1987; Dittmar, 1997; Kibby & Long, 1997; Lezak, 1988b). Without adequate information, relatives are likely to become frustrated with these injured persons when they have difficulty resuming preinjury activities and responsibilities. Information about the possible effects of mild TBI can give family members realistic expectations for the patient and enhance their awareness of the patient's changing status (Sohlberg, Glang, & Todis, 1998).

In our experience most family members are interested in better understanding their relative's problems and appreciate suggestions that will improve the situation. A smaller proportion want an opportunity to express and deal with their own reactions. Children with a TBI sibling or parent also frequently need counseling and supportive care. Counseling these children at a level appropriate to their understanding and situation can challenge even experienced clinicians who normally work with adults. Sachs (1991, pp. 130–133) offered further discussion of this important topic.

Relatives' difficulty appreciating the severity of a loved one's deficits also contributes to conflict between family members and rehabilitation staff and hampers the process of setting attainable rehabilitation goals (Rosenthal & Young, 1988). Different values, philosophies, or cultural backgrounds between providers and families also can make collaboration and family treatment difficult (Cavallo & Saucedo, 1995; Kreutzer, Sander, & Fernandez, 1997). Insufficient time to build relationships or to support families, lack of training in working with families, and pressure to elicit change quickly can further impede the process of helping families (Malec, 1996). Clinicians may respond constructively to these potential obstacles by (a) attempting to understand and respect differences in values or philosophies, (b) acknowledging differences of opinion or perspective when they arise, (c) addressing adverse emotional reactions with relatives when possible, (d) acknowledging program or service limitations, and (e) focusing on goals or areas of common ground.

Family Therapy

Although a distinction between family counseling and therapy is somewhat arbitrary, the terms are used separately here to acknowledge that some families require more intensive and sophisticated therapy to facilitate maximal adjustment. Also, the family unit or specific relationships within the family are the focus of treatment, rather than the TBI individual's problems. Family therapy includes strategies that focus on family structure, roles, communication, or operational rules for problem solving and behavioral control (e.g., Maitz & Sachs, 1995). Families may require therapy when (a) demands placed on the family exceed resources, (b) significant and often long-standing relationship problems exist between family members, (c) issues of guilt or blame disrupt the family, or (d) individuation/separation is being considered (Maitz & Sachs, 1995; Zarski & DePompei, 1991). Moreover, because many survivors tend to improve—and only a few deteriorate—family members may benefit from a periodic review of the patient's status and their roles and expectations. For example, once family members have initially shifted roles to compensate for the injured person's disability, they may resist changing again even when the survivor is ready to assume more responsibilities. In other cases, appropriate roles are not shifted initially, and the needs of family members may go significantly unmet unless the family is helped to restructure.

When setting goals for treatment, clinicians must consider the injured person's capabilities and limitations to assist with an appropriate restructuring within the family and to decide whether or how to include the brain-injured person in these sessions. Some writers suggest that family therapy may not benefit persons with significant cognitive, emotional, or communicative deficits, or those whose behaviors are maladaptive or poorly controlled (e.g., Rollin, 1987). Zarski and DePompei argued that, "the final decision for including the person in the family therapy session may be made on the basis of the therapist's knowledge of appropriate functional levels of the person as they are revealed in the context of the family" (1991, p. 287). Whenever possible, clinicians providing family therapy should have substantial training in family functioning and treatment so they can work effectively with these often challenging families. Several writers have applied family systems theory to work with TBI families (e.g., Maitz & Sachs, 1995; Miller, 1993; Sachs, 1991).

Research addressing the efficacy of family therapy with TBI families is sparse. Perlesz and O'Loughlan (1998) attempted to measure the impact of family therapy on relatives' stress and burden. Fifteen families of severely injured persons (aged 12 to 55 years) who voluntarily sought treatment were studied. Assessment took place before counseling and 12 and 24 months posttreatment. Measures of subjective burden, overall health, mood disturbance, social adjustment, and family functioning were employed. An average of 8.4 sessions was reported, with attendance ranging from 1 to 22 sessions. Unfortunately, the nature of the therapy provided was not described, and 10 different therapists were involved. Nevertheless, the authors reported positive findings, including decreased distress for both survivors and relatives, decreased burden, and some improvements in family functioning. Follow-up data (24 months after injury) suggested that reported levels of anger increased and marital adjustment returned to baseline levels.

Marital therapy/sexual counseling can be considered as one aspect of family therapy. Research highlights the challenges presented by brain injury to marital or intimate partner relationships and the likelihood that many (even premorbidly stable) relationships will fail. However, when both partners are committed to remaining together, therapy addressing marital and sexual issues may be useful. In some cases, genital competency will have been compromised, and medical or physiatric assistance is required (Zasler & Horn, 1990). Libido sometimes increases after brain injury, but more often it decreases, often significantly (Lishman, 1973). Injured persons who have become less sensitive to others may be impaired in the interpersonal aspects of sexual relationships. Depression and other emotional reactions also can affect sexuality adversely. A few excellent published discussions have addressed sexual dysfunction after TBI, treatment, and (more rarely) the impact on marital relationships (Rosenthal & Young, 1988; Zasler & Horn, 1990; Zasler & Kreutzer, 1991).

Family Training Programs

Uomoto and Brockway (1992) described an outpatient training program that targeted anger problems for TBI patients and their families. Treatment required 8 to 12 sessions and usually included both the injured person and family. Treatment included teaching patients self-control strategies for anger and teaching relatives behavioral modification techniques. The two case reports included in this article provided a detailed description of the training involved. This approach appears to offer a promising method for improving difficult TBI-related behaviors. Both teaching survivors emotional self-management strategies and including them in setting treatment goals likely contributed to the reported success of these behavioral programs.

Carnevale (1996) evaluated a caregiver training program for families of both adolescent and adult survivors of brain injury. The Natural Setting Behavior Management project brought education, counseling, and training techniques to TBI survivors and their caregivers within home, school, and work settings. Treatment was offered over the course of a year. Families were monitored over a second year. This innovative project used a mobile treatment team of two therapists and a videotape for assessment, consultation, and treatment planning. Families individually received information about the consequences of TBI and behavioral assessment and modification techniques. The team taught relatives the skills they needed by modeling and role playing. When feasible, survivors were given control over their programs. Behaviors most often targeted were verbal or physical aggressive outbursts, although other types of disinhibited or inappropriate behavior were dealt with as well. Target behaviors improved 82% from baseline. The greatest improvement occurred during the education phase (51%), and an additional increment of 27% occurred during treatment.

These two studies are examples of successful attempts to train family members and caregivers to use behavioral-management techniques. Important factors included the presence of intact, consistent caregiver systems, young TBI survivors who were attached to the family system, and targeting clearly specified excess behaviors rather than deficits. In contrast, Quine, Lyle, and Pierce (1993) trained family members to act as therapists, an effort that did not prove feasible. Family members were trained to provide coma-stimulation therapy, which was acknowledged to be of uncertain benefit as well as extremely time-consuming for the relatives. The authors, who were social workers charged with monitoring caregivers' stress for ethical reasons, highlighted the stressfulness of this situation for relatives and did not support continuation of the planned project after this pilot. This article underscored the importance of monitoring relatives' reactions when they serve as cotherapists or lay therapists. Additionally, some writers have noted that having family members serve as therapists runs counter to the philosophy of helping TBI survivors live as normal a life as possible (e.g., Wilson, 1999).

To support their brain-injured family member effectively, caregivers often need to advocate for services and thus essentially serve as case managers (Blosser & DePompei, 1995). Relatives not only need to understand the effects of brain injury and the nature of rehabilitation services, they also need skills in gathering information and in interacting effectively with physicians, lawyers, and financial advisors and with community agencies such as schools and state social security and vocational rehabilitation division offices. Blosser and DePompei encouraged the development and evaluation of professional-to-family-member mentoring programs while acknowledging that other types of mentoring relationships, such as family-to-family training in case management or advocacy skills, also may be beneficial.

Social and Community Support

Family support groups, which may be offered through local chapters of brain injury associations, offer newcomers the opportunity to benefit from knowledge gained by family members with greater experience. Participants typically benefit from sharing experiences, reactions, and possible solutions (Miller, 1992; Rosenthal & Young, 1988). Participation in a support group also can be highly effective in reducing relatives' sense of isolation.

Another potentially useful approach to solidifying and maintaining a family's social support is called *social network intervention*. Initially developed for families with a mentally ill member for whom periodic crises were likely, this approach has been effective with TBI families (Rogers & Kreutzer, 1984). Typically, clinicians are involved in setting up and initially facilitating meetings in which relatives, friends, and acquaintances of the TBI survivor are brought together. Members of the network can volunteer to help the TBI person or family in specific ways while each is protected from feeling overwhelmed. The goal is for the social network team to continue indefinitely, meeting periodically to coordinate efforts, to offer mutual support, and to change the group's composition as needed.

Research Evaluating Combined or Comparative Family Services

Smith and Godfrey (1995) offered a sample program-evaluation study addressing comprehensive family services. This New Zealand program included a series of educational sessions for individual TBI families tailored to the survivor's particular problems, and then a series of follow-up "case monitoring" visits. In-home services included education, advice about particular problems, instruction in implementing behavioral-management strategies, relationship therapy when needed, and assistance accessing community resources. Families received an average of 27.6 hours of service. For these participants, distress about their family member's residual symptoms *decreased* between 6 and 24 months after the injury. In contrast, distress about survivors' problems *increased* for control group families who received standard hospital care, which offered little if any follow-up service. Slightly lower levels of depression, higher ratings of self-esteem, and increased consumer satisfaction were found for program participants. TBI survivors' ratings also tended to be more positive for those involved in the family-based rehabilitation. Although specific information regarding cost-effectiveness was not reported, the researchers noted that the amount of service required was far less than typical inpatient or day-treatment rehabilitation programs.

Man (1999) presented a program-evaluation study of a community-based "empowerment" program. Based on his description of the family program, it appears that education, coping skills training (specific to brain injury-related problems), and family-to-family support were all components of the 8-week program. Professionals and family members worked jointly to develop the session themes. Based on pre-, post-, and 3-month assessments, the program was found to be effective in increasing participant ratings of different aspects of empowerment (knowledge, efficacy, support, and aspiration). Ratings on measures of psychological well-being, subjective burden, self-efficacy, and use of support systems also improved.

Singer and colleagues (1994) compared a parent informational support group to a family group designed to improve parents' coping skills. A heterogenous group of children with acquired brain injuries comprised their fairly small sample. Nevertheless, the coping skills group was more effective in reducing parents' distress levels than the informational group. Unfortunately, few studies have evaluated the effectiveness of family services or compared different types or amounts of family services.

Summary of Clinical Utility of Psychological Services for Family Members After TBI

The preceding sections reviewed the literature pertaining to family reactions to TBI and the family's influence on rehabilitation outcome, and also discussed the range of services typically considered appropriate for these relatives. Table 5.3 provides a summary of the major findings in support of providing services to families with a TBI member. Although much of the evidence provides indirect support of family services, research directly examining the benefits and outcomes associated with family interventions is beginning to accumulate.

☐ Managed Health Care and Cost Outcome Comparisons

Hosack and Rocchio (1995) cited the general effects of the increasing presence of managed care in rehabilitation as including the following: (a) greater limitations on lengths of stay in a particular setting, (b) a heightened need for early discharge planning, (c) lack of coverage for family services and social services, and (d) involvement of external case managers. The combination of these factors translates into increased pressure to make decisions quickly and less time for relatives to prepare for their roles as caregivers and advocates. Providers and programs are pressured to "develop effective and efficient family service programs; serve families more quickly and more intensely; prioritize family treatment goals, plans, and services; and ensure that families are referred to follow-up community practitioners after discharge" (Hosack & Rocchio, 1995, p. 58). Family members and rehabilitation clinicians must quickly reach an agreement about which rehabilitation goals to pursue—not always an easy feat to accomplish.

TABLE 5.3. Summary of the Utility of the Services Provided by Neuropsychologists to Family Members After TBI: Studies of Efficacy

1. The importance of neuropsychological services for families of persons with TBI is evident from:
   a. evidence that families provide the gist of long-term care and support for their brain-injured relatives (Finset et al., 1995; Jacobs 1988);
   b. high prevalence rates of caregiver distress and unhealthy family functioning (e.g., Brooks et al., 1986; Kreutzer et al., 1994a; Rivara et al., 1996);
   c. family members' reports of ongoing need for information and services for years after their relatives' TBI (McCaffrey et al., 1987; McMordie et al., 1991; Serio et al., 1995);
   d. findings that emotional, behavioral, and cognitive problems are more closely related to caregiver and family functioning than measures of physical problems or disability (e.g., Kreutzer et al., 1994b; Rosenbaum & Najenson, 1976).
2. Improving or supporting families is important because family functioning predicts neurobehavioral outcome for persons with TBI. This finding is well documented in the pediatric literature (Rivara et al., 1996; Wade et al., 1998) and likely holds true for many adult TBI patients as well (e.g., Leach et al., 1994).
3. Relatives' adverse emotional reactions and conflicts between rehabilitation staff and families have been observed to hamper the process of identifying appropriate treatment goals and making progress toward these goals (Lezak, 1996; Rosenthal & Young, 1998; Shaw & McMahon, 1990).
4. Programs that include family education and intervention report excellent return-to-work statistics, and the alliance with families is predictive of positive outcomes (Cohadon et al., 1998; Klonoff et al., 1998; Prigatano et al., 1994).
5. Education is an important intervention for family members, as most people have little or no former experience with TBI (Lezak, 1996; McMordie et al., 1991). Providing information is relatively inexpensive, and extensive resources are available (e.g., see Holland & Shigaki, 1998).
6. Counseling that provides a forum for family members to express their loss, concerns, and frustrations helps relatives go through the necessary reorientation process so that they can respond appropriately to their loved one's altered abilities and behavior (Lezak, 1986; Prigatano, 1999).
7. Training family members in behavioral strategies is effective in improving behavioral management of anger or other disruptive behaviors in TBI patients (Carnevale, 1996; Uomato and Brockway, 1992).
8. Family/marital therapy provides more intense and sophisticated therapies to facilitate maximum adjustment. Indirect evidence suggests such therapy can reduce distress in TBI patients and their relatives and, in some instances, improve family functioning (Perlesz & O'Laughlan, 1998).
9. Community support groups for families with persons who have a TBI reduce the social isolation experienced by family members and provide various types of support (Miller, 1992; Rosenthal & Young, 1988). As neuropsychologists may primarily be involved in referring families to these groups or providing time-limited assistance, this represents another inexpensive means for providing help to families.
10. One comprehensive family program—which included education, counseling, and help with accessing community resources, clearly demonstrated the utility of providing services to families (Smith & Godfrey, 1995). Benefits included a decrease in family members' distress about the patient's residual symptoms, in contrast to an increase in distress for family members receiving "standard care." Better emotional

(Continued)

TABLE 5.3. Continued

functioning, fewer physician visits, and increased consumer satisfaction for family member participants also were documented. On the average, 27.6 hours of professional support per family was required to achieve these results.

11. For persons sustaining mild brain injuries, family education and support are an essential part of rehabilitation. Counseling in this situation can prevent adjustment problems for both the injured person and the family (Casey et al., 1987; Kibby & Long 1997; Lezak 1988b).

Hosack and Rocchio (1995) offered several strategies that may help prepare families in an expeditious manner. They urge the following: (a) physician encouragement of family involvement in rehabilitation, (b) starting discharge planning upon entry to the program, (c) helping families understand the importance of providing enough structure and support for the injured family member ("environmental engineering"), (d) providing guidance to the family about what activities the patient may reasonably and safely undertake, and (e) assisting families in arranging for longer-term community resources.

Another change with the advent of managed care has been increased attention to the cost-effectiveness of psychological services. The several types of equations for examining costs in relation to various indices of benefit or outcome are referred to as cost–outcome comparisons (see Chapter 1 of this text for an introduction to the concepts and terminology). At this point, cost–outcome data specific to family services in TBI rehabilitation are almost nonexistent. This situation is unfortunate because data supporting the allocation of resources for family services are needed to demonstrate to insurance providers, policy makers, administrators, and other consumers (patients and families) that these services are worth the expenses incurred. Such data also would help service providers involved in program development and management to offer the most effective family services in as affordable a manner as possible to those who need and can benefit from them. This section reviews major types of cost–outcome comparisons as they might be explored in relation to family services in TBI rehabilitation.

Table 5.4 provides sample cost–outcome comparisons of potential relevance to serving families with TBI members. For the sake of simplicity, cost in this example is defined as the charge-based expenses for typical family services (estimated at an average of $140 per hour for individual services). Costs also might be calculated in terms of what the service actually costs the consumer (i.e., the amount reimbursed by the insurer or the patient/family). Clinical program administrators, however, might be more interested in examining costs in terms of salaries of staff and the overhead associated with providing the services. Calculating costs is a complex issue, and the interested reader is referred to Wolff, Helminiak, and Tebes (1997) for an in-depth discussion of the cost side of the equation.

Outcomes can be defined in terms of dollar savings or other indicators of the value of these services. Most practitioners are loathe to define the value of their services in terms of money saved, but insurers and public agencies providing long-term support to persons with TBI would find such comparisons compelling. As is true for other health-care and psychological services, the primary intended benefits typically are to improve

TABLE 5.4. Toward Demonstrating Cost-Effectiveness of Services Provided by Neuropsychologists to Family Members After a TBI: Sample Cost Outcome Comparisons

Type and Cost of Service*	Potential Savings and Value
Education $50 × 8 group sessions = $400 $140 × 4 individual sessions = $560	*Savings*: Minimize time spent with physician specialists educating the family. *Value*: Increase relatives' informed cooperation in patient's rehabilitation; prepare relatives to provide care for patient outside of or after rehabilitation program; minimize relationship strain due to gross misunderstanding of patient's problems.
Counseling of family members $140 ×15 to 25 sessions/year = $2100 to $3500/year	*Savings:* Addressing relatives' emotional reactions and stressors can decrease their own medical problems or need for treatment (medical offset). *Value*: Decreased emotional distress; improved ability to provide appropriate support for the TBI family member.
Family/marital counseling $140 x 15 to 25 sessions/year = $2,100 to $3,500/year	*Savings*: Fewer costs due to separation or divorce; decreased need for professional support or paid attendant care for family member with TBI. *Value*: Improve marital adjustment or satisfaction; ensure adequate safety and care of children in the home.
Training families in behavioral strategies to decrease TBI-related aggressive or other clearly inappropriate behaviors $140 × 20 sessions/year = $2,800/year	*Savings*: Maintain person with TBI at home rather than placing in expensive program or alternate housing; may decrease costs due to property destruction, calls to police, injury. *Value*: Improve well-being of patient and family; increase access to community and decrease isolation of family.
Establishment of a good working alliance with families within the context of neuropsychologically oriented milieu program (as described by Prigatano et al., 1986) $140 × 4 to 6 hours/month = $560 to $840/month or course of rehabilitation	*Savings*: Increase likelihood that person with TBI will be productively involved in competitive employment or voluntary work; family members need to invest less time supervising the patient, and an attendant may not be needed. *Value*: Decreased stress/conflict between family and rehabilitation staff; increased participation of patient in program and/or improved outcome (e.g., more efficient completion, patient/family satisfaction).

*For purposes of illustration, a charge-based model of defining cost was used, estimated at $140 per hour; charges are expected to vary based on locale and differences among programs or providers.

the health or well-being of recipients, not to save money. As Table 5.4 depicts, there are many possible ways to demonstrate that the services provided to family members result in a measurable benefit. The importance given to these benefits is likely to depend on the nature of one's involvement in rehabilitation services (i.e., clinician vs. insurer vs. family member).

Table 5.5 offers possible research questions corresponding to the major categories of cost–outcome comparisons as outlined in Chapter 1. Only the *cost–benefit analysis* considers costs and outcomes strictly in terms of dollars saved. A related concept, *medical cost offset*, has been of major importance to clinical psychology, as research has demonstrated that savings in health-care expenditures can be realized through provision of focused psychological intervention (e.g., Thomas & Cummings, 2000). Extrapolating from this literature, it may similarly be expected that providing appropriate psychological intervention to family members will reduce expenses associated with their own unnecessary medical appointments, use of prescription drugs, or severity of stress-related chronic illnesses. Providing initial support for this hypothesis, Smith and Godfrey (1995) found that family members participating in their program had fewer physician visits than a comparison group.

TABLE 5.5. Sample Research Questions Addressing Cost Outcome Comparisons when Providing Neuropsychological Services to Family Members of TBI Patients

1. Research addressing economic benefits of providing family services:

When feasible, assess *cost–benefit* ratios associated with family services or family-oriented rehabilitation. Does providing family services result in any dollar savings, such as lower amounts of lost income for the family or decreased expenditures for attendant care?

Evaluate *medical offset cost changes* associated with neuropsychological services for family members (i.e., number of physician visits, prescription medications, health problems for relatives with and without family intervention or before and after course of intervention).

2. Research addressing costs in relation to nonmonetary aspects of outcome:

Answer questions of *cost-effectiveness or cost-efficiency,* such as these:

What is the least costly intervention that still results in a satisfactory outcome (or in comparable outcomes)?

How does regular family counseling compare with a multifamily group counseling on measures of family functioning, relatives' emotional/physical symptoms, ratings of distress or ability to cope with the patients' problem behaviors/deficits?

Does family counseling result in more rapid improvements compared to "spontaneous" improvement? (Refer to McNeilly and Howard, 1991, for effectiveness of psychotherapy in general.)

How many sessions are needed to produce a meaningful change in relatives' affective status (see Howard et al., 1999; dose-response model)?

Does providing family education and support increase the patient's compliance with medical-rehabilitation protocols?

Are vocational rehabilitation outcomes enhanced when the family is included in rehabilitation?

Cost-efficiency analyses, which emphasize determining the most economical way to achieve the desired outcome, seem particularly relevant to rehabilitation efforts. Such comparisons would likely be of interest to providers, insurers, and families alike.

Cost-effectiveness studies examine whether interventions—as typically provided—produce the intended result. Whether the result is achieved more quickly than spontaneous improvement occurs also could be compared. For example, relatives may eventually work their way through stages of denial, anger, grieving, and reorientation to their injured family member. Facilitating this process via therapy, however, is likely to lead to earlier resolution for the family member, which in turn is helpful in terms of the nature and extent of support they may offer the injured person.

Finally, *cost–utility* analyses expand the definition of outcome to include multiple measures of outcome. The idea of evaluating quality of life as one measure of outcome has been discussed in the context of cost–utility analysis. For example, in health care this variable has been examined by looking at years gained at a certain quality of life. Development of measures to examine such aspects of outcome now allow study of this potentially important variable (e.g., Quality of Well-Being Scale; Kaplan, & Anderson, 1988). In TBI rehabilitation, assessment of outcome might include multiple perspectives (e.g., ratings from family members as well as case managers) or multiple aspects of outcome (e.g., consumer satisfaction with services along with measures of improved psychological health).

Although research addressing cost–outcome analyses in relation to serving families of TBI persons is lacking, such research is beginning to accumulate for other populations. Gabbard, Lazar, Hornberger, and Spiegel (1997) analyzed 18 studies that addressed the economic benefits of psychotherapeutic interventions for persons with a severe psychiatric disorder. One clear area of benefit was providing consultation to families with a schizophrenic member. Specifically, educating and supporting family members and otherwise mobilizing a patient's support network appeared to reduce exacerbations of the mental illness and the subsequent need for hospitalization. Despite the obvious differences between schizophrenia and TBI (e.g., the main cost saving for mentally ill persons was fewer days of inpatient hospitalization), similar research could be conducted with TBI families. We hope the examples provided in Tables 5.4 and 5.5, along with research accumulating for other patient groups, will help generate ideas for cost–outcome studies among those who provide or evaluate family services within TBI rehabilitation programs.

☐ Conclusions

Clinical experience and research with TBI families indicate that many relatives experience considerable distress and, at one time or another, suffer adverse emotional, physical, psychosocial, and financial consequences when a family member sustains a significant brain injury. At the same time, survivors' adaptation to brain injury depends partly on the ability of caregivers and families to sustain them. Ethically, morally, and rationally it makes sense to offer whatever assistance we can to help these families adapt—as best they can—to the challenges presented by the patient's brain injury. Economical considerations also suggest that, as a society, we should pay full attention to bolstering the family to provide this support when feasible. Inadequate levels of service to families may lead to more severe psychological disorders, such as depression, substance abuse, and stress-related health problems for both patients and family members, thereby creating additional health-care costs. Patients who do not make an adequate adjustment at home may end up in more expensive settings, such as residential rehabilitation programs, foster care, or institutions (e.g., jails or psychiatric facilities).

Informing families about TBI effects and treatments and providing some level of counseling for involved or interested relatives should be considered basic and necessary services in the rehabilitation of all severities of TBI. More intensive forms of therapy for relatives, couples, or families; training to assist family members in implementing behavior management strategies; teaching case-management skills to relatives; and directly promoting the family's support network are all potentially useful interventions that should be initiated when appropriate. Both the extent of neurobehavioral problems demonstrated by the TBI patient and the extent of caregiver or family resources available will influence the need for more intensive services to families. Future development and evaluation of family services should focus on further clarifying the effectiveness and relative costs of various treatment options. To allow continuation of adequate care, researchers are urged to assess the costs of treatment and to document the benefits obtained, including economic savings when feasible. Clinicians also are encouraged to work with TBI families on advocacy efforts, whether to help develop adequate services in a particular community or to attempt to influence legislation and insurance coverage requirements that might permit a more favorable environment for TBI rehabilitation.

References

Abidin, R. R. (1995). *Parenting stress index* (manual). Odessa, FL: Psychological Assessment Resources.

Abidin, R. R., & Konold, T. R. (1999). *Parenting alliance measure* (manual). Odessa, FL: Psychological Assessment Resources.

Acorn, S. (1995). Assisting families of head-injured survivors through a family support programme. *Journal of Advanced Nursing, 21*(5), 872–877.

Anderson, V. A., Morse, S. A., & Klug, G. (1997). Predicting recovery from head injury in young children: A prospective analysis. *Journal of the International Neuropsychology Society, 3*(6), 568–80.

Annegers, J. F. (1983). The epidemiology of head trauma in children. In K. Shapiro (Ed.), *Pediatric head trauma* (pp. 1–10). New York: Futura.

Blosser, J., & DePompei, R. (1995). Fostering effective family involvement through mentoring. *Journal of Head Trauma Rehabilitation, 10*(2), 46–56.

Broman, S. H., & Michel, M. E. (Eds.) (1995). *Traumatic head injury in children*. New York: Oxford University Press.

Brooks, N., Campsie, L., Symington, C., Beattie, A., & McKinlay, W. (1987). The effects of severe head injury on patient and relative within seven years of injury. *Journal of Head Trauma Rehabilitation, 2*(3), 1–13.

Brooks, N., Campsie, L., Symington, C., Beattie, A., & McKinlay, W. (1986). The five year outcome of severe blunt head injury: A relative's view. *Journal of Neurology, Neurosurgery, and Psychiatry, 49*, 764–770.

Camplair, P. S., Kreutzer, J. S., & Doherty, K. (1990). Family outcome following adult traumatic brain injury: A critical review of the literature. In J. S. Kreutzer & P. Wehman (Eds.), *Community integration following traumatic brain injury* (pp. 207–223). Baltimore: Paul H. Brookes.

Carnevale, G. J. (1996). Natural-setting behavior management for individuals with traumatic brain injury: Results of a three-year caregiver training program. *Journal of Head Trauma Rehabilitation, 11*(1), 27–38.

Casey, R., Ludwig, S., & McCormick, M. C. (1987). Minor head trauma in children: An intervention to decrease functional morbidity. *Pediatrics, 80,* 159–164.

Cavallo, M. M., & Saucedo, C. (1995). Traumatic brain injury in families from culturally diverse populations. *Journal of Head Trauma Rehabilitation, 10*(2), 66–77.

Cavatorta, S., Cattelani, R., Lombardi, F., et al. (2000). Sexual and couple relationship dysfunctions following traumatic brain injury. In A.-L. Christensen & B. P. Uzzell (Eds.), *International handbook of neuropsychological rehabilitation* (pp. 308–309). New York: Kluwer Academic/Plenum.

Cohadon, F., Castel, J.-P., Richer, E., Mdazaux, J.-M., & Loiseau, H. (1998). *Les traumatises craniens de l'accident a la reinsertion.* Velizy-Villacoublay, France: Arnette Initiatives Sante.

Conoley, J. C., & Sheridan, S. M. (1996). Pediatric traumatic brain injury: Challenges and interventions for families. *Journal of Learning Disabilities, 29*(6), 662–669.

DePompei, R., & Zarski, J. J. (1991). Assessment of the family. In J. M. Williams & T. Kay (Eds.), *Head injury: A family matter* (pp. 101–120). Baltimore: Paul H. Brookes.

Dittmar, C. (1997). Outpatient rehabilitation programs for clients with persisting mild to moderate symptoms following traumatic brain injury. *Applied Neuropsychology, 4*(1), 50–54.

Douglas, J. M., & Spellacy, F. J. (1996). Indicators of long-term family functioning following severe traumatic brain injury in adults. *Brain Injury, 10*(11), 819–839.

Epstein, N. B., Baldwin, L. M., & Bishop, D. S. (1983). The McMaster Family Assessment Device. *Journal of Marital and Family Therapy, 9*(2), 171–180.

Finset, A., Dyrnes, S., Krogstad, J. M., & Berstad, J. (1995). Self-reported social networks and interpersonal support 2 years after severe traumatic brain injury. *Brain Injury, 9*(2), 141–150.

Florian, V., Katz, S., & Lahav, V. (1989). Impact of traumatic brain damage on family dynamics and functioning: A review. *Brain Injury 3*(3), 219–233.

Gabbard, G. O., Lazar, S. G., Hornberger, J., & Spiegel, D. (1997). The economic impact of psychotherapy: A review. *American Journal of Psychiatry, 154*(2), 147–155.

Gillen, R., Tennen, H., Affleck, G., & Steinpreis, R. (1998). Distress, depressive symptoms, and depressive disorder among caregivers of patients with brain injury. *Journal of Head Trauma Rehabilitation, 13*(3), 31–43.

Groom, K. N., Shaw, T. G., O'Connor, M. E., Howard, N. I., & Pickens, A. (1998). Neurobehavioral Symptoms and Family Functioning in Traumatically Brain-Injured Adults. *Archives of Clinical Neuropsychology, 13*(8), 695–711.

Holland, D., & Shigaki, C. L. (1998). Educating families and caretakers of traumatically brain injured patients in the new health care environment: A three phase model and bibliography. *Brain Injury, 12*(12), 993–1009.

Hosack, K. R., & Rocchio, C. A. (1995). Serving families of persons with severe brain injury in an era of managed care. *Journal of Head Trauma Rehabilitation, 10*(2), 57–65.

Howard, K. I., Lueger, R. J., Martinovich, Z., & Lutz, W. (1999). The cost-effectiveness of psychotherapy: Dose-response and phase models. In N. E. Miller & K. M. Magruder (Eds.), *Cost-effectiveness of psychotherapy: A guide for practitioners, researchers, and policymakers* (pp. 143–152) . New York: Oxford University.

Jacobs, H. E. (1988). The Los Angeles Head Injury Survey: Procedures and initial findings. *Archives of Physical Medicine and Rehabilitation, 69,* 425–431.

Kaplan, R. M., & Anderson, J. P. (1988). A general health policy model: Update and applications. *Health Services Research, 23*(2), 203–235.

Kazak, A. E., Stuber, M. L., Barakat, L. P., Meeske, K., Guthrie, D., & Meadows, A. T. (1998). Predicting posttraumatic stress symptoms in mothers and fathers of survivors of childhood cancers. *Journal of the American Academy of Child & Adolescent Psychiatry, 37*(8), 823–831.

Kibby, M. Y., & Long, C. J. (1997). Effective treatment of minor head injury and understanding its neurological consequences. *Applied Neuropsychology, 4*(1), 34–42.

Klonoff, P., Lamb, D. G., Henderson, S. W., & Shepherd, J. (1998). Outcome assessment after milieu-oriented rehabilitation: New considerations. *Archives of Physical Medicine and Rehabilitation, 79,* 684–690.

Kraus, J. F. (1995). Epidemiological features of brain injury in children: Occurrence, children at risk, causes and manner of injury, severity and outcomes. In S. H. Broman & M. E. Michel ME (Eds.), *Traumatic head injury in children* (pp. 22–39). New York: Oxford University Press.

Kreutzer, J. S., Gervasio, A. H., & Camplair, P. S. (1994a). Primary caregivers' psychological status and family functioning after traumatic brain injury. *Brain Injury, 8*(3), 197–210.

Kreutzer, J. S., Gervasio, A. H., & Camplair, P. S. (1994b) Patient correlates of caregivers' distress and family functioning after traumatic brain injury. *Brain Injury, 8*(3), 211–230.

Kreutzer, J. S., Marwitz, J. H., & Kepler, K. (1992). Traumatic brain injury: Family response and outcome. *Archives of Physical Medicine and Rehabilitation, 73*, 771–778.

Kreutzer, J. S., Sander, A. M., & Fernandez, C. C. (1997). Misperceptions, mishaps, and pitfalls in working with families after traumatic brain injury. *Journal of Head Trauma Rehabilitation, 12*(6), 63–73.

Leach, L. R., Frank, R. G., Bouman, D. E., & Farmer, J. (1994). Family functioning, social support and depression after traumatic brain injury. *Brain Injury, 8*(7), 599–606.

Lezak, M. (1996). Family perceptions and family reactions: Reconsidering "denial." In H. S. Levin, A. L. Benton, J. P. Muizelaar, & H. M. Eisenberg (Eds.), *Catastrophic brain injury* (pp. 175–182). New York: Oxford University Press.

Lezak, M. (1988a). Brain damage is a family affair. *Journal of Clinical & Experimental Neuropsychology, 10*(1), 111–123.

Lezak, M. (1988b). The walking wounded of head injury: When subtle deficits can be disabling. *Trends in Rehabilitation, 3*(3), 4–9.

Lezak, M. (1986). Psychological implications of traumatic brain damage for the patient's family. *Rehabilitation Psychology, 31*(4), 241–250.

Lezak, M. (1978). Living with the characterologically altered brain injured patient. *Journal of Clinical Psychiatry, 39*, 592–598.

Light, R., Asarnow, R., Satz, P., Zaucha, K., McCleary, C., & Lewis, R. (1998). Mild closed-head injury in children and adolescents: Behavior problems and academic outcomes. *Journal of Consulting and Clinical Psychology, 66*(6), 1023–1029.

Linn, R. T., Allen, K., & Willer, B. S. (1994). Affective symptoms in the chronic stage of traumatic brain injury: A study of married couples. *Brain Injury, 8*(2), 135–147.

Lishman, W. A. (1973). The psychiatric sequelae of head injury: A review. *Psychololgical Medicine, 3*, 304–318.

Livingston, M. G. (1985). Families who care. *British Medical Journal, 291*, 919–920.

Maitz, E. A., & Sachs, P. R. (1995). Treating families of individuals with traumatic brain injury from a family systems perspective. *Journal of Head Trauma Rehabilitation, 10*(2), 1–11.

Malec, J. F. (1996). Ethical conflict resolution based on an ethics of relationships for brain injury rehabilitation. *Brain Injury, 10*(11), 781–795.

Man, D. (1999). Community-based empowerment programme for families with a brain injured survivor: an outcome study. *Brain Injury, 13*(6), 433–445.

Max, J. E., Roberts, M. A., Koele, S. L., Lindgren, S. D., Robin, D. A., Arndt, S., Smith, W. L., & Sato, Y. (1999). Cognitive outcome in children and adolescents following severe traumatic brain injury: Influences of psychosocial, psychiatric, and injury-related variables. *Journal of the International Neuropsychology Society, 5*, 58–68.

Mazzucchi, A., Cattelani, R., Gugliotta, M., Brianti, R., & Janelli, G. (2000). Family experiences in the long-term care of severely head-injured patients. In A.-L. Christensen & B. P. Uzzell (Eds.), *International handbook of neuropsychological rehabilitation* (pp. 303–304). New York: Kluwer Academic/Plenum.

McCaffrey, R. J., Pollock, J., & Burns, P. (1987). An archival analysis of the needs of head injured survivors in New York State: Preliminary findings. *Archival Analysis, 4*, 174–177.

McCubbin, H. I., Larsen, A., & Olson, D. H. (1985). Family Crisis Oriented Personal Evaluation Scales. In D. H. Olson, H. I. McCubbin, & H. Barnes, et al. (Eds.), *Family inventories: Inventories used in a national survey of families across the life cycle* (pp. 143–159). St. Paul, MN: University of Minnesota, Family Social Science.

McMordie, W. R., Rogers, K. F., & Barker, S. L. (1991). Consumer satisfaction with services provided to head-injured patients and their families. *Brain Injury, 5*(1), 43–51.

McNeilly, C., & K. I. Howard (1991). The effects of psychotherapy: A reevaluation based on dosage. *Psychotherapy Research, 1,* 74–78.

Miller, L. (1993). Family therapy of brain injury: Syndromes, strategies, and solutions. *The American Journal of Family Therapy, 21*(2), 111–121.

Miller, L. (1992). When the best help is self-help, or, everything you always wanted to know about brain injury support groups. *Journal of Cognitive Rehabilitation, 10*(6), 14–17.

Moos, R. H., & Moos, B. S. (1994). *Family Environment Scale manual* (3rd ed.). Palo Alto, CA: Consulting Psychologists Press.

Mulhern, R. K., Carpentieri, S., Shema, S., Stone, P., & Fairclough, D. (1993). Factors associated with social and behavioral problems among children recently diagnosed with brain tumor. *Journal of Pediatric Psychology, 18*(3), 339–350.

Oddy, M., Humphrey, M., & Uttley, D. (1978). Stresses upon the relatives of head-injured patients. *British Journal of Psychiatry, 133,* 507–513.

Orsillo, S. M., McCaffrey, R. J., & Fisher, J. M. (1993). Siblings of head-injured individuals: A population at risk. *Journal of Head Trauma Rehabilitation, 8,* 102–115.

Panting, A., & Merry, P. H. (1972). The long-term rehabilitation of severe head injuries with particular reference to the need for social and medical support for the patient's family. *Rehabilitation, 38,* 33–37.

Perlesz, A., & O'Loughlan, M. (1998). Changes in stress and burden in families seeking therapy following traumatic brain injury: A follow-up study. *International Journal of Rehabilitation Research, 21*(4), 339–354.

Pessar, L. F., Coad, M. L., Linn, R. T., & Willer, B. S. (1993). The effects of parental traumatic brain injury on the behavior of parents and children. *Brain Injury, 7*(3), 231–240.

Peters, L. C., Stambrook, M., Moore, A. D., & Esses, L. (1990). Psychosocial sequelae of closed head injury: Effects on the marital relationship. *Brain Injury, 4*(1), 39–47.

Pino, C. J., Simons, N., & Slawinowski, M. J. (1995). *The Children's Version of the Family Environment Scale* (manual). East Aurora, NY: Slosson Educational Publications.

Prigatano, G. P. (1999). *Principles of neuropsychological rehabilitation.* New York: Oxford University Press.

Prigatano, G. P., Fordyce, D. J., Zeiner, H. K., Roueche, J. R., Pepping, M., & Wood, B. C. (1986). *Neuropsychological rehabilitation after brain injury.* Baltimore: The John Hopkins University Press.

Prigatano, G. P., Klonoff, P. S., O'Brien, K. P., Altman, I. M., Amin, K., Chiapello, D., et al. (1994). Productivity after neuropsychologically oriented milieu rehabilitation. *Journal of Head Trauma Rehabilitation 9,* 91–102.

Quine, S., Lyle, D., & Pierce, J. (1993). Stressors experienced by relatives of patients in an innovative rehabilitation program. *Health and Social Work, 18*(2), 114–122.

Reeber, B. J. (1992). Evaluating the effects of a family education intervention. *Rehabilitation Nursing, 17*(6), 332–336.

Riggio, R. E. (1989). *Social Skills Inventory (manual).* Palo Alto, CA: Consulting Psychologists Press.

Rivara, J. B., Jaffe, K. M., Polissar, L. N., Fay, G. C., Liao, S., & Martin, K. M. (1996). Predictors of family functioning and change three years after traumatic brain injury in children. *Archives of Physical Medicine and Rehabilitation, 77,* 754–764.

Rogers, P. M., & Kreutzer, J. S. (1984). Family crises following head injury: A network intervention strategy. *Journal of Neurosurgical Nursing, 16,* 343–346.

Rollin, W. (1987). *The psychology of communication disorders in individuals and their families.* Englewood Cliffs: NJ, Prentice-Hall.

Romano, M. D. (1974). Family response to traumatic brain injury. *Scandinavian Journal of Rehabilitation Medicine, 6,* 1–4.

Rosenbaum, M., & Najenson, T. (1976). Changes in life patterns and symptoms of low mood as reported by wives of severely brain injured soldiers. *Journal of Consulting and Clinical Psychology, 44*(6), 881–888.

Rosenthal, M., & Young, T. (1988). Effective family intervention after traumatic brain injury: Theory and practice. *Journal of Head Trauma Rehabilitation, 3*(4), 42–50.

Sachs, P. R. (1991). *Treating families of brain injury survivors*. New York: Springer Publishing.

Sahler, O. J., Roghmann, K. J., Carpenter, P. J., Mulhern, R. K., Dolgin, M. J., Sargent, J. R., Barbarin, O. A., Copeland, D. R., & Zeltzer, L. K. (1994). Sibling adaptation to childhood cancer collaborative study: Prevalence of sibling distress and definition of adaptation levels. *Journal of Developmental & Behavioral Pediatriatrics, 15*(5), 353–366.

Sander, A. M., High, W. M., Hannay, H. J., & Sherer, M. (1997). Predictors of psychological health in caregivers of patients with closed head injury. *Brain Injury, 11*(4), 235–249.

Satz, P., Zaucha, K., McCleary, C., Light, R., Asarnow, R., & Becker, D. (1997). Mild head injury in children and adolescents: A review of studies (1970–1995). *Psychological Bulletin, 122*(2), 107–131.

Sawyer, M. G., Streiner, D. L., Antoniou, G., Toogood, I., & Rice, M. (1998). Influence of parental and family adjustment on the later psychological adjustment of children treated for cancer. *Journal of the American Academy of Child & Adolescent Psychiatry, 37*(8), 815–822.

Serio, C. D., Kreutzer, J. S., & Gervasio, A. H. (1995). Predicting family needs after brain injury: Implications for intervention. *Journal of Head Trauma Rehabilitation, 10*(2), 32–45.

Shaw, L. R. & McMahon, B. T. (1990). Family-staff conflict in the rehabilitation setting: causes, consequences, and implications. *Brain Injury, 4*(1), 87–93.

Sheras, P. L., Abidin, R. R., & Konold, T. R. (1998). *Stress Index for Parents of Adolescents (manual)*. Odessa, FL: Psychological Assessment Resources.

Singer, G. H. S., Glang, A., Nixon, C., Cooley, E., Kerns, K. A, Williams, D., & Powers, L. E. (1994). A comparison of two psychosocial interventions for parents of children with acquired brain injury: An exploratory study. *Journal of Head Trauma Rehabilitation, 9*(4), 8–49.

Smith, L. M., & Godfrey, H. P. D. (1995). *Family support programs and rehabilitation: A cognitive-behavioral approach to traumatic brain injury*. New York: Plenum Press.

Snyder, D. K. (1997). *Marital Satisfaction Inventory-Revised (manual)*. Odessa, FL: Western Psychological Services.

Sohlberg, M. M., Glang, A., & Todis, B. (1998). Improvement during baseline: Three case studies encouraging collaborative research when evaluating caregiver training. *Brain Injury, 12*, 333–346.

Taylor, H. G., Yeates, K. O., Wade, S. L., Drotar, D., Klein, S. K., & Stancin, T. (1999). Influences on first-year recovery from traumatic brain injury in children. *Neuropsychology, 13*(1), 76–89.

Taylor, R. M., & Morrison, L. P. (1996). *Taylor-Johnson Temperament Analysis (manual)*. Los Angeles: Psychological Publications.

Tennant, A., MacDermott, N., & Neary, D. (1995). The long-term outcome of head injury: Implications for service planning. *Brain Injury, 9*(6), 595–605.

Thomas, J. L., & Cummings, J. L. (Eds.) (2000). *The collected papers of Nicholas A. Cummings, Volume 1: The value of psychological treatment*. Phoenix, AZ: Zeig, Tucker.

Thomsen, I. V. (1984). Late outcome of very severe blunt head trauma: A 10–15 year second follow-up. *Journal of Neurology, Neurosurgery, and Psychiatry, 47*, 260–268.

Uomoto, J. M., & Brockway, J. A. (1992). Anger management training for brain injured patients and their family members. *Archives of Physical Medicine and Rehabilitation, 73*, 674–679.

Uysal, S., Hibbard, M. R., Robillard, D., Pappadopulos, E., & Jaffe, M. (1998). The effect of parental traumatic brain injury on parenting and child behavior. *Journal of Head Trauma Rehabilitation, 13*(6), 57–71.

Wade, S. L., Taylor, H. G., Drotar, D., Stancin, T., & Yeates, K. O. (1998). Family burden and adaptation during the initial year after traumatic brain injury in children. *Pediatrics, 102*(1), 110–116.

Wilson, B. A. (1999). *Case studies in neuropsychological rehabilitation*. New York: Oxford University Press.

Wolff, N., Helminiak, T. W., & Tebes, J. K. (1997). Getting the cost right in cost-effectiveness analyses. *American Journal of Psychiatry, 154*(6), 736–743.

Wood, R. L., & Yurdakul, L. K. (1997). Change in relationship status following traumatic brain injury. *Brain Injury, 11*(7), 491–501.

Wrightson, P., McGinn, V., & Gronwall, D. (1995). Mild head injury in preschool children: Evidence that it can be associated with persisting cognitive defect. *Journal of Neurology, Neurosurgery, and Psychiatry, 59,* 375–380.

Yeates, K. O., Taylor, H. G., Drotar, D., Wade, S. L., Klein, S., Stancin, T., & Schatschneider, C. (1997). Preinjury family environment as a determinant of recovery from traumatic brain injuries in school-age children. *Journal of the International Neuropsychology Society, 3,* 617–630.

Zasler, N. D., & Horn, L. J. (1990). Rehabilitative management of sexual dysfunction. *Journal of Head Trauma Rehabilitation, 5*(2), 14–24.

Zasler, N. D., & Kreutzer, J. S. (1991). Family and sexuality after traumatic brain injury. In J. M. Williams & T. Kay (Eds.), *Head injury: A family matter* (pp. 253–270). Baltimore: Paul H. Brookes.

Zarski, J. J., & DePompei, R. (1991). Family therapy as applied to head injury. In J. M. Williams & T. Kay (Eds.), *Head injury: A family matter* (pp. 283–297). Baltimore: Paul H. Brookes.

PART

II

CEREBRAL VASCULAR DISORDERS

6

CHAPTER

Neil H. Pliskin
Lisa A. Sworowski

Neuropsychological Assessment of Patients with Cerebrovascular Accidents

Introduction

The preceding chapters focused on neuropsychological services for patients with traumatic brain injury (TBI) and those with residual postconcussional disturbances. The value of working with family members of individuals who suffered TBI was highlighted in Chapter 5. We will now discuss the value of neuropsychological assessment in persons who suffer a cerebral vascular accident (CVA) or stroke. We will begin with a review of medical information, followed by the economics of stroke. We will then discuss in some detail the role of the neuropsychologist in the care of stroke patients and the scientific studies documenting the value of neuropsychological services for this patient group. The impact of neuropsychological services on the economics of stroke will be considered as well as its potential value for the patient, the family, the physician, and the hospital that provides these services. Suggestions for future cost outcome research will also be considered with specific examples.

Medical Considerations

A CVA, or stroke, is defined as rapidly developing clinical signs of focal (or global) disturbance of cerebral function, with symptoms lasting 24 hours or longer or leading to death, with no apparent cause other than vascular origin (World Health Organization, 1984). Strokes in which there is altered circulation due to an occlusion affecting a limited region of the cerebral hemispheres, brain stem, or cerebellum are considered *ischemic*. Occlusions of large cerebral vessels often are caused by either atherosclerotic plaques or cardiac embolisms, whereas occlusions of smaller vessels resulting in lacunes often are associated with hypertension and diabetes (Fieschi, Falcou, Sacchetti, & Toni, 1998). *Hemorrhagic* strokes are associated with hypertension, ruptured micro-aneurysms, arteriosclerosis, necrosis of vessels, arteriovenous malformations, ruptured highly vascularized tumors, and hematological disorders. Subarachnoid hemorrhages are often the result of ruptured congenital aneurysms and arteriovenous malformations as well as drug abuse (e.g., cocaine) or trauma that causes bleeding into the parenchyma or meninges. The most common forms of stroke include cerebral infarction (86%), primary (or spontaneous) intracerebral hemorrhage (9%), and subarachnoid hemorrhage (5%; Sudlow & Warlow, 1997). The occurrence of type stroke varies according to a number of demographic, physical, and lifestyle factors. Hemorrhagic stroke patients typically are younger, are more often African-American, have poorer outcomes (i.e., medical complications leading to greater disability), and have greater mortality rates during early phases of recovery relative to patients who suffer an ischemic event (Hankey et al., 2000).

A number of biological and lifestyle factors have been studied to determine the possible risk factors for developing ischemic stroke. Hypertension is the major risk factor for stroke in both sexes, in which both elevated systolic and elevated diastolic blood pressure are strongly associated with stroke incidence (Fieschi et al., 1998). In one large epidemiological investigation, for example (the Framingham study), 80.8% of stroke patients had hypertension, 32.7% had coronary artery disease, 14.5% had previous cardiac failure, 14.5% had atrial fibrillation, and only 13.6% had none of these (White, 1991). Additional risk factors–including obesity, cigarette smoking, diabetes, alcohol consumption, and parental history of stroke–have all been shown to increase an individual's risk for developing a stroke (Donnelly, Ernslie-Smith, Gardner, & Morris, 2000; Fieschi et al., 1998; Morrison, Fornage, Liao, & Boerwinkle, 2000).

The average annual incidence of stroke (i.e., first-ever stroke occurring in 1 year) rises exponentially with age, with a 100-fold increase in rates from about 3 per 10,000 people in the third and fourth decades of life to almost 300 in the eighth and ninth decades (Bergman, van der Meulen, Limburg, & Habbeman, 1995; Bonita, Beaglehole, & North, 1984; Sudlow & Warlow, 1997). In one large-scale epidemiological study conducted in Rochester, Minnesota, the annual incidence of stroke was 1,378 per 100,000 for those over the age of 75 (Sudlow & Warlow, 1997). Differences in stroke incidence vary significantly by gender and race. Specifically, 1 in 10 men and 1 in 15 women aged 45 may experience a stroke in their subsequent 30 years of life (Bonita et al., 1984). Although the lifetime risk of having a stroke is higher in men, the lifetime risk of dying from stroke is actually higher in women (i.e., 16% vs. 8%), perhaps due to longer life expectancy in women (World Health Organization, 1989). Studies examining differences in stroke incidence among people with different racial backgrounds have found that stroke rates are approximately twice as high in U.S. Blacks compared to U.S. Whites for individuals ages 35 to 74 years, and approximately three to four times higher in younger Blacks between 33 and 44 years of age (Cooper, 1987). Additionally, the relative risk for U.S. Black women is significantly higher than for U.S. White women, except in women between the ages of 65 and 74 (Gaines & Burke, 1995). Like the distribution of overall stroke incidence, the occurrence of various subtypes of stroke differs between people with different racial backgrounds. Among U.S. Blacks, the incidence of intracerebral hemorrhage and subarachnoid hemorrhage is higher than for U.S. Whites, and there is a greater incidence of extracranial obstructive vascular disease that occurs in U.S. Whites (Cooper, 1987).

Throughout the world, stroke is the second most common cause of death (behind ischemic heart disease), causing 4.4 million (9%) of a total of 50.5 million deaths each year (Murray & Lopez, 1997); in Western countries, stroke accounts for about 12% of all deaths (666 per million per year; Hankey, 1999). In general, patients with cardioembolic strokes have a higher mortality rate (i.e., 2.5 times more likely) at 5 years after stroke when compared to individuals with other stroke subtypes (Petty et al., 2000). The risk of death from stroke also varies with regard to age, gender, and among individuals with different racial backgrounds. Approximately 88% of deaths attributed to stroke occur in people older than 65 years (Bonita et al., 1984; Holroyd-Leduc, Kapral, Austin, & Tu, 2000). However, the relative risk of dying is greater for younger individuals and subsequently decreases with age. Patients younger than 45 years have about a 200-fold higher risk of dying than individuals of the same age and sex in the general population, whereas the relative risk of dying among patients older than 85 years is 3.2 times greater than individuals of the same age and sex in the general population (Hankey et al., 2000). In younger patients, there is no sex difference in short-term and long-term mortality rates, but in elderly patient groups, men have higher mortality rates than older women (Holroyd-Leduc et al., 2000). With regard to race, stroke is the cause of death in about 11% of Caucasian-Americans and 13% of African-Americans (Gaines & Burke, 1995). At 3 years following either cerebral infarctions or cerebral hemorrhages, US Caucasians have been shown to have slightly better survival rates than African-Americans. A study of 4,559 consecutive autopsies showed that aneurysms (ruptured or unruptured) were found more frequently among Black males (1.4%) than among White males (0.6%), and that fatal hypertensive hemorrhage and cerebral arteriolar necrosis were higher in Black males than in White males (Gaines & Burke, 1995).

During the past immediate decade, there has been a considerable deceleration in the rate of decline in stroke mortality such that in some Western countries stroke mortality rates are stabilizing, despite the increasing number of incident stroke cases as the population becomes older (Hankey, 1999; Sudlow & Warlow, 1997). Many stroke patients now survive who wouldn't have 20 years ago, thanks to improved management of hypertension as well as new and emerging treatments for acute ischemic stroke, including intravenous thrombolytic drugs (e.g., r-TPA), carotid endarterectomy, oral anticoagulants, and antiplatelet aggregating drugs (e.g., anti-ICAM-1). Thus, the number of stroke survivors, as well as people disabled by stroke, is increasing. Studies that examine the economic, physical, cognitive, and emotional burden of stroke have been crucial for determining the needs of patients and caregivers, as well as for determining the most appropriate, cost-effective medical care to help patients adjust to disability and to prevent stroke recurrence.

☐ The Economics of Stroke

Stroke is the single most important cause of disability in Western populations (Murray & Lopez, 1997). There have been numerous studies examining the cost of stroke for medical care during the acute phase of stroke recovery, long-term care involving rehabilitation services or nursing care, and number of days lost from work. The numbers are substantial. For the estimated 390,000 first-time strokes that occurred in 1990, the accumulated lifetime cost due to these strokes is $406 billion, or $103,576 per patient (Taylor et al., 1996). Furthermore, the economic burden of stroke in the United States was estimated to be $30 billion in 1993, of which $17 billion accounted for *direct* medical costs (i.e., cost of resource use such as medical care, nursing home care, rehabilitation, etc.) and $13 billion accounted for *indirect* costs (i.e., lost earnings due to morbidity and premature death after stroke; Matchar & Duncan, 1994). A third set of costs relate to the impact on a patient's cognitive functioning, depression and anxiety on daily functioning, quality of life, and social relationships. Progress continues to be made in measuring these dimensions, although their full impact on the cost of stroke is undetermined. Capturing the value of reducing these costs is essential in demonstrating the utility and cost–benefits of neuropsychological services.

Many studies conducted in Sweden, Canada, Europe, and the United States have focused on acute hospitalizations, which are a substantial portion of the direct costs, for determining the proportion of medical care costs allocated for stroke. Holloway, Witter, Lawton, Lipscomb, and Samsa (1996) showed that, across five academic medical centers in the United States, the cost of hospitalizations for stroke differed considerably according to CVA subtype (see Table 6.1).

The cost of care for patients with subarachnoid hemorrhage was most expensive, because the length of hospitalization was longer than for other patients and they required more costly services, such as surgical and intensive care services. In another population-based prospective study estimating direct costs for stroke patients including both inpatient and outpatient care (Leibson et al., 1996), costs of care in the first month following the stroke comprised more than half of the total acute care costs in the year after stroke ($3,304,715 in the first 30 days, and $6,284,471 in the first 12 months). The total charges for inpatient and outpatient acute care activity in the first 30 days after stroke were $3,304,715, in which patients with subarachnoid hemorrhage was on average the most costly stroke, followed by intracerebral hemorrhage, severe cerebral infarctions, and mild cerebral infarctions. Not surprisingly, patients discharged to home were approximately half as expensive as those discharged to another facility (nursing homes, rehabilitation facility); for example, subarachnoid hemorrhage patients who were discharged to their home had an average hospitalization cost of $29,576, whereas the average cost for those discharged to another facility was $60,426 (Holloway et al., 1996).

Inpatient rehabilitation accounts for approximately 5% of overall direct stroke costs ($850 million annually), and 10% to 15% of stroke survivors receive these services (Dobkin, 1995). About 70% of patients receive inpatient or outpatient rehabilitative services within 90 days of stroke. Granger and Hamilton (1992) showed that, of 25,000 stroke patients in a rehabilitation facility, mean length of stay was 29 days, compared to a mean length of stay for nursing home admissions due to stroke of 432 days. Given

TABLE 6.1. Acute Care Cost of Strokes (in Dollars)

	Hospitalizations	Costs per Day
Subarachnoid hemorrhage	40,000	2,215
Intracerebral hemorrhage	20,000	1,396
Ischemic stroke	10,000	1,036
Transient ischemic attack	5,000	1,117

From Holloway et al. (1996). Reprinted with permission.

that Dobkin (1995) estimated that inpatient rehabilitation services accounted for 5% of direct costs due to stroke ($850 million) and about 40,000 patients receive these services each year, the annual cost of inpatient rehabilitation can be estimated as $21,250 per patient receiving inpatient rehabilitative treatment.

Of all stroke survivors combined, 15% to 30% are placed in nursing homes after acute hospitalization, 5% to 20% are admitted to rehabilitation units, and 35% to 60% are discharged home (Dobkin, 1995). Epidemiological data from an incidence-based study (i.e., in which costs calculated are lifetime costs, and the accumulated costs from stroke to death are referred to the year of stroke) indicate that nursing home costs for patients with stroke as a primary diagnosis were $2.9 billion in 1990, and accounted for approximately 17% of direct costs attributable to stroke (Taylor et al., 1996). The actual number of nursing home admissions due to stroke in 1990 was estimated as 101,900, and the average cost per person was $29,296 (Taylor et al., 1996).

In summary, there are significant costs associated with the acute and postacute care of stroke patients. Patients suffering from more severe strokes require more expensive acute care and have a higher likelihood of having severe disability, resulting in greater dependency and a need for supervised, long-term care. Exactly how clinical neuropsychological services impact overall costs associated with stroke and contribute to the functional recovery/outcome of stroke patients is the focus of the remainder of this chapter.

The Role of the Neuropsychologist in the Care of Stroke Patients

The clinical neuropsychologist works with stroke patients in a variety of ways and clinical settings. A neuropsychologist might be asked to evaluate a poststroke patient in the acute care hospital setting to determine what aftercare and level of rehabilitation services are needed. According to the American Heart Association guidelines (1997), the rehabilitation process for stroke patients should include six major areas of focus:

1. management of comorbid illness and medical complications;
2. training for maximum independence;
3. facilitation of maximum psychosocial coping by the patient and family;
4. prevention of secondary disability by promoting resumption of home, family, recreational, and vocational activities;
5. enhancement of quality of life in view of residual disability; and
6. prevention of recurrent stroke and other vascular conditions.

They also suggest that, because the clinical manifestations of stroke are multifaceted and complex, and that a team of rehabilitation professionals coordinating treatment efforts is an optimal approach to helping patients maximize functional independence goals.

Neuropsychologists play a critical role in realizing many of these goals by serving as part of the rehabilitation treatment team and by assessing and diagnosing cognitive dysfunction and emotional disturbance that may impede rehabilitation progress and attainment of functional goals. Accurate assessment and reassessment of physical, emotional, and cognitive deficits during rehabilitation and after return to the community are strongly recommended to evaluate each patient's progress, need for special accommodations in their environment, and potential need for additional, postdischarge treatment (Agency for Health Care Policy and Research Post-stroke Rehabilitation Guidelines, 1995). Thus, neuropsychologists commonly provide assessment and treatment services to poststroke patients in private or group outpatient practices as well.

☐ Cognitive Disorders and Neurobehavioral Disorder Associated with Stroke

What are the cost and associated values of having the input and expertise of a neuropsychologist as part of the standard of care for stroke victims? In order to understand this, one needs to first consider the neuropsychological sequelae and neurobehavioral syndromes that often occur following stroke and how they can substantially affect a patient's functional outcome.

Stroke patients can experience a variety of neuropsychological impairments in one or more cognitive domains–including attentional capacity, information processing speed, memory, language, visuospatial processing, and executive functioning–that can affect a patient's functional outcome considerably. *Attention* deficits associated with stroke often involve decreased alertness, especially during the acute phase of stroke recovery. As a result of brain stem lesions or compression from edema, the stroke patient may be at the lowest level of tonic arousal and, therefore, be comatose and unable to respond to the environment. Individuals with less severe levels of impairment in attention may appear disoriented, confused, and unable to respond effectively to environmental cues. Impairments in the ability to selectively attend to environment stimuli, shift attentional sets, and sustain attentional focus also may occur. The ability to process information rapidly often is affected by stroke and can reduce an individual's cognitive efficiency, impacting one's ability to perform adequately in vocational and leisure activities. A study examining cognitive deficits among 229 stroke patients, ages 18 to 70, found that approximately 70% of patients showed difficulty in performing adequately under conditions of time pressure, in which they were required to process information quickly (Hochstenbach, Mulder, van Limbeek, Donders, & Schoonderwaldt, 1998). Specifically, the majority of stroke survivors' speed of performance was impaired (i.e., two or more standard deviations below the control subjects' mean) on a number of measures assessing simple and complex attention including tests such as Trails A and B, WAIS-R Digit Symbol, WAIS-R Block Design, and a letter cancellation task. Compared to other deficits observed (i.e., left-sided neglect, impaired visuospatial functioning, impaired language functioning, and impaired memory functioning) in the stroke patient group, general cognitive and motor slowing, decreased information processing speed, and attention deficits were the most prominent.

Impairments in *memory* functioning characterized by an amnestic syndrome can occur in stroke survivors, especially among individuals who have experienced an occlusion of the posterior cerebral artery, which affects blood supply to the mesial temporal lobes, a thalamic infarct or lesion that affects other diencephalic structures, or a bleed involving the anterior communicating artery that affects basal forebrain structures (Delaney & Ravdin, 1997; Tranel, 1993). Individuals with multiple subcortical ischemic infarcts more frequently demonstrate memory impairment involving retrieval processes in which spontaneous recall of information initially encoded is deficient but, when a recognition paradigm is used, memory performance is within normal limits or only minimally impaired. The ability to recall modality-specific material, such as visual or verbal information, may be affected and is somewhat dependent on location of the vascular lesion and the structures involved. For example, left temporal-limbic damage, such that as associated with a left middle cerebral artery infarction, likely will produce a partial amnestic syndrome that primarily affects auditory-verbal information, whereas memory for nonverbal material is likely to be preserved (Tranel, 1993). Stroke patients with a unilateral cortical stroke involving the middle cerebral artery may not complain of memory difficulties; however, on formal testing, impairments in short-term recall and learning efficiency may be evident (Delaney & Ravdin, 1997).

On formal evaluation of memory functioning, Hochstenbach and associates (1998) found that 30% of their sample of 229 stroke patients (i.e., 199 ischemic and 30 hemorrhagic) demonstrated deficiencies (i.e., more than two standard deviations below the mean of the control group) in memory. More specifically, performances on delayed recall of organized (i.e., stories) and randomly organized (i.e., AVLT list words) words were more impaired than performances on immediate recall tasks, and recognition memory was normal or only minimally affected. Differences in type of deficits observed in this sample did not significantly vary according to several factors, including lesion location (i.e., cortical vs. subcortical), number of strokes, level of consciousness upon admission to the hospital, the presence of risk factors, paresis of the hand, or time between stroke onset and neuropsychological assessment. Accurate assessment and identification of the specific types of memory problems experienced by stroke patients allow for remediation techniques to be targeted to each patient's specific deficits, thus decreasing the impact of acquired memory dysfunction on daily functioning.

Language disturbance is common in stroke patients, and at least 20% to 30% of all CVAs result in aphasia (Leske, 1981). Aphasic patients have difficulty either comprehending language or formulating language, or both. Difficulties with language fluency, comprehension, repetition, and naming often occur. Patients with a global aphasia (i.e., language disruption affecting both expressive and receptive functions) evidence the most severe language impairments and have poorer functional outcomes than patients with language dysfunction affecting primarily expressive speech (e.g., Broca's aphasia) or auditory-verbal comprehension (e.g., Wernicke's aphasia). Other aphasia variants include transcortical sensory aphasia (i.e., resembles Wernicke's aphasia but repetition is intact), transcortical motor aphasia (i.e., resembles Broca's aphasia but repetition is intact), subcortical aphasia (i.e., an atypical aphasia in which auditory comprehension may be impaired and dysarthria may be present), and aprosodia (i.e., disturbances of prosody, associated with right-hemisphere lesions in structures homologous to the language-related structures of the left hemisphere; Tranel, 1993). Given that aphasia frequently occurs among patients with CVA, a clear assessment of the type of language dysfunction, as well as relative strengths and weaknesses through neuropsychological or speech evaluation, is necessary for the development of an effective rehabilitation plan.

A prospective study of 881 acute stroke patients (i.e., the Copenhagen Study) conducted by Pedersen, Jorgensen, Nakayama, Raaschou, & Olsen, 1995 showed that 38% of individuals in their sample had some type of aphasia upon hospitalization for stroke. Twelve percent of the aphasic patients had mild aphasia, 6% were moderately affected, 20% had severe aphasia, and an additional 6% had dysarthria. The severity of aphasia was associated with higher mortality rates in the early phases of recovery. Specifically, 47% of patients (81 individuals) with severe aphasia died during their hospitalization.

Overall, 31% of patients who showed any evidence of aphasia died before being discharged from the hospital. Fifty percent of the stroke patients with initial aphasia also had aphasia at 6-month follow-up. Complete recovery occurred in only 8% of the patients with severe aphasia, 32% of the patients with moderate aphasia, and 54% of the patients with mild aphasia. Eighty percent of patents displaying any evidence of aphasia had reached stationary language function within 2 weeks after stroke onset, and a total of 95% of patients within 6 weeks following the event. Because no significant change in aphasia score was found between discharge and the 6-month follow-up, it can be assumed that only a few patients will experience clinically significant change in language function later than 1.5 months following stroke. In this study, aphasia from a right-sided lesion did not have a better prognosis than aphasia from a left-sided lesion.

Stroke patients may display difficulties in *visual-spatial functioning* due to disruption in sensory systems, perceptual systems, or both. Sensation involves the reception of information by the different senses (e.g., sight, taste), whereas perception involves the active processing of information received through the senses (Pliskin, Cunningham, Wall, & Cassisi, 1996). An example of a specific sensory deficit is cortical blindness, which occurs as a result of bilateral occipital lobe infarcts. Disorders of perception often involve the right hemisphere, in which more complex visual perceptual operations are believed to occur in the right parietal lobe (Hier, Mondlock, & Caplan, 1983; Vallar & Perrani, 1986). There are a number of neuropsychological manifestations of impaired perception that involve only one sensory system. Focusing on the visual modality, three common perceptual disorders among stroke patients are visual agnosia, Balint syndrome, and visual neglect (Tranel, 1993). *Visual agnosia* is a disturbance of recognition in which patients lose the ability to recognize visual stimuli. Lesions resulting in visual agnosia typically affect the occipital or temporal cortices, or both. One of the more common visual agnosias is prosopagnosia, or the inability to recognize familiar faces. *Balint syndrome* also may occur and manifests as a constellation of three symptoms—specifically, simultanagnosia (i.e., the inability to attend to only a limited portion of the visual field at any point in time), ocular apraxia (i.e., the inability to direct gaze toward a stimulus located in peripheral vision), and optic ataxia (i.e., the inability to point accurately at a target, under visual guidance). *Visual neglect* also may ensue; patients with this perceptual disturbance fail to attend to visual stimuli from the hemispace contralateral to their lesion.

Perceptual disorders also can involve multiple sensory systems, including auditory, visual, and somatosensory functions. For example, *left hemi-imperception* (or neglect) includes deficits of both the somatosensory and visual systems. Patients with this impairment will have difficulty perceiving physical and visual stimuli on their left side and may not even recognize that the left side is part of their own body. Hemispatial neglect frequently occurs following right-hemisphere strokes, with the perceptual disturbance and inattention expressed more predominantly in contralateral space, although the presentation of the neglect syndrome is quite variable (Delaney & Ravdin, 1997). In a study determining the cognitive deficits among 229 stroke survivors, nearly 50% of the sample displayed left-sided neglect (Hochstenbach et al., 1998).

Another deficit commonly observed among stroke patients is classical *apraxia,* which results from impairments in sensory perception and motor integration (Delaney & Ravdin, 1997). Apraxia is the inability to carry out learned, purposeful motor activities in the absence of primary motor or sensory impairments or deficits in motivation, memory, or comprehension, and it appears to be one of the more frequent impairments after a left-hemisphere stroke (Donkervoort, Dekker, van den Ende, Stehmann-Saris, & Deelman, 2000; Lezak, 1995). Donkervoort et al. (2000) showed that among 492 patients suffering a first-ever stroke involving the left hemisphere, 28% of patients residing at rehabilitation centers had apraxia and 37% of stroke patients in nursing homes had a diagnosis of apraxia. Of the individuals with recurrent stroke (n = 108), 30% of rehabilitation patients and 55% of nursing home patients had apraxia. In their sample, the prevalence of apraxia was not associated with gender, age, or type of stroke.

A number of cognitive abilities come under the term *executive function,* and there is debate in this field about whether this is the best term to use. However, for purposes of simplicity we will use this term with the full understanding that there are many potential neuropsychological disturbances that fall under this category. Vascular lesions affecting subcortical/frontal systems may result in a variety of cognitive deficits reflecting executive dysfunction, and deficits in planning, judgment, organization, problem solving, self-control, awareness of difficulties, and personality changes may be especially prominent. Executive deficits impair an individual's ability to function independently in vocation and novel self-care activities, and can negatively impact social relationships, resulting in isolation from others. For example, strokes affecting the frontal lobe-subcortical-limbic circuitry can lead to significant apathy and amotivation. Caregivers often complain that the patient is unmotivated or depressed. These impairments may go unrecognized without formal neuropsychological evaluation in which tests designed to assess executive abilities (as well as a clinical interview with the patient and family members) are conducted. Patients with executive dysfunction secondary to frontal-subcortical strokes also may display defective autonomic responses to emotionally heightened situations ("acquired sociopathy"), exhibit mental and motor perseveration (i.e., continue responding to contingencies that are no longer operative in their environment), have a loss of cognitive fluency, and demonstrate deficiencies in prospective memory (i.e., "remembering to remember"; Tranel, 1993). Intact executive functioning guides complex human behaviors, and if impairments in this cognitive domain are at least moderately severe, the likelihood of maintaining functional independence is substantially decreased.

The risk of developing *dementia*—commonly vascular dementia or Alzheimer's disease, in which significant memory disturbance and additional cognitive disturbances (e.g., aphasia, apraxia, agnosia, executive dysfunction) are present—also is increased substantially among stroke patients. Pohjasvaara and colleagues (1998) found that, among 377 patients with ischemic stroke, dementia was present in 107 individuals (31.8%). In a geriatric rehabilitation population, the rate of dementia for stroke patients was 34.7%, which is much higher than community base rates of dementia for individuals ages 65 to 74 (2%) and 75 to 84 years (18%) (Mast, MacNeill, & Lichtenberg, 1999). Stroke patients with dementia tend to be older and often are less educated (< 6 years) than stroke patients without dementia (Pohjasvaara et al., 1998). Some vascular risk factors also have been associated with higher rates of dementia among stroke survivors, including current smoking and cardiac failure (Pohjasvaara et al., 1998). Additionally, a history of prior cerebrovascular disease or prior ischemic stroke (but not transient ischemic attack) is more frequent in demented versus nondemented stroke patients. The relative risk of dementia for stroke patients compared with stroke-free control subjects has been shown to be as high as 3.1, and risk for dementia is especially high within 3 months of stroke onset (Tatemichi et al., 1994). When studied prospectively and after adjusting for demographic factors, the relative risk for dementia increases to 5.5. After 52 months of follow-up, Tatemichi et al. (1994) demonstrated that the cumulative proportion of stroke patients in their sample surviving without dementia was 66.3, and it was 90.3 for stroke-free control subjects. Importantly, stroke patients with dementia often evidence a progressive course of cognitive decline in the absence of newly acquired vascular lesions, possibly suggesting that more than one etiological factor contributes to their dementia.

An increased prevalence of *depression* has long been a problem associated with poststroke difficulties experienced by CVA patients. The reported prevalence of depression following stroke varies widely, from 25% to 60% (Robinson, Starr, Kubos, Rao, & Price, 1983). Population-based studies show that about 40% to 53% of stroke survivors who are able to communicate reliably will develop poststroke depression within the first year, and half of these patients will suffer from major depression (Andersen, 1997; Kauhanen et al., 1999). This reported rate of depression is much higher than that of elderly people in community samples, in which 1% of individuals suffer from major depression and 19% of older adults acknowledge dysphoric mood (Mast et al., 1999). Depression commonly develops in the acute phase of stroke recovery, with approximately half of patients being diagnosed in the first month following their CVA and a further 80% in the subsequent 2 to 3 months. Nearly 50% of the patients diagnosed with depression early in the stages of recovery will experience remission of their depressive symptoms within a few months of stroke onset. Kauhanen and colleagues (1999) showed that antidepressant medication was used in 36% of the depressed patients in their sample at 3 months and in 36% of the depressed patients and 8% of the nondepressed patients at 12 months. At 1 year after stroke, newly diagnosed poststroke depression does not differ significantly from the general population (Andersen, 1997).

Several factors influence both the course and severity of poststroke depression, including age, time since stroke, severity of cognitive impairment, social support, past history of depression, and lesion location (Andersen, Vestergaard, Ingermann-Nielsen, & Lauritzen, 1995; Angeleri et al., 1997; Chemerinski & Robinson, 2000; House et al., 1991; Rao, 2000; Robinson, Bolduc, & Price, 1987). Recent studies suggest that side of the vascular lesion may not significantly contribute to the likelihood of developing poststroke depression. In fact, there is no strong evidence that poststroke depression relates to the side of the lesion; however, patients with left-hemisphere strokes tend to develop depressive symptoms earlier in the course of their recovery when compared to patients with right-sided lesions. Over time, however, this difference diminishes (Angeleri et al., 1997; Astrom, Adolfsson, & Asplund, 1993; Chemerinski & Robinson, 2000). Structural and functional imaging studies have largely supported the hypothesis that vascular lesions affecting frontal and subcortical regions are more often associated with depression than lesions affecting other regions (Rao, 2000; Chemerinski & Robinson, 2000). Although the cause of poststroke depression remains unclear, one hypothesized mechanism for this relationship involves the depletion of monoaminergic amines resulting from lesions occurring in frontal regions or the basal ganglia (Chemerinski & Robinson, 2000).

The interaction between poststroke depression and cognitive dysfunction in stroke patients is somewhat complex, but in general, patients with cognitive deficits and depressive symptoms tend to have poorer prognoses and functional outcomes. Results from Kauhanen et al. (1999) indicated that depressed stroke patients' scores were significantly inferior to those of stroke patients without depression on tests assessing all cognitive domains. When examining patients with dysphasia specifically, they found a main effect of depression on nonverbal problem solving, verbal and visual memory, attention, and psychomotor speed. At the time of the 1-year assessment, 25% of the patients with dysphasia had minor depression and 35% had major depression; overall, the presence of dysphasia was associated with more severe depression. Gender was not related to the development of depression, although depressed patients were older and more dependent in their daily activities at both 3 months and 12 months after the stroke (Kauhanen et al., 1999). Some longitudinal studies have suggested that the association between cognitive impairment and poststroke depression declines over time. For example, Downhill & Robinson (1994) demonstrated that stroke patients with major depression had greater cognitive impairment relative to nondepressed stroke survivors during hospitalization and at 6-month and 12-month follow-up, but did not show greater cognitive impairment at the 2-year follow-up assessment.

In this section we described the significant changes in cognitive abilities, emotional functioning, and even personality that occur after stroke. Neuropsychologists play a critical role in the detection of these disorders through use of standardized, valid, and reliable assessment techniques sensitive to the effects of cognitive impairment, and through their experience and training as clinical psychologists. Thorough neuropsychological assessment and reassessment conducted with stroke patients also can improve rehabilitative treatment by targeting interventions to minimize specific cognitive deficits; it also can provide meaningful information regarding progress in attaining rehabilitation goals, preparing discharge plans, and anticipating functional outcomes and adjustment to poststroke living.

Clinical Utility of Neuropsychological Assessment in Stroke Populations

We have described the role of the neuropsychologist and neuropsychological services in evaluating and treating the stroke survivor, highlighted the types of cognitive disorders commonly encountered after stroke, and discussed the unique role of the neuropsychologist in evaluating and treating poststroke cognitive disorders. But what empirical evidence exists in the literature that *scientifically* supports the clinical utility of neuropsychological assessment in stroke populations?

One area to consider relates to identification of factors associated with prediction of functional outcome (i.e., likelihood of being discharged home following rehabilitation). Some studies have documented that brief but focused neuropsychological findings can predict outcomes from inpatient neurorehabiliation (Prigatano & Wong, 1999). In a study examining differences among stroke patients discharged to home or to an assisted living facility (Lofgren, Gustafson & Nyberg, 2000), the most significant predictors of returning to home status included four factors, one of which was a cognitive factor. Specifically, patients who had postural stability, were living with a caregiver, were younger, and did not exhibit perceptual disturbances were more likely to return to prestroke living arrangements than individuals who did not possess these characteristics (Lofgren & Guftafson, 2000). As noted earlier, neuropsychological assessment typically includes a thorough evaluation of perceptual functioning.

Assessment of global cognitive functioning in 541 stroke patients was shown to have a significant predictive value on functional outcome in both ability to perform activities of daily living (ADL) at discharge and the likelihood of returning to independent living after discharge (Pedersen, Jorgensen, Nakayama, Raaschou, & Olsen, 1996). In this study, using the Mini Mental State Exam (MMSE), a higher score (i.e., greater than 24) was found to be a better predictor of independent living than a discharge score on a basic functional measure (i.e., Barthel Index score), probably because responsibilities associated with independent living place higher demands on cognitive functioning than the basic ADL functions measured by the Barthel Index. It is well understood that the MMSE is a screening instrument that has limited sensitivity (Lezak, 1995; McHeith, 1992) and, indeed, the authors of this study suggested that a neurocognitive assessment, more complete than the screening properties of the MMSE, would likely predict discharge status even more accurately.

The assessment of specific cognitive deficits has been shown to have significant prognostic value for stroke recovery and functional outcomes. For example, patients with Broca's aphasia tend to experience minimal or no effect on their level of functioning in daily activities or overall mobility (Paolucci et al., 1996). Patients with perceptual disorders such as neglect, however, do demonstrate significant functional impairment. Specifically, hemi-neglect is the best predictor of poor functional outcome in daily activities and mobility (Paolucci et al., 1996). Although recovery from neglect often occurs within the first 6 months following stroke, patients with chronic neglect are less aware of their impairments, and this can limit progress in rehabilitation therapy and independent adaptive function. A neuropsychological evaluation designed to identify the presence of perceptual disorders can help direct intervention planning to avert obstacles to making treatment gains in rehabilitation. Moreover, accurate identification of neglect among stroke patients is an important first step to educating caregivers and assisting with accommodations for those individuals discharged to home.

The utility of conducting a neuropsychological exam that evaluates executive functioning is extremely important in stroke patients. Rehabilitation staff and caregivers do not always easily recognize executive deficits, yet their impact on the patient's ability to function independently is crucial. Patients exhibiting a specific type of executive dysfunction, such as response inflexibility (assessed by the Wisconsin Card Sorting Test), are more likely to have lower scores on the Functional Independence Measure (FIM) upon discharge from rehabilitation (Greve, Bianchini, Hartley, & Adams, 1999). Patients with greater cognitive flexibility determined by neuropsychological assessment are judged by health-care providers to have a greater capacity for self-care, overall better mobility, and better cognitive functioning in general. Studies also have found particular relevance of intact executive skills on progress in rehabilitation. For example, one study showed that nonverbal problem solving, error correction, and cognitive flexibility were related to functional recovery of a hemiplegic upper limb (Barreca, Finlayson, Gowland, & Basmajian, 1999). Specifically, an initial upper extremity analysis function test (UEFT) score, initial Halstead Category Test score (a common neuropsychological test of executive function), and clinical ratings of dyspraxia explained 86.5% of the variance of the discharge UEFT score after completing either an integrated behavioral treatment program with EMG biofeedback or a traditional physiotherapy exercise program. Discharge Category Test scores also correlated with discharge UEFT scores and were associated with independent ratings of intact cortex on CT scans. Barreca and colleagues (1999) suggested that inherent in the type of persistent, intensive rehabilitation presented in their study is the client's proficiency to concentrate, recognize an incorrect action, adapt the original motor message, and subsequently elicit a correct movement. The mental operations necessary for progress in this type of rehabilitation are assessed by neuropsychological tests of executive function, such as the Category Test.

Determining stroke patients' insight into their cognitive deficits also can be achieved through neuropsychological evaluation and clinical interview and has important implications for adjustment to poststroke living (Prigatano, 1991). Unawareness of cognitive deficit (anosognosia) commonly occurs among patients with neurological disability, including stroke survivors. Wagner and Cushman (1994) showed that anosognosia occurred in approximately 40% of stroke patients in a rehabilitation facility. The unawareness of deficit presents a major challenge to rehabilitation treatment, but it also has implications for safety awareness and possible impairments in social adaptation. The inability to perceive one's impairments in cognition influences one's ability to adjust to living arrangements that were maintained prestroke.

Traditional screening measures (e.g., MMSE) and functional outcome assessments (e.g., FIM) underestimate the impact of subtle cognitive deficits on independent living. Among stroke patients who were judged to evidence a "good outcome" according to physical capabilities at the time of discharge from rehabilitation, between 40% and 50% reported cognitive difficulties and required assistance with shopping, meal preparation, housework, and personal finances (Hackett & Anderson, 2000). Although the majority of the patients participated in social activities, only 56% drove themselves or traveled outside of the home on a daily basis. Despite the high level of physical independence in basic ADLs, there was a high rate of rehospitalization and persistent cognitive/social impairment and disability in this sample (39% of patients). Caregivers of patients with cognitive deficits also report that stroke survivors have poorer functional outcome. For example, stroke patients with visual-spatial deficits were rated by caregivers as having greater cognitive decline and lower Barthel Index scores (Starr, Nicolson, Anderson, & Dennis, 2000). Patients with similarly impaired verbal abilities were rated as higher-functioning individuals at discharge. Overall, the accurate assessment of neurocognitive functioning is essential for implementing effective rehabilitation treatments; monitoring physical, emotional, and cognitive changes; identifying cognitive strengths, as well as weaknesses in which the patient may require assistance; and predicting functional outcome to provide caregivers with realistic expectations for recovery and accommodations for poststroke living.

Neuropsychological assessment of patients also is useful for determining whether a patient who suffered an acute CVA demonstrates cognitive deficits associated with a degenerative dementia. Recently, Mast and colleagues (2000) designed a study to determine the clinical utility of a brief battery in differentiating patients with possible vascular dementia from cognitively intact geriatric patients of a racially mixed sample. They selected 86 cognitively intact, elderly, urban medical patients and 65 urban dementia patients who were admitted to a rehabilitation hospital due to stroke. Their battery was composed of the Dementia Rating Scale, the Fuld Object Memory Exam, Logical Memory subtests from the WMS-R, the Visual Form Discrimination Test, and the Hooper Visual Organization Test. Functional status was rated on the FIM by a multidisciplinary team of rehabilitation specialists, and these raters were blind to patients' neuropsychological test scores. Results indicated that the neuropsychological test battery demonstrated a sensitivity of 78.69% and a specificity of 87.21%. Additionally, the positive predictive power for the battery was 81.36%, and the negative predictive value was 85.23%, indicating that the utility of the NSRP battery for detecting dementia among stroke patients, distinguishing them from cognitively intact elderly medical patients, was realized. It is clear that conducting a neuropsychological assessment to evaluate not only specific deficits related to stroke but also progressive cognitive decline associated with a vascular dementia provides essential information for a patient's outcome regarding cognitive skills, functional abilities, and appropriateness for rehabilitation.

In sum, studies in the scientific literature document the efficacy of cognitive testing in predicting stroke recovery and functional outcome, recognizing executive dysfunction and unawareness in stroke patients, and diagnosing comorbid dementia syndromes. Although further studies are needed to clarify the nature of cognitive impairment associated with stroke, there is also a progressive realization that studies need to be conducted on the clinical utility and cost outcomes associated with neuropsychological assessment of CVAs.

☐ Toward Assessing Cost Outcome Research for Neuropsychological Services in Stroke Patients

Health-care economists have helped clarify the distinction between efficacy studies and cost-effectiveness studies. As scientists, we have just reviewed studies that deal with efficacy. But we must make the bridge into studies that deal with cost-effectiveness. How is this done? By combining what we know scientifically with our clinical experience to guide research on the potential values of neuropsychological services and estimating the cost of those values.

What are the costs and associated values of having the input and expertise of a neuropsychologist as part of the standard of care for stroke victims? This question can be answered from a number of perspectives. Table 6.2 lists possible indices of both objective and subjective markers of value that can be realized and studied.

From the hospital's perspective, provision of neuropsychological services provides

TABLE 6. 2. Possible Objective and Subjective Markers of Value of Neuropsychological Services in Stroke Treatment

Hospital
Objective: CARF accreditation vs. no CARF accreditation
Subjective: Patient satisfaction after being seen by a neuropsychologist
Physician
Objective: Knowledge on which to base medical decisions
Subjective: Patient satisfaction after being seen by a neuropsychologist
Patient
Objective: Fewer accidents
Subjective: Reduced confusion and frustration
Family
Objective: Documentation of needs to get the necessary medical care
Subjective: Sense of burden is reduced
Third-Party Payer
Objective: Cost minimization for necessary services
Subjective: Insured is happy with their coverage

for a continuum of care. This can lead to obtaining and maintaining appropriate accreditations. Accreditations from such organizations as the Council for Accreditation of Rehabilitation Facilities often requires neuropsychologists to attend to patients. Obtaining this accreditation can affect reimbursement and therefore can be measured as an objective marker of value. In addition to this objective marker, institutions obviously enjoy a positive reputation in their community if their services are recognized by appropriate accreditation committees and if families are pleased with the services they receive. This latter point will be discussed below, but it is important to note that hospitals again benefit from neuropsychological services in a variety of ways, and innovative methods should be developed to assess both the objective and subjective markers of value for such institutions when neuropsychologists provide services in that setting.

The attending physician also benefits from neuropsychological services. This is perhaps most easily seen when the information provided by the neuropsychologist provides for a clear statement as to the nature of higher cerebral dysfunction in a given patient. For example, the ability to detect a progressive dementia in a CVA patient may have a profound impact on medical care. Physicians have progressively recognized the value of neuropsychological testing in aiding them in their medical decision making, as recently reflected by the American Academy of Neurology Task Force on the value of neuropsychological assessment in the diagnosis and treatment of patients with neurological disturbances.

Another objective marker of value for a physician may be seen in the usefulness of neuropsychological reports in protecting them from lawsuits and expensive litigation. A neuropsychologist's report often can clarify what may be unsafe behaviors for a patient, and the physician having that documentation can make appropriate decisions.

There also may be subjective markers of value for the physician to have a neuropsychologist see his or her patient. Patient and family satisfaction with psychological services reflects well upon physicians and can enhance reputations.

Because of the potential nature of the brain disorder, the patient may have the least understanding of how neuropsychological evaluation may help. An objective marker of value to the patient can ultimately be measured in terms of how his or her quality of life has been enhanced and how various complications have been avoided. Patients indirectly benefit if a comprehensive neuropsychological evaluation places them in a safe environment and helps them make choices that avoid potentially catastrophic consequences, such as driving a car prematurely or returning to work when the cognitive skills for carrying out a demanding job are not present. Obviously, if such individuals are allowed to go back to work without careful evaluation, all involved in their care are open to litigation.

In the case of the aphasic patient, the neuropsychological examination frequently can identify areas of preserved higher cerebral functions. Patients may then be able to use those preserved functions to compensate for their obvious language impairment. In some instances, this allows individuals to function independently in their homes and may also allow them to return to some level of productivity. Clarification of a patient's poststroke condition clearly facilitates treatment and dispositional planning that then enhances the patient's safety and leads to potentially fewer accidents, as noted above.

Although the consequences of all of these interventions can be measured clearly in their economic impact, there are subjective markers of value for the patient as well. Certainly, helping patients reduce their confusion and frustration and allowing them to function to maximum capacity can provide some sense of psychological relief, which is difficult but not impossible to measure.

An objective marker of value for the family includes the use of neuropsychological test findings to clearly document what their family member needs by way of further care. This can be crucial when getting third-party payers to pay for rehabilitation services, as well as when court-appointed guardianship is needed. Information derived from the neuropsychological evaluation frequently can help family members gain a much better understanding as to their relative's cognitive and emotional changes and how they need to plan for the future. This, again, is a subjective marker of value for them.

Finally, third-party payers clearly have different interests than the other parties discussed above, but they too can benefit from a neuropsychological evaluation. One way to document objectively the value of a neuropsychological examination for this group is to conduct studies that demonstrate what are the most efficient ways of providing neuropsychological assessments. These types of cost-minimization studies need to be done and will strengthen, not weaken, our field.

Third-party payers also benefit from neuropsychological services in prolonged recovery and increased service utilization. Moreover, the development of a focus treatment plan that takes into account the patient's cognitive and emotional status allows for patient care to be conducted in a cost-effective manner. Although these studies have yet to be done, we clearly can begin to outline the necessary steps to carry out this research.

In addition to the value of neuropsychological assessment for the hospital, the physician, the patient, and the family, neuropsychological assessment is an important tool in clinical research trials. Measuring patients' cognitive functioning can help determine the efficacy of new treatments designed to reduce the morbidity in stroke populations (Helgason & Wolf, 1997). They also can be used to study more thoroughly the effectiveness of various forms of medical intervention, such as carotid endarterectomy.

The financial and cost-containment measures brought on by the managed care mandate that neuropsychologists conduct studies that demonstrate their utility, value, and efficiency are often reacted to negatively in our field. Yet, they do force us to take a close look at what we are doing and to enhance the quality of services provided. In that spirit, we now propose three studies that potentially could measure the cost–outcomes of neuropsychological assessment. Although it might be obvious, there may be instances in which such studies will demonstrate that certain forms of neuropsychological services are not cost-effective. This should not discourage us. It should only allow us to think through more carefully how we can improve what we do. This is the true spirit of scientific investigation that has now been brought into focus in the marketplace.

Study 1: How Safe Is It for Stroke Patients with Hemi-Neglect to Be Home Alone?

The subjects for this study are 100 stroke patients suffering from hemi-neglect, which has already been noted to adversely affect functional outcome. Fifty patients are given a neuropsychological examination as part of their standard of stroke care, and 50 receive no neuropsychological evaluation. Over a 24-month period, the number of patient accidents is recorded, as is the cost of their care and subjective reports of emotional distress in the family. The empirical question is this: Did the neuropsychological input for the group of 50 patients who received it affect their functional outcome? Put in economic terms, if it cost $600 for the neuropsychological evaluation ($150 × 4 hours), what was the effect on patient outcome and associated costs (e.g., additional hospitalizations, falls, emergency room admissions, danger to others, familial distress) to have the input of the neuropsychologist early in the course of treatment? What was actually saved by not obtaining neuropsychological consultation?

This is a cost–utilization study. Note that it includes many measures of outcome, including potential dollars saved, psychometric estimates of improvement in quality of life, and subjective estimates of decreased emotional distress. Many studies that will involve neuropsychologists in the future will actually include cost–utility studies, not just cost-efficiency studies.

Study 2: Patient and Family Satisfaction with Rehabilitation Services for Stroke Patients

Two rehabilitation facilities would be the focus of this study: one setting that routinely uses a neuropsychologist to provide information to the patient and family services, and the other a setting that cannot afford a neuropsychologist to do so. In the second setting, it will become the responsibility of the physician to provide information to the patient and family. The study would examine patient and family satisfaction levels with the services they receive in rehabilitation. Specifically, does familial level of satisfaction with the quality of rehabilitation services differ between the two facilities? Would the family refer a friend to that facility? What is the level of family distress when they have information from the neuropsychologist versus when they don't receive it?

This is a cost-effectiveness study for two reasons. One is measuring the outcome in nondollar terms. The second is comparing the relative costs and benefits of two parallel forms of intervention. This needs to be kept in mind when designing such cost-effectiveness studies.

Study 3: Prediction of Safe Driving Capacity After Right-Hemisphere Stroke

The subjects for this study will be stroke patients who have suffered from right-hemisphere stroke. The empirical question would be, what is the value of neuropsychological evaluations in the first 6 months following stroke in predicting who is safe to operate a motor vehicle? Patients would be classified into three conditions: those at high risk, moderate risk, and low risk for motor vehicle accidents based on (a) physician input only; (b) combined physician and occupational therapist input; or (c) combined physician, occupational therapist, and neuropsychologist input.

Using local department of motor vehicle records to determine the number of accidents that have occurred over a 1-year period poststroke, a calculation of the total costs associated with those accidents could be compared to the costs of the physician's time, the cost of the combined times of the physician and occupational therapist, and the added cost of the neuropsychological evaluations.

This latter study is also a cost-effectiveness study. Note in this case, one is actually comparing three forms of parallel interventions. One would then assess the actual economic costs associated with providing those interventions and what were the benefits as measured by reduction in accidents. If one goes on to further assess not just the reduction in accidents but the actual dollar values saved, this study would become a cost–utility study. Thus, depending on the dependent measures used in such investigations, any given study potentially could be a purely cost-minimization study versus a cost–benefit study versus a cost-efficiency study versus a cost–utilization study. The challenge in the field is to determine what are the best outcome measures and what are the best comparisons to deal with important problems faced in the care of neurological patients.

References

Agency for Health Care Policy and Research Post-stroke Rehabilitation Guidelines. (1995).

American Heart Association Guidelines. (1997).

Anderson, C. (1994). Baseline measures and outcome predictions. *Neuroepidemiology, 13,* 283–289.

Andersen, G. (1997). Post-stroke depression: Diagnosis and incidence. *European Psychiatry, 12*(Suppl. 3), 255s–260s.

Andersen, G., Vestergaard, K., & Ingeman-Nielsen, M. (1995). Post-stroke pathological crying-frequency and correlation to depression. *European Journal of Neurology, 2,* 45–50.

Andersen, G., Vestergaard, K., & Ingeman-Nielsen, M., & Lauritzen, P. (1995). Risk factors for post-stroke depression. *Acta Psychiatria Scandinavia, 94,* 272–278.

Angleri, F., Angeleri, V., Foschi, N., Giaquinto, S., Nolfe, G., Saginario, A., Signorino, M. (1997). Depression after stroke: An inventigation through catamnesis. *Journal of Clinical Psychiatry, 58*(6), 261–265.

Astrom, M., Adolfsson, R., & Asplund, K. (1993). Major depression in stroke patients: A 3-year longitudinal study. *Stroke, 24,* 976–982.

Barreca, S. R., Finlayson, M. A. J., Gowland, C. A., & Basmajian, J. V. (1999). Use of the Halstead Category Test as a cognitive predictor of functional recovery in the hemiplegic upper limb: A cross-validation study. *The Clinical Neuropsychologist, 13*(2), 171–181.

Bergman, L., van der Meulen, J., Limburg, M., & Habbema, D. F. (1995). Cost of medical care after first-ever stroke in the Netherlands. *Stroke, 26,*1830–1836.

Bonita, R., Beaglehole, R., & North, J. (1984). Event, incidence, and case-fatality rates of cerebrovascular disease in Auckland, New Zealand. *American Journal of Epidemiology, 120,* 236–243.

Brown, R. D., Whisnant, J. P., Sicks, J. D., O'Fallon, W. M., & Wiebers, D. O. (1996). Stroke incidence, prevalence and survival: Secular trends in Rochester, Minnesota, through 1989. *Stroke, 27*(3) 373–380.

Caetano, C., & Christensen, A. L. (1999). Outpatient/day patient rehabilitation at the centre for rehabilitation of brain injury, Copenhagen, Denmark. *Neuropsychological Rehabilitation, 9*(3/4), 447–456.

Chemerinski, E., & Robinson, R. G. (2000). The neuropsychiatry of stroke. *Psychosomatics, 41,* 5–14.

Cooper, E. (1987). Clinical cerebrovascular disease in hypertensive blacks. *Journal of Clinical Hypertension, 3*(Suppl), 79–84.

Delaney, R. C. & Ravdin, L. D. (1997). The neuropsychology of stroke. In P. D. Nussbaum (Ed.), *Handbook of neuropsychology and aging* (pp. 315–329). New York: Plenum Press.

Desmond, D. W., Moroney, J. T., Bagiella, E., Sano, M., & Stern, Y. (1998). Dementia as a predictor of adverse outcomes following stroke: An evaluation of diagnostic methods. *Stroke, 29,* 69–74.

Dobkin, B. (1995). The economic impact of stroke. *Neurology, 45* (Suppl 1), S6–S9.

Dombovy, M. L., Drew-Cates, J., & Serdans, R. (1998). Recovery and rehabilitation following subarachnoid haemorrhage: Part II long-term follow-up. *Brain Injury, 12*(10), 887–894.

Donkervoort, M., Dekker, J., van den Ende, E., Stehmann-Saris, J. C., & Deelman, B. G. (2000). Prevalence of apraxia among patients with a first left hemisphere stroke in rehabilitation centres and nursing homes. *Clinical Rehabilitation, 14,*130–136.

Donnelly, R., Ernslie-Smith, A. M., Gardner, I. D., & Morris, A. D. (2000). ABC of arterial and venous disease: Vascular complications of diabetes. *British Medical Journal, 320,* 1062–1066.

Doornhein, K., & De Haan, E. (1998). Cognitive training for memory deficits in stroke patients. *Neuropsychological Rehabilitation, 8*(4), 393–400.

Downhill, D. E., & Robinson, R. G. (1994). Longitudinal assessment of depression and cognitive impairment following stroke. *Neurosurgical Clinics of North America, 182,* 425–431.

Evers, S., Engel, G., & Ament, A. (1997). Cost of stroke in the Netherlands from a societal perspective. *Stroke, 28,* 1375–1381.

Fieschi, C., Falcou, A., Sacchetti, M. L., & Toni, D. (1998). Pathogenesis, diagnosis, and epidemiology of stroke. *CNS Drugs, 9,* 1–9.

Gaines, K., & Burke, G. (1995). Ethnic differences in stroke: Black-white differences in the united states population. *Neuroepidemiology, 14,* 209–239.

Gold, M. R., Siegel, J. E., Russell, L. B., & Weinstein, M. C. (Eds.). (1996). *Cost-effectiveness in health and medicine.* New York: Oxford University Press.

Granger, C. & Hamilton, B. (1990). Measurement of stroke rehabilitation: Outcome in the 1980s. *Stroke, 21* (Suppl. 2), 46–47.

Greve, K. W., Bianchini, K. J., Hartley, S. M., & Adams, D. (1999). The Wisconsin card sorting test in stroke rehabilitation: Factor structure and relationship to outcome. *Archives of Clinical Neuropsychology, 14*(6), 497–509.

Hackett, M. L., & Anderson, C. S. (2000). Health outcomes 1 year after subarachnoid hemorrhage: An international population-based study. *Neurology, 55,* 658–662.

Hankey, G. J. (1999). Stroke: how large a public health problem, and how can the neurologist help. *Archives of Neurology, 56*(6), 748–754.

Hankey, G. J., Jamrozik, K., Broadhurst, R. J., Forbes, S., Burvill, P. W., Anderson, C. S., & Stewart-Wayne, E. G. (2000). Five-year survival after first-ever stroke and related prognostic factors in the Perth community stroke study. *Stroke, 31*(9), 2080–2086.

Helgason, C. M., & Wolf, P. A. (1997). American Heart Association prevention conference IV: Prevention and rehabilitation of stroke. *Circulation, 96,* 701–707.

Henon, H., Pasquier, F., Durieu, I., Pruvo, J. P ., & Leys, D. (1998). Medial temporal lobe atrophy in stroke patients: Relation to pre-existing dementia. *Journal of Neurology, Neurosurgery, and Psychiatry, 65*(5), 641–647.

Hier, D. B., Mondlock, J., & Caplan, L. R. (1983). Recovery of behavioral abnormalities after right hemisphere CVA. *Neurology, 33,* 345–350.

Hochstenbach, J., Mulder, T., van Limbeek, J., Donders, R., & Schoonderwaldt, H. (1998). Cognitive decline following stroke: A comprehensive study of cognitive decline following stroke. *Journal of Clinical and Experimental Neuropsychology, 20*(4), 503–517.

Holloway, R. G., Witter, D. M., Lawton, K. B., Lipscomb, J., & Samsa, G. (1996). Inpatient costs of specific cerebrovascular events at five academic medical centers. *Neurology, 46,* 854–860.

Holmqvist, L., Widen, R.., von Koch, L., Kostulas, V., Holm, M., Widsell, G., Tegler, H., Johansson, K., Almazan, J., & de Pedro-Cuesta, J. (1998). A randomized controlled trial of rehabilitation at home after stroke in southwest Stockholm. *Stroke, 29*(3), 591–597.

Holroyd-Leduc, J. M., Kapral, M. K., Austin, P. C., & Tu, J. V. (2000). Sex differences and similarities in the management and outcome of stroke patients. *Stroke, 31*(8), 1833–1837.

House, A., Dennis, M., Moridge, L., Warlow, C., Hawton, K., & Jones, L. (1991). Mood disorders in the year after first stroke. *British Journal of Psychiatry, 158,* 83–92.

Isard, P., & Forbes, F. (1992). The cost of stroke to the national health service in Scotland. *Cerebrovascular Diseases, 2,* 47–50.

Jorgensen, H. S., Nakayama, H., Raaschou, H. O., & Olsen, T. S. (1997). Acute stroke care and rehabilitation: an analysis of the direct cost and its clinical and social determinants: The Copenhagen stroke study. *Stroke, 28,* 1138–1141.

Kauhanen, M., Korpelainen, J. T., Hiltunen, P., Brusin, E., Mononen, H., Maatta, R., Nieminen, P., Sotaniemi, K. A., & Myllyla, V. V. (1999). Poststroke depression correlates with cognitive impairment and neurological deficits. *Stroke, 30*(9), 1875–1880.

Kavanagh, S., & Knapp, M. (1999). Cognitive disability and direct care costs for elderly people. *British Journal of Psychiatry, 174*(6), 539–546.

Kwakkel, G., Wagenaar, R., Koelman, T., Lankhorst, G., & Koetsier, J. C. (1997). Effects of intensity of rehabilitation after stroke: A research synthesis. *Stroke, 28*(8), 1550–1556.

Leibson, C. L., Hu, T., Brown, M. D., Hass, S. L., O'Fallon, W. M., & Whisnant, J. P. (1996). Utilization of acute care services in the year before and after first stroke: A population based study. *Neurology, 46,* 861–869.

Leske, M. C. (1981). Prevalence estimates of communication disorders in the United States: Language, hearing, and vestibular disorders. *AHSA, 23,* 229–237.

Lezak, M. (1995). *Neuropsychological assessment.* New York: Oxford University Press.

Lindenstrom, E., Boysen, G., & Nyboe, J. (1993). Risk factors for stroke in Copenhagen, Denmark II: Life-style factors. *Neuroepidemiology, 12,* 43–50.

Lofgren, B., Gustafson, Y., & Nyberg, L. (2000). Cross-validation of a model predicting discharge home after stroke rehabilitation. *Cerebrovascular Diseases, 10,* 118–125.

Lofgren, B., Nyberg, L., Osterlind, P., Mattsson, M., & Gustafson, Y. (1997). Stroke rehabilitation-discharge predictors. *Cerebrovascular Diseases, 7,* 168–174.

Mamoli, A., Censori, B., Casto, L., Sileo, C., Cesana, B., & Camerlingo, M. (1999). An analysis of the costs of ischemic stroke in an Italian stroke unit. *Neurology, 53,* 112–116.

Mast, B. T., MacNeill, S. E., & Lichtenberg, P. A. (2000). Clinical utility of the normative studies research project test battery among vascular dementia patients. *The Clinical Neuropsychologist, 14*(2), 173–180.

Mast, B. T., MacNeill, S. E., & Lichtenberg, P. A. (1999). Geropsychological problems in medical rehabilitation: Dementia and depression among stroke and lower extremity fracture patients. *Journal of Gerontology, 54A*(2), M607–M612.

Matchar, D., & Duncan, S. (1994). Cost of stroke. *Stroke Clinical Updates, 5,* 9–12.

Morrison, A. C., Fornage, M., Liao, D., & Boerwinkle, E. (2000). Parental history of stroke predicts subclinical but not clinical stroke: The atherosclerosis risk in communities study. *Stroke, 31*(9), 2098–2102.

Murray, C., & Lopez, A. (1994). Global and regional cause of death patterns in 1990. *Bulletin of the World Health Organization, 72,* 447–480.

Nord, E. (1999). *Cost-value analysis in health care: Making sense out of QALYs.* Cambridge: UK: Cambridge Press.

Office of Disease Prevention and Health Promotion, Office of Public Health and Science, U.S. Department of Health and Human Services. (1996). *Cost-effectiveness in health and medicine.* Rockville, MD: Author.

Paolucci, S., Antonucci, G., Gialloreti, L. E., Traballesi, M., Lubich, S., Pratesi, L., & Palombi, L. (1996). Predicting stroke inpatient rehabilitation outcome: The prominent role of neuropsychological disorders. *European Neurology, 36,* 385–390.

Paolucci, S., Grasso, M. G., Antonucci, G., Troisi, E., Morelli, D., Coiro, P., & Bragoni, M. (2000). One-year follow-up in stroke patients discharged from rehabilitation hospital. *Cerebrovascular Diseases, 10,* 25–32.

Pedersen, P. M., Jorgensen, H. S., Nakayama, H., Raaschou, H. O., & Olsen, T. S. (1996). General cognitive function in acute stroke: The Copenhagen stroke study. *Journal of Neurological Rehabilitation, 10*(3), 153–158.

Pedersen, P. M., Jorgensen, H. S., Nakayama, H., Raaschou, H. O., & Olsen, T. S. (1995). Aphasia in acute stroke: Incidence, determinants, and recovery. *Annals of Neurology, 38,* 659–666.

Petty, G., Brown, R., Whisnant, J., Sicks, J., O'Fallon, W., Wiebers, D. (1998). Survival and recurrence after first cerebral infarction: A population-based study in Rochester, Minnesota, 1975 through 1989. *Neurology, 50,* 208–216.

Pliskin, N. H., Cunningham, J. M., Wall, J. R., & Cassisi, J. E. (1996). Cognitive rehabilitation for cerebrovascular accidents and Alzheimer's disease. In P. W. Corrigan & S. C. Yudofsky (Eds.),

Cognitive rehabilitation for neuropsychiatric disorders (pp. 193–222). Washington, DC: American Psychiatric Press.

Pohjasvaara, T., Leppavuori, A., Siira, I., Vataja, R., Kaste, M., & Erkinjuntti, T. (1998). Frequency and clinical determinants of poststroke depression. *Stroke, 29,* 2311–2317.

Porsdal, V., & Boysen, G. (1997). Cost-of-illness studies of stroke. *Cerebrovascular Diseases, 7,* 258–263.

Prigatano, G. P. (1991). Disturbances of self-awareness of deficit after traumatic brain injury. In G. P. Prigatano & D. L. Schacter (Eds.), *Awareness of deficit after brain injury: Theoretical and clinical issues* (pp. 111–126). New York: Oxford University.

Prigatano, G. P., & Wong, J. L. (1999). Cognitive and affective improvement in brain dysfunctional patients who achieve inpatient rehabilitation goals. *Archives of Physical Medicine and Rehabilitation, 80,* 77–84.

Rao, R. (2000). Cerebrovascular disease and late life depression: An age old association revisited. *International Journal of Geriatric Psychiatry, 15,* 419–433.

Robinson, R. G., Bolduc, P. L., & Price, T. R. (1987). A two-year longitudinal study of poststroke mood disorders: Diagnosis and outcome at one and two years. *Stroke, 18,* 837–843.

Robinson, R., Starr, L., Kubos, K., Rao, K., & Price, T. (1983). A two-year longitudinal study of post-stroke mood disorders: Findings during the initial evaluation. *Stroke, 14,* 736–741.

Ryan, C., & Hendrickson, R. (1998). Evaluating the effects of treatment for medical disorders: Has the value of neuropsychological assessment been fully realized? *Applied Neuropsychology, 5*(4), 209–219.

Smurawska, L. T., Alexandrov, A. V., Bladin, C. F., & Norris, J. W. (1994). Cost of acute stroke care in Toronto, Canada. *Stroke, 25,* 1628–1631.

Starr, J. M., Nicolson, C., Anderson, K., & Dennis, M. S. (2000). Correlates of informant-rated cognitive decline after stroke. *Cerebrovascular Diseases, 10,* 214–229.

Sudlow, C. L. M., & Warlow, C. P. (1997). Comparable studies of the incidence of stroke and its pathological types: Results from an international collaboration. *Stroke, 28*(3), 491–499.

Sulch, D., Perez, I., Melbourn, A., & Kalra, L. (2000). Randomized controlled trial of integrated (managed) care pathway for stroke rehabilitation. *Stroke, 31*(8), 1929–1934.

Tatemichi, T. K., Paik, M., Bagiella, E., Desmond, D. W., Stern, Y., Sano, M., Hauser, W. A., & Mayeux, R. (1994). Risk of dementia after stroke in a hospitalized cohort: Results of a longitudinal study. *Neurology, 44,* 1885–1891.

Taylor, T. N., Davis, P. H., Torner, J. C., Holmes, J., Meyer, J. W., & Jacobson, M. F. (1996). Lifetime cost of stroke in the United States. *Stroke, 27,* 1459–1466.

Tranel, D. (1993). The role of neuropsychology in the diagnosis and management of cerebrovascular disease. In H. P. Adams (Ed.), *Handbook of cerebrovascular diseases* (pp. 613–635). New York: Marcel Dekker.

Turner-Stokes, L. (1999). Outcome measures for inpatient neurorehabilitation settings. *Neuropsychological Rehabilitation, 9*(3/4), 329–343.

U.S. Department of Health and Human Services, Public Health Service, Agency for Health Care Policy and Research. (1995). *Post-stroke rehabilitation* (AHCPR Publication No. 95-0663). Rockville, MD: Author.

Vallar, G., & Perrani, D. (1986). The anatomy of unilateral neglect after right-hemisphere stroke lesions: a clinical/CT scan correlation study in man. *Neuropsychologia, 24,* 609–622.

Van Heugten, C. M., Dekker, J., Deelman, B. G., Stehmann-Saris, F. C., & Kinebanian, A. (1999). A diagnostic test for apraxia in stroke patients: Internal; consistency and diagnostic value. *The Clinical Neuropsychologist, 13*(2), 182–192.

Wagner, M. T. & Cushman, L. A. (1994). Neuroanatomic and neuropsychological predictors of unawareness of cognitive deficit in the vascular population. *Archives of Clinical Neuropsychology, 9,* 57–69.

White, M. (1991). Reducing cardiovascular risk factors in the United States—An overview of the National Educational Programs. *Cardiovascular Risk Factors, 1,* 277.

World Health Organization. (1987). *International classification of diseases* (10th ed.). Geneva: Author.

World Health Organization statistics annual (1989). Geneva: WHO.

7

CHAPTER

John DeLuca
Maria T. Schultheis

Neuropsychological Assessment of Patients Who Have Undergone Surgical Repair of Anterior Communicating Artery Aneurysms

Introduction

In Chapter 6, the broad topic of neuropsychological services for patients who suffered a CVA or stroke was considered. In the present chapter, we focus on the "typical" middle-aged adult who suffers a subarachnoid hemorrhage (SAH) and is found to have a ruptured aneurysm of the anterior communicating artery (ACoA). Due to advancements in technology, particularly techniques of surgical interventions, the survival rate following surgery for cerebral aneurysms has increased dramatically. As a result, issues regarding the quality of life of these individuals have become a major focus of research with surviving patients. As we will see, ACoA patients can present with formidable cognitive, behavioral, and personality changes, even without showing frank neurological deficits (Bornstein, Weir, Petruk, & Disney, 1987; DeLuca & Diamond, 1995). These cognitive, behavioral, and personality problems may range from no impairment to subtle cognitive and emotional problems to profound amnesia, confabulation, or abulic states (Bottger, Prosiegel, Steiger, & Yassouridis, 1998; D'Esposito, Alexander, Fischer, McGlinchey-Berroth, & O'Connor, 1996; Ogden, Mee, & Henning, 1993). Consequently, ACoA patients are frequently referred for neuropsychological evaluation.

In addition to the increased understanding of the range of neurobehavioral difficulties following ACoA aneurysm, recent progress in ACoA research has begun to refine the identification of the neuropathological underpinnings of the major behavioral problems associated with these aneurysms (e.g., D'Esposito et al., 1996; Tidswell, Dias, Sagar, Mayes, & Battersby, 1995). However, research on the course of recovery, effectiveness of rehabilitation, and cost-effectiveness of interventions has lagged behind.

In this chapter we provide a brief overview of the neurobehavioral and neuroanatomical features associated with ACoA aneurysm rupture (see DeLuca & Diamond, 1995, for more details). The clinical utility of neuropsychological services for this patient population is then considered. Potential studies dealing with cost–outcomes research of neuropsychological services for ACoA patients are also presented.

Medical Considerations

An aneurysm is an abnormal enlargement of a blood vessel resulting from a flaw in the blood vessel wall. Cerebral aneurysm is fairly common, with a prevalence of 2.3% to 5% in adults (McCormick, 1984; Rinkel, Djibuti, Algra, & van Gijn, 1998) and incidence of approximately 5.5 per 100,000 (Roos et al., 2000). The highest incidence of cerebral rupture occurs between the ages of 40 and 70 (McCormick, 1984) and occurs more frequently in females (Adams & Biller, 1992). Subarachnoid hemorrhage following aneurysm rupture is common and a major cause of death. Poor outcome is associated most with severity of initial bleeding, rebleeding, and the presence of cerebral ischemia (Roos et al, 2000). Although congenital defects have been identified as the most common cause of aneurysms, other factors (e.g., suspected pituitary adenomas, polycystic kidney disease, and degenerative vessel disease) also have been identified as potential etiologies of cerebral aneurysms (Rinkel et al., 1998). Increased risk for rupture has been associated with age, debility, family history of SAH, hypertension, and alcohol use (Rinkel et al., 1998; Saveland, 1992)

The ACoA is one of the most common sites of cerebral aneurysm in humans and one of the most frequent site of cerebral infarct following aneurysm rupture (McCormick, 1984, Rinkel et al., 1998). As seen in Figure 7.1, the ACoA lies at the anterior portion of the Circle of Willis, interconnecting the two anterior cerebral arteries just rostral to the optic chiasm. Despite its relatively small size, the ACoA has significant arterial branches (Crowell & Morawetz, 1977; Dunker & Harris, 1976), which perfuse the paraterminal gyrus (including the septal nuclei), the genu of the corpus callosum, anterior cingulum, optic chiasm, columns of the fornix, substantia inominata, anterior hypothalamus, the mesial anterior commissure, and the nucleus basalis of Meynert (Tatu, Moulin, Bogousslavsky, & Duvernoy, 1998). Vasospasm (constriction of the arterial vessel that limits blood flow) is a major cause of cerebral infarcts. Infarcts often are observed along the distribution of the anterior cerebral arteries and the small perforating arterial branches directly off of the ACoA itself (Alexander & Freedman, 1984; Gade, 1982). Several authors have suggested that the neurobehavioral changes commonly observed following ACoA aneurysm may be a direct result of infarction to these areas (Alexander & Freedman, 1984; Damasio et al., 1985; Gade, 1982). Little is known about the incidence of severe neuropsychological difficulties following ACoA aneurysm, but estimates range from 1% to 60% (see DeLuca & Diamond, 1995).

Modern treatment for cerebral aneurysms typically involves placing a clip at the neck of the aneurysm to prevent further bleeding (see Figure 7.2). Clipping requires the need for a craniotomy, which itself has complications and risk factors. More recently, a coiling procedure has been developed that diminishes the need for a craniotomy. With this procedure, a catheter is inserted, usually into the femoral artery, and then guided to the site of the aneurysm. At the site, a mild current then releases the coil, which acts to close the ruptured vessel.

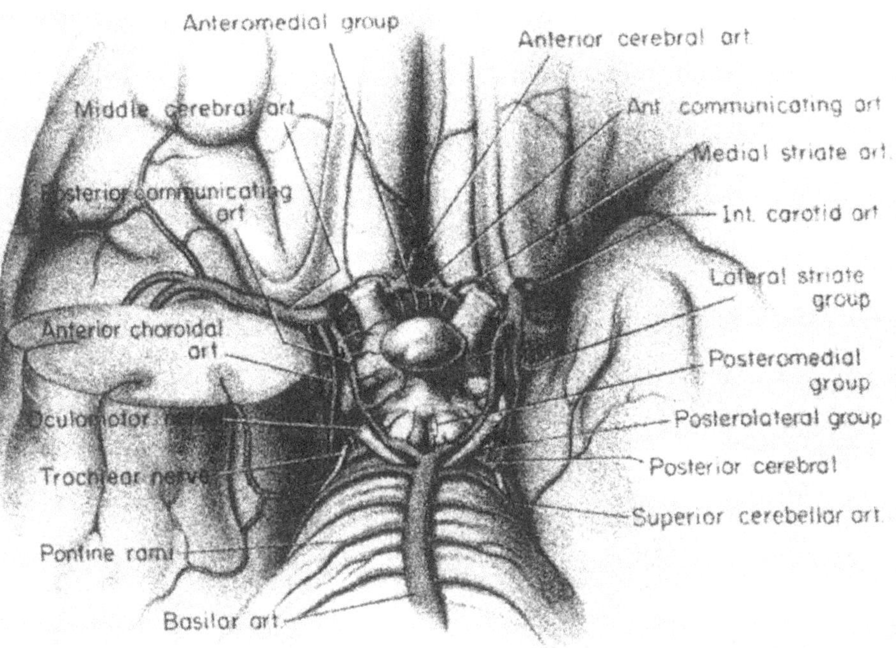

FIGURE 7.1. Cerebral vasculature at the Circle of Willis at the base of the brain. Note the relatively small size of the ACoA. Also note the arterial branches off the ACoA. Lack of perfusion through these small arterial branches is thought to result in amnesia secondary to basal forebrain damage. (Carpenter, 1991, reproduced by permission of Lippincott, Williams, & Wilkins.)

☐ General Neuropsychological Profile Following ACoA Rupture and Repair

It is now well known that rupture at the ACoA appears to be particularly susceptible to neurobehavioral impairments (Bornstein et al., 1987; Larsson et al., 1989; Sonesson, Ljunggren, Saveland, & Brandt, 1987). These include a memory deficit often described as Korsakoff-like in nature, confabulation, and significant personality changes (see DeLuca & Diamond, 1995, for a review). These neurobehavioral changes have been collectively referred to as the *ACoA syndrome* (Alexander & Freedman, 1984; Damasio et al., 1985). However, not all ACoA patients present with a unitary constellation of neurobehavioral impairments, and this singular syndrome does not adequately describe the variety of cognitive and behavioral changes following ACoA aneurysm. For example, executive impairments also have been identified as a major consequence following ACoA aneurysm (Diamond, DeLuca, & Kellety, 1997; DeLuca & Locker, 1996). ACoA patients exhibit a wide range of cognitive, behavioral, and social difficulties, ranging from few to many, mild to severe, and transient to long-lasting, with relatively few patients exhibiting a full-blown ACoA syndrome. As such, reference to an ACoA syndrome is of little clinical utility today (see DeLuca & Chiaravalloti, in press, for details).

The following section provides a brief description of specific neuropsychological deficits commonly observed in ACoA survivors. It should be emphasized that not all ACoA patients will present with difficulties in all domains discussed below. Readers

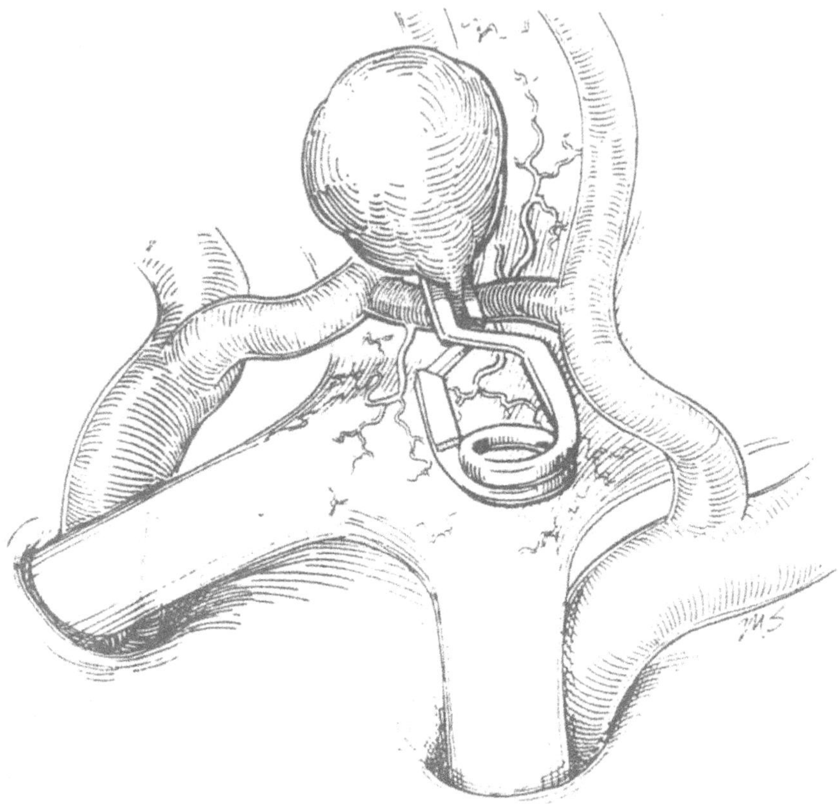

FIGURE 7.2. Clipping the ACoA aneurysm at its neck is the most common surgical intervention. Note that the small perforating arteries off the ACoA are spared with the clipping procedure. (Drumm, Greene, & Marciano, 1993, reproduced by permission of Barrow Neurological Institute.)

are referred to DeLuca and Diamond (1995) for a more detailed description of neuropsychological sequelae.

Memory

Early work documenting the existence of memory deficits following ACoA rupture discussed the presence of a Korsakoff-like amnesia (Lindqvist & Norlen, 1966; Talland, Sweet, & Ballantine, 1967). It was originally hypothesized that the amnesia resulted from lesions of the same diencephalic structures as demonstrated in Korsakoff patients. However, with the identification of the various perforating branches from the ACoA, including its perfusion of the basal forebrain, it was hypothesized that the impaired memory was due to involvement of the basal forebrain (Gade, 1982), the reciprocal connections of the basal forebrain with the hippocampus (Abe, Inokawa, Kashiwagi, & Yanagihara, 1998; Damasio et al., 1985), or both. With the advent of neuroimaging techniques such as CT scans, case report studies of ACoA patients showed discrete lesions in the basal forebrain, which were attributed to the amnesic condition (Abe et al., 1998).

Memory functioning in ACoA patients ranges from amnesic, to moderate–mild impairment, to normal performance. In general, immediate recall is far less impaired (if any) than delayed recall, even among amnesic ACoA patients. There is some suggestion that ACoA patients show particular difficulty in discriminating temporal context during recall. Relatively few studies have examined retrograde memory, yielding mixed results. Although the results of some studies suggested that the degree of retrograde memory impairment is significantly less than that observed in diencephalic or mesial temporal amnesics, one study found no group differences (Gade & Mortensen, 1990). D'Esposito and colleagues showed that retrograde memory impairments resulted from severe executive dysfunction secondary to bifrontal lesions (D'Esposito et al., 1996). The few studies examining implicit memory reported intact performance in ACoA patients (Bondi, Kaszniak, Rapcsak, & Butters, 1993).

Confabulation

Confabulation is not uncommon among ACoA patients in acute rehabilitation. It can be defined as statements or actions that involve unintentional but obvious distortions of memory (Moscovitch & Melo, 1997). This distortion often is described as spontaneous or provoked, which some have argued represent two distinct forms of confabulation (Schnider, von Daniken, & Gutbrod, 1996), whereas others argue that these two descriptors represent differences in degree and not kind (e.g., DeLuca & Cicerone, 1991). Several studies have found a significant relationship between the severity of confabulation and deficits in executive functioning (e.g., DeLuca, 1993; Kapur & Coughlan, 1980; Stenhouse, Knight, Longmore, & Bishara, 1991). However, DeLuca (1993) and others (e.g., Fischer, Alexander, D'Esposito, & Otto, 1995) have shown that spontaneous confabulation is observed only among amnesic ACoA patients who had frontal/executive impairments as well as basal forebrain lesions. This "dual-lesion" hypothesis of both basal forebrain/memory impairment and frontal/executive dysfunction has been suggested in ACoA subjects (DeLuca, 1993) and also suggested as a mechanism for confabulation in non-ACoA patients with basal forebrain and frontal lesions (Hashimoto, Tanaka, & Nakano, 2000; Squire, Shimamura, & Graf, 1987).

Executive Functions

Deficits in executive control functions constitute a major difficulty among ACoA patients. Specifically, executive impairments such as reduced cognitive flexibility, poor concept formation, and poor planning have been reported by several authors, across a variety of subsets of ACoA patients, particularly among amnesics (e.g., Bottger et al., 1998; Ljunggren, Sonesson, Saveland, & Brandt, 1985; Sonesson et al., 1987; DeLuca, 1992). Preliminary studies suggest that executive dysfunction is more severe among ACoA amnesics than in other amnesic etiologies, such as temporal lobe resection or herpes encephalitis (Corkin et al., 1985; Shoqeirat, Mayes, MacDonald, Meudell, & Pickering, 1990). Also, outcome parameters such as return to work in ACoA patients have been associated with improvements in executive functioning (e.g., DeLuca & Locker, 1996).

Executive dysfunction also plays a significant role in the memory abilities of ACoA patients. For instance, Diamond, DeLuca, and Kelley (1997) showed that anterograde memory was significantly improved when ACoA subjects used an organizational strategy to facilitate encoding on the Rey Complex Figure Test. These authors found that organizational strategy facilitated both immediate and delayed recall in the amnesic group to the level observed in nonamnesic ACoA subjects. The ability to utilize an organizational intervention to improve memory appeared to be related to the degree of executive impairment, as measured by the Wisconsin Card Sorting Test (WCST).

Intellectual Functions

Most studies show that intelligence is largely preserved following ACoA aneurysm (e.g., Bottger et al., 1998; DeLuca, 1992; Stenhouse et al., 1991), although select patients can show mild impairment (e.g., Irle, Wowra, Kumert, Hample, & Kunze, 1992). Performance IQ is often decreased compared to relatively intact Verbal IQ, (DeLuca & Cicerone, 1989; DeLuca & Locker, 1996), although this is not always the case (e.g., Alexander & Freedman, 1984; Irle et al., 1992). The few studies estimating premorbid intelligence report that ACoA patients show a decrease in postinjury overall intelligence compared with a premorbid estimate (i.e., National Adult Reading Test) of intelligence, despite performance remaining generally within the normal range (Parkin, Leng, Stanhope, & Smith, 1988; Stenhouse et al., 1991).

Attention and Concentration

Generally speaking, simple attentional skills remain relatively intact or mildly diminished in ACoA patients. Multiple studies have shown that most ACoA patients score within the normal range on measures such as the Digit Span and Mental Control subtests of the Wechsler Memory Scale (see DeLuca & Diamond, 1995). More difficulty has been observed in some ACoA patients on tests of complex concentration, such as the Stroop and Trail Making Test.

In contrast, ACoA patients show a significant susceptibility to interference, with several studies documenting increased susceptibility and release from proactive interference (e.g., Leng & Parkin, 1988; Volpe & Hirst, 1983) and impaired performance on the Brown-Peterson distractor task (e.g., Parkin et al., 1988).

Visuospatial/Perceptual and Constructional Abilities

Visual–perceptual functions are generally reported to be intact following ACoA aneurysm. Yet, select studies have reported some visuoconstructional disorganization and impaired visuoperceptual abilities following ACoA aneurysm (Laiacona et al., 1989; Ljunggren et al., 1985; Sonesson et al., 1987).

Language

Language functions (i.e., expressive, receptive, naming, repetition, reading, writing) have been shown to be preserved in the amnesic ACoA case study literature (see DeLuca & Diamond, 1995, for a review). Some studies have reported deficient spontaneous speech, impaired speech initiation (e.g., Alexander & Freedman, 1984; Vilkki, 1985), or, rarely, akinetic mutism (Lindqvist & Norlen, 1966). Paraphasic or neologistic speech errors have not been reported. The only area of language that more consistently reveals defective performance is verbal fluency. However, this deficit is primarily attributable to initiation deficits (i.e., executive), as opposed to language system dysfunction.

Motor and Other Impairments

A less frequent symptom following ACoA aneurysm is "alien hand syndrome" (AHS). AHS is marked by apparently purposeful but uncontrollable movements of one hand (usually the left), which often interferes with the actions of the other hand. Although rare, several reports of AHS following ACoA aneurysm have been reported (e.g., Banks et al., 1989; Starkstein, Berthier, & Leiguarda, 1988). The exact neurological mechanism in AHS is as yet undetermined, but various regions have been postulated, including a combination of mesial frontal lesions (Banks et al., 1989), involvement of the anterior corpus callosum (Chan & Liu, 1999), or both.

Also rare following rupture of the ACoA is akinesia, or absence of movement, presumed to be due to damage to the dopamine system or its projections (Tanaka, Bachman, & Miyazaki, 1991; see also Okawa, Maeda, Nukui, & Kawafuchi, 1980). Sudden paraplegia or paresis has been documented following ACoA aneurysm but is also extremely rare (Maiuri, Gangemi, Correiro, & D'Andrea, 1986; Ohno, Masaoka, Suzuki, Monma, & Matsushima, 1991), whereas ideomotor dysfunction generally has not been reported (Laiacona et al., 1989).

Personality

Personality changes following ACoA aneurysm have been documented in the literature since the 1950s. Changes in personality vary dramatically among patients; some, for instance, show decreased initiation, apathy, lack of concern, and flattened affect, whereas others may display increased irritability, socially inappropriate behavior, and unpredictable aggression (Alexander & Freedman, 1984; Logue, Durward, Pratt, Piercy, & Nixon, 1968). Other documented changes include an increase in emotional lability, talkativeness, selfishness, euphoria, childlike behavior, laziness, and indifference following ACoA aneurysm (Okawa et al., 1980). Importantly, several investigators have noted that personality change can occur in the absence of confabulation or amnesia.

Studies investigating personality changes following ACoA aneurysm have been relatively sparse for a number of reasons, perhaps most notably due to the limited tools available for assessing change in personality from premorbid status. The few studies that have been completed have methodological limitations and allow for few inferences to be drawn.

As with amnesia and confabulation, early studies attributed personality changes to diencephalic regions because of similarities with Korsakoff's syndrome (e.g., Talland et al., 1967). More recent studies have examined the relationship between alteration of personality and changes within the mediobasal region of the frontal lobes commonly affected by ACoA (Luria, 1973; 1980). The important role of orbital frontal regions in altered personality following ACoA aneurysm has been well documented over the years (e.g., Blumer & Benson, 1975; Damasio et al., 1985).

Several investigators have noted that personality alterations often were chronic and resistant to change, resulting in long-term management problems and the most significant obstacle to successful social reintegration (Okawa et al., 1980; Steinman & Bigler, 1986). Additionally, chronic, persistent personality changes have been shown to lead to poorer outcome in terms of employment status, return to the home (Alexander & Freedman, 1984), and intellectual performance (Sengupta, Chiu, & Brierley, 1975).

Summary of General Outcome Following ACoA

Despite the variability in pattern and degree of impairment following ACoA, some general conclusions can be drawn regarding outcome and recovery following ACoA aneurysm.

Although it was believed that ACoA aneurysms result in particularly poor cognitive outcomes, results of recent studies examining cognitive recovery following ACoA have produced varying results. Some studies have reported that during the first three months following ACoA, significant recovery in specific cognitive functions (such as retrograde amnesia and executive functions; D'Esposito et al., 1996) and confabulation can be observed (Okawa et al., 1980). Others have noted that most cognitive gains occur within the first 6 weeks postsurgically (Richardson, 1991), with little change noted between the 6-week and 6-month postoperative assessment. Despite the difference in timeframe for recovery, these authors noted that cognitive recovery appeared to move from broad cognitive impairments to specific cognitive deficits over time (Richardson, 1991).

In contrast to these studies, many researchers have reported the presence of long-term cognitive deficits following ACoA. For example, on a 12 to 84 month postsurgical assessment, Stenhouse et al. (1991) reported that approximately 41% of the ACoA patients returned to their premorbid level of functioning; however, other individuals demonstrated persistent intellectual and memory impairment as compared with a control group. Alexander and Freedman (1984) reported that ACoA patients demonstrated continued improvement for months following lesion, during which time confabulation, denial, and confusion cleared.

Studies examining vocation issues have reported that up to 84% of ACoA patients return to work (Hori & Suzuki, 1979; Teissier du Cros & Lhermitte, 1984;). However, such numbers should be viewed cautiously, as it is well documented that SAH patients with little to no neurological deficits (i.e., good outcome) have significant neuropsychological, emotional, and psychosocial disturbances (Ljunggren et al., 1985; Sonesson et al., 1987). Such deficits have been found to be most prominent among ACoA patients (Sonesson et al., 1987).

In fact, more recent studies that examined return to work as an outcome measure reported that multiple factors–including cognitive, emotional and behavioral factors—can influence an individual's ability to return to work (Vilkki, Holst, Ohman, Servo, & Heiskanen, 1990). Studies have identified several premorbid factors, such as employment status and work environment to which the individual is returning to, that also can affect this outcome. For example, Storey (1970) reported that ACoA individuals returning to work in large corporations were better able to transition to the workplace than those returning to a self-employed status. Others have reported successful return to work of ACoA patients on a part-time basis (Vilkki, 1985). However, neurobehavioral difficulties, including memory and attentional processes, generally have been found to be significantly related to both general measures of outcome, such as the Glasgow Coma Scale (GCS), and return to work (Bottger et al., 1998; Vilkki et al., 1990). As such, the neuropsychologist should play a primary role in issues related to return to work with ACoA patients.

Personality changes following ACoA also have been demonstrated to affect outcome.

Specifically, researchers have reported that personality alterations frequently were chronic and resistant to change, often resulting in long-term management problems and serving as a significant problem to successful return to home (Alexander & Freedman, 1984), social reintegration (Steinman & Bigler, 1986), and poorer outcome in terms of employment status (Alexander & Freedman, 1984). These authors also noted that patients who demonstrated significant personality changes, such as apathy and disinhibition, had a poorer prognosis for outcome.

☐ Utility of Neuropsychological Services

The importance of the neuropsychological evaluation should not be underestimated. This evaluation provides critical information regarding the direct consequences of brain damage that the standard neurological evaluation does not provide. As such, the results of the neuropsychological evaluation are critical to the physician, treatment team, and family (see Table 7.1).

The services provided by a neuropsychologist in the treatment of ACoA survivors can vary significantly, depending on the stage of treatment when services are initiated. In general, relevant neuropsychological contributions to treatment can begin as early as prerupture or presurgical intervention for ACoA patients.

Prerupture/Presurgical

Although treatment for ACoA is most commonly initiated following rupture of the aneurysm, many individuals do not experience rupture. However, if identified prior to rupture, patients and their families often must decide whether to proceed with surgical intervention (i.e., clipping of the aneurysm). In these cases, neuropsychological assessment can provide important information to the family and surgeon regarding treatment decisions. The following case provides an illustration.

> KP was a 79-year-old male ACoA patient, referred by his neurosurgeon to evaluate the possibility of a dementia syndrome independent of an identified unruptured ACoA aneurysm. This information was deemed important in making a decision of whether to perform surgical intervention for the aneurysm. The family reported subtle balance difficulties, progressive cognitive decline over a number of years, and many examples of impaired memory and functioning, most of which were denied by the patient. Results of the neuropsychological evaluation showed deficits in specific areas of cognitive function from estimates of premorbid intellectual abilities. These were in language abilities, simple nonverbal visuoperceptual abilities, attention/concentration abilities, and verbal/nonverbal new learning memory. The pattern of test performance was not consistent with diffuse or generalized cognitive dysfunction typically associated with an advanced dementia syndrome (i.e., DAT). Rather, a circumscribed pattern of cognitive deficits was noted, consistent with dysfunction of brain systems subserved by the frontal lobes, perhaps representing the effects of the ACoA aneurysm, with possible resultant frontal vascular ischemic compromise and/or mass effect. Given the questionable source of the cognitive decline documented by the neuropsychological evaluation, the neurosurgeon opted not to perform the aneurysmal clipping.

Further discussion of the utility and cost-effectiveness benefits of neuropsychological findings for the determination of surgical intervention will be discussed later in this chapter.

TABLE 7.1. Key Descriptors of Usefulness of Neuropsychological Services in ACoA Patients

Value to the Medical Team
- Presurgical consultation concerning neuropsychological status
- Monitoring course of acute recovery (e.g., abulia, confabulation, amnesia)
- Objective monitoring of potential benefits of medication trials (e.g., abulia, attention)
- Contribute to acute discharge planning (e.g., home vs. rehabilitation hospital)

Value to the Rehabilitation Team
- Educate team on cognitive/emotional/personality issues (e.g., alien hand syndrome)
- Monitor course of recovery (e.g., confabulation, amnesia, personality, abulia)
- Differentiate between "organic" vs. "psychiatric" interpretations of behavior
  - Depression vs. diminished initiation
  - Confabulation vs. delusion or psychosis
- Contribute in discharge planning
  - Return to work
  - Discharge to home vs. assisted living
  - Need for continued rehabilitation services
- Design and monitor rehabilitation interventions
  - Confabulation behavioral treatment plan
  - Awareness training plan
  - Cognitive rehabilitation

Value to the Family
- Educate family regarding expected cognitive/behavioral changes (e.g., personality)
- Educate family regarding expected course of recovery
- Provide instructions and support for addressing difficulties at home
  - Deal with a confabulator
  - Issue regarding changed personality

Acute Hospital

For many neuropsychologists, the first contact with an ACoA patient is immediately following surgery in the acute hospital. Although the main priority during this period may be the medical stabilization of the patient, neuropsychologists with a working knowledge of the type of cognitive and behavioral problems that can be observed following ACoA aneurysm can significantly contribute to care of the patient. For instance, understanding that confabulation is common in acute ACoA patients, neuropsychologists can aid physicians in determining appropriate treatment and help to differentiate confabulatory behavior from other postsurgery complications (e.g., delirium) or psychiatric interpretations (e.g., psychosis). Neuropsychologists with a working knowledge of risk factors for cognitive decline such as hydrocephalus, vasospasm, or rebleeding can aid the treating physicians by closely monitoring the patient's mental status, which could suggest postsurgical complications. Knowledge of less well-known neurobehavioral consequences of ACoA aneurysm (e.g., alien hand syndrome [AHS]) could be immediately beneficial to the treatment team and family.

The benefits of identifying and monitoring cognitive process at this early stage are not only pertinent to immediate treatment decisions but also could aid in the determination of follow-up care of ACoA survivors, such as consideration for rehabilitation. By providing a thorough evaluation of the patients' cognitive, emotional, and behavioral status, neuropsychologists can play a key role in determining various treatment decisions—for instance, whether ACoA patients can be discharged to home or require rehabilitation services; whether the patient should return to work and, if so, full-time or part time; if rehabilitation is required, should it be inpatient or outpatient, full-time or part-time, and so on. The role of the neuropsychologist in these important decisions should not be underestimated, as it is well known that survivors from cerebral aneurysms who are discharged from the acute hospital with little or no obvious physical or neurological deficits, even those who are described as having "good or excellent" recoveries, can have significant problems in cognitive, emotional, vocational, and social functioning in everyday life (Ljunggren et al., 1985; Sonesson et al., 1987). Such individuals likely receive little to no interventions acutely.

Inpatient Rehabilitation Setting

For many ACoA patients, the next step in treatment and recovery is inpatient rehabilitation. Although the decision-making process by which patients are sent to inpatient rehabilitation services is not clear, it is likely that only ACoA patients with significant cognitive and/or physical disabilities are referred. The net effect of such decision making is that a large segment of the ACoA population (e.g., those who are discharged to home) will be lost to the neuropsychologist.

During inpatient rehabilitation, therapeutic and functional goals typically are set and addressed by a rehabilitation team. Because physical difficulties are fairly rare or relatively minor following ACoA aneurysm rupture, the cognitive and behavioral difficulties become the primary focus of treatment. Thus, most ACoA patients are admitted to inpatient rehabilitation primarily due to significant cognitive difficulties, abulia, or both. The neuropsychologist plays a key role in both circumstances. Working with the team to address family concerns and family education also is a key responsibility. Each of these roles is described more fully below.

Working Within the Interdisciplinary Team. Because addressing cognitive and behavioral problems often is the primary treatment goal with ACoA patients in acute rehabilitation, the neuropsychologist should take a leadership role within the team when working with ACoA patients. This role needs to expand beyond basic assessment of cognitive strengths and weaknesses and addressing emotional needs. First, the neuropsychologist should educate members of the team who are not familiar with ACoA patients with the types of behavioral, cognitive, and personality difficulties that can be observed. These include abulic states, confabulation, unawareness of deficit, apathetic or disinhibited behavior (often interpreted as personality change), amnesia, and AHS. Understanding the nature of these problems can have significant treatment implications. For instance, "classic" neurobehavioral symptoms resulting from ACoA aneurysm can be misinterpreted as psychiatric conditions, which could result in unnecessary and potentially hindering psychiatric treatment (i.e., medication). The most notable example of this is confabulation, which can be misinterpreted as delusions, disorientation, acute confusional states, or even psychotic states. Diminished initiative (often referred to as apathy) can be misinterpreted as depression or reduced compliance with treatment goals. Finally, working with the family, both during inpatient rehabilitation and postacute rehabilitation (e.g., for family education, training for behavioral management, understanding cognitive and emotional difficulties), is a key role for the neuropsychologist (see below).

Assessment and Interventions. With respect to assessment, the neuropsychologist treating ACoA patients has at least two major responsibilities: (a) assessing of cognitive, behavioral, emotional, and personality problems; and (b) designing and implementing rehabilitation interventions. Interventions include not only designing and implementing a traditional cognitive rehabilitation plan for the patient, but possibly behavioral management (e.g., for disinhibited behavior), behavioral monitoring (e.g., of behavioral changes following pharmacological interventions to treat abulia), and designing and implementing a program to diminish confabulation and increase awareness of deficit (DeLuca, 1992).

ACoA patients within acute rehabilitation settings may demonstrate a wide range of neurobehavioral deficits, ranging from profound impairments at admission to minimal deficits at time of discharge. Subsequently, traditional neuropsychological assessment may vary from monitoring mental status to completion of full neuropsychological evaluations.

ACoA patients with difficulties such as abulia, mutism, disorientation, severe amnesia, or severe confabulation may not be able to tolerate an extensive, more traditional neuropsychological evaluation. As a result, neuropsychological evaluations may be limited to monitoring mental status and behavioral changes, orientation, and simple comprehension and expression. This initial evaluation can provide adequate information for the development of early treatment planning while minimizing the elaborate assessment of functions that are likely to improve. As recovery progresses and for those ACoA patients presenting without profound neurobehavioral difficulties, more traditional approaches to the assessment of cognitive skills may be possible.

Abulia is one reason for referral to inpatient rehabilitation for ACoA patients. In cases of abulia, ACoA patients show significantly reduced initiative or drive, which may be severe enough to result in akinetic mutism. Such patients appear awake, but fail to respond to commands or do so only after very long delays. Physicians often treat abulic states with pharmacological agents such as Amantadine, Bromocriptine, and Sinemet. During such trials, the neuropsychologist plays a critical role in quantifying behavioral improvement. This can be accomplished by establishing a behavioral monitoring program in which specific target behaviors (e.g., latency to respond to set questions, number of words to respond) are established and quantified. Measuring behavioral improvement from baseline performance can aid significantly in judging medication effectiveness.

Pharmacological agents often are used to treat cognitive factors following brain injury during acute inpatient rehabilitation (McDowell, Whyte, & D'Espositio, 1998; Whyte et al., 1997). Because many of the most profound neurobehavioral consequences of ACoA (i.e., severe amnesia and confabulation) are commonly observed at the acute level, pharmacological agents may be suggested for these patients as well. The influence of medication on cognitive functioning should always be a prime concern for the neuropsychologist on the rehabilitation team. Examples of pharmacological interventions at this stage of recovery can include the use of stimulants to address abulic behavior and the use of medications designed to increase attention and concentration to help minimize amnestic symptoms (Whyte et al., 1997). It should be recognized that the effectiveness of such medications with ACoA patients is unknown. The neuropsychologist should play a key role in determining whether to include pharmacological agents into a patient's treatment, and should consider what impact such medication may have on other symptoms (e.g., confabulation).

Although medical issues may not be the primary focus during inpatient rehabilitation, knowledge by the neuropsychologist of how secondary complications (such as hydrocephalus and vasospasm) may affect functioning and recovery can significantly aid the treating physician in the overall management of the ACoA patient. The following is an illustration of an ACoA patient whom the author knew for many years prior to the aneurysm and whose course of her recovery he has followed closely for several years.

> Patient DG is a 60-year-old female who presented with significant abulia and apathy after surgery for clipping of an ACoA aneurysm rupture. Her surgical treatment was uncomplicated. Serial postoperative CT scans showed decreasing intracerebral blood over time, but moderate ventricular enlargement. After surgery, DG was very slow to respond to questions, if she responded at all. Her verbal responses were brief, and she showed little to no verbal or behavioral initiation. Motorically, she was slow and sluggish, but able to move all extremities with full range, although she was weak. She showed little to no improvement over a period of about 3 months, despite attempts by the acute rehabilitation team to employ several behavioral and pharmacological interventions. Because of familiarity with ACoA patients, the neuropsychologist suggested that a ventricular peritoneal (VP) shunt might decrease the ventricular enlargement and potentially improve the patient's mental status. The neurosurgeon was reluctant, because spinal taps yielded essentially normal CSF pressure. However, the neurosurgeon eventually agreed and a VP shunt was placed. Within hours, the patient was markedly more alert, was conversing with family in full, clear sentences, and showed dramatic improvement in initiation, motor functions, and cognition. She was soon discharged and now lives a normal life in her community.

This case example illustrates how a neuropsychologist's familiarity with medical issues surrounding ACoA aneurysm complication and course can have a significant impact not only in improving cognitive functioning but in all aspects of quality of life.

Another prominent symptom in many ACoA patients during acute rehabilitation is confabulation. It is now well established that unawareness of deficit is a key factor in confabulation. That is, as awareness of deficit improves, confabulation diminishes (Mercer, Wapner, Gardner, & Benson, 1977; Stuss, Alexander, Lieberman, & Levine, 1978). DeLuca (1992) described an interdisciplinary approach to the treatment of confabulation in ACoA patients, based on levels of unawareness following brain damage. Such a behavioral intervention should be designed by the neuropsychologist and requires the cooperation of the entire treatment team, as well as other staff (e.g., nursing). Briefly, unawareness of one's own deficit (i.e., anosognosia) is not a unitary phenomenon. According to Crosson and colleagues (1989), deficits in awareness can be classified according to three interdependent levels: intellectual awareness, which is the patient's ability to understand that a particular function is impaired (e.g., confabulation); emergent awareness, which is the patient's ability to recognize a problem when it is actually occurring; and anticipatory awareness, which is the ability to anticipate that a problem can occur in advance of its occurrence. These three levels are hierarchical in nature, with attainment of the lower level as a prerequisite to achieving the subsequent level.

Using this theoretical approach allows the treatment of confabulation to be specific to the particular needs of the patient at each stage of unawareness (see DeLuca, 1992, for details). For instance, treatment to improve intellectual awareness could include the use of videotaping or gently confronting the patient with errors in his or her statements or beliefs. These early interventions can serve as a foundation for later outpatient rehabilitation strategies.

Behavioral interventions may be of benefit in addressing changes in personality, which are commonly observed following ACoA rupture. These changes–which commonly result from the involvement of the frontal lobes, often from anterior cerebral artery vasospasm–can range from a severely apathetic presentation to the presence of disinhibited and impulsive behavior. Regardless of which end of the spectrum is being presented, these behaviors can directly impact progress in treatment. For example, disinhibited and impulsive behavior may disrupt participation in therapies and be mistakenly viewed as noncompliance or refusal to participate. Neuropsychological interventions providing education to other team members about the etiology of the behavior, and developing intervention approaches that can be consistently employed by all team members are critical contributions to improving treatment progress in the presence of these behavioral difficulties.

On the other extreme, severe apathy, which may result in patients being unable to initiate even the most basic of activities required for participation in therapies, also can significantly interfere with treatment progress. Apathy can be mistakenly viewed as noncompliance or as a sign of depression. The latter is a differentiation that should not be minimized, given the potential contraindicated effects of commonly used antidepressant medications. Neuropsychological interventions for apathy-like states should include coordinated treatment with the physician to identify and monitor pharmacological interventions to increase arousal, in addition to behavioral monitoring.

Family Education. The cognitive and behavioral difficulties observed in survivors of ACoA can be particularly devastating to family members. The family frequently experiences difficulties in understanding the observed changes (e.g., "How can my loved one remember something from 5 years ago [often an accurate confabulatory response displaced temporally] and not remember what he or she did this morning?"), and often require both support and education. Although services provided by the social worker on the rehabilitation team can offer guidance and support for family members, it is the neuropsychologist, serving as the behavioral expert on the rehabilitation team, who can work with the family as the primary educator to explain the neurobehavioral sequelae.

In general, at the acute rehabilitation stage family members benefit most from education regarding brain–behavior relationships (e.g., understanding confabulation), course of recovery (e.g., how long will confabulation last), and rationale for compensatory strategies (e.g., when to involve and not involve the family in treatment).

Regarding brain–behavior relations, it is often difficult for family members to understand behavioral changes (i.e., why the patient confabulates, how this is different from amnesia), and they often cope poorly with the observed changes in the patient's personality. As with the rehabilitation team, differentiation of neurobehavioral symptoms resulting from ACoA rupture versus psychiatric processes often helps in alleviating some family concerns. Education regarding the commonly observed process of recovery from neurobehavioral symptoms, in combination with reports of observed and documented changes of the patient's progress, provides family members with a clearer understanding of the treatment plan, progress, and prognosis.

Finally, because family members often serve as "primary caregivers" following discharge from acute rehabilitation, inclusion of family members in treatment interventions (e.g., confabulation) can improve carry-over of treatment benefits to the home setting. The neuropsychologist can coordinate training and education regarding specific behavior interventions that may be developed during acute rehabilitation.

Outpatient Rehabilitation

Although acute rehabilitation services may provide much of the initial groundwork for cognitive remediation following ACoA rupture and repair, continued neuropsychological treatment can be critical for successful reintegration into society. ACoA patients usually are discharged from acute rehabilitation to either home or assisted living settings. Many patients receive outpatient cognitive rehabilitation services, whereas others do not. Unfortunately, the decision for follow-up rehabilitation often is not made on clinical need. The neuropsychologist should play a central role in the cognitive and behavioral management of the ACoA patient after discharge. Particular areas of concern include issues of self-awareness, vocational issues, and emotional adjustment (patient and family).

Because ACoA patients discharged to home may still be confabulating, family members usually are in significant need for strategies to cope. Approaches and examples of treatment for confabulation (and unawareness of deficit) and strategies for how the family can be incorporated into treatment upon return to home are outlined elsewhere (DeLuca, 1992; DeLuca & Locker, 1996). The type of intervention applied by the family (e.g., how does the family respond to a confabulation?) will depend on the level of unawareness of the patient (see Figure 7.1). As such, a close relationship with the neuropsychologist will not only serve to apply and monitor the appropriate intervention, but also diminish circumstances that could be destabling for the patient and family ("Why does my dad say things that are wrong?"). As awareness of deficit increases, confabulation decreases. However, with increased awareness, one often finds increased depression and anxiety. This can have significant consequences for family dynamic (or work or other social circumstances).

Neuropsychologists working with ACoA patients at this stage in recovery also should focus on the identification of specific cognitive deficits and the development of strategies to compensate for these deficits. Although initial efforts may be introduced at the inpatient level, often these strategies require reevaluation and modification, in order to be applicable to the patient's new environment and schedule.

Vocational. Often, ACoA survivors are relatively young. As such, returning to competitive employment is a major factor for the patient, family, and employer. In ACoA patients who receive outpatient rehabilitation, the neuropsychologist plays a pivotal role in treatment planning, providing therapy, monitoring progress, and discharge planning. The comprehensive neuropsychological evaluation is the traditional first step in vocational planning. In particular, neuropsychological findings can document the extent and nature of cognitive impairment and provide a more comprehensive understanding of that individual's ability to return to work. Such objective information can be invaluable in making decisions regarding returning to work. (Should the patient return to work at all, return to the same or different job, at the same or different capacity? What aids may be required?)

Other members of the rehabilitation team also gather information, which will contribute to vocational planning. For instance, the occupational therapist may work directly with the employer to learn about the ACoA patient's work environment, exact duties, and tasks required to perform the job duties. This team information, in conjunction with the results of the neuropsychological evaluation, is then used to develop the vocational plan. For instance, simulated work scenarios often are implemented during outpatient rehabilitation to prepare and monitor the patient's potential return to employment (DeLuca & Locker, 1996). In this model, the neuropsychologist works with the rehabilitation team as well as the employer in designing an appropriate simulated work scenario (e.g., preparing and teaching a lecture). Scientific training makes the neuropsychologist particularly qualified to design such trials and to apply the results to the specific psychosocial and vocational needs of the ACoA patient.

The results of the simulated work-study will provide needed information about the ACoA patient's ability to return to work. Deciding whether modifications to the work environment are required, educating the employer about the patients cognitive and behavioral status (e.g., despite personality changes, he or she is still able to perform the job duties), and educating employers about job coaching and mentoring are all responsibilities of the neuropsychologist and the rehabilitation team.

Emotional. Leaving the hospital and returning to the home environment marks the point at which medical needs are minimal and, subsequently, departure from the safety of the hospital environment can be an emotionally challenging transition. For many ACoA patients and their families, returning to the home environment commonly involves continued coping with neurobehavioral symptoms, such as memory difficulties, confabulation, or changes in personality. In addition, returning to the home environment involves new challenges, such as providing continued care without the support of on-site medical personnel and addressing issues that were not applicable in the hospital setting (i.e., facing questions of returning to driving or returning to work).

As mentioned, as recovery progresses and survivors develop increased awareness of the cognitive and behavioral consequences of their ACoA rupture, it can be anticipated that behavioral and emotional difficulties may develop. In addition, the emotional concerns of the family may become more prominent at this stage (e.g., "He is not the same dad I used to have.").

☐ Cost-Effectiveness/Outcome Issues Following ACoA Aneurysm

As explained in Chapters 1 and 2, few studies have examined the cost-effective benefits of neuropsychological services and rehabilitation services. To our knowledge, no studies exist on the cost-effectiveness of neuropsychological services with ACoA patients. Cost-effectiveness studies often compare the costs of an intervention using non-dollar outcome measures (see Chapters 1 and 2). Only a handful of case studies have reported some overall benefits of neuropsychological assessment or cognitive rehabilitation efforts with ACoA patients. This section will outline issues of cost-effectiveness in ACoA patients and present research ideas to begin to address the question of cost-effectiveness of neuropsychological services with ACoA patients.

Cost-Effectiveness

Reports of cost and intervention efficacy for ACoA patients are embedded within studies reporting overall estimations for stroke and SAH populations (e.g., annual report of the National Stroke Association). However, drawing conclusions regarding cost and effectiveness among ACoA individuals from these studies can present significant problems, as ACoA patients may have very different neuropsychological and rehabilitation needs from, for instance, those with ischemic stroke. For example, reports examining cost and type of treatment among stroke patients may be based on physical or speech-related services, which are frequent areas of disability following stroke (see Chapter 6). However, for ACoA patients this may provide an inaccurate estimation of cost and effectiveness, as many ACoA patients do not experience significant physical disabilities or traditional speech-related impairments. Similarly, ischemic stroke patients typically are elderly adults, which may influence both the type of interventions selected and overall treatment goals. By contrast, ACoA patients often are younger adults, so treatment goals may focus on different aspects, such as returning to work. Thus, extrapolating cost-effectiveness from stroke or SAH studies can be misleading.

Given the lack of studies examining cost-effectiveness of neuropsychological services for ACoA patients, the need for specific research in this area is clear. One way to examine cost-effectiveness data in ACoA is to use data obtained from the traumatic brain injury (TBI) population. Given that the salient deficits in ACoA patients are cognitive and behavioral, with minimal physical limitations, ACoA patients traditionally are admitted to brain-injury rehabilitation units and not stroke rehabilitation units. Therefore, it can be argued that cost and effectiveness of treatment in ACoA may be more comparable to that of patients with TBI. However, there are some differences with TBI that need to be addressed as well. For instance, unlike TBI, the ACoA population tends to be primarily female. As such, issues that may be gender-sensitive need to be taken into account in any such studies. Nonetheless, using this approach in conjunction with the objective markers of value suggested by Prigatano et al. (see Chapter 2), some predictions can be made regarding the benefits of neuropsychological services in ACoA patients, and areas for future investigation can be discussed.

Cost-Benefit Ratio. The first objective marker suggested by Prigatano et al. (see Chapter 2) is the cost–benefit ratio calculated as a result of objectively describing a patient's higher cerebral functioning. Although there is ample research to document the nature and severity of potential cognitive problems after ACoA aneurysm, there are no studies relating this to cost–benefit analysis. However, anecdotal evidence can be found in most clinics and practices. For instance, in the previous description of patient DG, the cost savings resulting from the information provided by the neuropsychologist are clearly apparent. If the VP shunt was never inserted and patient DG remained in her abulic state, the likelihood of being discharged to a nursing home rather than home to her family would have increased dramatically. In monetary value, a saving of approximately $1,458,750 can be estimated. That is, given the current life expectancy (approximately 79 years for a White female) and current cost of both subacute rehabilitation (approximately $400 per day) and long-term care ($215 per day), follow-up care for 60-year-old DG would have cost $72,000 (for 6 months of subacute) and $1,386,750 (for 18.6 years of long-term care). This cost savings (financial) alone is significant, not to mention the psychosocial well-being costs for the patient and family. The same is true for the case study by DeLuca and Locker (1996) of an ACoA amnesic who, after receiving intensive cognitive rehabilitation for over a year, was able to return to a lifestyle similar to his premorbid level, including returning to work part-time as a college professor. The cost savings associated with not going on disability and remaining a productive member of society are significant. From the TBI literature, we know that early and accurate objective measurement of cognitive difficulties can provide targeted interventions that can reduce length of stay, minimize secondary complications, and improve functional level/outcome at discharge (Morgan, Chapman, & Tokarski, 1988). However, although seemingly a logical extension from TBI, the effectiveness of such early interventions on ACoA outcome is unknown.

Effectiveness of Services. A second recommended objective marker of value for neuropsychological services is determining the effectiveness and guidance of various treatments. Reports of the effectiveness of neuropsychological interventions in ACoA patients are almost nonexistent. They are limited to anecdotal reports of patients being able to return to work following "rehabilitation" treatment (Vilkki, 1985) and patients demonstrating "fairly substantial improvement" at evaluation 5 to 10 years later, after receiving cognitive rehabilitation (Wilson, 1991). In the only case that clearly documented effectiveness (DeLuca & Locker, 1996) reported on an ACoA amnesic who, after receiving intensive cognitive rehabilitation for over a year, was able to return to a lifestyle similar to his premorbid level, including returning to work part-time as a college professor. In the theoretical intervention program for the treatment of confabulation following ACoA aneurysm by DeLuca (1992) outlined above, a few case studies on effectiveness were presented.

Although such case studies and theoretical treatment approaches serve as examples in support of rehabilitation efforts in ACoA patients, they do not provide specific evidence for the cost-effective benefits of neuropsychological and rehabilitative services. What is truly needed is systematic documentation that such an intervention is successful, followed by randomized controlled clinical trials. For example, among the TBI population the utility of neuropsychological services has been established by studies demonstrating that neuropsychologically oriented rehabilitation results in better outcome than traditional rehabilitation treatment (Prigatano et al., 1994). Although it would be tempting to assume that such treatment would be effective for ACoA patients, only clinical research trials can truly address such important questions.

Some objective benefits of the neuropsychological assessment in the guidance of the medical and surgical management of the ACoA patient have been illustrated. For patient KP (described earlier), the neuropsychologist was able to provide critically useful information to the neurosurgeon and family to help in deciding whether surgery for clipping of the ACoA aneurysm was appropriate. In this sense, the cost (not just financial) of the surgical intervention was assessed with the aid of the neuropsychological information provided.

Another example of treatment direction benefiting from neuropsychological services is with pharmacological interventions. Clinically, it is not uncommon for physicians to use pharmacological agents to address various cognitive and behavioral changes. However, studies to guide such usage in ACoA patients are virtually nonexistent. Using TBI as a model, various studies have examined the effectiveness of specific pharmacological agents in relation to specific cognitive or behavioral impairments in TBI (McDowell, Whyte, & D'Esposito, 1998; Whyte et al., 1997). Although it is again tempting to generalize the knowledge from these TBI studies to those with ACoA aneurysm, caution is advised. Once again, examining the specific benefits of pharmacological intervention for specific ACoA symptoms (e.g., confabulation, apathy, and memory) and their relationship to rehabilitation performance is needed to address issues of efficacy and cost-effectiveness with ACoA patients. The role of the neuropsychologist in designing, measuring, and analyzing such studies is clear.

Providing the Continuum of Care. Continuum of care and improvement in quality of life also can serve as objective markers of value for neuropsychological services. Little is known about the continuum of care with ACoA patients. In general, we know that after acute inpatient care, a minority of ACoA patients are sent for rehabilitation services (interestingly, usually to brain-trauma units rather than stroke units). It is not clear where the other ACoA patients go after acute care, but locales include home and nursing homes. How decisions are made in determining the need for further rehabilitation is unclear. Traditionally, the decision for additional treatment is made on a case-by-case basis, and often is dependent on the treating physician's observations and experience. Studies examining neuropsychological variables and services at the acute level to help identify essential elements for determining rehabilitation eligibility would be fruitful. One idea for a research project is to retrospectively identify ACoA patients who have and have not attended postacute, inpatient rehabilitation services. Identifying medical variables (e.g., grade at presentation, the presence of vasospasm, and hydrocephalus), clinical variables (such as the acute presence of confabulation, amnesia, or personality change), and postdischarge psychosocial variables (e.g., return to work, social functioning) may yield important information on which variables may be critical in making discharge decisions from the acute hospital. One would expect that severity of cognitive difficulties would be a major factor, arguing for the need for such services early in the management and treatment of ACoA patients.

For those ACoA patients who receive inpatient rehabilitation services, much work is needed to fully examine the potential benefits of rehabilitation. For instance, among TBI patients the benefits of receiving inpatient rehabilitation have been demonstrated through better outcomes of self-care abilities, living arrangements, and vocational status compared to individuals who do not receive formal rehabilitation (Aronow, 1987). In general, vocation rehabilitation services have been demonstrated to be cost-effective in TBI and reportedly result in a reduction of dependency on public assistance (Abrams, Barker, Haffey, & Nelson, 1993). The value of such services for ACoA patients has not been adequately evaluated and is an open area for research. Relatedly, little is known about return to work among those ACoA patients who receive inpatient rehabilitation. Among TBI cost-effective studies, vocational and return-to-work variables are common and important outcome areas by which the success of rehabilitation programs are measured (Malec & Bashford, 1996; Wehman, West, Kregal, Sherron, & Zasler, 1995). Such studies have shown that a greater percentage of individuals who do not receive rehabilitation services suffer from long-term unemployment, compared to those who do receive services (Johnstone, Schopp, Harper, & Koscuilek, 1999; Malec & Bashford, 1996). Similar studies with ACoA patients would be helpful in understanding the impact of the continuum of care on functional outcome.

Impact on Physicians. The final source of value of the clinical neuropsychologist is the impact on physicians. Because cognitive difficulties are the primary problems observed after ACoA aneurysm, the clinical neuropsychologist is in a unique position to aid the physician and the treating team with regard to management and need for rehabilitation services. As illustrated with patient KP, the neuropsychologist can provide the surgeon with useful information, which can be used in making determinations of whether to perform surgical intervention. Similarly, patient DG's case illustrates how knowledge of course and potential interventions to improve functional status can have a substantial impact on clinical status, functional outcome, and financial burden. Designing programs for behavioral intervention (e.g., rehabilitation of confabulation) can become the central focus of rehabilitation. Lastly, objective assessment of cognitive and emotional processes is the key to making determinations for rehabilitation. As such, the neuropsychologist should play a major role in determining rehabilitation needs and effectiveness of the intervention.

Regarding potential research, because of the potential for pre- and postsurgical assessments, patients who are candidates for surgical interventions for repair of cerebral aneurysms provide a unique opportunity for the neuropsychologist to examine intervention effectiveness. We are unaware of any such studies. The information such a study would yield could have significant implications for the utility and cost-effectiveness of neuropsychological services in the assessment and treatment of ACoA aneurysm.

☐ Conclusion

The neuropsychologist can provide a variety of important and sometimes critical services in the treatment of ACoA survivors. Depending on which level of treatment the patient is receiving, these services vary significantly. The major role of the neuropsychologist remains documenting the cognitive, behavioral, and emotional strengths and weaknesses after ACoA aneurysm. However, given that these problems are the major issues for the ACoA population, the role of the neuropsychologist in treatment planning and posttreatment placement becomes essential. In general, a neuropsychologist with a good foundation and understanding of the neurobehavioral consequences of ACoA can provide important support for the patient, family, and other treating specialists. The need for outcome-oriented research demonstrating the cost-effectiveness of neuropsychological services is grossly lacking. Potential areas of research outlining the cost-effectiveness of neuropsychological services have been outlined. It is hoped that such ideas will help spawn a new area of research interest for neuropsychologists.

☐ References

Abe, K., Inokawa, M., Kashiwagi, A., & Yanagihara, T. (1998). Amnesia after a discrete basal forebrain lesion. *Journal of Neurology, Neurosurgery, and Psychiatry, 65,* 126–130.

Abrams, D., Barker, L. T., Haffey, W., & Nelson, H. (1993). The economics of return to work for survivors of traumatic brain injury: Vocational services are worth the investment. *Journal of Head Trauma Rehabilitation, 8,* 59–76.

Adams, H. P., & Biller, J. (1992). Hemorrhagic intracranial vascular disease. *Clinical Neurology, 2,* 1–64.

Alexander, M. P., & Freedman, M. (1984). Amnesia after anterior communicating artery aneurysm rupture. *Neurology, 34*(6), 752–757.

Aronow, H. U. (1987). Rehabilitation effectiveness with severe brain injury: Translating research into policy. *Journal of Head Trauma Rehabilitation, 2,* 24–34.

Banks, G., Short, P., Martinez, J., Latchaw, R., Ratcliff, G., & Boller, F. (1989). The alien hand syndrome: Clinical and postmortem findings. *Archives of Neurology, 46*(4), 456–459.

Blumer, D., & Benson, D. F. (1975). *Psychiatric aspects of neurological disease.* New York: Grune & Stratton.

Bondi, M. W., Kaszniak, A. W., Rapcsak, S. Z., & Butters, M. A. (1993). Implicit and explicit memory following anterior communicating artery aneurysm rupture. *Brain and Cognition, 22,* 213–229.

Bornstein, R. A., Weir, B. K., Petruk, K. C., & Disney, L. B. (1987). Neuropsychological function in patients after subarachnoid hemorrhage. *Neurosurgery, 21*(5), 651–654.

Bottger, S., Prosiegel, M., Steiger, H. J., & Yassouridis, A. (1998). Neurobehavioral disturbances, rehabilitation outcome, and lesion site in patients after rupture and repair of anterior communicating artery aneurysm. *Journal of Neurology, Neurosurgery, and Psychiatry, 65*(1), 93–102.

Carpenter, M. B. (1991). Blood supply of the central nervous system. In T. S. Satterfield (Ed.), *Core Text of Neuroanatomy, 4th ed.* (p. 444). Baltimore: Williams & Wilkins.

Chan, J.-L., & Liu, A.-B. (1999). Anatomical correlates of alien hand syndromes. *Neuropsychiatry, Neuropsychology, and Behavioral Neurology, 12,* 149–155.

Corkin, S., Cohen, N. J., Sullivan, E. V., Clegg, R. A., Rosen, T. J., & Ackerman, R. H. (1985). Analyses of global memory impairments of different etiologies. *Annals of the New York Academy Sciences, 444,* 10–40.

Crowell, R. M., & Morawetz, R. B. (1977). The anterior communicating artery has significant branches. *Stroke, 8*(2), 272–273.

Crosson, B., Poeschel Barco, P., Velozo, C. A., et al. (1989). Awareness and compensation in postacute head injury rehabilitation. *Journal of Head Trauma Rehabilitation, 4,* 46–54.

D'Esposito, M., Alexander, M. P., Fischer, R., McGlinchey-Berroth, R., & O'Connor, M. (1996). Recovery of memory and executive function following anterior communicating artery aneurysm rupture. *Journal of the International Neuropsychological Society, 2*(6), 565–570.

Damasio, A. R., Graff-Radford, N. R., Eslinger, P. J., Damasio, H., & Kassell, N. (1985). Amnesia following basal forebrain lesions. *Archives of Neurology, 42*(3), 263–271.

DeLuca, J. (1992). Cognitive dysfunction after aneurysm of the anterior communicating artery. *Journal of Clinical and Experimental Neuropsychology, 14*(6), 924–934.

DeLuca, J. (1993). Predicting neurobehavioral patterns following anterior communicating artery aneurysm. *Cortex, 29*(4), 639–647.

DeLuca, J., & Chiaravalloti, N. D. (in press). Neuropsychological consequences of ruptured aneurysms of the anterior communicating artery. In J. E. Harrison & A. M. Owen (Eds.), *Cognitive deficits in brain disorders* (pp. 00–00). London: Martin Duntz.

DeLuca, J., & Cicerone, K. D. (1989). Cognitive impairments following anterior communicating artery aneurysm. *Journal of Clinical and Experimental Neuropsychology, 11,* 47.

DeLuca, J., & Cicerone, K. D. (1991). Confabulation following aneurysm of the anterior communicating artery. *Cortex, 27*(3), 417–423.

DeLuca, J., & Diamond, B. J. (1995). Aneurysm of the anterior communicating artery: A review of neuroanatomical and neuropsychological sequelae. *Journal of Clinical and Experimental Neuropsychology, 17*(1), 100–121.

DeLuca, J., & Locker, R. (1996). Cognitive rehabilitation following anterior communicating artery aneurysm bleeding: a case report. *Disability and Rehabilitation, 18*(5), 265–272.

Diamond, B. J., DeLuca, J., & Kelley, S. M. (1997). Memory and executive functions in amnesic and non-amnesic patients with aneurysms of the anterior communicating artery. *Brain, 120*(6), 1015–1025.

Drumm, D. A., Greene, K. A., & Marciano, F. F. (1993). Neurobehavioral deficits following rupture of the arterior communicating artery (ACoA): The ACoA aneurysm syndrome. *BNI Quarterly, 9*, 9.

Dunker, R. O., & Harris, A. B. (1976). Surgical anatomy of the proximal anterior cerebral artery. *Journal of Neurosurgery, 44*(3), 359–367.

Fischer, R. S., Alexander, M. P., D'Esposito, M., & Otto, R. (1995). Neuropsychological and neuroanatomical correlates of confabulation. *Journal of Clinical and Experimental Neuropsychology, 17*(1), 20–28.

Gade, A. (1982). Amnesia after operations on aneurysms of the anterior communicating artery. *Surgical Neurology, 18*(1), 46–49.

Gade, A., & Mortensen, E. L. (1990). Temporal gradient in the remote memory impairment of amnesic patients with lesions in the basal forebrain. *Neuropsychologia, 9*, 985–1001.

Hashimoto, R., Tanaka, Y., & Nakano, I. (2000). Amnesic confabulatory syndrome after focal basal forebrain damage. *Neurology, 54*, 978–980.

Hori, S., & Suzuki, J. (1979). Early and late results of intracranial direct surgery of anterior communicating artery aneurysms. *Journal of Neurosurgery, 50*(4), 433–440.

Irle, E,. Wowra, B., Kunert, H. J., Hampl, J., & Kunze, S. (1992). Memory disturbances following anterior communicating artery rupture. *Annals of Neurology, 31*(5), 473–480.

Johnstone, B., Schopp, L. H., Harper, J., & Koscuilek, J. (1999). Neuropsychological impairments, vocational outcome and financial costs for individuals with traumatic brain injury receiving state vocational rehabilitation services. *Journal of Head Trauma Rehabilitation, 4*, 220–232.

Kapur, N., & Coughlan, A. K. (1980). Confabulation and frontal lobe dysfunction. *Journal of Neurology, Neurosurgery, and Psychiatry, 43*(5), 461–463.

Laiacona, M., De Santis, A., Barbarotto, R., Basso, A., Spagnoli, D., & Capitani, E. (1989). Neuropsychological follow-up of patients operated for aneurysms of anterior communicating artery. *Cortex, 25*(2), 261–273.

Larsson, C., Ronnberg, J., Forssell, A., Nilsson, L. G., Lindberg, M., & Angquist, K. A. (1989). Verbal memory function after subarachnoid haemorrhage determined by the localization of the ruptured aneurysm. *British Journal of Neurosurgery, 3*(5), 549–560.

Leng, N. R., & Parkin, A. J. (1988). Amnesic patients can benefit from instructions to use imagery: Evidence against the cognitive mediation hypothesis. *Cortex, 24*(1), 33–39.

Lindqvist, G., & Norlen, G. (1966). Korsakoff's syndrome after operation on ruptured aneurysm of the anterior communicating artery. *Acta Psychiatrica Scandinavia, 42*(1), 24–34.

Ljunggren, B., Sonesson, B., Saveland, H., & Brandt, L. (1985). Cognitive impairment and adjustment in patients without neurological deficits after aneurysmal SAH and early operation. *Journal of Neurosurgery, 62*(5), 673–679.

Logue, V., Durward, M., Pratt, R. T., Piercy, M., & Nixon, W. L. (1968). The quality of survival after rupture of an anterior cerebral aneurysm. *British Journal of Psychiatry, 114*(507), 137–160.

Luria, A. R. (1973). *The working brain*. New York: Basic Books.

Luria, A. R. (1980). *Higher cortical functions in man*. New York: Basic Books.

Maiuri, F., Gangemi, M., Corriero, G., & D'Andrea, F. (1986). Anterior communicating artery aneurysm presenting with sudden paraplegia. *Surgical Neurology, 25*(4), 397–398.

Malec, J. F., & Bashford, J. S. (1996). Post acute brain injury rehabilitation. *Archives of Physical Medicine and Rehabilitation, 77*, 198–207.

McCormick, W. F. (1984). Pathology and pathogenesis of intracranial saccular aneurysms. *Seminars in Neurology, 4*(3), 291–303.

McDowell, S., Whyte, J., & D' Esposito, M. (1998). Differential effect of dopaminergic agonist on prefrontal function of traumatic brain injury patients. *Brain, 121*, 1155–1164.

Mercer, B., Wapner, W., Gardner, H., & Benson, D. F. (1977). A study of confabulation. *Archives of Neurology, 34*(7), 429–433.

Morgan, A. S., Chapman, P., & Tokarski, L. (1988, January). *Improved care for the traumatically brain injured.* Paper presented at the Easter Association for Surgery of Trauma, First Annual Conference, Longboat Key, FL.

Moscovitch, M., & Melo, B. (1997). Strategic retrieval and the frontal lobes: Evidence from confabulation and amnesia. *Neuropsychologia, 35*(7), 1017–1034.

Ogden, J. A., Mee, E. W., & Henning, M. (1993). A prospective study of impairment of cognition and memory and recovery after subarachnoid hemorrhage. *Neurosurgery, 33*(4), 572–586.

Ohno, K., Masaoka, H., Suzuki, R., Monma, S., & Matsushima, Y. (1991). Symptomatic cerebral vasospasm of unusually late onset after aneurysm rupture. *Acta Neurochirurgica, 108*(3–4), 163–166.

Okawa, M., Maeda, S., Nukui, H., & Kawafuchi, J. (1980). Psychiatric symptoms in ruptured anterior communicating aneurysms: Social prognosis. *Acta Psychiatrica Scandinavica, 61*(4), 306–312.

Parkin, A. J., Leng, N. R., Stanhope, N., & Smith, A. P. (1988). Memory impairment following ruptured aneurysm of the anterior communicating artery. *Brain and Cognition, 7*(2), 231–243.

Prigatano, G. P., Klonoff, P. S., O'Brien, K. P., Altman, I. M., Amin, K., Chiapello, D., Shepherd, J., Cunningham, M., & Mora, M. (1994). Productivity after neuropsychological oriented milieu rehabilitation. *Journal of Head Trauma Rehabilitation, 9*, 91–102.

Richardson, J. T. (1991). Cognitive performance following rupture and repair of intracranial aneurysm. *Acta Neurologica Scandinavica, 83*(2), 10–22.

Rinkel, G., Djibuti, M., Algra, A., & van Gijn, J. (1998). Prevalence and risk of rupture of intracranial aneurysms: A systematic review. *Stroke, 29*, 251–256.

Roos, Y. B., deHaan, R. J., Beenen, L. F., Groen, R. J., Albrecht, K. W., & Vermeulen, M. (2000). Complications and outcome in patients with aneurysmal subarachnoid haemorrhage: A prospective hospital based cohort study in the Netherlands. *Journal of Neurology, Neurosurgery, and Psychiatry, 68*, 337–341.

Saveland, H. (1992). Overall outcome in aneurysmal subarachnoid hemorrhage. A prospective study from neurosurgical units in Sweden during a 1-year period. *Journal of Neurosurgery, 6*, 729–734.

Schnider, A., von Daniken, C., & Gutbrod, K. (1996). The mechanisms of spontaneous and provoked confabulations. *Brain, 119*, 1365–1375.

Sengupta, R. P., Chiu, J. S. P., & Brierley, H. (1975). Quality of survival following direct surgery for anterior communicating artery aneurysms. *Journal of Neurosurgery, 43*(1), 58–64.

Shoqeirat, M. A., Mayes, A., MacDonald, C., Meudell, P., & Pickering, A. (1990). Performance on tests sensitive to frontal lobe lesions by patients with organic amnesia: Leng & Parkin revisited [comment]. *British Journal of Clinical Psychology, 29*(4), 401–408.

Sonesson, B., Ljunggren, B., Saveland, H., & Brandt, L. (1987). Cognition and adjustment after late and early operation for ruptured aneurysm. *Neurosurgery, 21*(3), 279–287.

Squire, L. R., Shimamura, A. P., & Graf, P. (1987). Strength and duration of priming effects in normal subjects and amnesic patients. *Neuropsychologia, 25*(1B), 195–210.

Starkstein, S. E., Berthier, M. L., & Leiguarda, R. (1988). Disconnection syndrome in a right-handed patient with right hemispheric speech dominance. *European Neurology, 28*(4), 187–190.

Steinman, S. E., & Bigler, E. D. (1986). Neuropsychological sequelae of ruptured anterior communicating artery aneurysm. *International Journal of Clinical Neuropsychology, 8*, 135–140.

Stenhouse, L. M., Knight, R. G., Longmore, B. E., & Bishara, S. N. (1991). Long-term cognitive deficits in patients after surgery on aneurysms of the anterior communicating artery. *Journal of Neurology, Neurosurgery, and Psychiatry, 54*(10), 909–914.

Storey, P. B. (1970). Brain damage and personality change after subarachnoid haemorrhage. *British Journal of Psychiatry, 117*, 129–142.

Stuss, D. T., Alexander, M. P., Lieberman, A., & Levine, H. (1978). An extraordinary form of confabulation. *Neurology, 28*(11), 1166–1172.

Talland, G. A., Sweet, W. H., & Ballantine, H. T., Jr. (1967). Amnesic syndrome with anterior communicating artery aneurysm. *Journal of Nervous Mental Disease, 145*(3), 179–192.

Tanaka, Y., Bachman, D. L., & Miyazaki, M. (1991). Pharmacotherapy for akinesia following anterior communicating artery aneurysm hemorrhage. *Japanese Journal of Medicine, 30*(6), 542–544.

Tatu, L., Moulin, T., Bogousslavsky, J., & Duvernoy, H. (1998). Arterial territories of the human brain: cerebral hemispheres. *Neurology, 50*(6), 1699–1708.

Teissier du Cros, J., & Lhermitte, F. (1984). Neuropsychological analysis of ruptured saccular aneurysms of the anterior communicating artery after radical therapy (32 cases). *Surgical Neurology,* 22(4), 353–359.

Tidswell P., Dias, P. S., Sagar, H. J., Mayes, A. R., & Battersby, R. D. (1995). Cognitive outcome after aneurysm rupture: relationship to aneurysm site and perioperative complications. *Neurology 45*(5), 875–882.

Vilkki, J. (1985). Amnesic syndromes after surgery of anterior communicating artery aneurysms. *Cortex, 21*(3), 431–444.

Vilkki, J., Holst, P., Ohman, J., Servo, A., & Heiskanen, O. (1990). Social outcome related to cognitive performance and computed tomographic findings after surgery for a ruptured intracranial aneurysm. *Neurosurgery, 26*(4), 579–584.

Volpe, B. T., & Hirst, W. (1983). Amnesia following the rupture and repair of an anterior communicating artery aneurysm. *Journal of Neurology, Neurosurgery, and Psychiatry, 46*(8), 704–709.

Wehman, P., West, M. D., Kregal, J., Sherron, P., & Zasler, N. (1995). Return to work for person with severe traumatic brain injury: a data-based approach to program development. *Journal of Head Trauma Rehabilitation, 10,* 27–39.

Wilson, B. W. (1991). Long-term prognosis of patients with severe memory disorders. *Neuropsychology Rehabilitation, 1,* 117–134.

Whyte, J., Hart, T., Schuster, K., Fleming, M., Polansky, M, & Coslett, B. H. (1997). Effects of methylphenidate on attentional function after traumatic brain injury: A randomized, placebo-controlled trial. *American Journal of Physical Medicine and Rehabilitation, 76,* 440–450.

PART

III

NEOPLASMS

8 CHAPTER

Christina A. Meyers
Scott B. Cantor

Neuropsychological Assessment and Treatment of Patients with Malignant Brain Tumors

Introduction

The clinical utility and cost-effectiveness of neuropsychological services for patients with diseases that progress relatively rapidly to death are controversial. Until recently, neuropsychological services for patients with malignant brain tumors were rarely performed, because their value was assumed to be minimal compared to their cost. However, the value of such services is increasingly being recognized. Part of this recognition stems from the improved survival of certain brain-tumor patients, with the resulting need for disability evaluations, rehabilitation, and other typical uses of neuropsychological services outlined in Chapter 2. However, it has been increasingly recognized that neuropsychological evaluations are of value in medical decision making, in palliative as well as rehabilitative interventions, and in evaluating the risks versus benefits of new anticancer treatments and technologies. Primary brain cancer continues to be a highly serious health problem for which there is no effective cure. However, neuropsychological services can have a major impact on the ability to reduce symptoms and improve the physical and psychological health of these individuals.

Primary Malignant Brain Tumors

The incidence of primary malignant brain tumors is small compared to other cancers. Although approximately 14,800 new cases of malignant glioma are diagnosed in the United States per year, these tumors are associated with significant morbidity and mortality and account for 13,000 deaths per year (Wrensch, Minn, & Bondy, 2000). In fact, death from brain tumors is the second leading cause of death from neurologic disease after stroke (Radhakrishnan, Bonen, & Kurland, 1994). Estimated 2- and 5-year relative survival rates for all types of CNS tumors and 36% and 27%, respectively (Davis, McCarthy, Freels, Kupelian, & Bondy, 1999). However, there is a strong influence of age and specific histologic type of tumor on survival. Over the past 20 years, there has been no improvement in survival for patients with glioblastoma multiforme or those whose age exceeds 65 at diagnosis. Seventy-two percent of younger patients (under 44 years) with anaplastic astrocytomas survive 2 years, compared to 2% of older patients with glioblastoma multiforme and 7% of older patients with anaplastic astrocytoma (Wrensch et al., 2000). Further, tumors in the majority of patients diagnosed with "benign" low-grade gliomas will undergo malignant transformation as some point. Thus, the median survival for most patients diagnosed with this supposedly nonmalignant tumor is 4 to 7 years, with a 10-year survival rate of only 15% to 45% of patients—hardly a benign process (Bernstein & Bampoe, 2000).

In addition to primary brain tumors, there are more than 100,000 new cases of brain tumors that are metastatic from other sites in the body each year (Lang, Wildrick, & Sawaya, 2000). Most new cases develop from lung cancer, but patients with melanoma are at the highest risk (40% to 60%) for developing brain metastases. Many patients have multiple metastatic sites in the brain. Similar to primary-brain-tumor patients, these patients also suffer from the effects of expanding mass lesions as well as neurotoxic side effects of CNS treatment. Thus, there are considerable numbers of cancer patients who have brain involvement with resulting neurocognitive impairment.

Even though primary brain tumors are relatively rare, they account for a great deal of disability. In a global burden of disease study, it was found that neurologic and psychiatric illnesses accounted for only 1.4% of all deaths but 28% of all disabilities (cited in Holden, 2000).

Brain dysfunction caused by brain tumors is multifactorial and related to lesion site, lesion momentum, and treatment effects. Impairments due to tumor site are typically cortical in nature and follow usual brain-behavior patterns (e.g., patients with temporal lobe tumors generally experience difficulties with memory). However, primary brain tumors grow by infiltrating normal brain tissue, and thus site-related deficits tend to be milder and more variable than focal lesions that are of sudden onset (Anderson, Damasio, & Tranel, 1990). Lesion momentum is a critical factor in the manifestation of cognitive deficits. Rapidly progressing tumors may cause devastating neurocognitive impairments due to increased intracranial pressure and inability of the brain to adapt, whereas slowly growing tumors may allow for considerable cerebral plasticity and reorganization of function. For example, Figure 8.1 shows the brain CT scan of a 25-year-old individual who underwent resection of an extensive left-hemisphere tumor. The resection included portions of the left frontal, temporal, and parietal lobes down to the brain stem. Postoperatively, the patient had no detectable cognitive impairments, with total preservation of verbal memory and language function. Of note, this person switched hand dominance rather suddenly at age 5½, from right- to left-handed (Meyers, Berman, Hayman, & Evankovick, 1992). In contrast, Figure 8.2 displays the MRI scan of a somewhat smaller lesion in the same area. This individual developed a global aphasia, alexia, and agraphia over a 2-week period, suggesting a very rapidly growing tumor.

Treatment, particularly radiation therapy, tends to affect the subcortical white matter, causing impairments in cognitive speed, "executive" functions (e.g., apathy, perseveration), memory, sustained attention, and motor coordination. Some patients

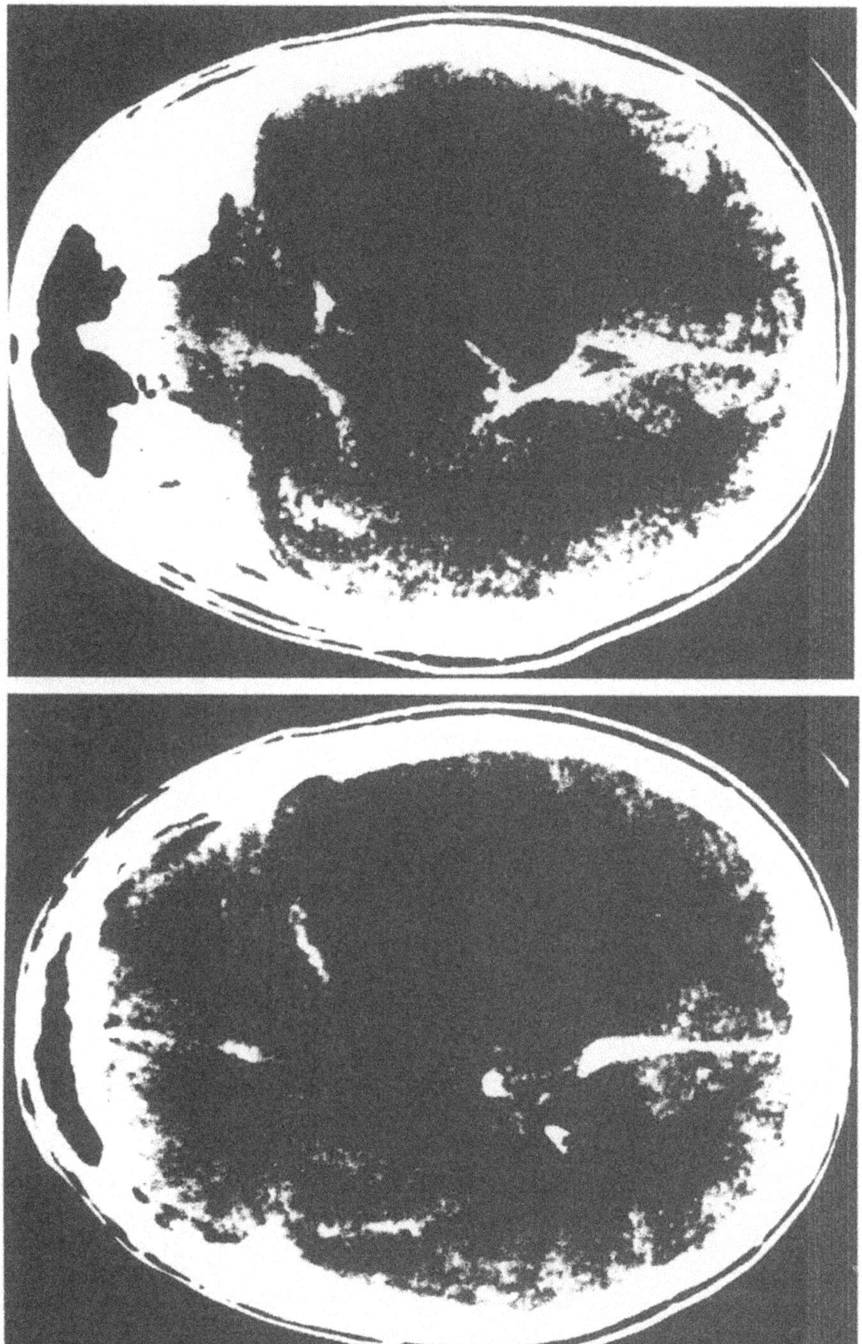

FIGURE 8.1. Preoperative CT scan of a huge tumor occupying the left temporal lobe extending into the frontal and parietal regions in patient with no detectable neurocognitive impairments.

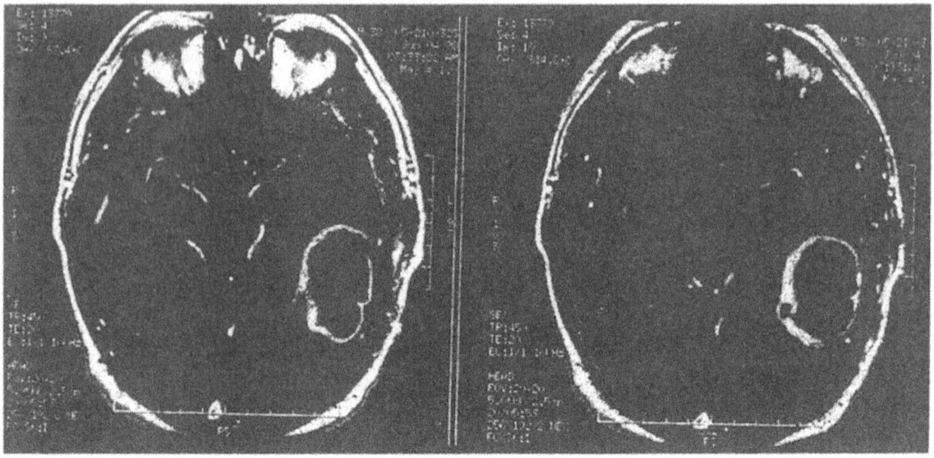

FIGURE 8.2. Preoperative MRI of a smaller lesion in a similar location. This patient had significant impairments of expressive speech, comprehension, reading, and writing.

develop an outright treatment-related dementia that may even lead to death (Meyers, Hess, Yung, & Levin, 2000). The adverse effects of chemotherapy are less well described and generally considered to be acute and reversible unless delivered intraventricularly. However, immunotherapy, such as treatment with interferon-alpha, may have profound effects on cognition and mood. These agents have effects on brain neurotransmitters, neuroendocrine function, and induction of neurotoxic proinflammatory cytokines (Valentine, Meyers, Kling, Richelson, & Hauser, 1998). Although not well studied as of yet, there also is concern that hormone ablation therapy (such as tamoxifen) will have adverse effects on cognitive function due to effects on neurotransmitter and cytokine systems. In addition, brain-tumor patients experience medical complications from treatment as well as side effects of adjuvant medications such as steroids. Steroids are used very frequently to control edema caused by the tumor and treatment. These medications may have significant effects on memory and mood, including emotional lability, major depression, mania, and delirium. Common medical complications include endocrine dysfunction; only 23% of treated brain-tumor patients have normal thyroid, gonadal, and adrenal hormone levels (Arlt et al., 1997). Another frequent medical complication is seizures. Seizures occur in 50% to 70% of patients at some time during the course of the disease. Persistent seizures reduce cognitive efficiency and exacerbate underlying cognitive deficits. Finally, most brain-tumor patients experience significant cancer-related fatigue. This fatigue is characterized by an unusual, persistent tiredness that does not respond much to rest. The mechanisms by which fatigue occurs in cancer patients is not known, but it is likely related to hemoglobin level, cytokines such as interleukin-6 that are secreted by the cancer cells and induced by treatment, and hormonal deficiencies (Cleeland, 2001). Many patients are nearly incapacitated by fatigue and as a consequence are severely limited in their daily activities, even when cognitive dysfunction is not prominent.

Resource Utilization for the Treatment of Malignant Brain Tumors

Most patients with brain tumors undergo surgical excision, radiotherapy, and chemotherapy. Many require reoperation due to tumor recurrence or radiation necrosis, and most need additional systemic treatment. These patients require frequent neuroimaging studies, as well as palliation of symptoms and terminal care. Even those patients with stable, low-grade tumors require frequent surveillance, due to the high risk of malignant transformation of the tumor. A cost-of-treatment model developed for a major pharmaceutical company in 1996 estimated that over a 12-month period patients with malignant tumors typically need 2 surgical procedures, 4 courses of chemotherapy, 11 months of monitoring (including 1 CT scan every 3 months), and 4.5 months of palliation. The estimated cost was approximately $138,500 (1995 dollars). This number underrepresents the current cost of usual care, which would include more frequent neuroimaging with magnetic resonance (MR) imaging as well as more chemotherapy treatments.

Monitoring that includes a brief neuropsychological assessment every 3 months would add only about $1,200 per year and yet provide more detailed evaluation of patient response to treatment, affecting medical decision making and providing information relevant to intervention strategies, palliation, and disability.

Brain cancer also has a significant impact on society. Costs to employers include absenteeism, lack of productivity, and need to pay for medical disability and drug costs (Menon & Assiff, 2000). The burdens to the caregiver include loss of caregiver's income in addition to the patient's loss of income, payment for assistance in the home, and other economic impacts.

Utility of Neuropsychological Assessment and Treatment for Brain-Tumor Patients

Table 8.1 summarizes the utility of neuropsychological services for brain-tumor patients. Neuropsychological assessment can improve clinical outcomes by helping to provide a more appropriate decision threshold for the treatment of brain-tumor patients (Swets, Daws, & Monhan, 2000). This includes the decision to continue or change antineoplastic treatment, whether interventions have efficacy, and whether new treatments offer more favorable risk–benefit ratios. Patients with stable, low-grade tumors that are undergoing malignant transformation can be flagged earlier, even before anatomic evidence of tumor progression. Other areas of impact include issues regarding differential diagnosis to assist patient management, rehabilitative and palliative interventions, and end-of-life care.

Assessment Issues

Although it is the standard practice of neurologists and other health-care professionals to rely on brief assessments of mental status, more extensive neuropsychological testing often is needed. Brain-tumor patients manifest different cognitive impairments

TABLE 8.1. Utility of Neuropsychological Services for Brain-Tumor Patients

- Differential diagnosis and treatment
  - Tumor versus treatment effects
  - Psychiatric/dynamic versus neuropsychological conditions
- Treatment decisions
  - Prediction of survival of survival, prognosis
  - Aggressiveness of neurosurgery
  - Change or continuation of current brain-tumor therapy
- Patient care
  - Rehabilitation
  - Pharmacologic interventions for symptoms
  - Disability determinations
  - End-of-life care
- Clinical research
  - New drug approval
  - Safety/toxicity monitoring on clinical trials for risk-benefit analysis

secondary to tumors in varying locations, and there are different patterns of cognitive decline related to tumor progression and treatment effects (Scheibel, Meyers & Levin, 1996). One study highlighted the potential pitfalls when neuropsychological assessment is not utilized appropriately. The authors used the Mini Mental State Exam (MMSE) to monitor cognitive function in patients with high-grade gliomas undergoing radiation therapy and reported that no cognitive decline was observed (Taylor et al., 1998), despite the extensive literature contradicting this assertion. Brief examinations such as the MMSE only detect moderate to severe global cognitive impairment and are not sensitive or specific to deficits related to brain tumors or brain-tumor therapy. In another study, the MMSE was not able to detect significant declines in memory functioning related to a toxic new cancer treatment (Meyers et al., 1998). There is substantial risk that patients with true disability resulting from cognitive impairments would not be identified and offered appropriate interventions when an insensitive screening tool is used in the place of a neuropsychological assessment.

Furthermore, insensitive assessment tools may provide misleading information from clinical trials. For example, Chataway, Bleehen, Stenning, and Grant (1999) found that different outcome measures significantly altered the interpretation of a randomized clinical trial. When a World Health Organization (WHO) performance status scale was used to determine progression of disease, the difference between two doses of radiation therapy was highly significant ($p = 0.04$). When a scale specifically designed to measure neurologic status was utilized, there was no difference between the groups ($p = 0.94$).

Utility for Treatment Decisions

Neuropsychological assessments currently are used to monitor the functional status of brain-tumor patients to assist the primary treatment team in clinical decision making. For instance, neurocognitive tests are independent predictors of survival in brain-tumor patients (Meyers et al., 2000) and decline nearly a month in advance of neuroimaging evidence of tumor progression (Meyers et al., 1996). Thus, the decision as to whether to keep a patient on a specific treatment needs to consider his or her neurocognitive status as well as neuroimaging findings.

One common use for neuropsychological assessment is for neurosurgical planning. For instance, at our comprehensive cancer center, a young patient with a very large left temporal tumor was referred for preoperative neuropsychological assessment, functional MR imaging (fMRI), and the WADA procedure to help the neurosurgeon make decisions about the aggressiveness of the operative approach. Neuropsychological testing revealed impaired verbal memory but no evidence of receptive or expressive language disturbance. WADA testing revealed right hemisphere contributions to language, and fMRI also revealed bilateral expressive speech activation. Because the patient already had a severe memory deficit and the other assessments all pointed to bilateral speech representation, the surgeon decided to be aggressive and performed a total resection of the tumor. Postoperatively, the patient had no expressive speech disturbance.

Neuropsychological examinations also can be used to screen neurosurgical patients for cognitive deterioration postoperatively to detect early signs of complications. Cammermeyer and Evans (1998) reported that such evaluations expedited the diagnosis of treatable complications such as increased intracranial pressure, thus reducing the potential morbidity had the patients developed more severe and advanced symptoms. Another study found that preoperative language disturbance as assessed by neuropsychological testing was highly correlated with worsened language function postbiopsy, whereas patients without preoperative language dysfunction were a low risk for posttreatment dysphasia (Thomson, Taylor, Fraser, & Whittle, 1997). Thus, screening of brain-tumor patients presurgically can have a large impact on their postsurgical management.

Utility for Patient Care

Differential diagnosis of patient complaints and subjective symptoms is critical for effective palliation. For instance, many patients complain of "forgetfulness." This subjective complaint may be due to (a) restricted worrying memory capacity that limits the amount of information the patient can process, (b) problems with memory consolidation due to compromise of hippocampal structures and systems, (c) distractibility, (d) inefficient language comprehension, (e) a major mood disorder, or (f) sensory impairment such as loss of hearing. The interventions for each of these potential impairments might be quite different. Neuropsychological testing of functional status also is used to determine the suitability of pharmacologic and behavioral interventions and to monitor the efficacy of those interventions. For instance, methylphenidate has proved to be very helpful in improving cognitive functioning and functional status in primary brain-tumor patients, even in the setting of tumor progression and worsening radiation injury (Meyers, Weitzner, et al., 1998). These gains can be directly tied to lessened need for caregiving; some patients had improved gait with reduced risk of falls, others had more motivation to participate in their self-care activities, and one had increased bladder control that relieved her caregiver of assisting with toileting. Those patients who were working were better able to handle a full workload. The majority of patients also were able to reduce their glucocorticoid dose, thus cutting costs of medication and adverse side effects of steroids.

Cognitive rehabilitation only recently has been applied to brain-tumor patients because of the perceived dire prognosis and limited length of life. However, such interventions can prove to be beneficial and cost-effective both in the short run as well as in patients who are long-term survivors. For instance, postacute rehabilitation has been effective in selected brain-tumor patients. Sherer, Meyers, and Bergloff (1997) found that gains made in community independence and employment outcomes were maintained 8 months postdischarge, which is particularly impressive as most brain-tumor patients deteriorate over time due to disease progression or adverse effects of treatment. In addition, the treatment proved to be cost-effective; the average cost and length of stay was significantly less than is usual for a traumatic brain injured (TBI) population. The TBI patients required nearly twice as much treatment (length of stay 4.3 months compared to 2.6 months for the brain-tumor patients). The brain-tumor patients who graduated from this program also had increased financial independence, which requires less caregiver services and decreased reliance on social service programs and governmental assistance.

For those patients who have subtle impairments that impede their work efficiency but who may not require formal rehabilitation, neuropsychological assessment and intervention with employers to adapt the workplace environment is of benefit. We have found that patients were able to maintain gainful employment for a longer period of time with simple accommodations such as reducing ambient noise, allowing flexible deadlines for projects, and allowing flexible work hours to accommodate fatigue.

Another aspect of patient care involves end-of-life issues. Brain-tumor patients and their families face a complex terminal phase that includes cognitive deterioration, psychiatric and dynamic issues, and spiritual issues. The neuropsychologist is in the unique position of understanding both the neurologic and psychiatric concerns and to provide psychotherapy and make pharmacologic treatment recommendations under these circumstances. Considerable harm has been done to patients and families when they received counseling from someone unaware of the disease process and the neuropsychological contributors to marital strain, inappropriate behavior, and other cognitive and social sequelae of brain injury.

☐ Utility of Neuropsychological Evaluations for Clinical Research

Neuropsychological evaluations are being used for safety monitoring in clinical trials of new anticancer agents and in new strategies employing traditional therapies. As defined by a working group composed of members of the Food and Drug Administration (FDA), National Cancer Institute (NCI), and the NCI Division of Cancer Treatment Board of Scientific Counselors, net clinical benefit of cancer therapy includes (a) survival benefit, (b) time to treatment failure and disease-free survival, (c) complete response rate, (d) response rate, and (e) *beneficial effects on disease-related symptoms and/or quality of life* (O'Shaughnessy et al., 1991). In the case of brain cancer, which is characterized by progressive impairments of mental function, a beneficial treatment may be one that slows or stabilizes the progression of worsening symptoms, whether or not overall survival is extended.

Most new anticancer drugs for brain-tumor patients have very similar treatment outcomes (i.e., length of survival, time to tumor progression). Thus, a major rationale for choosing one over the other is the impact on neuropsychological function, such as rate of cognitive deterioration. Slowing cognitive deterioration also would save caregiving costs. This also applies to the analysis of new ways of delivering treatment. For example, radiation therapy continues to be the mainstay of brain-tumor treatment, and optimizing the efficacy of radiotherapy while minimizing the toxicity is a large area of clinical research. Altering fractionation (e.g., delivering the radiation more frequently) or dose and adding potential radiosensitizers are typical approaches. One study reported that children who received larger doses of radiation therapy for posterior fossa tumors had significanly poorer IQ scores and verbal comprehension than children who received lower doses, although long-term cognitive impairment occurred at all doses analyzed (Grill et al., 1999) Another study found that young children who received radiation therapy for brain tumors had not only cognitive decline but also growth and endocrine deficiencies that caused further morbidity, compared to children who did not receive radiation, and that survival was similar between the two groups (Moore, Ater, & Copeland, 1992). Serial neuropsychological evaluations also can determine the trajectory of treatment toxicity. For instance Vigliani, Sichez, Poisson, and Delattre (1996) found that patients with low-grade tumors suffered cognitive decline 6 months posttreatment, compared to nonradiated patients, but that these declines improved over the subsequent year to baseline levels, with only 1 in 17 irradiated patients suffering from continued cognitive deterioration over a 4-year interval. The careful evaluation of cognitive function in these trials is critical to determine risks and benefits of such manipulations (Groves et al., 1999).

☐ Objective and Subjective Indicators of Value

Objective markers of value of neuropsychological services include the reduction of other health costs because of improved management of patients with cognitive dysfunction. This includes trauma due to falls if the patient is unsupervised, inadvertent under- or overdosing of prescribed medications due to memory dysfunction, and management of comorbid conditions such as depression. Neuropsychological assessment also can assist with the appropriate differential diagnosis of conditions, such as frontal lobe apathy versus depression. The accurate diagnosis of such conditions is critical for appropriate treatment and patient safety.

Other objective markers of value include identifying patients who might be more vulnerable to developing adverse effects from their brain-tumor therapy because of preexisting conditions. For instance, elderly patients who develop brain tumors also may suffer from unrelated neurologic conditions such as Alzheimer's disease or cerebrovascular disease. Patients may have preexisting psychiatric disorders that compromise their ability to comply with their treatment regimen. Neuropsychological evaluations also contribute to the diagnostic decision process for disability determination.

Subjective markers of value for this patient population relate to quality of life, increased satisfaction at the workplace and at home, and ripple effects on the patient's family and social networks. Subjective value also relates to end-of-life care issues. At this stage of the disease, patients and families are frightened and confused. They often are more willing at this juncture than at any other time to spend money and resources on improving their quality of life and finding meaning in the process of dying. One study found that the burden associated with the morbidity induced by brain cancer was significant when a preference-based system for assessing health-related quality of life was used (Whitton, Rhydderch, Furlong, Feeny, & Barr, 1997). It was apparent from this study that the majority of brain-tumor patients have multiple problems that were not captured by their primary care physicians; in fact, only 1 patient in the sample of 50 reported no morbidity at all.

Education for patients and caregivers is essential to patient success and has the potential to reduce hospital visits and calls. Very early on, the results of the neuropsychological assessment are explained to the patient. Basic brain–behavior relationships are discussed, as well as the potential impact of the patient's impairments on his or daily life. Working in conjunction with the neuropsychologist, patients and family members are encouraged to set realistic goals and instructed in simple compensatory techniques to use at home (Anne Kayl, personal communication).

☐ Possible Outcome Studies for Neuropsychologists

Table 8.2 lists several examples of clinical problems that would benefit from various outcomes analyses. At this point, the value of neuropsychological services has not been sufficiently demonstrated to make them widely available to brain-tumor patients outside of major academic centers, where the value of clinical research is appreciated for itself. However, this will change in the next decade, as the plight of brain-tumor patients becomes a national priority. In July 2000, the Brain Tumor Progress Review Group, a committee jointly sponsored by the National Cancer Institute and the National Insti-

TABLE 8.2. Proposed Methodologies for the Clinical and Economic Assessment of Neuropsychological Interventions

- Efficacy of new pharmaceutical agents (hypothesis testing in randomized clinical trials)
  - Assessment of cost between two equivalent pharmaceutical agents—*cost-minimization analysis*
  - Assessment of impact of *toxic outcomes assessment*
  - Assessment of toxicity and cost between different techniques (e.g., radiosurgery vs. conventional surgery)—*cost-utility analysis*
  - Cost and clinical benefit of neuropsychological assessment vs. brief screening in clinical trials—*cost-effective analysis*
  - Evaluation of discriminative ability of new neuropsychological tests—*receiver operating characteristic curve (ROC) analysis*
- Efficacy of clinical services
  - Assessment of which individuals benefit from a given intervention—*regression analysis*
  - Assessment of cost-outcomes for intervening with family/caregiver-*cost-consequence analysis*
  - Cost-effectiveness of interventions for patients with short survival—*cost-effectiveness or cost-utility analysis*

tute of Neurological Disorders and Stroke, met to develop a national plan for the next decade of brain-tumor research. Prominent among the priorities was the expansion of research on the functional outcomes of brain-cancer patients and the development of interventions to enhance the functioning and quality of life of brain–tumor patients and their families (Brain Tumor Progress Review Group, November 2000). The report noted that cost-effectiveness of interventions needed to be built into research designs prospectively, in anticipation of eventual coverage of cost by third-party payers.

In the ideal scientific research paradigm, the utility of neuropsychological services (assessment, rehabilitation, education, etc.) in decreasing the disability experienced by brain-tumor patients would be evaluated by randomized clinical trials comparing such services to no treatment (i.e., the standard of care at most sites). However, it is highly unlikely that such randomized clinical trials should be performed. Therefore, decision analysis and cost-effectiveness analysis (Cantor, 1995) on neuropsychological services will need to be based on available clinical series to demonstrate the clinical and economic benefits of neuropsychological services.

Cost-Effectiveness of Neuropsychological Services: An Example

Figure 8.3 represents the decision tree for a hypothetical cost-effectiveness assessment of attention deficit by neuropsychological testing in a patient with a highly malignant brain tumor who is experiencing a poor quality of life, a common referral for cognitive testing in this patient population. In this simplified example, we are assuming that the patient has 1 year of life expectancy. The two clinical strategies are testing or no testing, represented by the square node, representing the decision. Should no testing occur, we would expect that the patient would have multiple neuropsychological deficits that are not well characterized, and thus be at additional risk of inappropriate management or inappropriate treatment.

The other branch represents the alternative of neuropsychological testing. The test battery is nearly perfect—that is, it has sensitivity and specificity close to one. If positive (attention deficits are uncovered), an intervention, including patient education

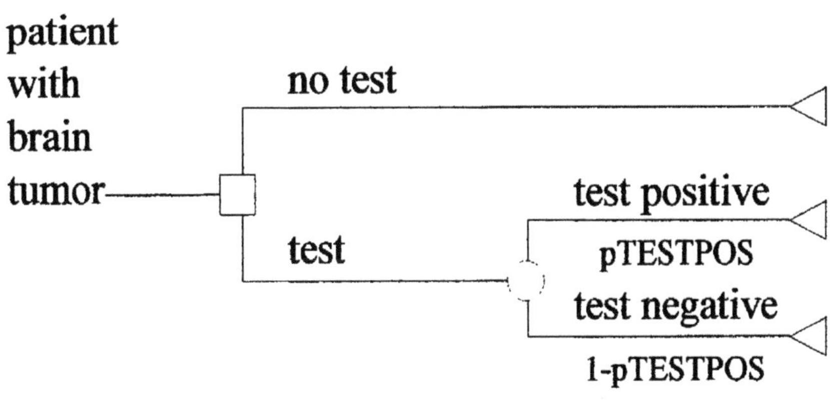

FIGURE 8.3. Decision tree model for determining cost-effectiveness of neuropsychological testing.

and medication, is indicated. In this case, it is expected that the patient will have improved quality of life, with no change in life expectancy. If the tests are negative (no attention deficits uncovered), then it is assumed that no intervention is required and that there is no change in quality of life. For this example, we will incorporate the following assumptions:

Base line costs of care = $1,000
Cost of neuropsychological testing = $100 (attention deficit component)
Treatment of attention deficit with methylphenidate = $600
Probability of positive test = 0.1
Baseline utility = 0.3
Utility posttreament = 0.5

The no-testing strategy costs $1,000, because of the baseline costs of care. Clinically, it yields 0.3 quality-adjusted life years (QALYs). The test strategy has two outcomes: With a probability 0.1, a positive test result will lead to treatment and improvement in quality-adjusted life expectancy to 0.5 QALYs; with complementary probability of 0.9, the test will be negative, and no further costs or benefits will accrue. Thus, the expected costs of the test strategy are 0.1 * (1000 + 100 + 600) + 0.9 * (1000 + 100) = $1160. The expected benefits of the test strategy (not incorporating discounting, given the short duration of life expectancy) are 0.1 * (0.5) + 0.9 * (0.3) = 0.32 QALYs. The incremental cost-effectiveness ratio (ICER) for testing compared to no testing can be computed as the difference in cost divided by the difference in effectiveness: ICER= ($1,160 – $1,000)/(0.32 – 0.30) = $160/(0.02) = $8,000 per QALY gained. Thus, the testing strategy costs $160 more than the no-testing strategy, but yields an additional 0.02 QALYs. The incremental cost-effectiveness ratio is $8,000 per QALY gained, which, compared to previously used thresholds for cost-effectiveness (ranging between $20,000 and $100,000 per QALY), is a cost-effective use of health-care resources.

This is a hypothetical, oversimplified example, but it illustrates the use of decision trees to structure the problem and the use of cost-effectiveness analysis to evaluate the economic costs and clinical benefits of the test intervention.

Cost-Effectiveness of Clinical Trial Batteries

It was reported that a more extensive neuropsychological battery provides more reliable data with fewer false negative results than a brief mental status screening. To prove this in a formal manner would require either a randomized clinical trial comparing the neuropsychological assessment results to those of a brief screening examination in brain-tumor patients, which might raise ethical issues, or including both assessments on the same patients in new clinical trials. This is actually going to be done in several upcoming Radiation Therapy Oncology Group (RTOG) trials of prophylactic brain radiation for patients with lung cancer and radiation therapy for brain metastases. In this way, comparison between a brief neurocognitive assessment and the Mini Mental State Examination (which has been used in all previous RTOG trials; cf. Choucair et al., 1997) will be performed to determine the potential clinical and economic benefits of these assessments, as well as the rate of false positive and false negative results. An ideal clinical trial battery needs to be brief, able to be administered by trained nonpsychologists at multiple sites, resistant to the effects of repeated exposure, sensi-

Table 8.3. Sample Neuropsychological Test Battery for Clinical Trials*

Cognitive Domain	Test	Time to administer (min)
Attention	Digit Span	5
Graphomotor Speed	Digit Symbol	5
Memory	Hopkins Verbal Learning Test	5
Verbal Fluency	Controlled Oral Word Association	5
Visual–Motor Speed	Trial Making Test Part A	3
"Executive" Function	Trial Making Test Part B	5
Fine Motor Dexterity	Grooved Pegboard	5
Activities of Daily Living	Functional Independence Measure	5
Symptoms	M. D. Anderson Symptom Inventory	2
Quality of Life	Functional Assessment of Cancer Therapy–Brain	5
		45 minutes

*For more detailed testing on an individual level, other tests are added. At the Department of Neuro-Oncology at The University of Texas M.D. Anderson Cancer Center, we generally include additional tests of intellectual function, expressive and receptive language, visual attention, visual–spatial functions, and so on for all brain-tumor patients at our site, with additional tests of executive function, academic achievement, and personality and mood depending on the referral question and the patient's level of function.

tive to changes in cognition yet not too difficult for impaired or ill individuals, and relatively inexpensive. There are a number of well-validated and reliable tests that could potentially be used. Table 8.3 describes the neuropsychological clinical trial battery that we are currently using in a number of multinational cancer research protocols. We supplement this battery with a variety of other assessment procedures when patients are seen for clinical purposes. The performance of patients with recurrent tumors on this clinical trial battery has been found to predict survival and time to tumor recurrence (Meyers et al., 1996; 2000). This research needs to be extended to newly diagnosed patients. If neuropsychological test performance at diagnosis was found to correlate with time to tumor progression and prognosis, the neuropsychological assessment would be justified as a standard-of-care diagnostic tool throughout the patient's disease course.

With respect to clinical trials of new agents, neuropsychological assessment is of clear relevance in equivalence trials in which the side effect and toxicity profile of two agents with similar efficacy is tested. However, the utility of neuropsychological assessment in other types of trials will involve the development of subjective assessments of trade-off between survival and quality of life, such as QALY approaches (Green, 1997). Finally, the degree to which institutions, payers, and society feel the added costs of neuropsychological services are worth the investment needs to be explored.

References

Anderson, S. W., Damasio, H., & Tranel, D. (1990). Neuorpsychological impairments associated with lesions caused by tumor or stroke. *Archives of Neurology, 47,* 397–405.

Arlt, W., Hove, U., Muller, B. et al., (1997). Frequent and frequently overlooked: Treatment-induced endocrine dysfunction in adult long-term survivors of primary brain tumors. *Neurology, 49,* 498–506.

Bernstein, M., & Bampoe, J. (2000). Low grade gliomas. In M. Bernstein & M. S. Berger (Eds.), *Neuro-oncology: The essentials* (pp.302–308). New York: Thieme Medical Publishers.

Brain Tumor Progress Review Group. (2000). November 2000 report. http://osp.nci.nih.gov/Prg_ssess/PRG/BTPRG.

Cammermeyer, M., & Evans, J. E. (1988). A brief neurobehavioral exam useful for early detection of postoperative complications in neurosurgical patients. *Journal of Neuroscience Nursing, 20,* 314–323.

Cantor, S. B. (1995). Decision analysis: Theory and applicationto medicine. *Primay Care, 22,* 261–270.

Chataway, J., Stenning, S., Bleehen, N., & Grant, R. (1999). Use of different outcome mesasures in randomized studies of malignant glioma can significantly alter the interpretation of time to progression: Reanalysis of the MCR BR2 study. *Journal of Neuro-Oncology, 43,* 87–92.

Choucair, A. K., Scott, C., Urtasun, R., Nelson, D., Mousas, B., Curran, W. (1997). Quality of life and neuropsychological evaluation for patients with malignant astrocytomas: RTOG 91-14. Radiation Therapy Oncology Group. *International Journal of Radiation Oncology Biology Physics, 38,* 9–20.

Cleeland, C. S. (2001). Cancer-related fatigue: New directions for research. *Cancer, 19,* 1657–1661.

Davis, F. G., McCarthy, B. J., Freels, S., Kupelian, V., & Bondy, M. L. (1999). The conditional probability of survival of patients with primary malignant brain tumors: Surveillance, epidemiology, and end results (SEER) data. *Cancer, 85,* 485–491.

Green, S. B. (1997). Does assessment of quality of life in comparative cancer trials make a difference? A discussion. *Controlled Clinical Trails, 18,* 306–310.

Grill, J., Renaux, V. K., Bulteau, C., Viguier, D., Levy-Piobois, C., Sante-Rose, C., Dellatolas, G., Raquin, M. A., Jampque, I., Kalifa, C. (1999). Long-term intellectual outcome in children with posterior foss tumors according to radiation doses and volumes. *International Journal of Radiation Oncology Biology Physics, 45,* 137–145.

Groves, M. D., Maor, M. H., Meyers, C., Kyritsis,, A. P. & Kevub, V. A. (1999). A phase II trial of high-dose bromodeoxyuridine with accelerated fractionation radiotherapy followed by procarbazine, lomustine, and vincristine for glioblastoma multifrome. *International Journal of Radiation Oncology Biology Physics, 45,* 127–135.

Holden, C. (2000). Global survey examines impact of depression. *Science, 288,* 39–40.

Lang, E. F., Wildrick, D. M., & Sawaya, R. (2000). Metastatic brain tumors. In M. Bernstein & M. S. Berger (Eds.), *Neuro-oncology: The essentials* (pp. 329–337). New York: Thieme Medical Publishers.

Menon, D. & Assiff, I. (2000). The burden of illness of employees on United States employers: A critical review of the ligerature. *Drug Information Journal, 34,* 47–58.

Meyers, C. A., Berman, S. A., Hayman, A., & Evankovich, K. (1992). Pathological left-handedness and preserved function associated with a slowly evolving brain tumor. *Developmental Medicine and Child Neurology, 34,* 1102–1117.

Meyers, C. A., Grous, J. J., Ford, K. M., et al. (1996). Multifaceted models for assessing quality of life in brain cancer therapy trials. *Drug Information Journal, 30,* 856–857 (abstr).

Meyers, C. A., Hess, K. R., Yung, W. K. A., & Levin, V. A. (2000). Cognitive function as a predictor of survival in patients with recurrent malignant glioma. *Journal of Clinical Oncology, 1*(18), 646–650.

Meyers, C. A., Kudelka, A. P., Conrad, C. A., Gelke, C. K., Grove, W., & Pazdur, R. (1998). Neurotoxicity of CI-980, a novel miotic inhibitor. *Clinical Cancer Research, 3,* 419–422.

Meyers, C. A., Weitzner, M. A., Valentine, S. D. & Levin, V. A. (1998). Methylphenidate therapy improves cognition, mood, and function of brain tumor patients. *Journal of Clinical Oncology, 16,* 2522–2527.

Moore, B. D., Alter, J., & Copeland, D. R. (1992). Improved neuropsychological outcome in children with brain tumors diagnosed during infancy and treated without cranial irradiation. *Journal of Child Neurology, 7,* 281–290.

O'Shaughnessy, J. A., Wittes, R. E., Burke, G., Friedman, M. A., Niederhuber, J. E., et al. (1991). Commentary concerning demonstration of safety and efficacy of investigational anticancer agents in clinical trial. *Journal of Clinical Oncology, 9,* 2225–2230.

Radhakrishnan, K., Bohnen, N. I., & Kurland, L. T. (1994). Epidemiology of Brain tumors. In R. A. Morantz & J. W. Walsh, (Eds.), *Brain tumors: A comprehensive text* (pp. 1–18). New York: Marcel Dekker.

Scheibel, R. S., Meyers, C. A., & Levin, V. A. (1996). Cognitive dysfunction following surgery for intracerebral glioma: Influence of histopathology, lesion location, and treatment. *Journal of Neuro-Oncology, 30,* 61–69.

Sherer, M., Meyers, C. A., & Gerloff, P. (1997). Efficacy of postacute brain injury rehabilitation for patients with primary malignant brain tumors. *Cancer, 80,* 250–257.

Swets, J. A., Dawes, R. M., & Monahan, J. (2000). Psychological science can improve diagnostic decisions. *Psychological Science in the Public Interest, 1,* 1–26.

Taylor, B. V., Buckner, J. C., Cascino, T. L., et al. (1998). Effects of radiation and chemotherapy on cognitive function in patients with high-grade glioma. *Journal of Clinical Oncology, 6,* 2195–2201.

Thomson, A. M., Taylor, R., Fraser, D., & Whittle, I. R. (1997). Sterotactic biopsy of nonpolar tumors in the dominant hemisphere: A prospective study of effects on language functions. *Journal of Neurosurgery, 86,* 923–926.

Valentine, A. D., Meyers, C. A., Kling, M. A., Richelson, E., & Hauser, P. (1998). Mood and cognitive side effects of interferon-alpha therapy. *Seminars in Oncology, 25,* 39–47.

Vigliani, M. C., Sichez, N., Poisson, M., Delattre, J. Y. (1996). A prospective study of cognitive functions following conventioal radiotheapy for supratentorial gliomas in young adults: 4-years results. *International Journal of Radiation Oncology Biology Physics, 35,* 527–533.

Whitton, A. C., Rhyddrech, H., Furlong, W., Feeny, D., Barr, R. D. (1997). Self-reported comprehensive health status of adult brain tumor patinets using the Health Utilities Index. *Cancer, 80,* 265–258.

Wrensch, M. R., Minn, Y., & Bondy, M. L. (2000). Epidemiology. In M. Bernstein & M. S. Berger (Eds.), *Neuro-oncology: The essentials* (pp. 2–17) New York: Thieme Medical Publishers.

PART

IV

DEMENTIA

9

CHAPTER

Kathleen A. Welsh-Bohmer
Deborah Koltai Attix
Douglas J. Mason

The Clinical Utility of Neuropsychological Evaluation of Patients with Known or Suspected Dementia

Introduction

Alzheimer's disease (AD) and related dementing disorders of aging are among the largest public health menaces facing the United States today. Advances in modern medicine have successfully reduced mortality in illnesses that have typically censured survival into late life. As a consequence, the number of individuals surviving into late life is growing at a staggering rate, and the projected future incidence of AD—with its attendant economic burden—threatens to overwhelm our current health-care system. To illustrate the magnitude of the problem, currently in the United States 5% to 10% of Americans over age 65 are affected by dementia (AHCPR, 1996). Of these, the vast majority of cases are accounted for by AD (nearly 60%; or approximately 4 million Americans; Small et al., 1997). This number is projected to triple in the next 50 years, to affect 7.5 to 14.3 million individuals by the year 2050 (Brookmeyer, Gray, & Kawas, 1998; Evans et al., 1990). The existing estimates of the economic burdens of AD care on our society vary tremendously. However midrange estimates suggest that the total cost of AD care in 1991 was $67 billion, with $21 billion attributable to direct costs for medical and nursing care, $13 billion attributed to indirect costs such as disability and premature mortality, and $33 billion for informal caregiving costs often provided and

This work was supported in part by grants from the National Institute on Aging (NIA Grants AG05128 & AG09997) and private donations to the Joseph and Kathleen Bryan Alzheimer's Disease Research Center.

absorbed by families (Ernst & Hay, 1994). Costing this out for care in the future suggests that costs will exceed $150 billion annually.

Developing an effective public policy to address the societal strain--both on the direct costs attributed to health care and the burden shouldered by care providers--challenges policy makers today. In the absence of effective treatments to prevent or cure these disorders, one approach to address the approaching health-care crisis is to design strategies to optimize function across the illness and to reduce disease comorbidities, thereby delaying transitions to major disability. The current evidence suggests that this may be effective in lowering some of the annual costs for the care of dementia patients. A number of studies have repeatedly demonstrated that costs are related to disease severity, with increased direct and indirect expenditures associated with the more severe stages of AD and with the transition from life in the community to life in the nursing home or other care institutions (see Small et al., 1997, for review).

As is true of many other medical conditions, identification of the illness very early in its course is a key feature of this "secondary" prevention strategy. The rationale is that acting early, before significant neural destruction has occurred, allows for the implementation of existing symptomatic therapies at a point that may be optimal in the illness course. Additionally, early identification allows better advanced planning, tracking, and management of comorbidities that can affect cognitive status and influence the patient's overall function and general quality of life. To this end, neuropsychology, with its demonstrated ability to advance early, reliable diagnosis of AD and other dementias, plays a strategic role in the medical management and ultimately in the prevention approaches to delay the occurrence of milestone events, such as nursing home placements (Welsh-Bohmer & Morgenlander, 1999). Although very few studies have examined the specific economic impact of neuropsychological assessment on dementia outcome, a number of studies have reported the critical importance of neuropsychology in the diagnosis of AD. In addition, converging lines of evidence suggest that there may be economic and management advantages to the early identification of AD. The purpose of this chapter is twofold. First, we highlight the role neuropsychology plays in the diagnosis of AD and other dementing illnesses. Second, we underscore the relative costs and benefits, both economical and quality of life, that are conferred by detecting the disease early in the elderly community at large. We propose that cognitive screening can be useful and can be practically applied in the majority of diagnostic settings, such as in the primary care doctor's practice. We further suggest that judicious use of neuropsychological referrals, reserved particularly for diagnostically challenging scenarios (e.g., ambiguous symptoms, medical or psychiatric confounding), can have large economic and practical benefits for patients, families affected by the disease, and society as a whole.

☐ Diagnosis of Alzheimer's Disease

In the last decade, notable advances have been made in understanding the pathogenesis of AD, suggesting new avenues to diagnosis and treatment within the near future. Despite this progress, there currently is no biological test allowing unequivocal diagnosis of the disorder. Genetic testing for point mutations on Chromosomes 1, 14, and 21 (Goate et al., 1991; Levy-Lahad et al., 1995; Sherrington et al., 1995) is generally conducted only in instances of young age of onset or in the presence of a compelling family history of dementia. Even then, the yield from such testing is relatively low, accounting for only 1% to 2% of the cases of AD dementia. A number of potential "susceptibility" genes for AD also have been suggested, which act to enhance risk but do not necessarily cause AD (Grodin & Laurie, 2000). Putative risk-enhancing genes include apolipoprotein E (Saunders et al., 1993a), alpha-2 macroglobulin (Blacker et al., 1998), interleukin 6 (Bagli et al., 2000), interleukin 1 (Nicoll et al., 2000), cathepsin D (Papassotiropoulos et al., 2000), and cystatin C (Finckh et al., 2000). The most well established of these is apolipoprotein E (APOE), a gene located on Chromosome 19 and involved in neuronal repair and cholesterol transport. The APOE gene has three common polymorphisms (apoe e2, e3, e4). Inheritance of the e4 allele increases risk of developing AD in a dose-dependent manner and reduces the age of disease onset (Corder et al., 1993). Consequently, routine genotyping for the APOE e4 polymorphism in symptomatic patients may be useful in verifying AD dementia, particularly in individuals under the age of 85 (Breitner et al., 1999). However, APOE genotype information in presymptomatic individuals is not clinically informative, given that it does not convey a certainty of the development of AD over the lifespan and therefore is not currently recommended for preclinical use (NIA/Alzheimer's Association Workgroup, 1996). This practice is likely to change as more is learned about the genetics of the illness, and certainly it will be important in the face of any effective treatment or prevention strategies that develop in the ensuing years.

In this absence of a biological test for AD, the diagnosis of AD and related dementing disorders continues to rest on clinical methods. Considerable progress has been made in this area to advance the clinical accuracy of the AD diagnosis, and neuropsychology has contributed importantly to this progress. Prior to the 1980s there was little consensus among clinicians regarding the clinical characteristics of AD, differential diagnosis, and natural history of the disorder. However, beginning in 1980 focused scientific funding initiatives through the National Institute of Aging allowed the study of AD and related dementias in the United States and have provided important advances in the diagnosis of the disorder. Among the most important contributions of that early effort were the careful articulation of diagnostic criteria for dementia (APA, 1980, 1987, 1994; see Table 9.1), and the delineation of criteria for the specific diagnosis of Alzheimer's disease (McKhann et al., 1984; see Table 9.2). The latter criteria, developed through a convened workgroup of dementia specialists from the National Institute of Neurological and Communicative Disorders and Stroke and the Alzheimer's Disease and Related Disorders Association (NINCDS-ADRDA), are the most commonly applied in clinical research settings.

It is frequently erroneously stated that AD is a diagnosis of exclusion. In fact, the diagnosis of AD requires first the presence of a number of inclusionary factors, based primarily on the neuropsychological features of the disorder (see Tables 9.1 and 9.2). A large neuropsychological literature over the last 20 years has allowed the careful characterization of the dementia of AD (Butters, Delis, & Lucas, 1995, for review). The clinical presentation of AD is now well recognized by a highly pronounced impairment in recent memory function (rapid forgetting) and impairments in intellectual and executive function, expressive language ability, motor praxis, and spatial judgment (see Welsh-Bohmer & Ogrocki, 1998, for review). Importantly, neuropsychological tests, particularly of learning and memory function, are able to reliably distinguish between early stage AD and normal aging in situations where other clinical methods, such as mental status testing, may fail (Bondi et al., 1994; Grober & Kawas, 1997; Howieson et

TABLE 9.1. *DSM-IV* Diagnostic Criteria for Dementia of the Alzheimer's Type

1) Cognitive Criteria: The development of multiple cognitive impairments including memory impairment, defined as impaired ability to learn new information, and at least one of the following cognitive disorders:
   a) impairment in language (*aphasia*)
   b) impairment in the execution of planned motor acts despite normal motor and sensory function *(apraxia)*
   c) failure to recognize or identify objects despite intact sensory function (*agnosia*)
   d) disturbance in higher intellectual and so-called "executive" functions. Typically this is manifest by impaired abstract thinking (e.g., similarities and differences), judgement, planning, organization, sequencing, and in ability to think flexibly and to "multitask" (attend to multiple competing task demands). This problem often leads to interpersonal problems, family issues, or job-related problems
2) Functional Criteria: The impairments interfere with social or occupational function
3) Course Criteria: Insidious onset with gradual and continual decline in cognitive function
4) Exclusionary Criteria:
   a) cognitive disorder cannot be attributable to some other central nervous system disorder known to have cognitive effects, such as cerebrovascular disease, Parkinson's disease, normal pressure hydrocephalus, tumor, subdural hematoma, etc.
   b) systemic conditions, known to cause dementia, are excluded as causal (e.g., hypothyroidism, B12 deficiency, neurosyphilis, etc.)
   c) substance abuse conditions are ruled out
   d) impairment is not due to delirium
   e) impairment is not due to another Axis I disorder (e.g., major depressive disorder, schizophrenia)

Modified from the American Psychiatric Association, *Diagnostic and Statistical Manual of Mental Disorders,* Fourth Edition (*DSM-IV*). Washington DC: American Psychiatric Society, 1994, pp. 142–143. Note the *DSM-IV* (1994) lists separately criteria for dementia by type or cause, unlike the previous version *DSM-III* that had a more generic description of dementia.

al., 1997; Katzman et al., 1989; Petersen et al., 1994; Welsh, Butters, Hughes, Mohs, & Heyman, 1991, 1992). Within the context of demonstrating the classic neuropsychological symptom complex of AD, medical exclusion factors must then be eliminated to arrive at a firm diagnosis.

Using the NINCDS-ADRDA criteria, a diagnosis of AD can be rendered reflecting the clinician's level of clinical certainty based both on the typicality of the clinical presentation and on the degree to which the condition is associated with other medical causation. A high level of confidence is conferred by a diagnosis of probable AD, which indicates a rather typical AD presentation and the evaluating clinician's view that no other medical etiology accounts for the disorder. A more conservative diagnosis of possible AD may be assigned if the clinical presentation deviates from the typical presentation or there is the presence of another existing brain disorder or medical explanation that could account for the dementia. Definite AD is reserved for situations in which *both* the clinical criteria are met and there is neuropathological verification of neurofibrillary plaques and tangles to support the AD diagnosis.

Adherence to the NINCDS-ADRDA criteria has resulted in increased accuracy of the

TABLE 9.2. NINCDS-ADRDA Criteria for Alzheimer's Disease

Probable Alzheimer's Disease
1. Dementia established by clinical examination and documented by mental status testing
2. Dementia confirmed by neuropsychological assessment
3. Deficits in two or more areas of cognition
4. Progression in symptoms over time
5. No disturbances in consciousness (no delirium)
6. Late onset and not developmentally acquired; onset between ages 40 and 90
7. Absence of other conditions that are capable of producing dementia

Possible Alzheimer's Disease
1. Atypical onset, presentation or progression of dementia symptoms, and/or
2. Presence of another systemic or other brain disease capable of producing dementia but not thought to be the cause in the case under consideration
3. Meets criteria for dementia as confirmed by clinical examination and neuropsychological testing
4. Progressive decline in symptoms over time
5. No disturbances in consciousness
6. Absence of other identifiable causes

Definite Alzheimer's Disease
1. Clinical criteria for Probable Alzheimer's disease are fulfilled
2. Histopathologic evidence of Alzheimer's disease by biopsy or postmortem examination

Summarized from the criteria of McKhann et al. (1984, pp. 939–944). These criteria were developed by a consensus panel of two joint groups from the National Institute of Neurological and Communicative Disorders (NINCDS) and the Alzheimer's Disease and Related Disorders Association (ADRDA).

clinical diagnosis of AD to over 80%, relative to neuropathological information, in most contemporary clinical series from specialty centers (Gearing et al., 1995; Lopez et al., 1999). When it does occur in these settings, misdiagnosis is most likely to happen in situations involving very early disease detection (i.e., before the clinical dementia syndrome is fully manifest) or in scenarios involving disease comorbidities such as AD and coexisting cerebrovascular disease or depression (Lopez et al., 2000b). Because many other medical comorbidities can, by themselves, cause cognitive problems and are potentially treatable, dementia may be ascribed to these other conditions when they are present rather than to AD (Lopez et al., 1999). Misclassifications of AD also can occur at the clinical interface of AD and similar neurodegenerative disorders, such as frontotemporal dementia (Lopez et al., 2000a; 2000b).

Neuropsychological assessment has been recognized as particularly useful in these diagnostically challenging scenarios (AHCPR, 1996; Cummings et al., 1996) and frequently is necessary in cases of early disease detection to allow verification of impairments in memory and other cognitive domains (Lopez et al., 2000a; 2000b; Welsh, Butters, Hughes, Mohs, & Heyman, 1992). These applications are described in further detail in sections that follow. In arriving at a firm diagnosis, additional sources of information—such as APOE genotype, considered together with neuropsychological testing (Tierney et al., 1996a; 1996b), or alone (Welsh-Bohmer, Gearing, Saunders, Roses, &

Mirra, 1997; Mayeux et al., 1998)—can enhance early AD detection. Detailed structural imaging of the medial temporal lobe (e.g., MRI) or consideration of functional brain activity (PET, SPECT, or fMRI) also can enhance diagnostic accuracy in early or atypical presentations of AD but are not yet typically used in standard dementia evaluations (Bookheimer et al., 2000; Hoffman et al., 2000; Small, Ercoli, et al., 2000).

Clinical Utility of Neuropsychology in the Diagnosis and Management of Dementia

The medical utility of neuropsychological assessment in the clinical evaluation of dementia is well recognized. Although not a requisite in each case of dementia, neuropsychology consultation is commonly sought in at least three common instances

1. First, consultation is requested to assist in arriving at a clinical diagnosis in medical situations in which neurocognitive impairment is suspected. Referrals may occur in the context of what is believed to be early stage Alzheimer's disease, as discussed above, but often arise in a number of other neurological conditions, psychiatric disorders, or in any of a variety of general medical conditions. Consequently, neuropsychological assessment is used both in the detection of dementia and in the differential diagnosis of disorders.
2. A second common referral issue is one in which a physician seeks an estimate of a patient's functional status. Related to this, referrals also are sought to inform competency assessment.
3. Finally, physicians may seek neuropsychology assistance for patient management, including cognitive intervention, psychotherapy, or behavioral management (see Koltai & Welsh-Bohmer, 2000, for review).

A summary appears in Table 9.3 and discussion of the specific utility of neuropsychology in each of the various applications follows.

Neuropsychology in the Identification and Differential Diagnosis of Dementia

Differential Diagnosis. The neuropsychological assessment plays a critical role in the differential diagnosis of dementia and can highlight inconsistencies suggestive of other confounding processes, such as medication effects, psychiatric symptoms, or depression. Distinctive profiles of cognitive impairment on neuropsychological examination permit clinical differentiation between normal aging, depression, AD, and the myriad of other similar neurodegenerative processes (see Koltai & Welsh-Bohmer, 2000, for review). The most common forms of dementia, beyond AD, include the vascular dementias, frontotemporal disorders (including Picks disease), and a diversity of disorders initially involving subcortical structures such as diffuse Lewy body dementia, corticobasal degeneration, and progressive supranuclear palsy. The profiles of neurocognitive impairment associated with each of these dementing disorders overlap to some extent, but there are some relatively distinctive features that permit useful differentiation.

For instance, in vascular dementia circumscribed defects on neuropsychological examination (such as aphasia) along with an abrupt onset of problems or a stepwise course

TABLE 9.3. Clinical Utility of Neuropsychological Evaluations of Patients with Known or Suspected Dementia

1. Documentation of cognitive compromise with standardized, objective instruments and use of norms accounting for the influence of age, education, and gender on performance
2. Delineation of specific areas of cognitive deficit critical to the differential diagnosis process, estimation of functional status, and intervention planning (e.g., rapid forgetting vs. aphasia)
3. Delineation of the overall constellation of neuropsychological findings for diagnosis (e.g., Alzheimer's disease vs. vascular dementia vs. frontotemporal dementia)
4. Ascertainment of the presence and degree of cognitive change resulting from various medical treatments
5. Documentation of the need for nonpharmacological interventions to improve function and adjustment
6. Determination of functional status to guide management decisions regarding limitations to ensure safety (e.g., driving, supervision) without needlessly restricting activities and acquisition of needed services (e.g., home health aides)
7. Determination of competency to guide management decisions regarding limitations to legal and everyday decision-making capacities (e.g., finances)

raise the possibility of large vessel stroke or multi-infarct dementia (Looi & Sachdev, 1999). A subcortical profile–with a retrieval memory deficit (partial forgetting on free recall testing, with better preserved recognition memory skills), executive dysfunction, and word retrieval deficits–is more commonly seen in small vessel types of vascular dementia, such as the lacunar state or Binswanger's (McPherson & Cummings, 1996).

By contrast, the neuropsychological profile of diffuse Lewy body dementia is characterized by evidence of mild Parkinsonism, prominent attentional fluctuation, severe visuospatial disturbances, and lesser memory disturbance than AD early on (Gnanalingham, Byrbe, Thornton, Sambrook, & Bannister, 1997; Hansen et al., 1990; Salmon et al., 1996). Frontal lobe dementias (Pick disease, frontotemporal lobe atrophy) typically present with a profile of marked changes in personality, social awareness, and behavior (e.g., disinhibition, compulsiveness, mood lability; Neary et al., 1998). This behavioral profile is accompanied by pronounced impairments on neuropsychological tests of executive function, including sequencing, cognitive flexibility, concept formation, abstraction, and judgment. Although less prominent, deficits also may be observed on tests of semantic memory, language, recent memory function, and visuospatial attention (Lindau et al., 1998; Moss, Albert, & Kemper, 1992; Pachana, Boone, Miller, Cummings, & Berman, 1996; Perry & Hodges, 2000).

There have been a number of studies examining neuropsychological discrimination between AD and these various other forms of dementia (for review see, Gnanalingham et al., 1997; Looi & Sachdev, 1999; Perry & Hodges, 2000; Pillon et al., 1995). A common finding is that discrimination can be achieved to some extent based on the neuropsychological information alone, but that there can be tremendous overlap in the neurocognitive profiles due to disease heterogeneity, imprecision in the clinical diagnostic standards applied, and potential presence of disease comordibities (e.g., AD and VaD often co-occur). Despite these limitations, use of very detailed neurocognitive analysis can be helpful in generating hypotheses of likely etiology for dementia, as was shown in one study involving carefully selected and well-matched patients with corticobasal degeneration, progressive supranuclear palsy, and AD (Pillon et al., 1995). In this study, distinctive neuropsychological profiles are reported on specific tests of dynamic motor execution, praxis, and use of semantic cues during the encoding and retrieval of new information. Knowledge such as this can be applied to diagnostically challenging scenarios to fully inform clinical diagnosis.

Neuropsychology services are perhaps most utilized when there is a clinical issue of comorbid depression in the setting of cognitive decline. Late-life depression is a prevalent but treatable problem. It is estimated that significant depressive disorders occur in approximately 15% of the elderly population overall (Blazer, 1994) and in a sizeable portion of the geriatric medical inpatient (40%) and institutionalized elderly (30% to 35+%) populations (see Koenig & Blazer, 1992, for review). Despite its prevalence, it often is unrecognized and is one of the largest sources of misdiagnosis among elderly patients (Kaszniak, 1987). In isolation, depression can result in cognitive impairments similar to those of AD, a condition historically referred to as *pseudodementia* and currently as the *dementia of depression*. More commonly, depressive symptoms cooccur within the setting of AD and other dementias (Migliorelli et al., 1995). Prevalence estimates of depressive disorders in AD highlight how common emotional distress attends cognitive dysfunction, with over half in some series meeting criteria for dysthymia or major depression (e.g., Migliorelli et al., 1995). In some instances, a significant depressive disorder can be the early preclinical sign of AD, predating the more ominous dementing process by a year or more (Steffens et al., 1997).

The importance of parcelling out the contribution of affective distress in the clinical presentation cannot be underscored enough. Depression is among the most common *treatable* sources of cognitive dysfunction (Albert, 1981; Clarfield, 1988). Thus, the potential to reduce "excess disability," or greater than warranted functional disability resulting from treatable factors (Brody, Kleban, Lawton, & Silverman, 1971), is evident. Although clearly delineating the presence and magnitude of deficits attributable to central nervous system dysfunction versus emotional distress is challenging, neuropsychological assessment is uniquely positioned to offer such a definition. A large body of research has offered insight into both the quantitative and qualitative types of performance errors made by the aforementioned subgroups on neuropsychological tests (Jones, Tranel, Benton, & Paulsen, 1992; Kaszniak, 1987; Silberman et al., 1983), and the typically observed pattern of impairment associated with the dementia of depression has been described (e.g., Koltai & Welsh-Bohmer, 2000). Because rational treatment rests on accurate diagnosis, neuropsychological consultation in such cases has the potential to lead to significant reductions in disability by clearly identifying factors amenable to treatment at the outset of medical management.

In short, the neuropsychological examination provides unique information to the diagnostic evaluation through its objective verification of the behavioral and cognitive complex under scrutiny. Used in the context of other attendant data—including the medical and neurological findings, the history of cognitive change, and other neurodiagnostic tests (e.g., brain imaging)—the results from the neuropsychological examination facilitate differential diagnosis of the dementia including the role of potential psychiatric comorbidities that may be interfering with cognition.

Early Detection. More recently, the role of neuropsychology in the early detection of AD has been addressed through systematic evaluation of the existing literature in individuals at risk of developing dementia because they evidence early cognitive changes suggestive of the disease (Petersen et al., 2001). A number of clinical and epidemiological studies of aging and dementia have demonstrated a continuum of cognitive change, including normal mentation, mild or ambiguous deficits perhaps reflective of brain disease, and dementia of varying severities (Breitner et al., 1999; Ritchie, Artero, & Touchon, 2001). The broad transitional zone, now referred to as *mild cognitive impairment (MCI)*, has gained general clinical acceptance as reflective of the prodromal state of AD. The results of longitudinal clinical series and pathological studies validate the notion of a continuum (e.g. Welsh-Bohmer et al., 2001). On average, the annual rates of conversion from MCI to AD (or dementia) in such cases followed in longitudinal clinical or cohort series is 6% to 25% (see Petersen et al., 2001, for review). This conversion rate is much higher than the annual incidence rates in the general population, where the rates range from 0.2% in the 65 to 69 years age range and 3.9% in the 85 to 89 years age range. This suggests that having mild memory or other cognitive impairment but not meeting clinical criteria for dementia or AD (i.e., MCI) significantly heightens the risk for the development of AD. Because of the ambiguity between memory change associated with pathological conditions and with normal aging of the nervous system, neuropsychological testing is commonly urged in cases of potential early stage disease to facilitate diagnosis. The development of diagnostic criteria for MCI also emphasizes

TABLE 9.4. Mild Cognitive Impairment Criteria

Proposed MCI Criteria
1. Memory complaint
2. Normal activities of daily living
3. Normal general cognitive function
4. Abnormal memory for age
5. Not demented
6. Late onset and not developmentally acquired; onset between ages 55 and 90
7. Absence of other conditions that are capable of producing cognitive impairment

Psychometric Refinements of the Criteria of the ADCS Alzheimer's Disease Cooperative Study
1. An obvious memory deficit that is confirmed by a friend or family member
2. Abnormal memory function documented by scoring below an education-adjusted cutoff on the Logical Memory II subscale of the Wechsler Memory Scale
3. Clinical Dementia Rating (CDR) Scale score of 0.5
4. A Mini-Mental State Exam (MMSE) score greater than or equal to 24

Supporting Evidence of MCI as Prodromal AD
1. Worsening of symptoms over time, as quantified by repeat testing/observation
2. Presence of at least one copy of the APOE e4 gene
3. MRI evidence of medial temporal lobe atrophy
4. PET/functional brain imaging evidence of temporal-parietal hypometabolism

Criteria are summarized from the publication of Petersen et al. (1999, pp. 303–308). Refinements in psychometric criteria obtained from the ADCS workgroup. Supporting evidence for prodromal AD from literature including Bookheimer et al. (2000), Reiman et al. (1996), Ritchie et al. (2001), Petersen et al. (1999), Small et al. (2000), Tierney et al. (1996 ; 1996b) neuropsychological testing by specifying suggested profiles of cognitive change for the condition (Petersen et al., 1999; see Table 9.4).

The medical utility of neuropsychological testing in the diagnosis of geriatric patients with dementia is supported by a number of well-designed case-control and cohort studies. Together these studies indicate that standalone use of neuropsychological assessments function well in detecting cases of dementia across a range of severity levels and ages compared to conventional diagnostic approaches (Bracco et al., 1990; Graham et al., 1996; Pittman et al., 1992; Stern et al., 1992; Tschanz et al., 2000). For instance, a recent prospective study of memory-impaired patients revealed that the use of memory test performance in conjunction with APOE genotyping predicted who developed AD over time better than the use of genotyping in isolation (92.5% vs. 73.8% accuracy; Tierney et al., 1996a, 1996b). Another recent population-based study of the very elderly examined the utility of a neuropsychological algorithm approach to the diagnosis of dementia in relation to clinical diagnostic procedures, history, neurological examination, neuropsychological testing, and laboratory studies (Tschanz et al., 2000). Using cognitive scores alone, the agreement between the two methods (conventional clinical diagnostic method and neuropsychological algorithmic) was reasonably high (79%, kappa = 0.57). The performance of the algorithmic approach improved to 90% (kappa of 0.76 between the two methods) when measures of functional ability were included with the cognitive measures (Tschanz et al., 2000). Generally the algorithm accurately identified participants without dementia, but was less apt to detect participants with very mild dementia, a problem likely offset by longitudinal observation in order to verify decline in function over time. In short, the results of this line of investigation suggest that neuropsychological methods form a critical part of the clinical diagnostic method, allowing for diagnostic accuracy that approximates that achieved with a full neurological examination and its attendant studies. Although this line of study was initiated in an effort to standardize epidemiological approaches, the results have direct implications for clinical practice. The findings suggest that neuropsychological assessment (even of a relatively limited scope, as in these epidemiological studies) may provide an efficient manner to screen for subjects at high and low risk for developing dementia. The method avoids problems of no informants, unreliable informants, and biases of self-report, and it circumvents ambiguities in clinical judgment (Tschanz et al., 2000).

Together the findings from these well-controlled observational studies support the use of neuropsychology for the screening of geriatric populations at risk of developing dementia. Practice parameters for the evaluation of dementia recently published by the Quality Standards Subcommittee of the American Academy of Neurology (Petersen et al., 2001) recommend the use of neuropsychological batteries for the identification of patients with dementia. Routine screening within geriatric practices also has been recommended by other groups (AHCPR, 1996). If applied routinely, it would serve as a mechanism for early detection of dementia, which might otherwise go undetected for extended periods of time.

Overall, the literature unequivocally supports the use of neuropsychological assessment in the detection and differential diagnosis of dementia. This has important implications for patient quality of life as well as health-care costs through its impact on health-care practices. Specifically, knowledge of a memory disorder facilitates appropriate management approaches. It permits the physician to identify comorbidities for reduction of secondary complications. It facilitates identification of appropriate candidates for cholinesterase-inhibiting agents. Likewise, such assessment clarifies the need for and appropriateness of nonpharmacological intervention approaches (see Chapter 10) during a time when patients are most likely to be able to effectively utilize various techniques. It may also provide closure to patients and families in diagnostically ambiguous situations, so that adjustment to the medical condition can begin, including advance planning and other types of decisions.

Functional Status and Competency Assessment

A common referral issue in geriatric neuropsychology practices is the assessment of a patient's functional status and capabilities, to guide decisions regarding supervision or independence in basic and instrumental activities of daily living. Frequently, neuropsychological assessments are requested to assist in the determination of work disability and competency or capacity to perform certain activities. Although neuropsychological tests were developed primarily to detect and differentiate brain illnesses rather than to predict function, converging lines of evidence suggest that cognitive performance relates directly to functional skills in daily life (Baum, Edwards, Yonan, & Srorandt, 1996; Diehl, Willis, & Schaie, 1995; Fitz & Teri, 1994; Greiner, Snowden, & Schmitt, 1996; Nadler et al., 1993). It is important to recognize that neuropsychological and functional assessments differ, measuring related but not identical constructs. However, the considerable shared variance between instruments used in these evaluations (see McCue, 1997, for review) indicates the utility of neuropsychological assessment in predicting functional status in some instances. Although additional research is warranted to further delineate the relationship between cognition and function, and caution must be exercised when predicting functional status, the potential for practical application is evident. For instance, preliminary pilot work has demonstrated the association between cognitive status and driving ability (Rebok, Keyl, Bylsma, Blaustein, & Tune, 1994). Thus, performance on cognitive measures may indicate the need for formal driving assessment or restriction of activities through limitations, supervision, or cessation of driving privileges in clear cases of impairment. In this manner, management often is guided by assessment results, with the goal of promoting independence and autonomy while ensuring safety.

Additionally, level of cognitive impairment is related to a number of important health outcomes, including utilization of services and institutionalization (Branch & Jette, 1982; Branch et al., 1988; Rockwood, Stolee, & McDowell, 1996; Willis & Marsiske, 1991). Data from the Canadian Study of Health and Aging (CSHA; Rockwood et al., 1996) indicate that cognitive impairment is an important predictor of admission into long-term care and that the severity of the impairment is related to institutionalization in a dose-dependent manner. For all stages of AD dementia, the unadjusted odds ratios for skilled care placement was 19.6. For mild AD, the odds ratio was very low, as might be predicted [0.62 (95% c.i. 0.44–0.84)]; but this increased dramatically as the level of impairment rose to the moderate level [6.1 (c.i. 2.7–8.9)] and for severe impairment [20.4 (c.i. 13.2–33.3)]. Because of the clear relationship between cognition and health-care utilization, assessment can be used to assist formal care planning in both individual and community settings. Neuropsychological results can be used to inform care decisions, so that pharmacotherapy or other management approaches can be implemented, with the aim of maintaining function and delaying admission to institutionalized care.

More recently, specific efforts have been devoted to developing methods tailored for predicting competency (see Koltai & Welsh-Bohmer, 2000, for further discussion). Although there are no clear standards at present for the evaluation of competence, there is a growing empirical literature supporting the use of neuropsychological data to predict various capacities (e.g., Marson, Ingram, Cody, & Harrell, 1995; Stanley, Stanley, Guido, & Garvin, 1988; Tymchuk, Ouslander, Rahbar, & Fitten, 1988). Decisions regarding competency based on general diagnoses such as "dementia" almost inevitably fail to capture true capabilities. They offer limited information about the functional capabilities of each individual (Scogin & Perry, 1986) and can lead to an unnecessary restriction of autonomy. An individual may be competent for social decisions, but not for complex matters, such as medical care decisions (Baker, 1987; Kloezen, Fitten, & Steinberg, 1988). The existence of different legal standards for specific legal competencies underscores that competency is not a unitary construct (Marson et al., 1994). Individuals benefit from viewing competency as a multifactorial concept, differentiating between personal, financial, and medical decision-making capacities.

Comprehensive neuropsychological evaluation often reveals the relative strengths and weaknesses of the individual, thus offering insight into which capacities may be preserved. The use of standardized tests to formally assess these various capacities is an area of growing application that shows promise by counteracting bias based on clinical impression alone (Steinberg, Fitten, & Kachuck, 1986). In this manner, neuropsychology expands its role beyond identification and diagnosis of neurological and psychiatric illnesses, by offering insight into estimated levels of functioning in various everyday capacities. The impact of such clinical care on quality of life and health-care variables again is obvious, as such information serves to improve the efficiency and accuracy of medical management strategies, with the potential results of increased autonomy and minimization of unnecessary care services.

Behavioral Management and Therapeutic Intervention

Neuropsychology frequently is called upon to provide therapeutic intervention in the form of cognitive retraining, psychotherapy, or behavior management in an effort to enhance patient functioning and overall quality of life. Because AD and other dementias are progressive, the approach taken will depend on the presenting problem and the severity of the condition. At all stages of dementia, interventions such as social support (e.g., support groups), family education, and environmental enhancement are commonly employed. In mild to moderately impaired patients, the approach may involve perceptual and cognitive interventions accompanied by more traditional forms of psychotherapy. The goals here are to assist in adjustment to the illness and to provide focused cognitive training related to tasks of daily living in an effort to postpone or prevent the need for formal care, reduce health-services utilization, and enhance patient autonomy and quality of life. In more severely impaired patients, the approach may include family education and behavioral management strategies to deal with problem behaviors (e.g., wandering or pacing). The overall goals are the same, although the level of autonomy that might be reasonably achieved is more limited. Evidence supporting the clinical efficacy of such interventions in the dementia population is growing, with promising outcomes shown in affective functioning, memory skills, and perception of memory functioning (e.g., Camp et al., 1996; Clare, Wilson, Breen, & Hodges, 1999; Koltai, Welsh-Bohmer, & Schmechel, 2001; McKitrick, Camp, & Black, 1992; Teri,

Logsdon, Uomoto, & McCurry, 1997). The potential for such interventions to reduce excess disability and enhance patient functioning is apparent.

Although evidence for improved cognition and patient well-being as a result of intervention is broadening, limited data exist at present regarding the impact of such intervention on functional health and health-service utilization outcomes. There are clear links in the literature between cognitive status and hospitalization, need for formal care, quality of life, and mortality in community-dwelling elderly (Branch & Jette, 1982; Kelman, Thomas, Kennedy, & Cheng, 1994; Swan, Carmelli, & LaRue, 1995). Given the clearly established relationship of cognitive and affective variables to functional and health status, a favorable impact on these secondary variables is conceivable (Koltai & Branch, 1998, 1999). For instance, preliminary lines of investigation suggest that interventions targeting cognitive and perceptual abilities can result in enhanced activities of daily living such as driving and medication recall (Ball et al., 1993; Leirer, Morrow, Pariante, & Sheikh, 1988). This is an area of ongoing research, and more information is likely to be forthcoming with the publication of the results of the NIA-sponsored ACTIVE trial. This 5-year cooperative study explores the effects of cognitive intervention on improving cognitive performance and activities of daily living in older adults at risk of loss of independence (Jobe et al., 2001).

The following chapter provides a review of various intervention approaches and a discussion of their clinical utility and potential impact on health-care costs. Neuropsychology is not only essential to the execution of such specialized interventions, but comprehensive neuropsychological evaluation often is indispensable to successful treatment planning (Koltai & Branch 1998, 1999; Prigatano, 1997). The neuropsychological evaluation is used to design interventions specific to the patient's level of functioning in various domains, and thus the results direct both the target of treatment as well as the techniques used. In this manner, neuropsychology further expands its role beyond identification and diagnosis of illness and estimating function, by providing data to inform and monitor the treatment process.

☐ Use of Neuropsychology in Primary Care Practice

Despite the acknowledged utility of neuropsychological testing in geriatric practice, cognitive assessment (even simple mental status screening) is not common in primary care practices (Siu, 1991). The reasons for this phenomenon are not entirely clear, but they appear to be due to a combination of factors including economic pressures imposed by managed care, physician burden, clinician knowledge of AD, perceptions regarding the practical utility of mental status testing, and availability of specialists to handle dementia referrals (Barrett, Haley, Harrell, & Powers, 1997; Brummel-Smith, 1998; Weiner et al., 1998). In one survey of 27 internists at the Mayo clinic, 65% felt that the MMSE rarely affected their diagnosis, and another 58% reported that mental status testing took too much time to complete (Tangalos et al., 1996). Another study examining knowledge of AD among primary care physicians, psychologists, nurses, and social workers showed deficits in fundamental knowledge of the illness across all four groups of generalists (Barrett et al., 1997). For example, in this survey only 40% of the sample of providers knew that AD was the most common cause of severe memory loss in people over age 65.

A challenge in today's climate of economic austerity and managed care is to find the appropriate balance between cost and accuracy of diagnosis. To this end, practice parameters for the evaluation of dementia have been put in place in an effort to provide a neutral, evidence-based mechanism for determining what tests to consider in diagnostic scenarios and for resolving conflicts about coverage under managed care (Report of the Quality Standards Subcommittee of the AAN, 1994). Practice parameters are divided into three levels of certainty: *standards* (strong certainty), *guidelines* (moderate certainty), and *options* (unclear certainty). Clinical evidence supporting the recommendations also are divided into three classifications based on scientific rigor. The strongest evidence is that of Class I, which is provided by one or more well-designed randomized controlled clinical trials. Class II evidence is provided by one or more well-designed clinical studies, such as case-control studies, observational studies, and the like. Class III evidence provides the weakest scientific support and is composed of expert opinion, case reports, or studies involving nonrandomized historical controls.

The practice recommendations of the Quality Standards Subcommittee for the diagnostic evaluation of AD recommended neurological examination, history, and mental status examination as essential *standard* components of the diagnostic evaluation (see Doody et al., 2001; Corey-Bloom et al., 1995; Knopman et al., 2001, for review). A number of laboratory studies of basic chemistry were suggested as *guidelines*, such as complete blood count, thyroid function tests, B12 levels, and syphilis serology. Neuropsychological tests, neuroimaging studies, and other laboratory tests were considered as *options*. With respect to the neuropsychological recommendations, the practice suggestions are fairly reasonable. As articulated, they underscore the importance of at least some minimal neurocognitive testing in all cases of suspected dementia, but they provide little guidance for when a more comprehensive neuropsychological referral should be sought.

To test the utility of the AAN practice parameters a recent study systematically analyzed the relative contribution of laboratory studies, neuropsychological testing, and neuroimaging studies to the diagnosis and management of dementia (Chui & Zhang, 1997). Using consecutive referrals to a specialty center for dementia, the first level of analysis examined diagnostic accuracy based on the recommended standards for the evaluation: history, mental status test, neurological, and physical examination. The next level of analysis examined the added benefit of the other optional studies.

The results of this study showed that neuropsychological assessment changed the diagnosis in 11% of the cases. The results of the neuropsychological testing were particularly important in differentiating mild cognitive impairment from early AD and in identifying depression comorbidity. Indeed, depression was diagnosed in 12% of the subjects, although this was not suspected after the standard history and examination. We suggest that, given the moderate cost of neuropsychological assessment and its "unique, but selective contribution," neuropsychological testing should be considered in cases of mild cognitive impairment or in atypical presentations, such as when secondary memory is not a dominant feature. These recommendations are more forcefully underscored by subsequent studies, which have examined the clinical accuracy of the AD diagnosis in the context of medical comorbidities (e.g., Lopez et al., 2000b).

As primary care physicians become more informed about the merit of early detection of dementia, availability of treatment options, and the effects that early treatment can have on immediate and long-term outcomes, trends in referrals for evaluation are likely to change. In addition, in-office screens informed and developed by neuropsychology also will also assist in early identification by making routine screening tenable.

Role of Neuropsychology in Emerging Trends of Primary and Secondary Prevention

The importance of neuropsychology in the diagnosis and management of dementia and its potential to positively contribute to favorable long-term outcomes are becoming apparent as a number of therapeutic and preventive therapies enter clinical practice. Neuropsychology plays a pivotal role in accurately diagnosing early cases of suspected dementia and in monitoring both large and subtle treatment effects on cognition. It also plays a critical role in ongoing epidemiological investigations of dementia and in primary and secondary prevention efforts.

Epidemiological studies of dementia have identified a variety of agents that may act to provoke or delay the occurrence of dementia. Factors include the use of nonsteroidal antiinflammatory drugs (Breitner et al., 1994), antioxidant agents such as vitamin E and C (Masaki et al., 2000), and estrogen replacement therapy in women (Kawas et al., 1997). What is becoming increasingly apparent is that AD likely is not caused in the majority of cases by a single gene or disease exposure. Rather, the illness likely is a genetically complex disease, provoked by a combination of gene–gene interactions (e.g., St George-Hyslop, McLachlan, Tuda, & Rogaev, 1994; Reynolds et al., 2000) and gene–environment interactions (e.g., Yaffe et al., 2000).

To test the hypotheses that these agents do act to influence the underlying pathological process to AD, a number of primary and secondary prevention trials are currently under way. The rationale underlying all of these studies is the observation that the neuropathogenic process of AD appears to be protracted, with changes occurring over a continuum and gradually over a period of many years and perhaps decades (Braak & Braak, 1991). Implementing therapy during the prodromal stage of AD (or so-called MCI) is likely to be advantageous. The critical role of neuropsychology instruments to detect small (as well as large) changes in cognition is apparent.

The importance of neuropsychology in assuring accurate diagnosis continues to grow as more medications enter the market for the treatment of symptoms of AD. To this end, there are currently four anticholinesterase medications available for patients with AD dementia: Cognex (tacrine; Knapp et al., 1994), Aricept (donepezil; Rogers et al., 1996), Exelon (rivistigamine; Corey-Bloom et al., 1998), and Reminyl (galantamine). New compounds also are under development targeting the underlying neurobiology of the illness (Schenk et al., 1999; Dovey et al., 2001). As more of these compounds move from the laboratory bench to the consumer market, it will become critical to begin treatments early in the disease process, before significant neural injury has occurred in the brain and while the chance of effective treatment is at its highest.

Economic Impact of Neuropsychological Diagnosis and Management of Dementia

The clinical utility of neuropsychological evaluation in dementia is apparent, as outlined above. Numerous lines of evidence support increased diagnostic accuracy in cases of early or ambiguous cognitive decline with neuropsychological assessment, as well as more precise differentiation between various competing diagnostic probabilities. The neuropsychological evaluation also guides the care process by providing information about functional status and informing the treatment process. Although at present there is a glaring absence of cost-analysis investigations involving neuropsychological assessment, the potential for demonstrating favorable economic impact with the use of neuropsychological services clearly exists. We anticipate that such studies will be forthcoming as the current trend of evidence-based medicine continues to direct care practices and reimbursement trends.

Examples of potential cost-analysis studies corresponding to the aforementioned utility areas can be found in Table 9.5. The first example highlights the potential long-term cost-savings of early identification. The independent variable is dollars spent and the dependent variable is dollars saved. In such a scenario, neuropsychological assessment identifies the likely presence of a neurodegenerative disease early during the course of illness, and thus facilitates the early introduction of anticholinesterase inhibitors. The mild increased costs during the early stage from neuropsychological evaluation and routine neurological follow-up are easily offset by the substantial long-term cost-savings of institutionalization being delayed. This *cost–benefits* analysis would focus on the relative cost of the two alternatives (i.e., examination with and without neuropsychological assessment), and would focus on the cost of two different forms of care.

The second example illustrates how assessment can result in a substantial gain in Quality Adjusted Years (QAYs) through the prediction of functions that affect competency decisions. Specifically, in this example the absence of assessment results in the diagnosis of dementia based on standard examination alone. Given that the patient presented with cognitive disturbance including memory loss, declined arithmetic skills, and diminished ability to handle household responsibilities (specifically, financial management), this diagnosis was reasonable. Based on the diagnosis, the patient was declared incompetent, and family members took over financial management responsibilities and medication management, and the patient's driving privileges were revoked. In contrast, the presence of assessment results in a markedly different outcome. Specifically, the patient is diagnosed with mild cognitive compromises secondary to subcortical vascular dysfunction. The profile suggests very circumscribed deficits characterized by a retrieval memory deficit and declined mathematical skills, occurring in the context of preserved intellectual, executive, language, and visual–spatial skills. Because there was no marked evidence suggesting that driving skills might be effected, restriction was not recommended, but formal evaluation of driving skills was in order to ensure safety. After passing this examination, the patient was allowed to retain driving privileges. The family was encouraged to assume responsibilities for fiscal matters and to assist in complex medication management as needed. In this example, neuropsychological assessment resulted in a more refined diagnosis, allowing for prediction of preserved versus affected skills. Doing so allowed for continued maximum autonomy and independence, as compared to a more global diagnosis leading to an unnecessary restriction of all complex activities. This *cost-effective* analysis would focus on the relative cost of the two alternatives in outcomes valued by individual and societal preferences. This would be valued as QAYs—in this example, defined years of functioning at maximum independence.

The third and final example highlights how neuropsychological assessment can promote the efficient delivery of intervention services. Specifically, this cost-analysis would

TABLE 9.5. Cost Analyses of Neuropsychological Assessment

Example 1: Cost–Benefits: Neuropsychological Assessment *Never* vs. *Present*

Initial Tests	Initial Costs ($)	Additional Costs (+$)	Benefit (-$)	Total Cost
Standard exam, laboratory tests	$500	$90,000 = 24 months nursing home (diagnosis uncertain; treatment delayed)	Low initial cost	$90,500

Initial Tests	Initial Costs ($)	Additional Costs (+$)	Benefit (-$)	Total Cost
Standard exam, laboratory tests, comprehensive neuropsychological examination	$1,500	$2,500 = cost of drug, MD visits (AD pattern on testing, drug prescribed)	$45,000 = Nursing home savings, patient stays home for 12 months	$49,000

Example 2: Cost-Effectiveness: Neuropsychological Prediction of Function *Never* vs. *Present*

Initial Tests	Initial Costs ($)	Outcome
Standard exam, laboratory tests	$500	Relative decrease in QAYs through unnecessary restriction of activities related to independence (i.e., driving)

Initial Tests	Initial Costs ($)	Outcome
Standard exam, laboratory tests, comprehensive neuropsychological examination	$1,500	Relative increase in QAYs through restriction of only activities related to isolated impairments identified on neuropsychological testing

Example 3: Cost-Efficiency (Minimization): Neuropsychological Assessment in Treatment Planning *Never* vs. *Present*

Initial Tests	Initial Costs ($)	Additional Costs (+$)	Benefit (-$)	Total Cost
Standard exam, laboratory tests	$500	$2,175 = 15 sessions of treatment needed to achieve positive treatment outcome	Low initial cost	$2,675

Initial Tests	Initial Costs ($)	Additional Costs (+$)	Benefit (-$)	Total Cost
Standard exam, laboratory tests, comprehensive neuropsychological examination	$1,500	$725 = 5 sessions of treatment needed to achieve positive treatment outcome	$450 cost savings with decreased therapy costs	$2,225

compare the cost of treatment with and without the benefit of being informed by neuropsychological data. Intervention strategies and techniques diverge in their complexity and reliance on intact underlying cognitive skill. With the test results, the therapist could easily identify the targets of treatment and the individually tailored treatment approach that would yield the greatest benefit based on the pattern of deficits versus spared areas cognition. Without such data, two or three techniques may be attempted before one is found that yields clinical benefit. This *cost-efficiency* (*minimization*) analysis would compare the relative costs of the two alternatives that had the same outcome, in this case improved adaptation and compensation to memory loss. It should be noted that although the cost-savings is offset minimally by the cost of the neuropsychological evaluation, benefits also would include the minimization of number of sessions for the patient and caregiver, and additional uses of the data (i.e., diagnosis, estimation of function). However, consideration of these last variables would require the use of a cost–benefit or cost–utility analysis, which allows for variation in the quality and magnitude of outcomes.

☐ Conclusions

The clinical utility of neuropsychological assessment is widely accepted in practice and is supported by empirical study. It is understood that comprehensive evaluation typically enhances diagnosis and management, and that this is particularly useful in cases involving ambiguous, early, or atypical cognitive change. The contribution of neuropsychological services in diagnostic, prognostic, and treatment services is reflected in the continued growth of the field. However, barriers to service utilization remain. These include lack of basic dementia education among practitioners, absence of familiarity with existing research indicating the unique contribution of neuropsychology to the diagnostic process (e.g., Tierney, 1996a; 1996b; Tschanz et al., 2000), limited access to services providing sensitive screens for routine use, and the absence of cost-analysis data to clearly demonstrate the potential gains of service utilization.

These limitations are to be expected, but they are not insurmountable. Additional efficacy data supporting the clinical utility of the various neuropsychological applications would be helpful in ameliorating a portion of these challenges, and such studies could serve as the foundation for cost-analysis investigations, which could then demonstrate outcomes in tangible units (e.g., fiscal savings, treatment efficiency, quality of life impact). Continued development and refinement of screening batteries for standard practice also would support rational, economically conservative approaches to assessment, with appropriate cases being referred for comprehensive evaluation when needed. As health-care practices continue to evolve around health-care policy, it is essential that empirical evidence of favorable clinical and cost outcomes become available to inform and shape that policy. It is with this awareness that research involving the neuropsychological assessment of early dementia should move forward. Neuropsychological studies can offer practical solutions to the primary care physician, supplying important tools for monitoring in a cost-effective manner the growing numbers of geriatric patients in their practices and providing a framework for when the referral of suspect cases for more detailed neuropsychological services may be helpful and warranted.

References

Agency for Health Care Policy and Research (AHCPR). (1996). *Early identification of Alzheimer's disease and related dementias.* Publication number 97-0703. Washington, DC: U.S. Department of Health and Human Services.

Albert, M. (1981). Geriatric neuropsychology. *Journal of Consulting and Clinical Psychology, 49,* 835–850.

American Psychiatric Association. (1994). *Diagnostic and statistical manual of mental disorders* (4th ed.). Washington DC: Author.

American Psychiatric Association. (1987). *Diagnostic and statistical manual of mental disorders* (3rd ed. rev.). Washington DC: Author.

American Psychiatric Association. (1980). Diagnostic and statistical manual of mental disorders (3rd ed.). Washington DC: Author.

Bagli, M., Papassotiropoulos, A., Jessen F., et al. (2000). Gene-gene interaction between interleukin-6 and alpha2- macroglobulin influences the risk for Alzheimer's disease. *Annals of Neurology, 47,* 138–139.

Baker, F. (1987). Competent for what? *Journal of the National Medical Association, 79,* 715–720.

Ball, K., Owsley, C., Sloane, M. E., Roenker, D. L., & Bruni, J. R. (1993). Visual attention problems as a predictor of vehicle crashes in older drivers. *Investigative Ophthalmology and Visual Science, 34,* 3110–3123.

Barrett, J. J., Haley, W. E., Harrell, L. E., & Powers, R. E. (1997). Knowledge about Alzheimer disease among primary care physicians, psychologists, nurses, and social workers. *Alzheimer's Disease and Associated Disorders, 11,* 99–106.

Baum, C., Edwards, D., Yonan, C, & Storandt, M. (1996). The relation of neuropsychological test performance to performance of functional tasks in dementia of the Alzheimer type. *Archives of Clinical Neuropsychology, 11,* 69–75.

Blacker, D., Wilcox, M. A., Laird, N. M., et al. (1998). Alpha-2 macroglobulin is genetically associated with Alzheimer disease. *Nature Genetics, 19,* 357–360.

Blazer, D. G. (1994). Dysthymia in community and clinical samples of older adults. *American Journal of Psychiatry, 151,* 1567–1569.

Bondi, M. W., Monsch, A. U., Galasko, D., Butters, N., Salmon, D. P., & Delis, D. C. (1994). Preclinical cognitive markers of Alzheimer's disease. *Neuropsychology, 8,* 374–384.

Bookheimer, S. Y., Strojwas, M. H., Cohen, M. S., Saunders, A. M., Pericak-Vance, M. A., Mazziotta, J. C., & Small, G. W. (2000). Patterns of brain activation in people at risk for Alzheimer's disease. *New England Journal of Medicine, 343,* 450–456.

Bracco, L., Amaducci, L., Pedone, D., Bino, G., Lazzaro, M. P., Carella, F., D'Antona, R., Gallato, R., & Denes, G. (1990). Italian Multicentre Study on Dementia (SMID): A neuropsychological test battery for assessing Alzheimer's disease. *Journal of Psychiatric Research, 24,* 213–226.

Braak, H., & Braak, E. (1991). Neuropathological staging of Alzheimer–related changes. *Acta Neuropathologica, 82,* 239–259.

Branch, L., & Jette, A. (1982). A prospective study of long-term care institutionalization among the aged. *American Journal of Public Health, 72,* 1373–1379.

Branch, L., Wetle, T., Scherr, P., Cook, N., Evans, D., Hebert, L., Masland, E., Keough, M., & Taylor, J. (1988). A prospective study of incident comprehensive medical home care use among the elderly. *American Journal of Public Health, 78,* 255–259.

Breitner J. C. S., Gau, B., Welsh, K. A., Plassman B., Helms M., & Anthony J. (1994). Inverse association between anti-inflammatory agents and Alzheimer's disease: Initial results of a co-twin control study. *Neurology, 44,* 227–232.

Breitner, J. C. S., Wyse, B. W., Anthony, J. C., Welsh-Bohmer, K. A., Steffens, D. C., Norton, M. C., Tschanz, J. D., Plassman, B. J., Meyer, M. R., Skoog, I., & Khatchaturian. (1999). APOE e4 predicts age when prevalence of Alzheimer's disease increases-then declines. *Neurology, 53,* 321–331.

Brody, E., Kleban, M., Lawton, M. P., & Silverman, H. (1971). Excess disabilities of mentally impaired aged: Impact of individualized treatment. *The Gerontologist* (Summer, Part 1), 124–133.

Brookmeyer, R. Gray, S., & Kawas, C. (1998). Projections of Alzheimer's disease in the U.S. and the public health impact of delaying disease onset. *American Journal of Public Health*, 88, 1337–1342.

Brummel-Smith, K. V. (1998). Alzheimer's disease and managed care: How much will it cost. *Journal of the American Geriatrics Society, 46,* 780–781.

Butters, N., Delis, D.C., Lucas, J. A. (1995). Clinical assessment of memory disorders in amnesia and dementia. *Annual Review of Psychology, 46,* 493–523.

Camp, C. J., Foss, J. W., O'Hanlon, A. M., & Stevens, A. B. (1996). Memory interventions for persons with dementia. *Applied Cognitive Psychology, 10,* 193–210.

Chui, H., & Zhang, Q. (1997). Evaluation of dementia: A systematic study of the usefulness of the American Academy of Neurology's Practice Parameters. *Neurology, 49,* 925–935.

Clare, L., Wilson, B., Breen, K., & Hodges, J. (1999). Errorless learning of face-name associations in early Alzheimer's disease. *Neurocase, 5,* 37–46.

Clarfield, A. (1988). The reversible dementias: Do they reverse? *Annals of Internal Medicine, 109,* 476–486.

Corder, E. H., Saunders, A. M., Strittmatter, W. J., et al. (1993). Gene dose of apolipoprotein E type 4 allele and the risk of Alzheimer's disease in late onset families. *Science, 261,* 921–923.

Corey-Bloom, J., Anand, R., & Veach, J. for the ENA 713 B352 Study Group. (1998). A randomized trial evaluating efficacy and safety of ENA 713 (rivistigmine tartrate), a new acetylcholinersterase inhibitor in patients with mild to moderately severe Alzheimer's disease. *International Journal of Geriatric Psychopharmacology, 1,* 55–65.

Cummings, J. L., & Therapeutics and Technology Assessment Subcommittee of the American Academy of Neurology. (1996). Assessment: Neuropsychological testing of adults: Considerations for neurologists. *Neurology, 47,* 592–599.

Diehl, M., Willis, S., & Schaie, K. (1995). Everyday problem solving in older adults: Observational assessment and cognitive correlates. *Psychology and Aging, 10,* 478–491.

Doody, R. S., Stevens, J. C., Beck, C., Dubinshy, R. M., Kaye, J. A., Gwyther, L., Mohs, R. C., Thal, L. J., Whitehouse, P. J., DeKosky, S. T., & Cummings, J. L. (2001). Practice parameter: Management of dementia (an evidence-based review). Report of the Quality Standards Subcommittee of the American Academy of Neurology. *Neurology, 56,* 1154–1166.

Dovey, H. F., Anderson, J. V., Chen, J. P., et al. (2001). Functional gamma-secretase inhibitors reduce beta-amyloid peptide levels in brain. *Journal of Neurochemistry, 76,* 173–181.

Ernst, R. L., & Hay, J. W. (1994). The U.S. economic and social costs of Alzheimer's disease revisited. *American Journal of Public Health, 84,* 1261–1264.

Evans, D. A., Scherr, P. A., Cook, N. R., et al. (1990). Estimated prevalence of Alzheimer's Disease in the United States. *Milbank Quarterly, 68,* 267–289.

Finckh, U., von der Kammer, H., Velden, J., et al. (2000). Genetic association of a cystatin C gene polymorphism with late onset Alzheimer's disease. *Archives of Neurology, 57,* 1579–1583.

Fitz, A., & Teri, L. (1994). Depression, cognition, and functional ability in patients with Alzheimer's disease. *Journal of the American Geriatrics Society, 42,* 186–191.

Gearing, M., Mirra, S. S., Hedreen, J. C., Sumi, S. M., Hansen, L. A., Heyman, A. (1995). The Consortium to Establish a Registry for Alzheimer's Disease (CERAD), Part X: Neuropathological confirmation of the clinical diagnosis of Alzheimer's disease. *Neurology, 45,* 461–466.

Gnanalingham, K. K., Byrne, E. J., Thornton, A., Sambrook, M. A., & Bannister, P. (1997). Motor and cognitive function in Lewy body dementia: Comparison with Alzheimer's disease and Parkinson's disease. *Journal of Neurology, Neurosurgery, and Psychiatry, 62,* 243–252.

Goate, A., Chartier, H. M., Mullan, J., et al. (1991). Segregation of a missense mutation in the amyloid precursor protein gene with familial Alzheimer's disease. *Nature, 349,* 704–706.

Graham, J. E., Rockwood, K., Beattie, B. L., McDowell, I., Eastwood, R., & Gauthier, S. (1996). Standardization of the diagnosis of dementia in the Canadian Study of Health and Aging. *Neuroepidemiology, 15,* 246–256.

Greiner, P., Snowdon, D., & Schmitt, F. (1996). The loss of independence in activities of daily living: The role of low normal cognitive function in elderly nuns. *American Journal of Public Health, 86,* 62–66.

Grober, E., & Kawas, C. (1997). Learning and retention in preclinical and early Alzheimer's disease. *Psychology & Aging, 12,* 183–188.

Grodin, M. A., & Laurie, G. T. (2000). Susceptibility genes and neurological disorders. *Neurology, 57,* 1569–1574.

Hansen, L., Salmon, D., Galasko, D., Masliah, E., Katzman, R., DeTeresa, R., Thal, L., Pay, M., Hofstetter, R., Klauber, M., Rice, V., Butters, N., & Alford, M. (1990). The Lewy body variant of Alzheimer's disease: A clinical and pathological entity. *Neurology, 40,* 1–8.

Hoffman, J. M., Welsh-Bohmer, K. A., Hanson, M., Crain, B., Hulette, C., Earl, N., & Coleman, R. E. (2000). Fluorodeoxyglucose (FDG) and positron emission tomography (PET) in pathologically verified dementia. *Journal of Nuclear Medicine, 41,* 1920–1928.

Howieson, D. B., Dame, A., Camicioli, R., Sexton, G., Payami, H., & Kaye, J. A. (1997). Cognitive markers preceding Alzheimer's dementia in the healthy oldest old. *Journal of the American Geriatric Society, 45,* 584–589.

Jobe, J. B., Smith, D. M., Ball, K., Tennstedt, S. L., Marsiske, M., Willis, S. L., Rebok, G. W., Morris, J. N., Helmers, K. F., Leveck, M. D., & Kleinman, K. (2001). ACTIVE: A cognitive intervention trial to promote independence in older adults. *Controlled Clinical Trials, 22,* 453–479.

Jones, R., Tranel, D., Benton, A., & Paulsen, J. (1992). Differentiating dementia from "pseudodementia" early in the clinical course: Utility of neuropsychological tests. *Neuropsychology, 6,* 13–21.

Katzman, R., Aronson, M., Fuld, P., Kawas, C., Brown, T., Morgenstern, H., Frishman, W., Gidez, L., Eder, H., & Ooi, W. L. (1989). Development of dementing illnesses in an 80-year-old volunteer cohort. *Annals of Neurology, 25,* 317–324.

Kawas, C., Resnick, S., Morrison, A., et al. (1997). A prospective study of estrogen replacement therapy and the risk for developing Alzheimer's disease: The Baltimore Longitudinal Study of Aging. *Neurology, 48,* 1517–1521.

Kaszniak, A. (1987). Neuropsychological consultation to geriatricians: Issues in the assessment of memory complaints. *The Clinical Neuropsychologist, 1,* 35–46.

Kelman, H. R., Thomas, C., Kennedy, G. J., & Cheng, J. (1994). Cognitive impairments and mortality in older community residents. *American Journal of Public Health, 84,* 1255–1260.

Kloezen, S., Fitten, L., & Steinberg, A. (1988). Assessment of treatment decision-making capacity in a medically ill patient. *Journal of the American Geriatrics Society, 36,* 1055–1058.

Knapp, M. J., Knopman, D. S., Solomon, P. R., Pendlebury, W. W., Davis, C. S., & Gracon, S. I. (1994). A 30-week randomized controlled trial of high-dose tacrine in patients with Alzheimer's disease: The Tacrine Study Group. *Journal of the American Medical Association, 271,* 985–991

Knopman, D. S., DeKosky, S. T., Cummings, J. L., Chui, H., Corey-Bloom, J., Relkin, N., Small, G. W., Miller, B., & Stevens, J. C. (2001). Practice parameter: Diagnosis of dementia (an evidence-based review). Report of the Quality Standards Subcommittee of the American Academy of Neurology. *Neurology, 56,* 1143–1153.

Koenig, H. G., & Blazer, D. G. (1992). Epidemiology of geriatric affective disorders. *Clinics in Geriatric Medicine, 8,* 235–251.

Koltai, D. C., & Branch, L. G. (1999). Cognitive and affective interventions to maximize abilities and adjustment in dementia. *Annals of Psychiatry: Basic and Clinical Neurosciences, 7,* 241–255.

Koltai, D. C., & Branch, L. G. (1998). Consideration of intervention alternatives to optimize independent functioning in the elderly. *Journal of Clinical Geropsychology, 4,* 333–349.

Koltai, D. C., & Welsh-Bohmer, K. A. (2000). Geriatric Neuropsychological Assessment. In R. D. Vanderploeg (Ed.), *Clinician's guide to neuropsychological assessment* (2nd ed., pp. 383–415). Mahwah, NJ: Lawrence Erlbaum.

Koltai, D., Welsh-Bohmer, K., & Schmechel, D. (2001). Influence of anosognosia on treatment outcome among dementia patients. *Neuropsychological Rehabilitation, 11,* 455–475.

Leirer, V. O., Morrow, D. G., Pariante, G. M., & Sheikh, J. I. (1988). Elders nonadherence, its assessment and computer assisted instruction for medication recall training. *Journal of the American Geriatrics Society, 36,* 877–884.

Levy-Lahad, E., Wasco, W., Poorkaj, P., et al. (1995). Candidate gene for the chromosome 1 familial AD locus. *Science, 269,* 973–977.

Lindau, M., Almkvist, O., Johansson, S. E., & Wahlund, L. O. (1998). Cognitive and behavioral differentiation of frontal lobe degeneration of the non-Alzheimer type and Alzheimer's disease. *Dementia & Geriatric Cognitive Disorders, 9,* 205–213.

Looi, J. C. L., Sachdev, P. S. (1999). Differentiation of vascular dementia from AD on neuropsychological tests. *Neurology, 53,* 670–678.

Lopez, O. L., Becker, J. T., Klunk, W., et al. (2000a). Research evaluation and diagnosis of possible Alzheimer's disease over the last two decades: I. *Neurology, 55,* 1854–1862.

Lopez, O. L., Becker, J. T., Klunk, W. et al. (2000b). Research evaluation and diagnosis of possible Alzheimer's disease over the last two decades: II. *Neurology, 55,* 1863–1869.

Lopez, O. L., Litvan, I., Catt, K. E. et al. (1999). Accuracy of four clinical diagnostic criteria for the diagnosis of neurodegenerative dementias. *Neurology, 53,* 1292–1299.

Marson, D., Schmitt, F., Ingram, K., & Harrell, L. (1994). Determining the competency of Alzheimer patients to consent to treatment and research. *Alzheimer Disease and Associated Disorders, 8,* 5–18.

Marson, D., Ingram, K., Cody, H., & Harrell, L. (1995). Assessing the competency of patients with Alzheimer's disease under different legal standards. *Archives of Neurology, 52,* 949–954.

Masaki, K. H., Losconczy, K. G., Izmirlian G., et al. (2000). Association of vitamin E and C supplement use with cognitive function and dementia in elderly men. *Neurology, 54,* 1265–1272.

McCue, M. (1997). The relationship between neuropsychology and functional assessment in the elderly. In: P. Nussbaum (Ed.), *Handbook of neuropsychology and aging* (pp. 394–408). New York: Plenum Press.

McKhann, G., Drachman, D. A., Folstein, M. F., Katzman, R., Price, D. L., & Stadlan, E. (1984). Clinical diagnosis of Alzheimer's disease: The report of the NINCDS-ADRDA Work Group under the auspices of the Department of Health and Human Services Task Force on Alzheimer's Disease. *Neurology, 34,* 939–944.

McKitrick, L., Camp, C., & Black, F. W. (1992). Prospective memory intervention in Alzheimer's disease. *Journal of Gerontology, 47,* P337–P343.

McPherson, S. E., & Cummings, J. L. (1996). Frontal-subcortical circuits and human behavior. *Brain & Cognition, 31,* 261–282.

Migliorelli, R., Teson, A., Sabe, L., Petracchi, M., Leiguarda, R., & Starkstein, S. (1995). Prevalence and correlates of dysthymia and major depression among patients with Alzheimer's disease. *American Journal of Psychiatry, 152,* 37–44.

Moss, M. B., Albert M. S., & Kemper, T. L. (1992). Neuropsychology of frontal lobe dementia. In R. F. White (Ed.), *Clinical syndromes in adult neuropsychology: The practitioner's handbook* (pp. 287–303). New York: Elsevier Press.

Nadler, J., Richardson, E., Malloy, P., Marran, M., & Hostetler Brinson, M. (1993). The ability of the Dementia Rating Scale to predict everyday functioning. *Archives of Clinical Neuropsychology, 8,* 449–460.

National Institute on Aging/Alzheimer's Association Working Group. (1996). Apolipoprotein E genotyping in Alzheimer's disease. *Lancet, 347,* 1091–1095.

Neary, D., Snowden, S., Gustafson, L., et al. (1998). Frontotemporal lobe degeneration: a consensus on clinical diagnostic criteria. *Neurology, 51,* 1546–1552.

Nicoll, J. A., Mrak, R. E., Graham, D. I., Stewart, J., Wilcock, G., MacGowan, S., Esiri, M. M., Murray, L. S., Dewar, D., Love, S., Moss, T., & Griffin, W. S. (2000). Association of interleukin-1 gene polymorphisms with Alzheimer's disease. *Annals of Neurology, 47,* 365–368.

Pachana, N. A., Boone, K. B., Miller, B. L., Cummings, J. L., & Berman, N. (1996). Comparison of neuropsychological functioning in Alzheimer's disease and frontotemporal dementia. *Journal of the International Neuropsychological Society, 2,* 1–6.

Papassotiropoulos, A., Bali, M., Kurz, A., et al. (2000). A genetic variation of cathepsin D is a major risk factor for Alzheimer's disease. *Annals of Neurology, 47,* 399–403.

Perry, R. J., & Hodges, J. R. (2000). Differentiating frontal and temporal variant frontotemporal dementia from Alzheimer's disease. *Neurology*, 54, 2277–2284.

Petersen, R. C., Smith, G. E., Ivnik, R. J., et al. (1994). Memory function in very early Alzheimer's disease. *Neurology, 44,* 867–872.

Petersen, R.C., Smith, G. E., Waring, S. C., et al. (1999). Mild cognitive impairment. Clinical characterization and outcome. *Archives of Neurology, 56,* 303–308.

Petersen, R. C., Stephens, J. C., Ganguli, M., Tangalos, E. G., Cummings, J. L., & DeKosky, S. T. (2001). Practice Parameter: Early detection of dementia: Mild cognitive impairment (an evidence based review). Report of the Quality Standards Subcommittee of the American Academy of Neurology. *Neurology, 56,* 1133–1142.

Pillon, B., Blin, J., Vidalhet, M., Deweer, B., Sirigu, A., Dubois, B., & Agid, Y. (1995). The neuropsychological pattern of corticobasal degeneration: Comparison with progressive supranuclear palsy and Alzheimer's disease. *Neurology, 45,* 1477–1483.

Pittman, J., Andrews, H., Tatemichi, T., Link, B., Struening, E., Stern, Y., & Mayeux, R. (1992). Diagnosis of dementia in a heterogeneous population. A comparison of paradigm-based diagnosis and physician's diagnosis. *Archives of Neurology, 49*, 461–467.

Prigatano, G. P. (1997). Learning from out successes and failures: Reflections and comments on "Cognitive rehabilitation: How it is and how it might be." *Journal of the International Neuropsychological Society, 3*, 497–499.

Rebok, G., Keyl, P., Bylsma, F., Blaustein, M., & Tune, L. (1994). The effects of Alzheimer disease on driving-related abilities. *Alzheimer Disease and Associated Disorders, 8*, 288–240.

Reiman, E. M., Caselli, R. J., Yun, L. S., Chen, K., Bandy, D., Minoshima, S., Thibodeau, S. N., & Osborne, D. (1996). Preclinical evidence of Alzheimer's disease in persons homozygous for the epsilon 4 allele for apolipoprotein E. *New England Journal of Medicine, 334*, 752–781.

Report of the Quality Standards Subcommittee of the American Academy of Neurology. (1994). Practice parameters for diagnosis and evaluation of dementia (summary statement). *Neurology, 44*, 2203–2206.

Reynolds, W. R., Hiltunen, M., Pirskanen, M., et al., (2000). MPO and APOEe4 polymorphisms interact to increase risk for AD in Finnish males. *Neurology, 55*, 1284–1290.

Ritchie, K., Artero, S., & Touchon, J. (2001). Classification criteria for mild cognitive impairment: A population based validation study. *Neurology, 56*, 37–42.

Rockwood, K., Stolee, P, & McDowell, I. (1996). Factors associated with institutionalization of older people in Canada: Testing a multi-factorial definition of frailty. *Journal of the American Geriatrics Society, 44*, 578–582.

Rogers, S. L., Friedhoff, L. T., et al. for the Donepezil Study Group. (1996). The efficacy and safety of donepezil in patients with Alzheimer's disease: Results of a US multicenter, randomized, double-blind, placebo-controlled trial. The Donepezil Study Group. *Dementia, 7*, 293–303.

Salmon, D. P., Galasko, D., Hansen, L. A., Masliah, E., et al. (1996). Neuropsychological deficits associated with diffuse Lewy body disease. *Brain & Cognition, 31*, 148–165.

Saunders, A. M., Schmader, K., Breitner, J. C., Benson, M. D., Brown, W. T., Goldfarb, L., Goldgaber, D., Manwaring, M. G., Szymanski, M. H., & McCown, N. (1993). Apolipoprotein E epsilon 4 allele distributions in late-onset Alzheimer's disease and in other amyloid-forming diseases. *Lancet, 342*, 710–711.

Scogin, F., & Perry, J. (1986). Guardianship proceedings with older adults: The role of functional assessment and gerontologists. *Law and Psychology Review, 10*, 123–128.

Sherrington, R., Rogaev, E., Liang, Y., et al. (1995). Cloning of a gene bearing mis-sense mutations in early onset Alzheimer's disease. *Nature, 375*, 754–760.

Silberman, E., Weingartner, H., Laraia, M., Byrnes, S., & Post, R. (1983). Processing of emotional properties of stimuli by depressed and normal subjects. *Journal of Neurological and Mental Disorders, 171*, 10–14.

Silverman, D. H., Gambhir, S. S., Huang, H. W., Schwimmer, J., Kim, S., Small, G. W., Chodosh, J., Czernin, J., & Phelps, M. E. (2002). Evaluating early dementia with and without assessment of regional cerebral metabolism by PET: A comparison of predicted costs and benefits. *Journal of Nuclear Medicine, 43*, 253–266.

Siu, A. L. (1991). Screening for dementia and investigating its causes. *Annals of Internal Medicine*, 115, 657–658.

Small, G. W., Ercoli, L. M., Silverman, D. H. S. et al. (2000). Cerebral metabolic and cognitive decline in persons at genetic risk for Alzheimer's disease. *PNAS, 97*, 6037–6042.

Small, G. W., Rabins, P. V., Barry, P. P., et al. (1997). Diagnosis and treatment of Alzheimer disease and related disorders: Consensus statement of the American Association for Geriatric Psychiatry, the Alzheimer's Association, and the American Geriatrics Society. *Journal of the American Medical Association, 278*, 1363–1371.

St. George-Hyslop, P., McLachlan, D. C., Tuda, T., & Rogaev, E. (1994). Alzheimer's disease and possible gene interactions. *Science, 263*, 537.

Stanley, B., Stanley, M., Guido, J., & Garvin L. (1988). The functional competency of elderly at risk. *Gerontologist, 28*, 53–58.

Steffens, D. C., Plassman, B. L., Helms, M. J., Welsh-Bohmer, K. A., Saunders, A. M., & Breitner, J. C. (1997). A twin study of late-onset depression and apolipoprotein E epsilon 4 as risk factors for Alzheimer's disease. *Biological Psychiatry, 41*, 851–856.

Steinberg, A., Fitten, L., & Kachuck, N. (1986). Patient participation in treatment decision-making in the nursing home: The issue of competence. *Gerontologist, 26,* 362–366.

Stern, Y., Andrews, H., Pittman, J., Sano, M., Tatemichi, T., Lantigua, R., & Mayeux, R. (1992). Diagnosis of dementia in a heterogeneous population: Development of a neuropsychological paradigm-based diagnosis of dementia and quantified correction for the effects of education. *Archives of Neurology, 49,* 453–460.

Swan, G. E., Carmelli, D., LaRue, A. (1995). Performance on the digit-symbol substitution test and five year morality in the Western Collaborative Group Study. *American Journal of Epidemiology, 141,* 32–40.

Tangalos, E. G., Smith, G. E., Ivnik, R. J., et al. (1996). The Mini-Mental State Examination in general medical practice: Clinical utility and acceptance. *Mayo Clinic Proceedings, 71,* 829–837.

Teri, L., Logsdon, R., Uomoto, J., & McCurry, S. (1997). Behavioral treatment of depression in dementia patients: A controlled clinical trial. *Journal of Gerontology, Psychological Sciences, 52B,* P159–P166.

Tierney, M. C., Szalai, J. P., Snow, W. G., Fisher, R. H., Tsuda, T., Chi, H., McLachlan, D. R., & St. George-Hyslop, P. H. (1996a). A prospective study of the clinical utility of ApoE genotype in the prediction of outcome in patients with memory impairment. *Neurology, 46,*149–154.

Tierney, M. C., Szalai, J. P., Snow, W. G., Fisher, R. H, Nores, A., Nadon, G., Dunn, E., & St.George-Hyslop, P. H. (1996b). Prediction of probable Alzheimer's disease in memory impaired patients: A prospective longitudinal study. *Neurology, 46,* 661–665.

Tschanz, J. T., Welsh-Bohmer, K. A., West, N., Norton, M. C., Wyse, B. W., Breitner, J. C. S., & Skoog, I. (2000). Identification of dementia cases derived from a neuropsychological algorithm: Comparisons with clinically derived diagnoses. *Neurology, 54,* 1290–1296.

Tymchuk, A., Ouslander, J., Rahbar, B., & Fitten, L. (1988). Medical decision-making among elderly people in long term care. *Gerontologist, 28,* 59–63.

Weiner, M., Powe, N. R., Weller, W. E., Shaffer, T. J., & Anderson, G. F. (1998). Alzheimer's disease under managed care: Implications from Medicare utilization and expenditure patterns. *Journal of the American Geriatrics Society, 46,* 762–770.

Welsh, K. A., Butters, N., Hughes, J. P., Mohs, R. C., & Heyman, A. (1991). Detection of abnormal memory decline in mild Alzheimer's disease using CERAD neuropsychological measures. *Archives of Neurology, 48,* 278–281.

Welsh, K. A., Butters, N., Hughes, J., Mohs, R., & Heyman, A. (1992). Detection and staging of dementia in Alzheimer's disease: Use of neuropsychological measures developed for the Consortium to Establish a Registry for Alzheimer's Disease (CERAD). *Archives of Neurology, 49,* 448–452.

Welsh-Bohmer, K. A., Gearing, M., Saunders, A. M., Roses, A. D., & Mirra, S. M. (1997). Apolipoprotein E genotypes in a neuropathological series from the Consortium to Establish a Registry for Alzheimer's Disease (CERAD). *Annals of Neurology, 42,* 319–325.

Welsh-Bohmer, K. A., & Morgenlander, J. C. (1999). Cognitive assessment of patients with suspected dementia: Mental status screening and neuropsychological assessment. *Postgraduate Medicine, 106,* 99–118.

Welsh-Bohmer, K. A., & Ogrocki, P. K. (1998). Clinical differentiation of memory disorders in neurodegenerative diseases. In A. I. Troster (Ed.), *Memory in neurodegenerative disease: Biological, cognitive, and clinical perspectives* (pp. 290–313). London: Cambridge University Press.

Welsh-Bohmer, K. A., Hulette, C., Schmechel, D., Burke, J., & Saunders, A. (2001). Neuropsychological detection of preclinical Alzheimer's disease: Results of a neuropathological series of "normal" controls. In K. Iqbal, S. S. Sisodia, & B. Winblad (Eds.), *Alzheimer's disease: Advances in etiology, pathogenesis and therapeutics. The Proceedings of the 7th International conference on Alzheimer's Disease and Related Disorders.* London: John Wiley & Sons, pp. 111–122.

Willis, S., & Marsiske, M. (1991). Life span perspective on practical intelligence. In D. Tupper & K. Cicerone (Eds.), *The neuropsychology of everyday life: Issues in development and rehabilitation* (pp. 183–198). Boston: Kluwer.

Yaffe, K., Haan, M., Byers, A., Tangen, C., & Kuller, L. (2000). Estrogen use, APOE, and cognitive decline. Evidence of gene-environment interaction. *Neurology, 54,* 1949–1953.

10
CHAPTER

Deborah Koltai Attix
Douglas J. Mason
Kathleen A. Welsh-Bohmer

Neuropsychological Consultation and Training of Family Members of Patients with Dementia

Introduction

Alzheimer's disease (AD) is a fatal neurodegenerative illness afflicting approximately 4 million people in the United States alone (Small et al., 1997). Families struggle as their loved ones confront steadily progressive, irreversible cognitive deterioration. The progressive destruction of intellectual capacity results in declining functional abilities and an increased need for assistance to carry out activities related to independence. Although estimates of the prevalence of AD vary considerably, a consistent finding is its responsibility for the majority of dementia cases in most series. AD accounts for approximately 45% to 67% of such cases, and less prevalent etiologies such as vascular dementia, Lewy-body disease, and Pick's disease account for the remainder (Cummings & Benson, 1992; Small et al., 1997).

Regardless of etiology, in most cases dementia robs its victim of the capacity to independently manage his or her own affairs. The family of the dementia patient thus becomes indispensable for the patient to effectively participate in everyday tasks, to ensure safety; and, in particular, to negotiate the health-care system. Typically, such assistance is essential to secure adequate heath care, including diagnosis and treatment to maximize functioning.

In this chapter, the role of the family in current neuropsychological practice will be outlined. The clinical utility of services involving family members of dementia patients will be reviewed. The potential cost impact of such services will be discussed through a review of examples of cost-analyses and considerations for future research.

☐ Consultation and Training of Family Members of Patients with Dementia: Current Practice

> Mrs. B is a 67-year-old female with 14 years of education who has recently sought medical evaluation at the encouragement of her family. She has a 2-year history of forgetfulness and has recently been repetitious and had difficulty carrying out activities of daily living requiring organization and reasoning. Despite these changes, she has managed to compensate relatively well and, with the assistance of her husband as well as her children, who visit frequently, she is able to participate in most of her previous activities and responsibilities. She is aware of her declining cognitive capacity and is reasonably concerned, given that these changes occur within the context of a strong family history of Alzheimer's disease. As once easily performed activities have become challenging, Mrs. B has shown increased withdrawal, tearfulness, and sadness. Her family is concerned that she is depressed.
>
> As part of her complete neurological examination, Mrs. B is referred for neuropsychological evaluation. Given that her findings support relatively intact insight and many spared abilities at this stage of the illness, the neurologist subsequently refers the patient for intervention. Based on the neuropsychological findings and the goals of the patient and her family, an intervention plan targeting mood and memory is agreed upon. In this particular case, the plan involves a behavioral approach to the patient's treatable depressive symptomatology and compensatory strategies to address her memory loss. The principal goal is to enhance present functioning to the maximal level of autonomy that can be executed without compromising safety.

For neuropsychologists, initial contact with family members of patients with dementia typically occurs when the patient is seen for neuropsychological evaluation. In this initial role, the family primarily serves as a source of collateral information. Evaluations that are completed without consideration of these family perspectives are at a distinct disadvantage, as there is clear evidence of increased diagnostic accuracy as a result of consideration of the history provided by an informant. Specifically, the accuracy of both dementia classification and prediction is enhanced through such collateral perspectives of patient functioning (Tierney, Szalai, Snow, & Fischer, 1996; Tschanz et al., 2000). Because the family often has also assumed the role of care manager at this time, it is important to consider family members' need to appreciate the purpose and utility of evaluation. For assessment as well as other neuropsychological services, it often is necessary for caregivers to grant consent and assume responsibility for services. In this sense, they become consumers. As an extension of this role, they also are involved as recipients of feedback, which addresses diagnosis, prognosis, and feasibility of intervention. (Chapter 9 of this text addressed the clinical utility of neuropsychological evaluation in patients with known or suspected dementia.)

Alternatively, contact may begin when patients and their families are referred for intervention services, with or without the benefit of neuropsychological data. Until recently, a longstanding bias existed against the use of memory training and psychotherapeutic interventions with dementia patients, due to a pervasive perception of their inability to benefit from such treatment. However, this ardent belief now appears to have been premature, as gains have been found as a result of memory training (e.g., Camp, Foss, O'Hanlon, & Stevens, 1996; Clare, Wilson, Breen, & Hodges, 1999; Koltai, Welsh-Bohmer, & Schmechel, 2001). The high prevalence of depression among dementia patients (Migliorelli et al., 1995) and promising findings of gain from intervention (Teri et al., 1997; Teri, Logsdon, Wagner, & Uomoto, 1994) also have served to motivate clinicians to target those aspects of patients' presentations that are amenable to treatment. As a result of an increasing awareness of both the feasibility and need to provide beneficial and ethical services to maximize functioning and quality of life, many dementia patients and their families are referred for neuropsychological services that extend beyond assessment. The initial roles of family members as informants and care managers during the diagnostic assessment process greatly expands with initiation of treatment. In most cases, benefit is contingent, in large part, upon their support and participation.

The Role of the Family During Neuropsyhological Interventions

Education and training in the geriatric dementia population takes numerous forms. It is determined by a number of factors, including the patient's presentation and the family's goals. It is recognized that this treatment does not directly affect the neuropathological process giving rise to the dementia. Rather, treatment has the potential to influence coping and everyday functioning at the time, with maintenance of gains being contingent on numerous patient- and illness-related variables. Most types of intervention target cognition, affect, or adaptive functioning, with the goal being to maximize abilities and adjustment. Family members are critical to both the formulation and evaluation of intervention, but they also directly effect efficacy. Caregivers typically play numerous roles during intervention, some of which are outlined in the sections that follow.

Neuropsychological Feedback and Dementia Education

Provision of accurate information to the patient and family struggling with dementia can be extremely useful. Of course, the actual fiscal valuation of feedback remains to be done. However, numerous potential clinical benefits are apparent. Review of the neuropsychological test results can enhance understanding of the sources of cognitive deficits and behavioral change; it also can elucidate preserved skill areas. The effect of both specific feedback and general dementia education on patient and family quality of life can manifest in many ways. Specifically, this information serves to guide caregivers in important care decisions, reduce the frequency of misunderstandings, promote healthy and safe interactions and participation in appropriate activities, and (at times) replace fatalistic or dangerously minimized perspectives with a realism that allows for adaptive actions to be taken.

Intervention Planning and Evaluation of Outcomes

When planning interventions, careful consideration of factors having the potential to impact outcomes enhances the likelihood and magnitude of benefit. Of course, neuropsychological and diagnostic data guide the selection and modification of techniques that capitalize on better preserved abilities to compensate for weaknesses and incorporate likely patterns of future cognitive, affective, and behavioral difficulties. However, other factors—such as the patient's goals, capacity for accurate self-appraisal, and motivation—are equally important in formulating an effective treatment plan (Koltai & Branch, 1999). These factors should be considered in light of family system goals and resources, with discrepancies resolved clearly and early in the treatment process. Family perception of intervention efficacy also is an important outcome, as it may differ considerably from that of the patient or therapist. For instance, one study found that patients' perceptions of gain from a treatment program varied according to whether or not they had insight, whereas caregivers perceived gain among treatment subjects relative to controls, regardless of patient insight status (Koltai et al., 2001). Because these perceptions can influence caregiver burden and decisions regarding continued care, it is essential that they be monitored throughout the treatment process.

Technique-Based Intervention

The role of the family is often critical in establishing any intervention requiring effort in the home. Even when techniques are patient-initiated and the patient can act relatively autonomously (e.g., a patient with very mild memory loss learning to use an appointment calendar or an association strategy), reminders from a caregiver often are needed initially to establish the new behavior. Many techniques with demonstrated efficacy require some degree of involvement from a caregiver. For instance, spaced retrieval is a technique involving repetition of target information, followed by recall at successively longer intervals, to increase the likelihood of storage. Evidence of gains by AD patients is promising and compelling (Camp et al., 1996; McKitrick, Camp, & Black, 1992). Although there is some evidence that patients with mild memory deficits can execute the spaced retrieval technique individually (Camp et al., 1996), in most cases someone else must cue retrieval at the appropriate interval until the information is successfully stored. Obviously, the caregiver offers a cost-effective alternative to a professional therapist in such roles. Other approaches require family participation as they necessitate consistency among those in close contact with the patient (e.g., consistent reinforcement contingencies during behavior modification).

☐ Clinical Utility of Intervention with Family of Dementia Patients

As in many illnesses, the families of dementia patients suffer with their loved ones. Their roles are pivotal throughout diagnosis and treatment and often determine the quality of patient adaptive functioning in everyday life. What follows is a review of the efficacy of interventions involving such families. Such outcome studies form the foundation of any analysis to determine the fiscal consumer and system costs of such services. Ultimately, these demonstrations likely will strongly influence the provision of care in the future.

Because of the previous bias against the use of interventions in this population, efficacy data have been somewhat sparse. In addition, there is an inherent challenge in conducting empirical investigations of therapies addressing concerns rooted in the individual's existence, which has been eloquently discussed by Yalom (1980). However, a number of factors are changing this situation, and systematic study of intervention outcomes with dementia patients and their families is now on the rise. First, there is increasing evidence of clinical utility, which serves to offset previous biases. Second, more instruments are available to capture and quantify aspects of experience and gain that previously eluded researchers, such as quality of life. Third, public policy has called for evidence-based practice, resulting in an increased need to make clinical doctrines and practices publicly verifiable.

Despite the emergence of favorable outcomes related to intervention with dementia patients and their families, empirical work is in its infancy. Of course, fiscal studies are even scarcer, as they ideally are carried out using data from well-designed efficacy studies. Translation of intervention outcomes to cost variables likely will become more frequent as the need for demonstration of efficacy and utility expands to include the fiscal dimension. When clinical utility is adequately established, formulation of cost-analyses can begin. What follows is a brief review of studies that highlight the clinical efficacy of various types of intervention.

Caregiver Intervention Programs

The value to the health-care system of working with families through caregiver intervention programs is becoming apparent, as strong evidence for impacting health-care utilization patterns emerge. Mittelman and colleagues (1996) found that a caregiver program involving counseling and support groups significantly delayed the time until institutionalization of AD patients, compared to controls. The program thus reduced the risk of placement, particularly in regard to patients with mild to moderate dementia, and resulted in increased in-home care. Another caregiver training program also revealed delayed institutionalization of dementia patients (Brodaty, Gresham, & Luscombe, 1997). The potential cost–benefits of such outcomes are obvious. In 1995, the National Institute of Health launched a 5-year initiative entitled Resources for Enhancing Alzheimer's Caregiver Health (REACH). This multisite investigation of social and behavioral interventions, which was designed to enhance family caregiving for AD and related disorders, utilizes various interventions. Although the primary outcome of interest is depressive symptomatology, its impact on health status, health practices, and health-care utilization also will be examined (REACH Website: http://www.edc.gsph.pitt.edu/REACH/). Various delivery methods for caregiver educational material also are being explored, and preliminary findings suggest that the timing and amount of information are critical in how the information is received and utilized (Gwyther, 2000, personal communication).

Memory Training Programs

Gains in memory functioning are of obvious import to dementia patients and their families. As noted, until recently few published reports of improved memory functioning existed, and some of these had significant methodological limitations. However, recent lines of inquiry have yielded promising results using techniques such as spaced retrieval and multiple-technique programs. These studies represent encouraging, pioneering efforts to identify effective interventions for dementia patients. Subjective perceptions of improvement by patients and their caregivers as a result of training have been shown (Koltai et al., 2001), having implications for both memory functioning and emotional well-being. In addition, specific techniques targeting distinct skills have proven effective at improving *actual* memory ability. For example, Camp and colleagues (1996) used spaced retrieval to teach patients with AD to use a calendar, and others have applied this strategy to teach AD patients to perform prospective memory tasks (McKitrick et. al, 1992). Errorless learning and associative techniques also have been used with dementia patients to improve learning or retention duration of face–name pairs (Clare et al., 1999; Hill, Evankovich, Sheikh, & Yesavage, 1987). Camp and colleagues (1996, p. 193) contended that "it is possible to design effective, pragmatically useful memory interventions" for this population. Through application of their theoretical and clinical expertise regarding the neuroanatomical correlates of behavior, neuropsychologists have the potential to uniquely contribute to the health-care system in the area of memory training.

Psychotherapeutic Interventions

Adaptive emotional adjustment also is a critical target of intervention, given that emotional factors often lead to "excess disability" or greater-than-warranted functional incapacity (Brody, Kleban, Lawton, & Silverman, 1971). Furthermore, affective distress is clearly treatable and potentially can impact cognition (Alexopoulos, Meyers, Young, Mattis, & Kakuma, 1993; Emery & Oxman, 1992; Lichtenberg, Ross, Millis, & Manning, 1995; Nussbaum, 1994). The high prevalence of depression among dementia patients is quite disquieting. Migliorelli and colleagues (1995) found that among AD patients, 28% had dysthymia and another 23% met criteria for major depression. Among behavior problems of special-care-unit demented patients, those related to emotional distress have been found to be second only to those related to memory dysfunction (Wagner, Teri, & Orr-Rainey, 1995). Even in the absence of clinical depression, patient reports of further reduced cognitive efficiency during periods of emotional distress highlight a potential target for improving function through affective intervention. Successful treatment of depression, even in the context of a progressive neurodegenerative illness, may optimize the use of residual capacities and delay the need for institutionalization. Studies have documented symptom mitigation and improved adjustment. Behavioral treatments have been shown to reduce both patient and caregiver depression (Teri et al., 1994; 1997; Teri & McCurry, 1994). Marriot, Donaldson, Tarrier, and Burns (2000) also demonstrated reduced distress and depression for AD caregivers and less patient behavioral disturbance as a result of a family intervention program. Others have emphasized the therapeutic potential of support groups for newly diagnosed AD patients, such as a decreased sense of isolation, facilitation of grief work, and the sharing of resources (Davies, Robinson, & Bevill, 1995; LaBarge & Trtanj, 1995; Yale, 1989). Suggested guidelines for psychotherapy, behavior management, and cognitive or environmental strategies have been put forth, as have necessary modifications to techniques (e.g., Greene, Ingram, & Johnson, 1993; Hausman, 1991; Jutagir, 1993; Solomon & Szwabo, 1992; Teri & Gallagher-Thompson, 1991; Teri et. al, 1994; Verwoerdt, 1981; Weiner, 1991; Whitehead, 1991).

The results of these investigations are promising, and continued demonstration of successful nonpharmacologic treatment of the behavioral symptoms associated with dementia will represent a major advance. There is a clear need to continue to formally measure the gains frequently observed by clinicians. Interventions are driven by the need to maximize functioning, promote the use of residual capacities, and improve quality of life for patients with dementia. The study of intervention is driven by the need to elucidate the gains and limits of such services and to form the basis of cost-analyses.

The interventions used with families of dementia patients offer numerous rich opportunities for study of outcomes and their relative costs. (Examples of interventions warranting investigation can be found in Table 10.1.)

TABLE 10.1. Intervention Approaches with Dementia Patients and Their Families

Interventions involving the family
Feedback from neuropsychological evaluation
Dementia education
Support group
Individual psychotherapy
Intervention program (e.g., REACH)
Assistance with resource management
Interventions involving the patient
Feedback from neuropsychological evaluation
Dementia education
Support group
Individual psychotherapy
Intervention program (e.g., memory and coping programs)

The clinical utility of interventions is evident, particularly when considering the multidimensional impact such treatment can make. Not only do patients demonstrate gains, frequently the benefit extends to caregivers through direct treatment effects, as well as through indirect gains from improved patient functioning. Table 10.2 outlines the potential clinical impact of interventions. This list is not exhaustive, but is constructed simply to illustrate the numerous varied outcomes related to such services. It is important to attempt to capture subjective as well as objective gains, as the valuation of these services from patient and family perspectives provides additional information regarding the utility of intervention. For instance, open-ended comments about par-

TABLE 10.2. Utility of Intervention with Family of Dementia Patients

Impact on patient: Reduction of disability
Reduction of depression and other affective distress
Increased subjective and objective memory functioning
Increased functional capacity
Reduction of physical effects (e.g., mortality)
Impact on family: Reduction of caregiver burden
Reduction of depression and other affective distress
Reduction of physical effects (e.g., immune suppression, mortality)
Increased adaptive management of dementia
Impact on health-care utilization: Reduction of use of services and costs
Reduction of both patient and caregiver "excess disability" associated costs
Reduced need for psychopharmacological and therapeutic treatments
Reduced health-care costs associated with depression (e.g., physician visits, length of hospitalization)
Increased home-based care; reduction of institutionalization costs
Reduced caregiver loss of work time and income

ticipation in the Memory and Coping Program at Duke University Medical Center suggested various perceived benefits. These included increased morale, sense of control, and memory functioning; better communication and interaction about cognitive compromise; decreased anxiety; and increased willingness to participate in appropriate activities while yielding others that could compromise safety. The potential outcomes highlighted in Table 10.2 can be applied to efficacy studies and also can be used in cost-analyses, as outlined in later sections.

Costs Related to Dementia Patients and Caregivers

The known health-care costs associated with dementia are astounding. Estimated direct and indirect costs of AD during 1991 were $20.6 and $67.3 billion, respectively (Ernst & Hay, 1994). Numerous factors are considered in such estimations, including costs related to diagnosis, nursing home placement, hospitalization, and physician visits. Also considered are caregiver-related costs, including costs associated with respite, loss of productive time, and increased medical care. There is evidence that caregivers of dementia patients make more physician visits, are hospitalized more, and use more prescription drugs than controls (George & Gwyther, 1986; Haley, Levine, Brown, Berry, & Hughes, 1987).

Considerable variance in cost estimates of AD and dementia are found in the literature, depending on the nature of the analysis. Schumock (1998) emphasized that costs depend on the perspective from which they are considered. The types of costs included in the analysis, the recipient of fiscal burden, and the study population all must be considered. Patient costs that might be included involve residential care, medications, physician and hospital services, community support services, and unpaid caregiver time (e.g., Hux et al., 1998). Contrasting studies highlight this variability. In 1998, total costs of each case of AD (including direct costs, unpaid caregiver costs, disability, and premature mortality costs) were estimated to be $194,698 (Schumock, 1998). In contrast, Leon and colleagues (1998) estimated the average annual total patient cost in 1996 at $27,672. An analysis of the costs of AD to Medicare in 1994 revealed costs of $6,021 per case (Taylor & Sloan, 2000), whereas average adjusted payments to Medicaid recipients with AD in 1995 were calculated at a far higher $20,618. Another study looking at the mean annualized total cost of dementia, rather than just AD, revealed a different figure of $13,487 (Gutterman, Markowitz, Lewis, & Fillit, 1999).

Despite the disparity between these figures, the fiscal burden of dementia is apparent. Findings also suggest that specific illness-related factors influence costs, again with variability as a function of cost perspective. Although one study showed that the cost of AD to Medicare decreases with year since diagnosis (Taylor & Sloan, 2000), another showed that the annual societal cost of AD increases with disease severity (Hux et al., 1998). As the disease progresses, a redistribution of costs occurs, with increases in some areas and decreases in others, again related to perspective. Not surprisingly, limitations in activities of daily living (ADLs) and poorer cognitive status result in increased costs (Taylor & Sloan, 2000). Gender also may be an important determinant (Kinosian et al., 2000). These potential cost modifiers–such as functional status, cognitive status, and level of behavioral disturbance, and how they influence various types of cost (Bianchetti, Frisoni, Ghisia, & Trabucchi, 1998; Ernst & Hay, 1998)–warrant further study.

A cost comparison across different types of dementia showed that institutional care accounted for the greatest part of total direct health-care costs across all subgroups (Murman, Colucci, Gelb, & Liang, 1998). It is clear that effective treatment of dementia would benefit patients and caregivers alike and could in turn affect both direct and indirect costs (Schumock, 1998). Cognitive and functional activities of daily living (ADL) deficits would be particularly useful to target, and treatment that could extend the time of in-home care would have substantial fiscal ramifications. Leon, Cheng, and Neumann (1998) recently estimated the costs of an AD sample in terms of formal and informal care, by disease severity and care-delivery setting. This pivotal study is an important landmark for future cost-analyses, as it provides a model by which cost savings related to treatment can be estimated. For example, an improvement in functional status of patients with mild dementia was estimated to save $3,264 per year (Leon et al., 1998).

Costs associated with depression and other affective disorders also warrant specific attention, as treatable emotional distress is often the target of intervention. Strong associations between depression and health-care service utilization have been shown in both middle-aged and elderly cohorts. For instance, a large medical-outcomes study compared outpatients with a depressive disorder or depressive symptoms to individuals with chronic medical conditions and individuals without chronic conditions (Wells et al., 1989). Patients with a depressive disorder or depressive symptomatology had worse physical, social, and role functioning; poorer perceived health; and more pain than those without chronic conditions. The poor functioning of the depressed patients was comparable to or worse than that of the medical patients in this study. Levenson, Hamer, and Rossiter (1990) also found that inpatients with depression, anxiety, cognitive dysfunction, or pain had significantly longer hospital stays, higher hospital costs, and more procedures done during hospitalization than inpatients who did not have these conditions. Elderly, depressed, primary-care patients also are more likely to rate their health as fair or poor and to have more emergency room visits, outpatient visits, and higher total outpatient charges than nondepressed patients (Callahan, Hui, Nienaber, Musick, & Tierney, 1994). Koenig, Shelp, Goli, Cohen, and Blazer (1989) also found that older, medically ill, depressed patients have longer inpatient stays and higher in-hospital mortality, and this excess resource utilization persists after discharge. Depression also was an independent risk factor for mortality in a large population-based sample of elders (Schulz et al., 2000).

Studies now are emerging (Unutzer et al., 1997) showing that the increased cost of medical services among depressed older adults are not accounted for by an increase in specialty mental-health care but, rather, by an increase for every component of health care. This is not surprising, given that dementia caregiving also has been associated with altered immunity. Specifically, chronic stress (particularly depression) and age have a negative impact on T cells, which may be associated with the higher risk of disease and mortality among dementia caregivers (Castle, Wilkins, Heck, Tanzy, & Fahey, 1995). Dementia caregivers' depression also directly impacts patient care decisions, as their depression and reaction to troublesome patient behaviors are predictors of nursing home placement (Mittelman, Ferris, Shulman, Steinberg, & Leven, 1996). A revealing study of elderly caregivers of patients with basic or instrumental ADL deficits showed that caregivers *experiencing mental or emotional strain* are at significantly higher risk for mortality than are noncaregiving controls. In contrast, those who are providing care but without strain, and those with disabled spouses who are not providing care, are *not* at increased risk for mortality (Schulz & Beach, 1999).

The impact of depression on dementia patients and their caregivers has been clearly documented. Equally informative is literature demonstrating the efficacy and cost-benefit of mental-health treatment. For example, Moos and Mertens (1996) examined the health-care patterns in mental-health and medical-service settings of a large cohort of patients with affective disorders. For both index medical and index mental-health patients, more intensive prior medical outpatient care was associated with shorter inpatient care. In addition, among index medical patients, a shorter inpatient episode also was predicted by more prior outpatient mental-health care. The authors suggest that inpatient care may be more timely when individuals are followed more closely on an outpatient basis, resulting in less need for later intensive care. In addition, outpatient mental-health care may specifically reduce the need for some medical care. In an 1991 essay, Cummings reviewed literature demonstrating that emotionally distressed persons who receive psychotherapy show significant declines in their excessive health-care utilization, and that these declines are maintained 5 years posttherapy termination. This cost offset through therapy has been replicated many times. Overall, many investigations have established the relationship between increased cost of health care in the context of depression and the potential reduction of subsequent service use and costs through adequate treatment.

☐ Future Directions: Analysys of the Economical Value of Consultation and Training of Family Members of Patients with Dementia

Economic evaluation in health care is conducted by selecting a cost-analysis type that is appropriate to the program alternatives being reviewed. Analysis types are differentiated primarily by their outcomes. For each alternative, cost components are examined, and outcomes are measured in monetary or utility terms. The objectives of cost-analyses typically are met by one of the following methods:

1. Cost-efficiency (or minimization) establishes which of two alternatives producing the same effect costs less.
2. Cost-efficiency determines which expenditure produces the greatest effect.
3. Cost–benefit determines to what degree the monetary benefit exceeds the investment of the program in each alternative.
4. Cost–utility determines the relative cost of each alternative in terms of the utility of each, as valued by individual or societal preferences.

Before reviewing the application of such analyses to neuropsychological intervention services, each analysis method is described briefly. These approaches are those reviewed in Chapter 1: cost-efficiency/minimization, effectiveness, benefit, and utility. They are also pragmatically delineated in Drummond, O'Brien, Stoddart, and Torrance's (1997) *Methods for the Economic Evaluation of Health Care Programmes*. In addition, Hargreaves, Shumway, Hu, and Cuffel's (1998) *Cost–Outcome Methods for Mental Health* also provided useful information about these methods, and Gold and colleagues (1996) offered critical guidelines regarding identifying and valuing outcomes.

The goal of the *efficiency (minimization) model* is to determine which of two programs results in the lowest cost. To use this type of analysis, outcomes must be identical: Programs with differences in outcomes in either magnitude or type cannot be compared. A simple example can be taken from grocery shopping: If we believe that two products taste identically, we will choose the product with the minimum cost.

In an *effectiveness model,* programs that have results varying only in magnitude are compared. Outcomes are valued in units. Dividing the program cost by its respective units of effectiveness then derives the unit cost of each approach. The more cost-effective program will have a lower cost per unit. An example of such an analysis from everyday life occurs when we choose between products that are used in the same way, but with different longevity. For instance, we may choose to purchase a brand of tires that has a longer predicted life for more dollars if we determine that the annual cost of those tires is less than for lower-cost tires with a shorter life.

A *cost–benefit model* allows for evaluation of programs with different or multiple benefits. In this type of analysis, benefits are valued in monetary terms. The objective of this analysis is to determine to what degree various treatment approaches are fiscally viable. The costs associated with each program are compared to the monetary value of its benefits. Benefits are discounted when they extend beyond a set timeframe. The program with the higher ratio of benefits to cost is considered more favorably. A simple life example involves choosing between a professional security system versus a self-defense class. The costs of each would be compared to the monetarily valued benefit of each, with these gains varying considerably (including potential level of protection, opportunity for physical exercise, and socialization).

A *utility model* involves comparison of the cost of treatment approaches with benefits valued in more natural terms, such as quality adjusted life years (QALYs). Outcomes of programs in this type of analysis may vary in type and magnitude. However, whereas gains in cost–benefit analyses are valued in terms of monetary gains, cost–utility analyses show value gains in terms of individual or societal preferences. In everyday life, we use this type of approach when we choose to purchase more expensive health foods because we feel they will increase our longevity.

Reliable cost-analyses investigations are based on rigorously designed intervention outcome studies. However, Drummond and colleagues (1997) noted that efficacy studies often are completed well before the cost-analyses approach is selected. Thus, formulation of efficacy studies should consider various cost-analysis plans. As Weinstein, Siegel, Gold, Kamlet, and Russell (1996, p. 1257) noted, "The quality and validity of a cost-effectiveness analysis depend crucially on the quality of the underlying data that describe the effectiveness of interventions and the course of illness without intervention." Target outcomes involving cognition, affect, behavior, or function should be clearly operationalized. Likewise, the intervention should be rigorously defined, with built-in demonstration of training acquisition and implementation to ensure that benefit is achieved.

The next challenge is to demonstrate empirically the relationship between positive treatment outcome and cost reduction. The options for study are ample. Any combination of intervention and outcomes, some of which are listed in Tables 10.1 and 10.2, could form the foundation of a cost-analysis study. One hypothetical example follows.

Cost-Effectiveness Analysis: Support Group Attendance vs. Patient–Caregiver Memory and Coping Program Attendance

The aim of this study was to determine the relative costs of two treatment alternatives for dementia patients: a support group versus a memory and coping program (MCP).

Preliminary data supported that these two alternatives had a common effect that differed only in magnitude on the particular outcome of interest, which in this case was reduction of patient depressive symptomatology. It should be noted that other outcomes–such as reduced caregiver depression, increased functioning, and less health-care utilization–also could be investigated.

Reduction in patient depression was operationalized as follows: *one unit per three-point reduction* on the Geriatric Depression Scale (GDS; Yesavage et al., 1983). In the preliminary efficacy study, patients–caregiver dyads were randomly assigned to support group and MCP conditions. Patients were pretested 2 weeks prior to participation, and both groups received weekly treatment for 8 weeks. Posttest change scores indicated an average 2-unit effect for MCP, and 1-unit effect for support group conditions.

The cost-analysis was conducted from the perspective of the consumer, and thus calculation of costs was restricted to patient–consumer costs and insurance costs, and did not include hospital, personnel, or administrative costs. Average cost of participation in the support group was estimated at $320, with $40 travel expenses per session, per dyad, and no cost to insurance. Average cost of participation in MCP was estimated at $440 for each dyad, with $40 travel expenses per session and an average $15 copayment per session. Costs of MCP to insurance was estimated at $376, which involved the remaining $47 per session (with clinical charges of $62 per person per session of group therapy). The outcome of this analysis resulted in the following data shown in Table 10.3.

As can be seen, the cost *per unit of effect* (i.e., three-point reduction on the GDS) for the patient–caregiver dyads is less for MCP than for support group participation, but the cost is greater for the average insurance provider.

This hypothetical illustration of a cost-effectiveness analysis is a simplified example of how such a study would be conducted. However, it effectively illustrates the goal of such studies, and how the selection of outcomes of interest and cost perspectives can influence results. Cost must be viewed considering the differential magnitude of each treatment, which is observed through its units of effect. Although the focus of such a study is the determination of cost-effectiveness of two treatments, clinical decision making and policy development should not neglect consideration of the value of the different treatment magnitudes to the consumer.

Given that efficacy studies on patient and family interventions in AD are only recently emerging, it is not surprising that few cost analyses of any treatment have been conducted. One investigation used a cost–benefit "willingness to pay" relative to expected cost approach to demonstrate that Donepezil is perceived by caregivers to be economically beneficial relative to no therapy (Lanctot, Oh, Risebrough, & Herrmann, 1999). In another preliminary report, pharmacological and nonpharmacological treatments were examined in terms of cost and quality adjusted life years, with results sug-

Table 10.3. Cost Per Unit of Effect to Dyads and Insurance

	Dyads	Insurance
MCP	$220	$188
Support group	$320	$0

gesting that pharmacological treatment of behavioral disorders is cost-effective in mild and moderate AD (Lanctot, Oh, Herrman, & Liu, 1997). Schumack (1998) offered a brief review of studies indirectly estimating the cost–benefit of treatment with tacrine, using delayed nursing home placement as a primary outcome. Schumack also commented on an interesting study showing that improved cognition with the cholinesterase inhibitor velnacrine was associated with a reduction in caregiver time relative to placebo—again highlighting an area of reduced indirect costs for further study. Another group used a cost-effectiveness approach, much like the example given above, to show that reality-orientation therapy might be an effective, low-cost therapeutic approach for mild to moderate AD patients (Zanetti, Bianchetti, & Trabucchi, 1998). Ernst and colleagues (1997) also provided a report of estimated annual cost savings in AD if treatment results in delayed decline or improved mental status.

An excellent example of economic evaluation by O'Brien and colleagues (1999) demonstrated that use of Donepezil for mild to moderate AD reduces 5-year costs relative to no treatment. Specifically, these investigators used the Canadian Study of Health and Aging data and found that Donepezil use was associated with a $929 (Canadian dollars) reduction in health-care costs per patient over 5 years, but increased caregiver costs of $48 per patient. Using the price of medication, these investigators determined that Donepezil use was supported from both cost and outcome perspectives. In a similar study, Neumann and colleagues (1999) demonstrated that the costs of Donepezil are partially offset by reduced cost of care related to enhanced cognition, as well as the delay of progression to more costly dementia stages and care settings. However, they noted that the degree of cost offset and the impact of treatment on health-related quality of life depended on their model's assumption about the duration of drug effect, for which data are presently lacking.

It is apparent that while some cost-analyses in dementia treatment exist, there are ample opportunities for further study, particularly in the area of neuropsychological interventions. Frequently used cost-analyses approaches are summarized in Table 10.4, with examples of potential applications among dementia patients and their families.

Economic evaluation is defined as "the comparative analysis of alternative courses of action in terms of both their costs and consequences" (Drummond et al., 1997; pp. 8–9). Caution must be exercised with cost–efficiency or minimization analyses. Although two treatment alternatives may yield the same benefit on the outcome of interest, other unmeasured outcomes may enhance or minimize the overall clinical utility of each program. For instance, for the example outlined in Table 10.4, caregivers may benefit from the social interaction provided by the seminar, be exposed to increased resources, and experience less isolation in addition to obtaining education about dementia. However, this type of analysis appears to be ideal for determination of the most cost-efficient manner of achieving a *specific* outcome. A similar caution applies to cost-effectiveness analysis, which also examines the cost of alternatives on a specific outcome of interest, although the magnitude of the effect may differ with different interventions. Cost–benefit and cost–utility analyses, although significantly more challenging, may be more appropriate methods of analyses for programs having numerous targets and outcomes. These analyses provide information regarding the absolute benefit of the alternatives by considering all relevant outcomes. Again, perspective defines both costs and outcomes.

As noted, it is not always possible to ascertain in advance which type of cost analyses will yield the most information. Efficacy data may not be available in advance of the

TABLE 10.4. Cost Analyses as Applied to Consultation and Training of Family Members of Patients with Dementia

Type of Cost Analysis	Goal	Example	Analysis Outcome Expressed
Efficiency (minimization)	To determine the relative cost of two alternatives *with identical outcomes;* requires efficacy data showing no difference in the outcome of interest	Determine cost of a dementia seminar series relative to cost of receiving pamphlets, with dementia education being the outcome of interest; requires data showing equivalent educational gain	Relative cost of each alternative Cost of production and distribution of pamphlets < cost of educational seminar
Effectiveness	To determine the relative cost of two alternatives *with a common effect, which may differ in magnitude*	Determine the relative cost and effects of support group versus caregiver intervention program participation, with the outcome of interest being length of time to patient institutionalization	Cost per unit of effect, or effects per unit of cost, for each alternative Cost of support group resulting in 2 years of home-care gain, relative to cost of intervention program resulting in 4 years home-care gain
Benefit	To determine the relative cost–benefit ratio of two alternatives, when *effects cannot be assumed to be common, achieved to the same degree, or when effects are multiple;* requires assigning value to effects	Determine benefit for cost of a patient–caregiver intervention program relative to no treatment	Cost–benefit ratio of each alternative Favorable intervention program cost–benefit ratio through delayed institutionalization and reduced depression, with fiscal gains offsetting program cost; although no treatment is less costly, it does not reduce costs through such gains
Utility	To determine the relative cost of alternatives, with outcomes valued by individual or societal preferences, when *effects cannot be assumed to be common, achieved to the same degree, or when they are multiple;* requires assigning a utility value to outcomes	Determine costs associated with individual therapy relative to no treatment, in terms of quality adjusted years (QAYs)	Cost per natural unit gained, such as QAYs or healthy days, for each alternative Cost of treatment yielding increased QAYs relative to cost of no treatment yielding less QAYs

study and different approaches might be combined, depending on the nature of the cost demonstration. Given this, data should be collected to facilitate application of the various cost-analyses techniques.

Given the paucity of efficacy data in this area, the near nonexistence of cost-analyses involving the treatment of families is not surprising. However, the cost-analysis literature provides numerous guidelines and examples to guide researchers. For example, Wolff, Helminiak, and Tebes (1997) outlined the potential errors that can be introduced by methodological choices in cost-effectiveness analysis involving mental-health treatments. The literature is a rich resource for such cautions and guidelines. Commonly used utility values and guidelines for determining resource value and estimating costs have been put forth (Gold et al., 1996; Hargreaves et al., 1998). The conceptualization and measurement of outcomes is critical to the analysis process (Hargreaves et al., 1998), and Gold and colleagues (1996) provided indispensable information and references in this area. Like the cost estimates of AD, these analyses are contingent on the study perspective (Drummond et al., 1997). For instance, various perspectives include costs related to society, patient and family, self-insured employer, public or private insurer, and managed care plans (Luce, Manning, Siegel, & Lipscomb, 1996). Clearly, progress in research demonstrating the efficacy and favorable cost–outcomes in neuropsychological assessment and intervention is essential. However, it is critical that such studies move forward in an informed manner, given their potential to affect patient functioning, caregiver burden, clinical practice, and health-care policy.

☐ References

Alexopoulos, G., Meyers, B., Young, R., Mattis, S., & Kakuma, T. (1993). The course of geriatric depression with reversible dementia: A controlled study. *American Journal of Psychiatry, 150,* 1693–1699.

Bianchetti, A., Frisoni, G., Ghisia, K., & Trabucchi, M. (1998). Clinical predictors of the indirect costs of Alzheimer's disease. *Archives of Neurology, 55*(letters), 130–131.

Blazer, D. C. (1994). Is depression more frequent in late life? An honest look at the evidence. *The American Journal of Geriattric Psychiatry, 3,* 193–199.

Bracco, L., Amaducci, L., Pedone, D., Bino, G., Lazzaro, M. P., Carella, F., D'Antona, R., Gallato, R., & Denes, G. (1990). Italian Multicentre Study on Dementia (SMID): A neuropsychological test battery for assessing Alzheimer's disease. *Journal of Psychiatric Research, 24,* 213–226.

Brodaty, H., Gresham, M., & Luscombe, G. (1997). The Prince Henry Hospital dementia caregivers' training programme. *International Journal of Geriatric Psychiatry, 12,* 183–192.

Brody, E., Kleban, M., Lawton, M. P., & Silverman, H. (1971). Excess disabilities of mentally impaired aged: Impact of individualized treatment. *The Gerontologist,* (Summer, Part I), 124–133.

Callahan, C., Hui, S., Nienaber, N., Musick, B., & Tierney, W. (1994). Longitudinal study of depression and health services use among elderly primary care patients. *Journal of the American Geriatrics Society, 42,* 833–838.

Camp, C., Foss, J., O'Hanlon, A., & Stevens, A. (1996). Memory Interventions for persons with dementia. *Applied Cognitive Psychology, 10,* 193–210.

Canadian Study of Health and Aging. (1994). The Canadian study of health and aging. Risk factors for Alzheimer's disease in Canada. *Neurology, 44,* 2073–2080.

Castle, S., Wilkins, S., Heck, E., Tanzy, K., & Fahey, J. (1995). Depression in caregivers of demented patients is associated with altered immunity: Impaired proliferative capacity, increased $CD8^+$, and a decline in lymphocytes with surface signal transduction molecules ($CD38^+$) and a cytotoxicity marker ($CD56^+$ $CD8^+$). *Clinical & Experimental Immunology, 101,* 487–493.

Clare, L.,Wilson, B., Breen, K., & Hodges, J. (1999). Errorless learning of face–name associations in early Alzheimer's disease. *Neurocase, 5,* 37–46.

Corey-Bloom, J., Thal, L. J., Galasko, D., Folstein, M., Drachman, D., Raskind, M., & Lanska, D. J. (1995). Diagnosis and evaluation of dementia. *Neurology, 45,* 211–218.

Cummings, J., & Benson, D. (1992). *Dementia: A critical approach.* Stoneham, MA: Butterworth-Heineman.

Cummings, N. (1991). Arguments for the financial efficacy of psychological services in health care settings. In J. Thomas & J. Cummings (Eds.), *The collected papers of Nicholas A. Cummings, Vol. 1: The value of psychological treatment* (pp. 225–247). Phoenix, AZ: Zeig, Tucker & Co.

Davies, H., Robinson, D., & Bevill, L. (1995). Supportive group experience for patients with early-stage Alzheimer's disease. *Journal of the American Geriatric Society, 43,* 1068–1069.

Drummond, M., O'Brien, B., Stoddart, G., & Torrance, G. (1997). *Methods for the economic evaluation of health care programmes.* New York: Oxford University Press.

Emery, V., & Oxman, T. (1992). Update on the dementia spectrum of depression. *American Journal of Psychiatry, 149,* 305–317.

Ernst, R., & Hay, J. (1998). Clinical predictors of the indirect costs of Alzheimer's disease. *Archives of Neurology, letters-reply, 55*(letters–reply), 131.

Ernst, R., & Hay, J. (1994). The US economic and social costs of Alzheimer's disease revisited. *American Journal of Public Health, 84,* 1261–1264.

Ernst, R., Hay, J., Fenn, C., Tinklenberg, J., & Yesavage, J. (1997). Cognitive function and the costs of Alzheimer disease. *Archives of Neurology, 54,* 687–693.

George, L., & Gwyther, L. (1986). Caregiver well-being: A multidimensional examination of family caregivers of demented adults. *Gerontologist, 26,* 253–259.

Gold, M., Patrick, D., Torrance, G., Fryback, D., Hadorn, D., Kamlet, M., Daniels, N., & Weinstein, M. (1996). Identifying and valuing outcomes. In M. Gold, J. Siegel, L. Russell, & M. Weinstein (Eds.), *Cost-effectiveness in health and medicine* (pp. 82–134). New York: Oxford University Press.

Greene, J., Ingram, T., & Johnson, W. (1993). Group psychotherapy for patients with dementia. *Southern Medical Journal, 86,* 1033–1035.

Gutterman, E., Markowitz, J., Lewis, B., & Fillit, H. (1999). Cost of Alzheimer's disease and related dementia in managed-Medicare. *Journal of the American Geriatrics Society, 47,* 1065–1071.

Haley, W., Levine, E., Brown, S. L., Berry, J., & Hughes, G. (1987). Psychological, social, and health consequences of caring for a relative with senile dementia. *Journal of the American Geriatrics Society, 35,* 405–411.

Hargreaves, W., Shumway, M., Hu, T., & Cuffel, B. (1998). *Cost–outcome methods for mental health.* San Diego: Academic Press.

Hausman, C. (1991). Dynamic psychotherapy with elderly demented patients. In G. Jones & B. Miesen (Eds.), *Caregiving in dementia* (pp. 181–198). Amsterdam: Routledge Publishers.

Hill, R., Evankovich, K., Sheikh, J., & Yesavage, J. (1987). Imagery mnemonic training in a patient with primary degenerative dementia. *Psychology and Aging, 2,* 204–205.

Hux, M., O'Brien, B., Iskedjien, M., Goeree, R., Gagnon, M., & Gauthier, S. (1998). Relation between severity of Alzheimer's disease and costs of caring. *Canadian Medical Association Journal, 159,* 457–465.

Kinosian, B., Stallard, E., Lee, J., Woodbury, M., Zbrozek, A., & Glick, H. (2000). Predicting 10-year care requirements for older people with suspected Alzheimer's disease. *Journal of the American Geriatrics Society, 48,* 631–638.

Koenig, H., Shelp, F., Goli, V., Cohen, H., & Blazer D. (1989). Survival and health care utilization in elderly medical inpatients with major depression. *Journal of the American Geriatrics Society, 37,* 599–606.

Koltai, D., & Branch, L. (1999). Cognitive and affective interventions to maximize abilities and adjustment in dementia. In F. Cacabelos & T. Giacobini (Eds.), *Annals of psychiatry: Basic and clinical neurosciences* (pp. 241–255). Barcelona, Spain: Prous Science Publisher.

Koltai, D., Welsh-Bohmer, K. & Schmechel, D. (2001). Influence of anosognosia on treatment outcome among dementia patients. *Neuropsychological Rehabilitation, 11*(3/4), 455–475.

Jutagir, R. (1993). Geropsychology and neuropsychological testing: Role in evaluation and treatment of patients with dementia. *Mount Sinai Journal of Medicine, 60,* 528–531.

LaBarge, E., & Trtanj, F. (1995). A support group for people in the early stages of dementia of the Alzheimer type. *Journal of Applied Gerontology, 14,* 289–301.

Lanctot, K., Oh, P., Herrmann, N., & Liu, B. (1997). Economic appraisal of pharmacologic therapy for behavioral disorders in dementia. *Clinical Pharmacology & Therapeutics, 61,* 173.

Lanctot, K., Oh, P., Risebrough, N., & Herrmann, N. (1999). Cost-benefit analysis of cholinesterase inhibitors in Alzheimer's disease. *Clinical Pharmacology & Therapeutics, 65,* 169.

Leon, J., Cheng, C., & Neumann, P. (1998). Alzheimer's disease care: Costs and potential savings. *Health Affairs, 17,* 206–216.

Levenson, J., Hamer, R., & Rossiter, L. (1990). Relation of psychopathology in general medical inpatients to use and cost of services. *American Journal of Psychiatry, 147,* 1498–1503.

Lichtenberg, P., Ross, T., Millis, S., & Manning, C. (1995). The relationship between depression and cognition in older adults: A cross-validation study. *Journal of Gerontology, 50,* P25–P32.

Lindau, M., Almkvist, O., Johansson, S. E., & Wahlund, L. O. (1998). Cognitive and behavioral differentiation of frontal lobe degeneration of the non-Alzheimer type and Alzheimer's disease. *Dementia & Geriatric Cognitive Disorders, 9,* 205–213.

Luce, B., Manning, W., Siegel, J., & Lipscomb, J. (1996). Estimating costs in cost-effectiveness analysis. In M. Gold, J. Siegel, L. Russell, & M. Weinstein (Eds.), *Cost-effectiveness in health and medicine* (pp. 176–213). New York: Oxford University Press.

Marriott, A., Donaldson, C., Tarrier, N., & Burns, A. (2000). Effectiveness of cognitive-behavioral family intervention in reducing the burden of care in carers of patients with Alzheimer's disease. *British Journal of Psychiatry, 176,* 557–562.

Mayeux, R., Saunders, A. M., Shea, S., Mirra, S., Evans, D., Roses, A. D., Hyman, B. T., Crain, B., Tang, M. X., & Phelps, C. H. (1998). Utility of the apolipoprotein E genotype in the diagnosis of Alzheimer's disease. Alzheimer's Disease Centers Consortium on Apolipoprotein E and Alzheimer's Disease. *New England Journal of Medicine, 338,* 506–511.

McKitrick, L., Camp, C., & Black, F. W. (1992). Prospective memory intervention in Alzheimer's disease. *Journal of Gerontology, 47,* P337–P343.

Menzin, J., Lang, K., & Friedman, M. (1999). The economic cost of Alzheimer's disease to a state Medicaid program. *Neurology, 52,* A8–A9.

Migliorelli, R., Teson, A., Sabe, L., Petracchi, M., Leiguarda, R., & Starkstein, S. (1995). Prevalence and correlates of dysthymia and major depression among patients with Alzheimer's disease. *American Journal of Psychiatry, 152,* 37–44.

Mittelman, M., Ferris, S., Shulman, E., Steinberg, G., & Levin, B. (1996). A family intervention to delay nursing home placement of patients with Alzheimer disease: A randomized controlled trial. *Journal of the American Medical Association, 276,* 1725–1731.

Moos, R., & Mertens, J. (1996). Patterns of diagnoses, comorbidities, and treatment in late-middle-aged and older affective disorder patients: Comparison of mental health and medical sectors. *Journal of the American Geriatrics Society, 44,* 682–688.

Murman, D., Colucci, P., Gelb, D., & Liang, J. (1998). Comparison of direct health care costs in degenerative dementias. *Neurology, 50,* A302–A303.

Neumann, P., Hermann, R., Kuntz, K., Araki, S., Duff, S., Leon, J., Berenbaum, P., Goldman, P., Williams, L., & Weinstein, M. (1999). Cost-effectivelness of Donepezil in the treatment of mild or moderate Alzheimer's disease. *Neurology, 52,* 1138–1145.

Nussbaum, P. (1994). Pseudodementia: A slow death. *Neuropsychology Review, 4,* 71–90.

O'Brien, B., Goeree, R., Hux, M., Iskedjian, M., Blackhouse, G., Gagnon, M., & Gauthier, S. (1999). Economic evaluation of donepezil for the treatment of Alzheimer's disease in Candada. *Journal of the American Geriatrics Society, 47,* 570–578.

Rockwood, K., Stolee, P., & McDowell, I. (1996). Factors associated with institutionalization of older people in Canada: Testing a multifactoral definition of frailty. *Journal of the American Geriatrics Society, 44,* 578–582.

Schulz, R., & Beach, S. (1999). Caregiving as a risk factor for mortality: The caregiver health effects study. *Journal of the American Medical Association, 282,* 2215–2219.

Schulz, R., Beach, S., Ives, D., Martire, L., Ariyo, A., & Kop, W. (2000). Association between depression and mortality in older adults: The cardiovascular health study. *Archives of Internal Medicine, 160,* 1761–1768.

Schumock, G. (1998). Economic considerations in the treatment and management of Alzheimer's disease. *American Journal of Health-System Pharmacy, 55*(21S), 17S–21S.

Small, G., Rabins, P., Barry, P., Buckholtz, N., Dekosky, S., Ferris, S., Findel, S., Gwyther, L., Khachaturian, Z., Lobowitz, B., McRae, T., Morris, J., Oakley, F., Schneider, L., Streim, J., Sunderland, T., Teri, L., & Tune, L. (1997). Diagnosis and treatment of Alzheimer's disease and related disorders. Consensus statement of the American Association for Geriatric Psychiatry, the Alzheimer's Association, and the American Geriatrics Society. *Journal of the American Medical Association, 278,* 1363–137.

Solomon, K., & Szwabo, P. (1992). Psychotherapy for patients with dementia. In J. Morley, R. Coe, R. Strong, & G. Grossberg (Eds.), *Memory function and aging-related disorders* (pp. 295–319). New York: Springer.

Steffens, D. C., Plassman, B. L., Helms, M. H., Welsh-Bohmer, K. A., Saunders, A. M., & Breitner, J. C. (1997). A twin study of late-onset depression and apolipoprotein E epsilon 4 as risk factors for Alzheimer's disease. *Biological Psychiatry, 41,* 851–856.

Taylor, D., & Sloan, F. (2000). How much do persons with Alzheimer's disease cost Medicare? *Journal of the American Geriatrics Society, 48,* 39–646.

Teri, L., Curtis, J., Gallagher-Thompson, D., & Thompson, L. (1994). Cognitive-behavior therapy with depressed older adults. In L. Schneider, C. Reynolds, B. Lebowtz, & A. Friedhoff (Eds.), *Diagnosis and treatment of depression late life: Results of the NIH Consensus Development Conference* (pp. 279–291). Washington DC: American Psychiatric Press.

Teri, L., & Gallagher-Thompson, D. (1991). Cognitive-behavioral interventions for treatment of depression in Alzheimer's patients. *Gerontologist, 31,* 413–416.

Teri, L., Logsdon, R., Wagner, A., & Uomoto, J. (1994). The caregiver role in behavioral treatment of depression in dementia patients. In: E. Light, G. Niederehe, & B. Lebowitz (Eds.), *Stress effects on family caregivers of Alzheimer's patients: Research and interventions* (pp. 185–204). New York: Springer.

Teri, L., & McCurry, S. (1994). Psychosocial therapies. In C. Coffey, J. Cummings, M. Lovell, & G. Pearlson (Eds.), *The American Psychiatric Press textbook of geriatric neuropsychiatry* (pp. 662–682). Washington, DC: American Psychiatric Press.

Teri, L., Logsdon, R., Uomoto, J., & McCurry, S. (1997). Behavioral treatment of depression in dementia patients: A controlled clinical trial. *Journal of Gerontology Series B-Psychological Sciences & Social Sciences, 52B*(4), P159–P166.

Tierney, M., Szalai, J., Snow, W., & Fisher, R. H. (1996). The prediction of Alzheimer disease: The role of patient and informant perceptions of cognitive deficits. *Archives of Neurology, 53,* 423–427.

Tschanz, J., Welsh-Bohmer, K. A., Skoog, I., West, N., Norton, M., Wyse, B., Nickles, R., & Breitner, J. C. (2000). Dementia diagnoses from clinical and neuropsychological data compared: The Cache County Study. *Neurology, 54,* 1290–1296.

Unutzer, J., Patrick, D., Simon, G., Grembowski, D., Walker, E., Rutter, C., & Katon, W. (1997). Depressive symptoms and the cost of health services in HMO patients aged 65 years and older: A 4-year prospective study. *Journal of the American Medical Association, 277,* 1618–1623.

Verwoerdt, A. (1981). Individual psychotherapy in senile dementia. In N. Miller & G. Cohen (Eds.), *Clinical aspects of Alzheimer's disease and senile dementia* (pp.187–208). New York: Raven Press.

Wagner, A., Teri, L., & Orr-Rainey, N. (1995). Behavior problems of residents with dementia in special care units. *Alzheimer Disease & Associated Disorders, 9,* 121–127.

Weiner, M. (1991). Psychological and behavioral management. In M. Weiner (Ed.), *The dementias: Diagnosis and management* (pp. 107–133). Washington, DC: American Psychiatric Press.

Weinstein, M., Siegel, J., Gold, M., Kamlet, M., & Russell, L. (1996). Recommendations of the panel on cost-effectiveness in health and medicine. *Journal of the American Medical Association, 276,* 1253–1258.

Wells, K., Stewart, A., Hays, R., Burnam, M., Rogers, W., Daniels, M., Berry, S., Greenfield, S., & Ware, J. (1989). The functioning and well-being of depressed patients: Results from the Medical Outcomes Study. *Journal of the American Medical Association, 262,* 914–919.

Welsh-Bohmer, K. A., Hulette, C., Schmechel, D., Burke, J., & Saunders, A. (2001). Neuropsychological detection of preclinical Alzheimer's disease: Results of a neuropathological series of "normal" controls. In K. Iqbal, S. S. Sisodia, & B. Winblad (Eds.), *Alzheimer's disease: Advances in etiology, pathogenesis and therapeutics. The Proceedings of the 7th International Conference on Alzheimer's Disease and Related Disorders"* (pp. 111–122). London: John Wiley & Sons.

Whitehead, A. (1991). Twenty years a-growing: Some current issues in behavioural psychotherapy with elderly people. *Behavioural Psychotherapy, 19,* 92–99.

Wolff, N., Helminiak, T., & Tebes, J. (1997). Getting the cost right in cost-effectiveness analyses. *American Journal of Psychiatry, 154,* 736–743.

Yale, R. (1989). Support groups for newly diagnosed Alzheimer's clients. *Clinical Gerontologist, 8,* 86–89.

Yalom, I. (1980). *Existential psychotherapy.* New York: Basic Books.

Yesavage, J., Brink, T., Rose, T., Lum, O., Huan, V., Adey, M., & Leirer, V. (1983). Development and validation of a geriatric depression screening scale: A preliminary report. *Journal of Psychiatric Research, 17,* 37–49.

Zanetti, O., Bianchetti, A., & Trabucchi, M. (1998). Cost-effectiveness of non-pharmacological interventions in Alzheimer's disease. *Journal of the American Geriatrics Society, 46,* 1481.

PART

V

EPILEPSY

11

CHAPTER

Carl B. Dodrill

Neuropsychological Evaluation of Patients with Epilepsy

Introduction to the Disorder of Epilepsy

Epilepsy refers to a disorder manifested by repeated unprovoked seizures. Seizures are sudden abnormal electrical alterations in brain functions with characteristic electrophysiological and behavioral changes. Epilepsy is a disorder that has existed for thousands of years, with clearly described cases in antiquity (Temkin, 1971). Despite improved medical and surgical treatment, the best evidence is that epilepsy has a prevalence rate of approximately two-thirds of 1%, even in technologically advanced societies such as the United States (Hauser & Hesdorffer, 1990). With the world's population at approximately 6.25 billion people at the time of this writing (U.S. Bureau of the Census, 2002), there are at least 42 million people in with world with epilepsy.

Types of Seizures

As has been known for many years, the types of seizures that people with epilepsy experience can be divided into two general categories (Commission on Classification and Terminology of the International League Against Epilepsy, 1981). The first of these are *partial seizures*, which include seizures that begin locally or focally. Among these are *simple partial seizures*, which typically have focal sensory and/or motor components but do not include impairment of consciousness. The other type of partial seizures is *complex partial seizures*, which can present in a variety of ways but involve some impairment of consciousness so that a person cannot respond efficiently and purposefully. Complex partial seizures most frequently arise from the temporal lobes; therefore, this group of attacks is sometimes called temporal lobe seizures or temporal lobe epilepsy. These terms are less preferred, and they are not technically correct, unless the patient(s) referred to have seizures that are truly of temporal lobe origin. Simple partial seizures may progress to complex partial seizures; complex partial seizures may progress to generalized tonic-clonic seizures. The latter are called *partial seizures secondarily generalized*.

The second type of seizures are *generalized seizures*. Instead of originating from a circumscribed area of the brain, these seizures are bilaterally symmetrical from the onset and involve most or all of the cerebral cortex throughout the attack. These seizures can be classified as *convulsive* or *nonconvulsive* by nature. Convulsive attacks most commonly include repetitive motor movements, such as in myoclonic and tonic-clonic seizures. Nonconvulsive seizures are exemplified by absence attacks, in which for a few seconds all activity stops. Although the person is not responsive during these episodes, there is typically a return to completely normal functioning a few seconds later.

By their nature, epileptic seizures are intermittent in appearance. In most cases, they also are unpredictable in their appearance, as only a portion of people with partial seizures have an aura or warning of an impending attack. This unpredictability has a substantial adverse impact not only on the person with seizures but also on other people with whom the individual with epilepsy is in contact. The fact that the patient with epilepsy appears to be entirely normal at times makes the sudden appearance of abnormalities in behavior even more striking and unnerving for everyone involved. It also creates special challenges in neuropsychological assessment, as one must be certain that one is evaluating enduring brain functions and not the effects of a recent attack.

The Costs of Epilepsy

In the United States, 2.3 million people have epilepsy, and the estimated annual cost of this disorder directly and indirectly is $12.5 billion. Furthermore, approximately 181,000 new cases of epilepsy appear each year, 10% of Americans will experience a seizure sometime in their lifetime, and 3% will develop epilepsy by age 75. These recent facts from the Epilepsy Foundation (1999) indicate that this disorder continues its widely destructive path with enormous costs on every level.

Although the economic costs are high, the costs in pain and suffering as well as stigma and ostracism cannot be calculated. People avoid identifying themselves with even the term epilepsy and often seek to use other terms, such as spells or seizures, in an effort to sidestep the stigma involved. Fundraising for epilepsy is unusually difficult, as telephoning and door-to-door campaigns are nearly impossible due to a lack of volunteers. In response to this situation, years ago I began to deliberately identify myself with epilepsy even ahead of neuropsychology when asked about the work in which I was engaged. Wearing lapel pins with epilepsy symbols, carrying briefcases with epilepsy-related markings, and even wearing a necktie depicting epileptiform discharges tend to further openness regarding epilepsy, as questions from strangers tend to arise from these items. The result is the chance to bring up epilepsy in conversation and to answer questions about it, clearing up misconceptions on many occasions.

In addition to the general stigma of the disorder, it is evident that there are important quality of life correlates of this neurological problem. In a community-based survey of some of these factors, for example, Fisher (2000) showed that marriage rates are diminished in epilepsy, that income is decreased in households with at least one person with epilepsy, and that unemployment among epilepsy patients is five times the rate of the general population. The great importance of such factors to human existence should not escape any reader. However, there are other factors of importance as well. When patients are asked the worst thing about having epilepsy, by far the most frequently mentioned factor is fear. This includes fear of dying, fear that others will witness a seizure, fear of losing employment, and fear of automobile accidents secondary to seizures. Furthermore, although progress has been made in seizure management over the years, only 50% of patients in Fisher's community-based sample considered their seizures to be under good control. In addition, side effects cited by a third or more of the sample included diminished energy level, memory, school performance, and overall quality of life as well as increased concern about having children.

Common Forms of Treatment for Epilepsy

By far the most common type of treatment for epileptic seizures is medication. Nearly all people receiving any type of treatment are treated with drugs, with very few exceptions. Traditionally used medications include phenobarbital (Luminol, Mebarol), phenytoin (Dilantin), carbamazepine (Tegretol), and valproic acid (Depakote). In recent years, these have been supplemented with gabapentin (Neurontin), tiagabine (Gabitril), lamotrigine (Lamictal), topiramate (Topamax), levetiracetam (Keppra), oxcarbazine (Trileptal), and zonisimide (Zonegran). Although the newer medications are of definite help for some patients, providing improved seizure control and reduced side effects, none has come close to making most patients with uncontrolled epilepsy free of their seizures, and the typical new medication is effective in making patients seizure-free in less than 10% of persons previously uncontrolled.

Surgery is a much more narrowly used treatment for epilepsy but one that is capable of producing a cure or near cure in many cases. The most common form of surgery is the lobectomy, which often is accomplished in connection with one or another of the temporal lobes. If the epileptic focus can be found in a circumscribed area of the brain and this area can be removed, the patient may be cured of the epilepsy and no longer have seizures. Furthermore, if the resection can be done without disturbing critical functions such as speech and memory, the return to the patient may be especially great. As will be detailed below, neuropsychologists can be of real value in the workup for epilepsy surgery and in follow-up after surgery as well.

Another surgically related procedure that has come into fairly common use is the implantation of a vagal nerve stimulator. This device is introduced into the upper chest wall on the left side and connected to the vagal nerve, which runs from the heart to the brain. Small electrical currents are thereby introduced into the brain at intervals, such as for 30-second periods every 5 minutes. With some people, seizures are diminished using this procedure, sometimes significantly so—but just as with the newer medications, rarely is a patient made completely seizure-free using this treatment.

Other techniques beyond the medical and surgical ones discussed here have been used in an effort to obtain control of epileptic seizures. For example, an operant conditioning approach has been used, and some amount of relief from seizures has been reported (Dahl, Brorson, & Melin, 1992; Dahl, Melin, & Leissner, 1988; Lantz & Sterman, 1988). However, the improvement in seizure frequency is not always sustained, and this finding (plus the considerable amount of effort involved in this technique) has lead to its use on an occasional basis only. Other techniques—such as the use of stress reduction therapy and the medical use of marijuana—have been reported as at least somewhat successful in temporarily reducing seizures.

Neuropsychological Services Commonly Provided

At the time of a seizure, the brain is unquestionably dysfunctional. As has been known for many years, however, abnormalities persist between attacks in the majority of persons with epilepsy, as is proven by interictal EEG studies, which often show both epileptiform (Wilkus & Dodrill, 1976) and nonepileptiform (Dodrill & Wilkus, 1978) changes. Were this not the case, the EEG would be of little value except during periods in which epileptic attacks are recorded. Because the brain is the basis for mental abilities and adaptive skills, it would be expected that decreased abilities would be found interictally in many persons with epilepsy, and this also has been established for many years (Dodrill, 1978). Furthermore, treatment for epilepsy–including medications and surgery–may themselves have significant iatrogenic cognitive effects.

This is far-reaching in its implications in terms of impacts on adjustment to everyday life and also in terms of economic impact. If the cognitive limitations observed are allowed to exert their toll unchecked, the economic effects of these problems can be enormous. However, by evaluating these cognitive limitations systematically, one can be appraised of the concerns that exist in individual people with epilepsy. One is then in a better position to take steps to minimize the economic effects of the cognitive concerns as well as to minimize effects on quality of life.

When there is attention to these factors, neuropsychologists provide a series of services of benefit to patients and professionals alike. These services are briefly indicated in Table 11.1.

Neuropsychological Evaluation

To adequately evaluate the variety of cognitive concerns that can exist in epilepsy, a broad battery of tests with demonstrated sensitivity to brain dysfunction is required. Although intelligence tests can be helpful, they were originally designed to predict performance in school and they are not systematically formulated to reflect adequacy of brain functions. Neuropsychological tests represent a far more adequate solution, providing (a) they have been shown to be sensitive to brain-related deficits, (b) they have been assembled on empirical grounds to reflect a broad range of brain functions, and (c) they take advantage of the strengths of a variety of methods of inference of brain condition. The Halstead-Reitan Battery for Adults (Reitan & Wolfson, 1985) is

TABLE 11.1. Services Provided by Neuropsychologists in the Context of Epilepsy

- Establish educational and vocational expectations based on a careful assessment of abilities
- Provide practical recommendations to assist the person with epilepsy in adjusting to the demands of everyday life
- Assist in the estimation of the cognitive effects of anti-epileptic drugs
- Confirm lateralization of the epileptic focus in cases being considered for surgery
- Provide definite evidence of side of speech in surgical cases
- Establish a baseline in functioning and then later provide objective evidence for changes from that baseline as a consequence of seizures or of a particular treatment
- Evaluate rehabilitation potential

one such battery that meets these conditions, and the Luria-Nebraska Neuropsychological Battery (Golden, 1981) is another with significant work in this direction. These tests have been used in a variety of contexts and with many different patient groups.

Beginning with the Halstead-Reitan approach, years ago I assembled a battery of tests specifically to meet the needs of adults with epilepsy (Dodrill, 1978). This group of tests meets the criteria established above, and it was assembled only after studies with it had been completed on topics of neuropsychological interest in epilepsy, including epileptiform and nonepileptiform EEG discharges, immediate and long-term effects of the attacks themselves, anti-epileptic drugs, and so on. The plea here is not for the use of one particular group of tests, but for the application of a carefully constructed battery that is well validated with respect to sensitivity to brain functions and directed toward the cognitive problems people with epilepsy frequently show. If this is done carefully, the tests can be of real value in a number of contexts, as detailed below.

Educational Evaluations. Sad but true is the fact that children with epilepsy often perform poorly in school. Key findings in the area have been summarized by Seidenberg and Clemmons (1997). Underlying brain dysfunction may be at the core of many of these problems. However, the subclinical epileptiform discharges that appear intermittently with many of these children can have the net effect of making the seating of memory traces difficult and otherwise result in diminished concentration. Also, the ever-present medications, designed to suppress seizures, can suppress general alertness and intellectual acuity. Neuropsychological evaluations can greatly assist in establishing appropriate expectations for individual children. Frequently, neither the parent nor the teacher really knows precisely what to expect, so genuine limitations in brain functions are misconstrued as motivational difficulties. Once appropriate expectations have been set for a given child, everyone is in a better position to assist in establishing an improved educational program that will help to utilize the child's strengths and sidestep weaknesses insofar as is possible. A better adjusted child may well be the result, one who is in a better position to maximize functioning in adult life.

Vocational Evaluations. As indicated, unemployment among epileptic persons can be as much as five times that found in the general population (Fisher, 2000). A return to work of a significant number of people with epilepsy is one of the clearest ways in which a fiscal return can be demonstrated for the health-care dollars expended. A good start toward this end is to study which neuropsychological variables actually distinguish between differing levels of unemployment. A second step is to evaluate people intensively before they begin to search for employment, and then to periodically check on their progress in finding and maintaining work. A third step is to test out predictors of employment in a proactive way within an intervention program to determine which people are likely to return to work with the investment of time and money in an intervention, and which are not likely to return to work even after such an investment. In the area of epilepsy, both of these steps have been taken, and samples of these efforts will be presented.

First, a number of neuropsychological tests have been shown to be effective discriminators between unemployed, underemployed, and fully employed persons with epilepsy; in fact, this was established many years ago. An example of this is a study (Batzel, Dodrill, & Fraser, 1980) in which 58 adults with epilepsy were classified as unemployed (less than 5 hours of work per week on average for the past 6 months), underemployed

(6 to 19 hours per week or sheltered work), and employed (20 or more hours per week). Students, homemakers, and retired persons were not included. Administration of Dodrill's (1978) neuropsychological battery revealed statistically significant differences on many measures, with an inverse relationship found between degree of employment and degree of cognitive impairment. For example, unemployed persons averaged 64% of neuropsychological tests being performed outside normal limits, underemployed individuals averaged 52%, and employed persons averaged only 31% ($p < .001$). The Wechsler Adult Intelligence Full Scale IQ score differentiated the groups ($p < .05$), but not as well as the neuropsychological test battery. Thus, the importance of administering specialized neuropsychological tests was evident.

The second step in studying the effectiveness of neuropsychological evaluations is to assess groups of people with epilepsy at critical life stages, and then to follow them for several years in terms of their ability to obtain and maintain employment. In one study (Clemmons & Dodrill, 1984) this was done with 40 adolescents with epilepsy who were near the end of their secondary school programs (ages 16 to 19) and who were followed up an average of 6.44 years later. At follow-up, it was noted that only 18 persons (45%) were actually employed 30 hours per week or more. Various neuropsychological test measures differentiated the groups at the time of the initial evaluation, with 44% of 16 neuropsychological tests (Dodrill, 1978) being outside normal limits among persons who ultimately obtained employment on their own and with 71% of scores being abnormal among persons who were unable to obtain and sustain such employment ($p < .01$).

The third step in evaluating the utility of neuropsychological variables is to test them prospectively in a formal study. An example of an investigation of this type is one by Fraser, Clemmons, Dodrill, Trejo, and Freelove (1986). In this study, 46 unemployed adults with epilepsy received an extensive neuropsychological evaluation prior to vocational counseling, and brain-related assets and deficits identified thereby were taken into account in the vocational planning program. This program included individual vocational counseling, vocational assessment of interests and aptitudes, and weekly job-finding club and job-seeking skills training. On average, the typical client participated in this intervention program for one year. Following an additional year of follow-up, participants were classified as employed if they had been employed full-time during that follow-up year (n = 22), or unemployed if they had not maintained full-time employment through that year (n = 24). Although basic biographical and seizure-history information did not distinguish between the groups, two neuropsychological variables (WAIS Digit Symbol and Name Writing Procedure from the neuropsychological battery) did make this differentiation, with better pretreatment scores indicating a greater likelihood of profiting from employment intervention. A predictive system was developed to identify in advance which people would and which would not profit from the employment training. This system was shown to be accurate in 75% of the cases.

In this study, it was evident that neuropsychological tests taking no more than 5 minutes to administer increased prediction of vocational training utility from 50% to 75%. If the year-long vocational intervention program cost an estimated $6,000 per client, and if the 5 minutes of testing cost an average of $50, a savings of 12,000% was experienced. Perhaps even more important, had the results of the study been applied to a similar group of patients, approximately 12 more likely successful responders to the vocational program could have been included, and these persons could have displaced 12 individuals who were unlikely to profit from the intervention. A substantial savings in the cost of this expensive intervention could have been realized. A related issue is the salary of successful program participants, as even if these persons had earned salaries of only $6 per hour during the follow-up year, a total of $144,000 would have been earned, which is much more than when they were unemployed. These savings do not include money that would have been spent on unemployment benefits and other financial subsistence during unemployment. Overall, it is believed that money spent on neuropsychological evaluations prior to directed vocational interventions is one of the best uses of funds that can be made to assist people with epilepsy.

Evaluations Conducted in Connection with Surgery for Epilepsy. Epilepsy surgery has enjoyed a tremendous increase in popularity in the last 20 years. The primary reason for this is that, when surgery can be utilized, it is much more likely to be effective in controlling epileptic seizures than is medication. In 1996, Spencer summarized the worldwide experience in reported lobectomies for epilepsy and reported that 68% of 3,579 temporal lobectomy candidates were seizure-free after their surgeries, and 45% of 805 extratemporal lobectomy cases were seizure-free. All of these patients had, by definition, failed anti-epileptic drug therapy, and the majority had failed multiple drugs

There are two basic activities in which neuropsychologists are involved in connection with surgery for epilepsy. Each of these is important, and in each case there are salient financial implications.

Pre- and postsurgical assessments. Neuropsychological evaluations before and after epilepsy surgery tend to be more directed than assessments conducted for other reasons. From a cognitive viewpoint, there is a particular need to evaluate those functions likely to be impacted by the surgery. In the vast majority of cases, surgery involves one or the other of the temporal lobes, and it is therefore essential that temporal lobe functioning be evaluated. Above all else, this means that capabilities pertaining to memory need to be assessed, and it is useful to think in terms of material-specific memory functions with verbal or language-related memory often relating to the left cerebral hemisphere and visual–spatial memory typically related to the right cerebral hemisphere. Another area of functioning commonly related to the temporal lobes pertains to language functions, and this certainly needs to be evaluated when surgery is on the same side as that associated with the production of speech. Finally, it is profitable to appraise general intellectual abilities from several perspectives. Although the inclusion of other areas may certainly be profitable for particular reasons, these areas need to be routinely examined.

Neuropsychological evaluations done preoperatively are routinely of help in a number of contexts. One of these is to use neuropsychology to help establish rehabilitation potential and expectations for level of functioning after surgery. Surgery and the workup for it are very expensive, and there needs to be a return when this amount of money is spent. Neuropsychological evaluation can be very useful in gauging ability to return to work and, with limited health-care resources, this can make a difference in determining if surgery is to be undertaken at all. In the cases in which surgery is to be undertaken, a neuropsychological evaluation can help to set realistic expectations for functional outcome, avoiding the unrealistic expectations commonly found. It is easy for unrealistic expectations to arise in connection with epilepsy surgery, which can be looked upon to solve a host of problems only indirectly related to seizure frequency. A neuropsychological evaluation can help prevent this by establishing appropriate expectations.

Other situations in which neuropsychological evaluation is especially helpful pertain to establishing a baseline against which changes in abilities can be compared, alerting the surgeon as to level of cognitive function which is associated with the area to be resected and which may become worse following the resection, and providing confirmation of dysfunction in the area targeted for removal.

Amobarbital testing for lateralization of language and memory. Of great concern to the surgeon is the possibility that cognitive functions may be adversely impacted after surgery. This is of concern particularly with respect to the functions of language and memory, as these are some of the most critical functions of the areas most commonly removed (temporal lobes). An indiscriminate removal of areas pertaining to these functions can result in persisting dysphasia and in a global amnestic syndrome in which short-term memory is almost completely obliterated. The result of either of these conditions is that functioning is markedly reduced, economic productivity is curtailed, and the person frequently requires expensive long-term care.

To avoid these calamitous circumstances, a test is commonly undertaken, which is called the Intracarotid Amobarbital Procedure (IAP) or Wada Test, after Juhn Wada, who originally developed the procedure. In this procedure, the middle portion of one hemisphere and then the other hemisphere are selectively anesthetized. During the few minutes in which the anesthesia is in effect, the neuropsychologist tests the critical functions of speech and memory and is able to determine what the patient can and cannot do without the portion of the brain that is temporarily dysfunctional due to the anesthesia. Based on this information, the neuropsychologist can make a reasonable prediction as to the likelihood of producing such a deficit after surgery.

The IAP is done at nearly every center in the world that performs epilepsy surgery, and it clearly represents the standard of care that has been used for many years. Some estimate of the adverse effects of omitting this procedure can be made by first estimating the number of cases that would be missed where critical functions might unexpectedly be disturbed by surgery and which might produce permanent disability. The second type of estimate that would need to be made is the dollar cost of the damage in the typical patient. Efforts will be made to do this below, but it should be realized that these efforts are best estimates rather than final figures.

First, one must estimate the number of cases in which there is risk for adverse cognitive change after surgery that would not be appreciated by the surgeon at the time the surgery is done. Data on exactly this point regarding the lateralization of speech currently are being assembled by the author and have already been reported in a preliminary way (Dodrill & Ojemann, 1999). As is well known, in the majority of cases basic speech and language functions are associated with the left hemisphere only. So the surgeon can be correct in assuming left speech in the majority of cases, especially if the patient is right-handed. The question arises, however, as to how often the surgeon will be *incorrect* in the assumption of left-hemisphere speech, with the result that there will be surgery on that side without the surgeon being aware of the possibility of permanently damaging communication skills. The answer to this question is found in Table 11.2 which presents the probabilities of speech *not* being on the left side only. The information in this table is based on 766 IAPs conducted over a 26-year period. As the table shows, there is at least a 4% chance of operating on the side of speech, even under conditions in which the most confident predictions can be made (right-handed with surgery on the right). If 1,000 surgeries are done for epilepsy per year (only an esti-

TABLE 11.2. Likelihood of Finding Atypical (Right Speech or Bilateral Speech) Representation Based on Handedness and Side of Surgery

	Side of surgery	
Handedness	Left	Right
Right (n = 617)	10%	4%
Left (n = 149)	53%	23%

mate, but a reasonable number), and if half are on the right side and half on the left, and if 80% of cases are right-handed (similar to our extensive experience reported in the table), then 400 of the cases would be right-handed and have surgery on the right. In 4% of these 400 cases (or 16 cases total), the surgeon would be operating on the side of speech without knowing it—and this represents the minimal risk condition. If the IAP were not done at all for any patient and the assumption of left speech was made in every case, 132 patients would be put at risk for language-related loss after surgery.

The dollar cost of the damage that might be produced by damaging the language-related parts of the brain is the second type of estimate that must be made to evaluate the cost-effectiveness of the neuropsychologist undertaking IAPs. This is difficult to determine for several reasons. First, at least a portion of the patients would not have resections likely including a speech-related area, and no deficits would be expected in those cases, regardless of the side of the operation. This would hold in perhaps 20% of the cases, in my experience. Second, when there is postoperative dysphasia, it may be transient and may not require treatment. Perhaps 60% of the remaining cases likely fall in this group and, although some of these people would continue to experience subtle language-related deficits probably impacting productivity slightly, such losses are difficult to document. In the final 20% are persons with persisting losses, some of whom are treated with rehabilitation efforts and some of whom are not. In the worst 5% would be persons requiring extensive rehabilitation with significantly diminished vocational productivity, unemployment, and the need for significantly increased care. If one considered only this worst 5% (6.6 persons out of 132 at risk) and estimated (a) the rehabilitation services need at $25,000 per person, (b) the loss of employment income at $30,000 per years for 30 years (based on surgery at about age 30), and (c) the need for subsistence funds at $12,000 per year for each of the 6.6 persons for 30 years each, the total damage in dollars for not doing the IAP would be $8,481,000. The cost for only the neuropsychologist doing the 1,000 IAPs would be approximately $750 per case, or $750,000. Not even considering either the human misery involved or cases beyond the worst 5%, the cost ($750,000) to savings ($8,481,000 less $750,000) ratio is 10.3. Thus, the money for this type of neuropsychological work is more than repaid.

Cost Outcome Studies in the Neuropsychology of Epilepsy

The dollar figures presented in the cost-savings illustrations are, by necessity, gross estimations that have limited importance. They are formed conservatively and, if anything, they underestimate the savings produced by neuropsychologists. In the future, a more accurate accounting of cost-effectiveness can be made by prospectively directing studies more specifically to cost–benefit issues. In addition, there are a number of areas in which studies could be done that would help to evaluate costs and how cost-effectiveness could be improved. Two ideas in this direction are sketched out in the following sections.

Immediate and Long-Term Needs of Children with Epilepsy

Except for the elderly with a first seizure, most people with epilepsy have their first seizure in childhood (Hauser & Hesdorffer, 1990), and this is an overarching fact that should not escape our attention. Many of these children require special educational assistance in childhood and special vocational assistance in adulthood. At the present time, however, the needs of these children are caught only as they become evident to parents and educational personnel, without a systemic effort to anticipate needs and to minimize their effects. A neuropsychological evaluation conducted with the typical child with epilepsy in the early elementary school years might be well repaid in a reduction in human misery, increased functioning as adults in society, and significantly reduced expenditures by the public. A randomized parallel group design could be applied to groups of children with epilepsy, with one group receiving a thorough neuropsychological assessment but with treatments otherwise being identical. The children could then be followed into adulthood, with attention to special services required and to important outcome variables including educational attainment, employment, and social adaptation. Such a study, never before undertaken, could do more than anything else to truly test whether neuropsychological practice can make a real difference in the long run for people with epilepsy.

Evaluation of Cognitive and Quality of Life (QOL) Effects of Antiepileptic Drugs

Although most epilepsy develops in childhood, most people with epilepsy live into senior adulthood. The consequence is that most people with epilepsy take medications for seizures for more than 50 years. Adverse cognitive and QOL effects of even small proportions have enormous costs over the years, but the likelihood of such effects is enhanced by important factors. Among these is the fact that drugs are designed to suppress certain functions of the brain (seizures). However, we also want the drugs to leave other functions (cognition, personality, etc.) intact. This is an exceedingly difficult demand, however, especially as most seizures involve the temporal lobes, which, of course, are involved in some of the most critical of human functions (such as language and memory). It is for these reasons and others that the majority of studies of the psychological effects of anti-epileptic drugs point to adverse cognitive and QOL effects of one type or another.

Thus far, the many studies done on the neurocognitive effects of these medications have provided important guidance to physicians who, on a daily basis, must make choices as to which drugs to administer. For example, the prescription of barbiturate drugs for long-term seizure control has been substantially curtailed by studies showing important adverse cognitive effects in most people. In epilepsy especially, there is a particular need for additional neuropsychological studies, as these medications often have similar levels of efficacy in terms of seizure control, and the result is that drug choice often must be made on the basis of toxicity considerations.

What is needed in this area now are studies that show the economic implications of the neuropsychological findings in studies of anti-epileptic drugs. At the moment, the emphasis is almost entirely on producing statistically significant results, but if a patient's response speed is diminished by about 12%, does it mean that about 1 hour less work gets accomplished on this drug per working day? Administering tests might be a shorthand way of predicting such changes; and by alerting physicians to such changes, productivity may be enhanced and major adverse situations (such as job loss) may be averted.

Additional studies with clear-cut cost-effectiveness ramifications can be easily envisioned. For example, the usual practice today is to include all patients in a drug study who meet certain medical criteria (seizure type, seizure frequency, etc.). Such a general practice ignores the fact that there is no anti-epileptic drug that is bad for every patient and no anti-epileptic drug that is good for every patient--even for the same seizure type. A subgrouping of patients based on neuropsychological criteria may be the best way to cast light on medications that seem similar when applied to large groups of patients. For example, the response of very bright patients to a certain medication may be quite different than that of a dull group of people, but the data are almost never evaluated in this manner. Neuropsychological tests can provide a basis for such a subgrouping which cannot be otherwise made. The result can be the identification of certain drugs for particular patients while avoiding others, with a consequent improvement in measurable functioning and a decrease in medical care required.

Conclusions

The information in this chapter underscores the important role neuropsychologists have in working with patients with epilepsy. To date, the economic value of this work has been documented only in a preliminary way. There is substantial value to this work, however, both from a cost-effectiveness viewpoint and from the viewpoint of human suffering. It is hoped this chapter will help to stimulate work in this area in the future, so that the value of neuropsychological work in this context can be better established and sharpened for improved productivity in the future.

References

Batzel, L. W., Dodrill, C. B., & Fraser. R. T. (1980). Further validation of the WPSI Vocational Scale: Comparisons with other correlates of employment in epilepsy. *Epilepsia, 21,* 235–242.

Clemmons, D. C., & Dodrill, C. B. (1984). Vocational outcomes of high school students with epilepsy and neuropsychological correlates with later vocational success. In R. J. Porter, R. H. Mattson, A. A. Ward, Jr., & M. Dam (Eds.), *Advances in Epileptology: XVth Epilepsy International Symposium* (pp. 611–614). New York: Raven Press.

Commission on Classification and Terminology of the International League Against Epilepsy. (1981). Proposal for revised clinical and electroencephalographic classification of epileptic seizures. *Epilepsia, 22,* 489–501.

Dahl, J. A., Brorson, L.-O., & Melin, L. (1992). Effects of a broad-spectrum behavioral medicine treatment program on children with refractory epileptic seizures: An 8-year follow-up. *Epilepsia, 33,* 98–102.

Dahl, J. A., Melin, L., & Leissner, P. (1988). Effects of a behavioral intervention on epileptic seizure behavior and paroxysmal activity: A systematic replication of three cases of children with intractable epilepsy. *Epilepsia, 29,* 172–183.

Dodrill, C. B. (1978). A neuropsychological battery for epilepsy. *Epilepsia, 19,* 611–623.

Dodrill, C. B., & Ojemann. G. A. (1999). Probability of atypical speech as a function of handedness and side of surgery. *Epilepsia, 40*(Suppl. 7), 83.

Dodrill, C. B., & Wilkus, R. J. (1978). Neuropsychological correlates of the electroencephalogram in epileptics. III: Generalized nonepileptiform abnormalities. *Epilepsia, 19,* 453–462.

Epilepsy Foundation. (1999). Epilepsy: A report to the nation. *Epilepsy USA,* as quoted on the Epilepsy Foundation Website.

Fisher, R. S. (2000). Epilepsy from the patient's perspective: Review of results from a community-based survey. *Epilepsy and Behavior, 1,* S9–S14.

Fraser, R. T., Clemmons, D. C., Dodrill, C. B., Trejo, W. R., & Freelove, C. (1986). The difficult-to-employ in epilepsy rehabilitation: Predictions of response to an intensive intervention. *Epilepsia, 27,* 220–224.

Golden, C. J. (1981). A standardized version of Luria's neuropsychological tests: A quantitative and qualitative approach to neuropsychological evaluation. In S. B. Filskov & T. J. Boll (Eds.), *Handbook of clinical neuropsychology* (pp. 608–642). New York: John Wiley.

Hauser, W. A., & Hesdorffer, D. C. (1990). *Epilepsy: Frequency, causes, and consequences.* New York: Demos Publications.

Lantz, D. L., & Sterman, M. B. (1988). Neuropsychological assessment of subjects with uncontrolled epilepsy: Effects of EEG feedback training. *Epilepsia, 29,* 163–171.

Reitan, R. M., & Wolfson, D. (1985). *The Halstead-Reitan Neuropsychological Test Battery,* Tucson: Neuropsychology Press.

Seidenberg, M., & Clemmons, D. C. (1997). Maximizing school functioning and the school-to-work transition. In J. Engel, Jr., & T. A. Pedley (Eds.), *Epilepsy: A comprehensive textbook* (pp. 2203–2209). Philadelphia: Lippincott-Raven.

Spencer, S. S. (1996). Long-term outcome after epilepsy surgery. *Epilepsia, 37,* 807–813.

Temkin, O. (1971). *The falling sickness: A history of epilepsy from the Greeks to the beginnings of modern neurology.* Baltimore: Johns Hopkins University Press.

U.S. Bureau of the Census. www.census.gov/2002.

Wilkus, R. J., & Dodrill. C. B. (1976). Neuropsychological correlates of the electroencephalogram in epileptics, I: Topographic distribution and average rate of epileptiform activity. *Epilepsia, 17,* 89–100.

12

CHAPTER

Roy Martin
Brian Bell
Bruce Hermann
Stephen Mennemeyer

Nonepileptic Seizures and Their Costs: The Role of Neuropsychology

☐ Introduction

Approximately 10% of all Americans will have at least one seizure at some point during their lives requiring medical evaluation and treatment. Epilepsy, defined as recurrent seizures, is a common neurological disorder affecting 0.6% to 1.0% of the population (Hauser & Hesdorffer, 1990). The annual number of office visits to neurologists for seizure-related conditions (i.e., ICD-9-M codes 780.3 [convulsions] and 345 [epilepsy]) is greater than 900,000, with over 80% receiving a diagnosis of convulsions (Schappert, 1995). Health-care costs associated with the treatment of epilepsy approach $3 billion for a single cohort year (Hauser & Hesdorffer, 1990). Total lifetime costs of epilepsy differ substantially according to point of seizure remission, with averaged per patient total dollar costs ranging from $4,272 for early seizure remission following initial drug treatment to $138,602 for patient cohorts with intractable seizures, which are defined as seizures that are uncontrolled with medications and that result in disability.

The possibility that a patient experiencing recurrent seizures does not have epilepsy but instead suffers from nonepileptic psychogenic seizures (NEPs) is one of the most challenging issues facing the clinician. Early identification of NEPs is critical, as the potential exists for misdiagnosis, iatrogenic hazards, and costly treatment over a protracted period of time. In addition, recent reports have indicated that the societal costs of NEPs may be considerable in terms of unemployment and disability rates, which may approximate those of intractable epilepsy (Krahn et al., 1997; Lepert & Schmitt, 1990).

This research was supported in part by NIH 37738 and NARSAD.

Between 5% and 20% of the 2 million persons treated yearly for epilepsy in the United States are estimated to have NEPs, with the overall prevalence of NEPs estimated at upward of 400,000 persons within the United States alone (Begley, Annegers, Lairson, Reynolds, & Hauser, 1994; Gates, Luciano, & Devinsky, 1991; Lesser, 1996). The lifetime dollar costs associated with the treatment of undiagnosed NEPs may approximate the lifetime dollar costs associated with the treatment of intractable epilepsy, which can be over $100,000 per patient. Lifetime dollars costs per patient cohort year for a NEPs group could range from $100 million to $600 million, because annual incidence rates of new cases of intractable epilepsy are approximately 150,000. To date, the medical and socioeconomic impact of the diagnosis and treatment of NEPs has not been formally established within the U.S. health-care system.

NEPs are etiologically rooted in psychiatric illnesses and primarily fall under the diagnostic rubric of somatoform disorders. Numerous studies have described the tremendous medical resource utilization of patients with coexisting psychiatric disorders who present to primary care providers (PCPs; Fink, 1992; Hollifield, Paine, Tuttle, & Kellner, 1999). The rate of primary care physician visits by patients with diagnosed mental disorders is twice that of other patients, with 50% to 70% of visits to PCPs primarily for psychologically based complaints and symptoms (Barsky & Borus, 1995). Given that NEPs are psychiatric phenomena, it is reasonable to predict similar increased utilization rates for patients with this condition.

Unfortunately, collection of medical care utilization data is lacking within the NEP population. Utilization data, if mentioned at all, typically involve general statements that repeated anti-epilepsy drug (AED) trials had been attempted or that serial outpatient EEGs had been negative or equivocal. A few studies have reported details of anti-epilepsy medication usage in NEP patients. Lancman, Brotherton, Asconape, and Penry (1993) reported that at the time of NEP diagnosis 54% of patients (n = 93) were taking AEDs, and that a total of 67% had taken AEDs at some time. Walczak et al. (1995) reported that 38 of 52 (73%) NEP patients were taking AEDs at the time of inpatient admission; but at follow-up contact after diagnosis, 50% were not taking any AEDs and 10 out of 38 (26%) had significant reduction in amount or number of AEDs. Moore, Baker, McDade, Chadwick, and Brown (1994) reported that 68% (13 of 19) of their NEP patients were taking AEDs at time of diagnosis, but no follow-up data were provided. Krahn et al. (1997) reported on a series of 94 consecutive NEP patients diagnosed by video-electroencephalographic (EEG) monitoring. AEDs had been either discontinued or reduced in 67% of the patients following diagnosis. No study has yet reported more specific drug information regarding type, dosage, or costs.

☐ Clinical Issues in the Diagnosis of NEPs

NEPs can be suggested by clinical observation of the patient's typical paroxysmal event (Chabolla, Krahn, So, & Rummans, 1996; Kuyk, Leijten, Meinard, Spinhoven, & Van Dyck, 1997). However, clinicians' predictive accuracy in identifying NEPs prior to inpatient video-EEG monitoring is approximately 50% (Kanner et al., 1990; King et al., 1982; Saygi, Katz, Marks, & Spencer, 1992). NEPs can be misdiagnosed as epilepsy in the outpatient clinic setting because there are many consistencies of clinical presentation between the two conditions (Brown, Levin, Ramsay, Katz, & Duchowny, 1991;

Henry & Drury, 1998). Confusing matters even more is the fact that more than of one-third of NEP patients may have coexisting epilepsy (Betts & Boden, 1992; Lempert & Schmidt, 1990).

Standard outpatient diagnostic testing for epilepsy (routine recording EEG or MRI) yields less than optimal diagnostic specificity (Morris et al., 1994). Ambulatory EEG monitoring is another outpatient technique that can aid in differential diagnosis. Although ambulatory EEG monitoring may have better diagnostic yield over routine EEG, only about one-third of recordings are diagnostically useful in terms of identifying epilepsy (Morris et al., 1994). In addition, certain seizure types, including frontal lobe seizures, are notoriously difficulty to distinguish from nonepileptic seizures without inpatient video-EEG monitoring (Kanner et al., 1990). Following negative routine EEG testing, initiation of AED therapy is not uncommon if there is a convincing report of clinical seizures. Remission rates for seizures following this first drug trial range from 30% to 70% (Hauser, Rich, Lee, Annegers, & Anderson, 1998; Mattson, 1998). However, if seizures are not controlled following that first drug trial, recurrence rates approach 80% to 90% following subsequent drug trials (Hauser et al., 1998).

Inpatient video-EEG seizure monitoring is considered the gold standard for definitive NEP diagnosis, but only a small fraction of persons with intractable seizure disorders receive such diagnostic assessment (Lesser, 1996). Video-EEG monitoring has been deemed a standard diagnostic tool for excluding nonepileptic seizures in the evaluation of potential epilepsy surgical candidates, according to a recent National Institutes of Health-sponsored consensus statement on epilepsy (NIH, 1990). Inpatient video-EEG monitoring can significantly impact diagnostic classification, treatment regime, and patient outcome (Gumnit, 1993; Sutula et al., 1981). The decision to use video-EEG monitoring in the evaluation of seizure disorders is based on multiple factors, including severity of illness, costs, availability, and prior success of outpatient treatment. However, the problem of misidentification of NEPs is highlighted by the fact that up to 40% of patients treated for epilepsy in an outpatient setting, prior to video-EEG seizure monitoring, are found to have NEPs upon subsequent inpatient admission (Devinsky et al., 1996; Gumnit, 1993; Ramani, Quesney, Olsen, & Gumnit, 1980; Synder, Rosenbaum, Rowan, & Strain, 1994; Thacker, Devinsky, Perrine, Alper, & Luciano 1997;). Published series of consecutive admissions to video-EEG seizure monitoring units commonly report that the average duration of NEPs prior to admission for monitoring approaches 7 years, and in some cases several decades. This finding suggests less than optimal diagnostic yield from available outpatient evaluation (Bowman & Markand, 1996; Martin, Gilliam, Kilgore, Faught, & Kuzniecky, 1998; Meierkord, Will, Fish, & Shorvon, 1991). Meierkord et al. (1991) cited data from their clinical population that showed the mean duration of NEPs prior to formal diagnosis was approximately 3 years, with a range of 1 to 20 years. A recent report by Bowman and Markand (1996) noted seizure disorder duration of 8.3 years, ranging from 1 month to 32 years in their sample of NEPs patients. Martin et al. (1998) reported an average NEPs duration of 6.8 years, with a range of 6 months to 33 years. Although inpatient monitoring is encouraged with patients presenting with intractable seizures—defined as seizures having not "been brought under acceptable control with the resources available to the primary care physician or neurologist" (NIH, 1990)—to date no empirically based data exist examining the impact on outcome of early video-EEG monitoring in the clinical course of the NEP disorder.

Several recent reports point to the frequent identification of nonepileptic seizures within the context of inpatient diagnostic monitoring. Westbrook, Devinsky, and Geocadin (1998) reported that over one-third of their patient sample had experienced NEPs for more than 10 years. Ramani et al. (1980) found that 20% of patients admitted to an inpatient epilepsy diagnostic unit had nonepileptic seizures instead. In a study of 387 consecutive admissions to an inpatient seizure-monitoring unit, 25% of the sample was found to have psychogenic seizures (Devinsky et al., 1996). A study of outpatient day monitoring seizure evaluations found that 62 of 262 patients had nonepileptic seizures rather than epileptic seizures (Synder et al., 1994). Thacker et al. (1997) found that 27% (103/375) of a consecutive series from an inpatient video-EEG seizure monitoring unit were diagnosed with psychogenic seizures. Finally, unpublished data from the University of Alabama at Birmingham inpatient video-EEG seizure-monitoring unit revealed that, over the 18-month period from January 1996 to June 1997 170 (28%) of 608 patients evaluated for possible seizure disorder had a discharge diagnosis of exclusively NEPs.

□ Clinical Outcomes for NEPs Following Inpatient Video/EEG Seizure Monitoring

In terms of clinical outcome, several longitudinal studies have reported that NEPs patients may experience improvement in nonepileptic seizure control as a result of definitive inpatient video-EEG monitoring-based diagnosis. Improved seizure control was exhibited in 15 of 34 (44%) NEP patients 5 years after inpatient video-EEG monitoring, whereas the remaining patients displayed no seizure frequency change (Krumholtz & Niedermeyer, 1983). Kristensen and Alving (1992) reported that 10 of 22 (45%) of NEP patients were seizure-free at 5-year median follow-up assessment, and that none reported worsened seizure outcome. Meierkord et al. (1991) reported that 40% (28 of 70) of their NEP patients became seizure-free within 6 months of inpatient video-EEG monitoring-based diagnosis. Lancman et al. (1993) reported that 5 years after definitive NEP diagnosis, 25% (16 of 63) of their patients were seizure-free, whereas 75% continued to experience seizures (frequency not specified). Walczak et al. (1995) presented 2-year or greater follow-up data on a sample of 51 NEP patients and found that 35% were seizure-free, 41% had experienced greater than 80% seizure frequency reduction, and 24% had experienced less than 80% reduction in seizure frequency. Lepert and Schmitt (1990) examined long-term outcome in 50 NEP patients and found that, of the 41 patients successfully contacted after diagnosis (mean interval = 24 months), 34% were seizure-free, 22% reported greater than 75% seizure reduction, and 41% (17 of 41) remained essentially unchanged. They also found that shorter prediagnosis seizure duration being employed at time of inpatient monitoring and absence of preexisting psychiatric diagnosis were significantly correlated with better "seizure" outcome following diagnosis, although other areas of outcome were not assessed. The overall impression from these studies is that freedom from nonepileptic seizures is a relatively frequent consequence of definitive inpatient video-EEG monitoring, but that the effect of duration of illness and other factors on outcome has yet to be fully examined.

Clinical Neuropsychological and MMPI Procedures and NEPs

We now turn to a review of the literature concerning the role of neuropsychological assessment in the diagnosis of NEPs. First, the literature pertaining to the neuropsychological status of patients with NEPs is reviewed. An attempt is made to determine whether neuropsychological (including intellectual) functioning in patients with NEPs differs from that of patients with epileptic seizures (ESs). If differences were found to exist, such findings might be of clinical utility in the evaluation of patients with suspected NEPs. Second, the literature examining personality characteristics of NEPs patients is discussed. Most of the data on this subject (particularly those emanating from the United States) come from the MMPI or MMPI-II; therefore, the following discussion focuses on work conducted with these instruments. Interest in this area has stemmed from reports that a particular subscale abnormality, the presence of a conversion profile, or the results of decision rules can discriminate NEPs from ES patients. The success with which the MMPI captures the distinction between ES and NEPs patients is reviewed.

Neuropsychological Discrimination of NEPs

There has been only a modest amount of formal inquiry into the neuropsychological characteristics of NEPs (Binder, Kinderman, Heaton, & Salinsky, 1998; Brown et al., 1991; Dodrill & Holmes, 2000; Kalogjera-Sackarelles & Sackallares, 1999; Risse, Mason, & Mercer, 2000; Sackellares et al., 1985; Swanson, Springer, Benbadis, & Morris, 2000; Wilkus & Dodrill, 1989; Wilkus, Dodrill, & Thompson, 1984). Variability in several cognitive characteristics, including intelligence, has been reported among patients with NEPs, although the general finding is that, at the group level, patients with NEPs often show some degree of cognitive impairment and do not differ significantly compared to patients with ESs on neuropsychological measures. The pertinent studies, and their hypotheses concerning the etiology of cognitive impairment in NEPs, are reviewed below.

Sackellares and colleagues (1985) examined patients admitted to the Diagnostic, Treatment, and Research Unit of the Comprehensive Epilepsy Program at the University of Virginia and the University of Michigan Epilepsy Laboratory. Using a strict set of inclusion and exclusion criteria, they obtained three groups of subjects: (a) patients with NEPs only (n = 19), (b) patients with ESs plus NEPs (n = 18), and (c) patients with documented generalized ESs only, who were randomly selected during the same period (n = 20). The patient groups were administered the Halstead-Reitan Neuropsychological Test Battery and allied procedures and the Wechsler Adult Intelligence Scale (WAIS). The authors found that patients with only NEPs had significantly higher mean WAIS IQ scores (FSIQ = 102, VIQ = 103, PIQ = 100) than both the mixed group (FSIQ = 90, VIQ = 90, PIQ = 90) and the generalized ES group (FSIQ = 86, VIQ = 90, PIQ = 83), although the latter two groups did not differ from one another. The Halstead-Reitan Impairment Index of the NEPs group (0.45) was significantly lower in comparison to the generalized ES group (0.71) and marginally lower (p = .08) than the mixed group (0.62), with the latter two groups again not differing from one another. Results of specific tests in the Halstead-Reitan Battery indicated that the NEPs group performed significantly better than the generalized ES group on the TPT test (total time, memory, and location), Category test, Seashore Rhythm test, and Speech Sounds Perception test. Compared to the mixed group, the NEPs patients performed significantly better on the TPT test (total time, memory, location) and Seashore Rhythm test and marginally better ($p = .08$) on the Speech Sounds Perception test. Again, there were no significant differences between the mixed and generalized ES groups. Although at first glance these results suggest that patients with NEPs had relatively intact neuropsychological function, Sackarelles et al. (1985) pointed out that the performance of NEPs patients on the neuropsychological tests was worse than that expected for "normal" individuals of similar intelligence. Their mean Impairment Index was in the range generally considered borderline between normal and impaired brain function. Interestingly, the authors raised the hypothesis that neurological impairment may play a role in the pathogenesis of NEPs.

In a more recent study of patients with either pseudoseizures or pseudoseizures and epilepsy Kalogjera-Sackarelles and Sackallares (1999) found the existence of a high frequency of neuropsychological impairment in both groups was predominant. For example, more than 50% of both groups scored in the impaired range on more than half the measures. In addition, across the entire sample of patients, the Full Scale IQ was in the low average or borderline impaired range in 41.5%, and the Halstead Impairment Index was in the impaired range in 63%. The authors also noted that these patients reported a history of a high incidence of accidents and physical trauma.

In a comprehensive study of NEPs, Wilkus et al. (1984) also evaluated the intellectual and neuropsychological status of patients (as well as personality functioning, to be discussed later in this chapter). Twenty-five patients with documented NEPs were compared to 25 patients with ESs who were comparable in age, sex, and level of education. The two groups were compared on the WAIS and Dodrill's Neuropsychological Battery for Epilepsy (NBE). The results were relatively straightforward. There were no differences between the groups on any of the WAIS subtests or IQ values, nor on any of the 16 measures from the NBE. Finally, there was no difference between the groups in the proportion of scores on the NBE that were outside of normal limits. Both groups demonstrated relatively elevated NBE scores (poorer performances). The NEPs group had 46% of their scores outside normal limits, compared to 51% of the scores for ES patients. The authors concluded that both groups exhibited evidence of brain damage or impairment of brain function. Citing this evidence, together with a high incidence of events that can cause CNS insult in the NEP group (e.g., history of trauma, disease), Wilkus et al. again raised the possibility that organic factors may, in some cases, contribute to the appearance of NEPs.

Although the results of Wilkus et al. (1984) appear to differ from those of Sackellares et al. (1985) in that the findings of the latter group suggest better cognitive function in NEPs patients compared to ES patients, both investigations reported comparable impairment indices (i.e., the proportion of test scores outside of normal limits) of 46% and 45%, respectively. In addition, the finding of frequent neuropsychological impairment among the pseudoseizure patients reported in Kalogjera-Sackallares & Sackallares (1999) is in accord with the data from Wilkus et al.

As part of a later investigation, Wilkus and Dodrill (1989) compared the neuropsychological findings reported in their previous study to those of other investigators. Specifically, they evaluated in detail the reasons for the different neuropsychological findings reported by Sackellares et al. (1985) and Wilkus et al. (1984). (MMPI findings from the investigation are reviewed later in this chapter.) Wilkus and Dodrill (1989) pointed out that their previous investigation (Wilkus et al., 1984) used groups of patients with ESs and NEPs that were matched for age, sex, and education. As reviewed above, they did not find differences in neuropsychological functioning between the two groups. On the other hand, the study by Sackellares et al. (1985) did not match their ES and NEP groups on these characteristics, and their generalized ES group had 2 years' less education, a significant difference. Wilkus and Dodrill (1989) speculated that the lack of matching in regard to education was responsible for the differences in the results of the two studies.

Four groups formed the basis for comparison in Wilkus and Dodrill's (1989) study: (a) the 25 NEP patients from their earlier study and three additional groups of 25 patients, each randomly selected from the neuropsychology lab files, including, (b) patients with partial ESs; (c) patients with generalized ESs matched to the NEP patients in terms of age, sex, and education; and (d) patients with generalized ESs who were matched to the NEP patients in terms of age and sex but not education (similar to Sackellares et al., 1985). The groups were compared on the WAIS and Dodrill's NBE. Comparing the age-, sex-, and education-matched groups of patients with NEPs, partial ESs, and generalized ESs revealed few differences. These results were similar to the findings in the original study by Wilkus et al. (1984). Only 2 of 22 comparisons reached statistical significance, and no discernible pattern was noted in the findings. On the other hand, when the NEP patients were compared to the group of patients with generalized ESs who were not matched on education, there were significant differences between the groups on 11 measures (3 IQ measures and 8 measures from the NBE). The NEPs groups performed in a less-impaired direction on all 11 measures. It should be remembered, however, that their overall performance was not within normal limits. Thus, controlling for educational level is an important consideration in these studies and can affect outcomes of group comparisons.

Recent studies comparing NEP and ES patients also have reported few if any neuropsychological differences between the two groups, with mildly abnormal performance being present at the group level in both disorders (Binder, Salinsky, & Smith, 1994; Brown et al., 1991; Dodrill & Holmes, 2000; Risse et al., 2000; Swanson et al., 2000). However, while continuing to acknowledge the possibility of an association between neuropsychological impairment and remote neurological insult in NEP patients, these recent studies have presented evidence that emotional and psychosocial factors may underlie the below-average neuropsychological profile of this group.

For example, in one study a qualitative analysis of neuropsychological data revealed unusual inconsistencies across neuropsychological scores, and between the level of neuropsychological functioning and level of overall functioning in everyday life, among some NEP patients. Similar inconsistencies were not observed within an ES group (Brown et al., 1991). Binder et al. (1994) reported that a NEP group performed significantly worse than ES patients on the Portland Digit Recognition Test (PDRT), a measure that is sensitive to level of motivation during test taking. In addition, there were statistically significant correlations between the PDRT and certain neuropsychological scores among the NEP patients. Swanson et al. (2000) found that groups of patients with ESs, NEPs, or somatoform disorders all performed similarly on a neuropsychological test battery. Based on the data from the latter group of patients, who had a psychiatric and no frank neurologic disorder, and because nearly one-half of their sample of NEP patients had undergone psychiatric hospitalization with histories of physical or sexual abuse in the majority, and evidence of more severe psychiatric symptomatology present in NEP compared to ES patients, Swanson et al. (2000) suggested that brain impairment does not have to be invoked to explain abnormal neuropsychological performance in groups of NEP patients. Although not excluding the possibility that brain impairment might contribute to the development of NEPs, they argued that psychiatric dysfunction in patients with this disorder may manifest as neuropsychological impairment as a result of a variable effort or a nonspecific attentional disturbance. Risse et al. (2000) offered a similar hypothesis. They suggested that NEP patients appear to be invested in their own dysfunction and might be prone to symptom exaggeration and reduced motivation during cognitive testing. Support for this hypothesis came from the finding in their study that the NEP group endorsed a high level of cognitive complaints but showed an absence of significant cognitive deficits on neuropsychological assessment. In a follow-up to previous studies from the Regional Epilepsy Center at the University of Washington in Seattle, Dodrill and Holmes (2000) examined the cognitive performance of 100 NEP patients, many of whom were included in the previous studies, and 100 demographically matched ES patients with lateralized seizures. Both groups generally performed below normal limits, but the NEP patients performed significantly better on Full Scale IQ and 4 of 16 other cognitive variables. As noted by the authors, the small group differences in those scores would be of no use when attempting to differentiate NEP from ES patients at the individual level. The authors concluded that compromised neuropsychological performance in NEP patients is likely due to both the neurological insults that are common in this population and to maladaptive response styles. As evidence for the latter, they cited the results of Binder et al. (1994) and a study in which NEP patients performed similarly to an ES group on the recall portion of a verbal memory test but showed a negative response bias, endorsing significantly fewer target items compared to the ES patients, in the recognition memory format (Bortz, Prigatano, Blum, & Fisher, 1995). The frequency (61%) of the finding of a negative response bias in NEP patients is consistent with the view that some of the neuropsychological deficits characteristic of this group might be attributable to factors other than neurological impairment.

Summary

These few controlled investigations suggest that it is not uncommon for patients with NEPs to exhibit at least mild signs of compromised brain function. However, although ES and NEP groups often do not show differences on standardized measures of neuropsychological status, there appears to be a growing consensus that emotional disturbance may contribute to the neuropsychological deficits in some NEP patients. This observation does not, of course, rule out the existence of genuine cognitive limitations in a subset of patients with NEPs, but it suggests that personality and motivational variables need to be considered in the interpretation of neuropsychological data in this group, and that the analysis of psychosocial and psychiatric history may aid attempts to differentiate NEPs and ESs and shed light on the etiologies of NEPs (Binder et al., 1998; Dodrill & Holmes, 2000; Swanson et al., 2000).

Although group data can be of limited utility to the clinician dealing with individuals, the studies reviewed suggest the following conclusions. The presence of impaired performance on neuropsychological examination does not rule out the possibility of

NEPs, just as the finding of normal cognitive ability does not rule out the presence of ESs. Impaired neuropsychological performance in an individual with NEPs, as in any patient, should be considered in the context of the patient's medical, psychiatric, and psychosocial history. Further, the neuropsychological profile should be examined for signs of inconsistencies or motivational issues. Because the studies cited above took place over the course of almost two decades, it also should also be pointed out that the frequency of impairment identified within ES and NEP groups will depend on the normative standards used, as many normative tables now include demographic corrections. Thus, the degree of success with which neuropsychological assessment ascertains the presence of NEPs versus ESs has been limited so far. The task of separating NEPs from ESs based on neuropsychological data is confounded by the use of anticonvulsant medications in NEP patients; the history of CNS insult in a sizable proportion of those patients; the vulnerability of ES patients to psychiatric disorders; and, perhaps especially, the frequency and diversity of emotional disturbance that may impact cognitive test performance in NEPs. Neuropsychological results, taking into account these considerations, can be integrated in treatment planning for NEP patients as they are with other patient groups (see Table 12.1). Finally, to our knowledge no study has yet compared patients' neuropsychological performance before and after the diagnosis of NEPs.

MMPI and NEPs

The evaluation of the MMPI literature is difficult for three major reasons. First, until relatively recently, interpretations (e.g., Nicholl, 1981; Ramani et al., 1980) rather than quantifications of the MMPI profiles often were reported in research articles. Second, the number of subjects included in many studies was quite low (studies of less than 10 subjects were not uncommon), limiting the generalizability of the findings. Third, inclusion and matching criteria for determining what constitute appropriate NEP patients and controls have differed across studies. These differences limit the ability to know the criteria by which the interpretation of conversion was made, the parameters (means and variability) of the results, and the comparability of experimental groups in order to make comparisons across studies. In general, MMPI studies may be categorized into three major types, according to the use of the instrument. These types include work with the pseudoneurologic (Pn) scale, conversion profiles, and decision rules. The development and utility of the findings in each of these three areas are reviewed. Before beginning, it is worth pointing out that a recent study provided evidence that among patients with ESs, seizure symptoms do not spuriously inflate psychopathology scales and alter the interpretation of MMPI-2 profiles (Derry, Harnadek, McLachlan, & Sontrop, 1997).

TABLE 12.1. The Role of Neuropsychological Assessment Within the NEPs Population

1. Determine overall level of neuropsychological and emotional functioning.
2. Determine contribution of emotional and motivational factors to neuropsychological performance.
3. Relate neuropsychological strengths and weaknesses and emotional status to educational, occupational, and psychological treatment planning.

Pn Scale

The first MMPI index reported to separate NEP and ES patients was the pseudoneurologic scale (Shaw & Matthews, 1965). The Pn scale was developed to differentiate neurologically impaired patients from patients with symptomatology suggestive of CNS dysfunction but without positive findings on neurological examination. The Pn scale consisted of 17 MMPI items derived from scales 1, 3, and 4. Patients endorsing 7 or more items in the expected direction were considered to have a nonneurological disorder. In the initial and subsequent validation studies, this cutoff correctly identified 81% and 67% of pseudoneurological patients, while misclassifying 25% and 22% of the patients with neurological disease.

Shaw (1966) later used the Pn scale to discriminate 15 NEP patients (a subgroup of all pseudoneurological patients) from 15 ES patients matched for age and sex. It is worth nothing that 13 NEP subjects in this study were identified as "pseudoseizures with concurrent epilepsy" and thus actually represented a mixed NEP/ES group, whereas only two NEP subjects were labeled as "pseudoseizures without concurrent epilepsy," representing pure NEPs. Discriminating patients with ESs from those with mixed ESs and NEPs is a difficult diagnostic challenge and, indeed, most current research excludes patients with combined ESs and NEPs. Nevertheless, Shaw correctly differentiated 73% (11 of 15) NEP from ES patients using the 7 or more items criterion; only 7% (1 of 15) of ES patients were misclassified, a significant difference.

Twenty-two years later, Henrichs, Tucker, Farha, and Novelly (1988) reexamined the utility of the Pn scale in discriminating NEP patients from ES patients. Their results indicated that the Pn scale correctly identified 68% of NEP patients but only 37% of patients with generalized ESs. They concluded that the Pn scale might not be a particularly helpful clinical tool with which to differentiate NEP from ES patients. To examine why the Pn scale was considered unsuccessful at capturing the NEP/ES distinction, the decision theory rules should be considered. Dichotomous decisions fall into the four categories of true positives, false positives, true negatives, and false negatives. Overall, these categorizations label not only how well a measure correctly identifies what it purports to identify but how often it appropriately excludes as well. As is known, true positives and true negatives are correct classifications ("hits") whereas false positives and false negatives are incorrect classifications ("misses"). Such an analysis of the Henrichs et al. (1988) MMPI Pn Scale data shows correct classifications [hit rate = hits/(hits + misses)] for 68% [21/(21 + 10)] of NEP and 37% [10/(10 + 17)] of ES patients, respectively. Thus, incorrect classifications occurred for 32% of NEP patients and 63% of ES patients, respectively. Using the concept of hit rate for each index, Henrichs et al. (1988) calculated that the hit rate was 55% [21/(21 + 17)] when predicting NEPs (by the 7-or-more cutoff rule) and 50% [10/(10 + 10)] when predicting ESs (not-NEPs by a less-than-7 cutoff rule). Therefore, although the correct identification of 68% of NEP patients is relatively high and actually quite close to the 73% identification rate originally found by Shaw (1966), the hit rate for the index is at the chance level.

Conversion Profiles

Studies of MMPI results in NEP patients often have examined the mean profiles for signs of neurotic or conversion symptomatology. The classic conversion profile includes a denial of psychological distress and a focus on somatic symptoms without evidence of significant depression or other psychopathology. Typically, this profile has been quantified by significant elevations ($T > 70$) on scales 1 (Hypochondriasis, Hs) and 3 (Hysteria, Hy), with both of these scales at least 10*T* higher than scale 2 (Depression, D), and no significant elevations on any other scales (Marks & Seeman, 1963).

Matthews, Shaw, and Klove (1966) found significant mean scale elevations on scale 3 but not on scale 1 in patients with pseudoneurological symptoms including (but not limited to) NEP patients relative to patients with unequivocal brain damage. Wurzman and Matthews (1982) found higher mean scales 1, 3, and 2 in NEP patients compared to ES patients. Wilkus et al. (1984) reported prominent elevations on scales 1 and 3 and less substantial but nonetheless significant elevations on scales 4 (Psychopathic Deviate, Pd) and 8 (Schizophrenia, Sc) in their NEP patients relative to ES patients. They suggest that their NEP profiles demonstrated MMPI patterns "seen in the conversion form of hysteria," although their mean scale 2 was only 2 to 4 *T*-scores lower than scales 1 and 3.

Wilkus and Dodrill (1989) attempted to refine NEP evaluations by classifying patients into subgroups based on characteristics of their behavior during their NEPs. This classification system dichotomized patients into independent subgroups based on

1. extent of *motor behavior,* including
   a. limited motor psychogenic seizures (the seizures resemble partial motor seizures with mild localized movements) or
   b. mostly motor psychogenic seizures (resembling generalized convulsive attacks with "vigorous, diffuse, tonic, and/or clonic motor activity," often with ictal unresponsiveness) and
2. extent of *affectual behavior,* including
   a. prominently affectual psychogenic seizures (behaviors include crying, choking, panic, and fear, among others) or
   b. limited no affectual psychogenic seizures (little affectual expression observed).

Wilkus and Dodrill (1989) reported that, when classified by this system, the MMPI profiles of NEP patients differed with respect to their "seizure" behavior. Specifically, they reported that the limited motor subgroup exhibited significant elevations on scales 1, 3, and 8, and the prominently affectual subgroup revealed elevations on scales 1, 3, 7, and 8, in comparison to ES patients with partial seizures. In contrast, the mostly-motor and limited/no affect subgroups did not differ from ES patients with generalized seizures. These findings suggest that MMPI differences can be found in some NEP patients. However, they do not appear to support suppositions that hysteria or conversion disorder is a specific form of psychopathology that consistently earmarks NEP patients as a group, at least from the standpoint of the classical MMPI conversion profile.

Decision Rules

In 1984, Wilkus and colleagues reported the development of a set of MMPI-based decision rules for discriminating patients with NEPs from those with ESs. These rules were defined empirically based on comparisons between groups of NEP and ES patients (n = 15 per group) matched for age, sex, and education. The rules are as follows:

1. Scale 1 or 3 is 70 or higher and is one of the two highest points, disregarding scales 5 and 0.

2. Scale 1 or 3 is 80 or higher, even though not one of the two highest points.
3. Scales 1 and 3 are both higher than 59, and both are at least 10 points higher than scale 2.

Patients meeting rule 1, 2, or 3 were called NEP. Wilkus et al. (1984) reported hit rates for discriminating groups by these decision rules of 92% [11/(11 + 1)] when predicting NEPs and 78% [14/(14 + 4)] when predicting ESs. The authors then used these decision rules to distinguish two additional groups of NEP and ES patients ($n = 10$ per group). Results of the cross-validation study indicated hit rates of 82% [9/(9 + 2)] when predicting NEP and 89% [8/(8 + 1)] when predicting ES by these rules. When the results of both groups of NEP and ES patients were combined, the hit rates were 81% [22/(22 + 5)] when predicting NEP and 87% [20/(20 + 3)] when predicting ESs. Thus, this system misclassified 19% of the NEP cases and 13% of the ES cases.

These results at the *group* level appear helpful, but it should be kept in mind that the frequency of misidentification of *individuals* is not trivial, perhaps too high for routine clinical use, especially considering the consequences of misclassification for ES patients. According to the criteria of Wilkus et al. (1984), nearly 20% of NEP patients would be misclassified as patients with actual seizures. Of course, misclassification of NEP patients as having true seizures carries its own caveats in terms of treatment initiation and maintenance.

Vanderzant, Giordani, Berent, Dreifuss, and Sackellares (1986) undertook a replication of the Wilkus et al. (1984) study with one major exception: Their NEP and ES patients were not matched demographically (i.e., according to age, sex, and education). These researchers found only a mildly elevated scale 8 in their NEPs group (mean T score = 71.2) and no statistically significant difference between the groups on any MMPI scale. There was no striking difference in the mean number of scales elevated between the groups (NEP = 3.4; ES = 2.4). Further, and similar to Wurzman and Matthews (1982), they reported that scale 2 elevations were almost as numerous in the NEP group as scale 1 elevations, and 5 of their 18 NEP patients had elevated scale 2 with "normal" ($30 > T$-score < 70) scales 1 and 3. They reported that only 37% (7 of 19) of NEP patients were correctly classified by the Wilkus et al. (1984) decision rules, whereas 10% (2 of 20) of ES patients were misclassified as having NEPs. From these data, index hit rates for their study are 78% [7/(7 + 2)] when predicting NEPs and 60% [18/(18 + 12)] when predicting ESs. Therefore, similar to Wilkus et al. (1984), 22% of the patients with NEPs were misclassified as having actual seizures. Further, 40% of ES patients were misclassified as having NEPs.

Henrichs et al. (1988) also attempted to replicate the Wilkus et al. (1984) findings using the MMPI decision rules. This study included a sample of 144 subjects, including 59 ESs with a left temporal focus, 27 ESs with a right temporal focus, 27 with primary generalized ESs, and 31 with NEP. Subjects were matched for age, education, age at onset of recurrent seizures, and duration of recurrent seizures (some gender differences were evident). Results indicated that 68% of NEP patients and 73% of ES patients were classified correctly by this system. Further, their index hit rates were only 41% [21/(21 + 30)] when predicting NEPs, although they were 89% (83/(83 + 10)] when predicting ESs. By these results, 59% of predictions would misclassify patients with actual seizures as having NEPs.

Across these studies, 19% to 59% of predictions by the Wilkus et al. (1984) decision rules misclassified patients with verified epilepsy as having NEPs. Wilkus and Dodrill's (1989) results from subtyping NEP patients suggest that refinement in the application of the decision rules might enhance their hit rates. For example, they argued that Vanderzant et al. (1986) failed to find MMPI differences in their NEP patients because of differences in their samples other than those derived from failure to match on demographics. They emphasized that Vanderzant et al. (1986) evaluated only NEP and ES patients with major motor displays in their "seizures," comparisons that also failed to yield significant findings in their own investigations, whereas their significant results stemmed from comparisons of NEP and ES patients with prominent affectual and limited motor behavior. They also suggest that the NEP patients in the Vanderzant et al. (1986) study probably closely resemble their own mostly-motor NEP subgroup.

Summary

These findings suggest that blinded use of the MMPI/MMPI-2 in isolation to discriminate NEP patients from ES patients comes with appreciable error. Although meta-analyses of published investigations indicate more favorable findings, application to individual patients obviously should be done with caution, and there should be little disagreement that each patient's history and current findings should be of value in coming to an opinion in such difficult cases. What should be evident from this review is that the discrimination of NEPs from ESs can be challenging if one is armed solely with neuropsychological tests and the MMPI. Part of the difficulty may be that the traditional approach to the problem has been too narrow. Perhaps, as originally suggested by Wilkus and Dodrill (1989), patients with NEPs are a heterogeneous group that may be characterized by a spectrum of identifiable neuropsychological and personality types—types that might differ either qualitatively or quantitatively from patients with epilepsy. In a creative approach to the problem, neuropsychologists at the University of Minnesota Epilepsy Center gathered a large number of patients with "nonepileptic events" and cluster-analyzed their neuropsychological and MMPI data. The findings, unpublished except in abstract form (Barrash, Gates, Heck, & Berriak, 1989), demonstrated that patients with NEPs were a heterogeneous group indeed, characterized by a variety of MMPI and neuropsychological profile types. Such information, in conjunction with an understanding of the distribution of similar profile types among patients with actual epilepsy, might eventually allow for more accurate probability statements regarding the presence of either epilepsy or NEPs. Following another promising statistical method, one group of investigators have suggested that the MMPI-2 may contribute to the differentiation of NEPs and ESs when it is used in combination with other predictors, including psychosocial and medical findings (Binder et al., 1994; Dodrill & Holmes, 2000; Storzbach, Binder, Salinsky, Campbell, & Mueller, 2000). Pertinent medical variables include EEG (a negative interictal EEG in isolation does not rule out ESs) and age of onset of the seizure disorder. Until these multivariate methods of classification undergo further development, ongoing collaborative efforts with neurological and psychiatric colleagues will help to reduce the error inherent in this difficult but important diagnostic task. Some of the potential benefits of an accurate NEP diagnosis are listed in Table 12.2.

It should be further noted that although present-day neuropsychological test procedures have limited value in separating NEP patients, the clinical neuropsychologist plays an important role on many epilepsy monitoring units (EMUs). The clinical neuropsychologist typically is the person who helps the NEP patient consider the role of possible psychiatric factors in producing symptoms. This is a delicate task and requires

TABLE 12.2. Some Potential Benefits of Accurate NEPs Diagnosis

1. *Decreased AED use*, with corresponding decrease in cost and risk of toxicity and neuropsychological impairment associated with AEDs.
2. *Access to psychological treatment* for issues possibly underlying NEPS, and less time and expense spent for neurological treatments.
3. *Increased quality of life*, including possible return to work and other activities, such as driving.

an ability to explain neuropsychological and personality findings in a manner that helps the patient find appropriate treatment. Without this input, many NEP patients leave EMU units discouraged and do not seek further psychiatric help.

Socioeconomic and Quality of Life Outcomes in NEPs

Information on occupational, social, and quality of life outcomes following NEP confirmed diagnosis through inpatient video-EEG monitoring is sparse. However, available studies indicate that detrimental socioeconomic and psychosocial outcomes are associated with undiagnosed NEP in terms of increased work absence, compensated medical disability, and psychiatric sequelae at time of NEP diagnosis (Sakamoto, Holthausen, & Noachtar, 1994; Walczak et al., 1995). Lepert and Schmitt (1990) reported on general emotional "well-being" outcome and change in occupational status. They found that 28% of NEP patients were employed at the time of diagnosis; 42% were unemployed or receiving disability payments; and 30% either were in school, were homemakers, or were pensioners. Occupational status changed for 15% of the sample, with 4 patients returning to school or work and 1 patient receiving permanent disability. Lancman et al. (1993) reported that 62 of 93 (67%) NEP patients were working prior to NEP onset, but that only 34 (37%) were working by time of definitive inpatient video-EEG monitoring-based diagnosis. No information was given about postdiagnostic occupational outcome. Westbrook et al. (1998) reported that 85% of their sample was working at the time of onset of nonepileptic seizures, but that disability and employment status one year after NEP diagnosis had not improved in 91% of those contacted. Of the contacted patients, 17 of 20 were receiving disability benefits. Further systematic data collection on these areas must be determined indirect societal costs are to be determined.

Only two studies have attempted to investigate issues related to health-care utilization and impact of inpatient video-EEG seizure monitoring. Krahn et al. (1997) identified 94 consecutive adult patients diagnosed via inpatient video-EEG monitoring with nonepileptic seizures of a physiological etiology (e.g., syncope). Of this group, 71 (50 female, 21 male) responded to investigators' request for information regarding health-care use and overall quality of life ratings. Median time for follow-up was 1.4 years (range 6 months to 3.1 years). Number of seizure-related visits within a 6-month period prior to seizure monitoring for mental health (psychiatrists/psychologists) and medical care (neurologists, PCPs, and other health-care providers) was reported. Although a substantial minority of patients did not respond to this question, of the responders over 30% reported four or more visits to a mental health provider, whereas approximately 20% reported four or more medical care contacts. Whether patients sought more than one type of service was not reported. At time of follow-up contact, over 50% of patients reported no further seizure-related hospitalizations, and 12 of 71 patients had three or fewer. Data on follow-up medical care visits was not provided; utilization data were gathered from questionnaire and medical chart review. In summary, Krahn et al. (1997) concluded that the majority of these patients who had a preexisting psychiatric disorder followed up with psychiatric intervention, and those who did reported improved quality of life and fewer seizures. Issues of specific utilization category change were not reported, nor were any data relevant to costs of such patients.

Martin et al. (1998) recently documented changes in health-care utilization patterns and costs in a sample of NEP patients definitively diagnosed through inpatient video-EEG seizure monitoring. Health-care resource utilization data was collected via questionnaire and medical chart review on a sample of 20 patients. Medication usage, outpatient visits, emergency room admission, and diagnostic testing over a 6-month prediagnosis and a 6-month postdiagnosis period were compared. Averaged prediagnosis health-care charges were over $8,000 per patient in the 6 months prior to inpatient video-EEG monitoring. Total medical charges for NEP patients in the 6-month prediagnosis period was over $170,000. Table 12.3 presents health-care utilization rates for the 6-month periods before and after NEP diagnosis. Seizure-related medical charges were reduced by an average of 84% following definitive NEP diagnosis. Average diagnostic testing charges declined 76%, average medication charges decreased 69%, outpatient clinic visits declined 80%, and emergency room visits were reduced by 97%.

This study demonstrated that a majority of patients with inpatient video-EEG monitoring-confirmed NEP diagnosis experienced substantial reductions in health-care utilization and dollar costs. Downward shifts in utilization rates (over 70%) were consistently found, including emergency room visits and outpatient clinic visits. Significant cost reductions also were noted. Martin et al. pointed out that utilization rates would not likely be as high for every 6-month time block, but that often inpatient monitoring is recommended only after extensive outpatient course. The long-term financial value of inpatient video-EEG monitoring is in the ability to make a definitive diagnosis. With this said, long-term costs associated with undiagnosed NEPs may approaches those of epilepsy patients with intractable seizures. Patients with intractable epilepsy contrib-

TABLE 12.3. Health-Care Utilization Rates Before and After NEPs Diagnosis

	Before Diagnosis			After Diagnosis		
	Patients Using Service	Total Utilization	Average Use (SE)	Patients Using Service	Total Utilization	Average Use (SE)
Outpatient visits	20	180	10.4 (1.8)	10	43	2.2 (.81)
Emergency room	15	126	6.3 (2.0)	2	4	.2 (.14)
Diagnostic procedures	18	56	2.9 (.52)	6	13	.7 (.30)
Laboratory tests	16	144	7.2 (31.5)	7	28	1.4 (.62)

ute more than 50% of the direct costs in population-based estimates of epilepsy cost (Begley et al., 1994). No information was provided on other nonseizure-related health or mental health-care utilization. As pointed out by Krahn et al. (1997), utilization for mental health-related services was common, and whether cost shifting from seizure related to psychiatric services would offset overall cost burden was not explored.

Impact of NEPS on Employment Status

With few exceptions, studies of NEP patients have focused on diagnosis and seizure outcome. Only a few studies mention the impact of NEPs on employment status. Retrospective chart review was conducted on 84 NEP patients diagnosed while on the UAB inpatient video-EEG monitoring unit between January 1997 and December 1997. Only patients with available information on employment status at time of NEP onset and employment status at time of UAB monitoring diagnosis were included. In addition, employment outcome was obtained in a sample of 24 of those 84 NEP patients contacted between 3 and 12 months postdiagnosis. Available follow-up data on those 24 cases were from an ongoing prospective outcome survey.

Employment status at NEP onset and time of diagnosis at follow-up is presented in Table 12.4. A dramatic shifting in employment status was found in NEP patients from time of first nonepileptic seizure to time of UAB inpatient video-EEG monitoring. At time of first NEP, 69% of our sample was employed; however, by time of video-EEG monitoring, only 20% were employed--81% of the sample was out of the workforce. From our smaller outcome sample, 17 patients were in the workforce at time of first seizure. Those patients returning to work were found to have had significantly shorter intervals from time of first NEP to video-EEG monitoring (see Table 12.5). This suggests a greater likelihood of return to work with early definitive video-EEG monitoring.

TABLE 12.4. Job Status at Time of First Seizure and Hospital Admission (n = 84)

	At Time of First Seizure	At Hospital Admission
Full-time	53 (63%)	13 (16%)
Part-time	5 (6%)	3 (4%)
Receiving disability benefits	8 (9%)	24 (29%)
Retired	1 (1%)	0 (0%)
Homemaker	9 (11%)	10 (12%)
Medical leave	0 (0%)	13 (16%)
Unemployed/not in work force	5 (6%)	19 (23%)
Never employed	3 (4%)	2 (2%)

☐ Psychotherapeutic Intervention Studies of NEPs

With definitive diagnosis, a dramatic shift of treatment modalities (e.g., antidepressant medication and psychotherapy) can be initiated, with focus on the more psychological/emotional aspects of the condition. Walczak et al. (1995) assessed outcome in a group of 51 patients with NEPs confirmed by video-EEG monitoring. Follow-up contact average 15 months after diagnosis with questions asking about extent of psychotherapeutic treatments. They found that 41 of the 51 patients had at least one therapy session, 31 had more than five sessions, and 23 were still in therapy at time of contact. However, they found no significant relationship between cessation of nonepileptic seizures and participation or extent of psychotherapy. However, this study did not detail the type of intervention or whether psychotropic medication was included. In observational, retrospective, nonrandomized study of 61 NEP patients, Aboukasm, Mahr, Gahry, Thomas, and Barkely (1998) examined the comparative effectiveness of a comprehensive epilepsy program (CEP)-based psychotherapy intervention, CEP physician care, non-CEP-based psychotherapy, or no feedback/no-intervention on "seizure" cessation and a single item overall quality of life rating (one question on 7-point Likert scale). They found that at time of follow-up contact (mean 22 months postdiagnosis), the no-intervention group had significantly poorer outcome in terms of both the overall quality of life rating and seizure frequency compared to the other three groups. The group receiving CEP-based psychotherapy experienced somewhat better quality of life ratings that the other intervention groups. Despite these initial efforts, no prospective investigation of psychotherapeutic or psychopharmacologic intervention has been reported within the NEP population. A few studies have reported the incidence of NEP patients entering into mental health care after diagnosis, but they lack information about length, type, and setting of intervention. No study to date has investigated whether mental health intervention impacts various aspects of NEP outcome other than seizure occurrence including return to work or quality of life. This is rather surprising, as considerable research has demonstrated the long-term cost-effectiveness of mental health care within the broader medical managed care domain (deGruy, Columbia, & Dickinson, 1987; Hellman, Budd, Borysenko, McClelland, & Benson, 1990; Kashner, Rost, Cohen, Anderson, & Smith, 1995; Strosahl & Sobel, 1996)

Cost-Effective NEP Modeling

What is the most cost-effective approach to obtaining a definitive diagnosis and seizure control for a patient with a history of uncontrolled seizures that might be due to epilepsy, NEPs, or possibly both? The answer depends on several issues: the prevalence of the conditions; the sensitivity, specificity, and costs of various diagnostic tests; and the probability of achieving control with a particular regimen of medication or counseling. More fundamental, however, is the viewpoint of the analysis: Are costs to be considered from the viewpoint of society, the individual, the employer, or the insurer?

TABLE 12.5. Employment Outcome as a Function of Time to NEPS Diagnosis (in Months)

	Full-Time to Full-Time Employment	FT/PT to Unemployment	Full-Time to Disability
Mean	14.0	141.0	169.7
SD	13.1	135.5	168.2
Minimum	1	12	24
Maximum	36	264	420
Median	12	144	60
n	5	4	8

Viewpoint

The narrowest perspective is that of the insurer. In the United States, the insurer is often a managed care organization (MCO) responsible for providing all necessary and appropriate treatment to the patient at a fixed annual premium. From a purely financial perspective, the MCO wants to provide sufficiently good care to keep the patient enrolled on a profitable basis. If diagnosis or treatment is sufficiently expensive, the MCO may be tempted to shed the patient. It can do this by rendering sufficiently poor service so that the patient quits the MCO in favor of another insurer. The other insurer might be the long-term disability system, which the patient would enter after losing his or her job because of uncontrolled seizures.

Individuals also may face mixed incentives Hadler, Carey, and Garrett (1995; 1996). A quick diagnosis with effective treatment may allow an individual to stay employed. For some jobs and salaries this may be attractive; for others, retirement with a full disability pension may be preferable financially, even if this involves occasional seizures. The attraction of retirement on disability may be offset by the inconvenience of losing a driver's license due to uncontrolled seizures. Recent legislation changes now allow disabled individuals to retain their Medicaid health insurance coverage if they reenter the workforce after qualifying for disability (U.S. Social Security Administration, 1999). This change should increase the incentive to return to work if seizures are eventually brought under control.

Employers generally have a strong interest in getting a rapid diagnosis and successful treatment in order to avoid lost productivity and the cost of replacing a trained worker. This is especially true if the costs of diagnosis and treatment have been assumed by the insurer for a fixed price.

The societal viewpoint takes a broader perspective, and it is often invoked as a gold standard. It wants to discover the regimen of diagnostic procedures and treatment that yields the best combination of cost and quality-adjusted life years. Cost is supposed to include all resources used by any element of society. Basically, this includes direct costs—essentially all relevant medical expenses—and all indirect costs, such as lost wages or traffic accident damages consequent from a seizure while driving. Note that payments by the disability system generally are not counted here because they merely transfer some income from those who still work and pay taxes to those who no longer work. The "real" loss from the societal viewpoint is the work that does not get done by the disabled worker (Gold, Siegel, Russell, & Weinstein, 1996; Mennemeyer, 1997).

Thus, viewpoint is important, because the cost-effectiveness of a particular approach to diagnosis and treatment depends on the perspective of who is paying the costs or enjoying the benefits. In the remainder of this section, we will consider the cost-effectiveness problem from the societal perspective that is usually used as the baseline.

Endpoint

The "endpoint" of the analysis also is important. What measures of cost and outcome are to define the problem? A simple way to view the cost-effectiveness problem is shown in Figure 12.1. The physician is confronted with a patient who has a history of epilepsy-like seizures that have not responded to at least one attempt at control by medication. The endpoint of the analysis occurs when either the seizures are controlled, the patient is referred for surgery, or the physician gives up and classifies the patient as uncontrollable. Thus, the problem focuses on the cost of reaching a final disposition—which may be "control," referral to surgery, or a final state of "uncontrolled seizures."

How might the physician decide to treat the seizure patient? One approach is to select a drug based on available diagnostic information, perhaps simply the history and physical exam. Empirical drug therapy can be viewed as an implicit diagnostic test. Subsequently, the patient's seizures may be controlled with the drug or they may continue. If seizures are controlled, the patient continues therapy indefinitely; if they are not controlled, the physician has to make a new decision about what to do. Direct costs of this approach are essentially the visit to the physician and the cost of the drug. An indirect cost might be the loss of employment if control is not achieved.

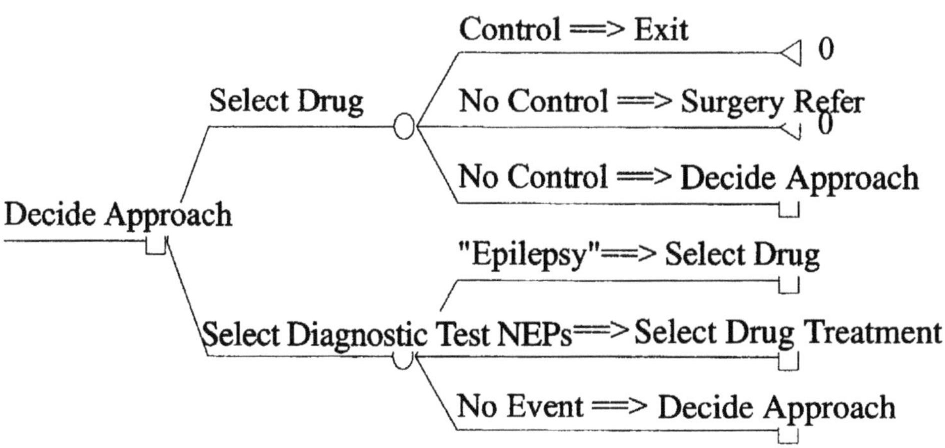

FIGURE 12.1. Example of endpoint analysis.

The alternative approach is to select a diagnostic test. This might be an outpatient EEG, video-EEG monitoring, or other diagnostic procedure. The diagnostic test may indicate epilepsy or NEPs, or it may be inconclusive. If epilepsy is indicated, the physician then selects an appropriate drug and waits to see if control is achieved. If NEPs are indicated, treatment will be counseling, periodic follow-up with neurology for continuity of care, and referral to psychiatry for possible medication. If the test is inconclusive, the physician has to decide again on whether to repeat the test, try another test, or try empirical treatment with a drug. Diagnostic tests are problematic, because their ability to correctly identify epilepsy or NEPs depends greatly on whether a seizure is observed during the test. Video-EEG has the advantage of being more likely to observe a seizure, because it may involve continuous observation for up to several days. Direct costs of the diagnostic testing approach include the physician visit, any counseling sessions, the expense of the test, and the expense of any drug that might be selected. Indirect costs again include the possibility of job loss if control is not achieved.

The figure hides the complexity of selecting from numerous drugs and several diagnostic tests. It also hides the time dimension of the problem: Trying different medications can be time-consuming if a physician typically allows 6 months before deciding if control has truly been achieved.

☐ Simulation Modeling

Economic theory recommends that decisions about what to do next should ignore costs that have already been incurred and focus on what needs to be spent next to achieve a goal. For the diagnosis of seizures, the cheapest solution from the insurer's viewpoint is always one more round of trying another drug. From the societal viewpoint, it is important to choose a route that has a high probability of achieving control before the patient loses a job and slips into disability.

Simulation modeling can be used to examine cost-effectiveness from the various perspectives. We have experimented with several formulations of Figure 12.1. One important issue in modeling is the prevalence of NEPs in the population relative to epilepsy. If a high proportion of the seizure population has only epilepsy, it often is cost-effective from a societal viewpoint to discover and treat these cases with antiepileptic drugs selected empirically or after outpatient diagnostic tests. This strategy avoids the expense of undertaking expensive diagnostic tests on cases that could be controlled successfully with epileptic drugs. After the population is restricted to persons who have not been successfully treated with early drug challenges, the proportion of persons with NEPs tends to rise, as does the cost savings of distinguishing NEP cases from epilepsy.

Using a societal viewpoint, our simulations have found that the largest cost in the problem is the possibility of job loss for a working person, especially if the seizures begin early in the working lifetime. For the employed person, it is cost-effective to undertake video-EEG monitoring in an early cycle of the decision process if there is a high probability that a seizure event will be observed during the test. Here the relatively high cost of the test is offset by the probability that a job loss can be avoided. Outpatient EEG monitoring is a thrifty substitute for video-EEG only if there is a high probability of observing a seizure during the comparatively brief office encounter. Multiple cycles of empirical drug treatment with little or no diagnostic testing are cost-effective only if the person is not in the labor force or if there is little chance that a seizure will be observed during a diagnostic test. This latter result, of course, depends crucially on how one values the time of a nonworking person. If the analysis is cast in terms of quality of life years, it becomes more attractive to undertake diagnostic testing for nonemployed persons early in the decision cycle.

References

Aboukasm, A., Mahr, G., Gahry, B. R., Thomas, A., & Barkely, G. L. (1998). Retrospective analysis of effects of psychotherapeutic interventions on outcome of psychogenic nonepileptic seizures. *Epilepsia, 39,* 470–473.

Barrash, I. Gates, I. R., Heck, D. G., & Berriak, T. E. (1989). MMPI subtypes among patients with nonepileptic events. *Epilepsia, 30,* 730.

Barsky, A. J., & Borus, J. F. (1995). Somatization and medicalization in the era of managed care. *Journal of the American Medical Association, 274,* 1931–1934.

Begley, C. E., Annegers, J. F., Lairson, D. R., Reynolds, T. F., & Hauser, W. A. (1994). Cost of epilepsy in the United States: A model based on incidence and prognosis. *Epilepsia, 35,* 1230–1243.

Betts, T., & Boden, S. (1992). Diagnosis, management and prognosis of a group of 128 patients with non-epileptic attack disorder, Part I. *Seizure, 1,* 19–26.

Binder, L., Kinderman, S., Heaton, R., & Salinsky, M. (1998). Neuropsychological impairment in patients with nonepileptic seizures. *Archives of Clinical Neuropsychology, 13,* 513–522.

Binder, L., Salinsky, M., & Smith, S. (1994). Psychological correlates of psychogenic seizures. *Journal of Clinical and Experimental Neuropsychology, 16,* 524–530.

Bortz, J., Prigatano, G., Blum, D., & Fisher, R. (1995). Differential response characteristics in nonepileptic and epileptic seizure patients on a test of verbal learning and memory. *Neurology, 45,* 2029–2034.

Bowman, E. S., & Markand, O. N. (1996). Psychodynamics and psychiatric diagnoses of pseudoseizure subjects. *American Journal of Psychiatry, 153,* 57–63.

Brown, M., Levin, B., Ramsay, R. E., Katz, D., & Duchowny, M. (1991). Characteristics of patients with nonepileptic seizures. *Journal of Epilepsy, 4,* 225–229.

Chabolla, D. R., Krahn, L. E., So, E. L., & Rummans, T. A. (1996). Psychogenic nonepileptic seizures. *Mayo Clinic Proceedings,* 71, 493–500.

deGruy, F., Columbia, L., & Dickinson, P. (1987). Somatization disorder in a family practice. *Journal of Family Practice, 25,* 45–51.

Derry, P., Harnadek, M., McLachlan, R., & Sontrop, J. (1997). Influence of seizure content on interpreting psychopathology on the MMPI-2 in patients with epilepsy. *Journal of Clinical and Experimental Neuropsychology, 19,* 396–404.

Devinsky, O., Sanchez-Villasenor, F., Vazquez, B., Kothari, M., Alper, K., & Luciano, D. (1996). Clinical profile of patients with epileptic and nonepileptic seizures. *Neurology, 46,* 1530–1533.

Dodrill, C., & Holmes, M. (2000). Part summary: Psychological and neuropsychological evaluation of the patient with non-epileptic seizures. In J. R. Gates & A. J. Rowan (Eds.), *Nonepileptic seizures* (2nd ed., pp. 169–181). Boston: Butterworth-Heinemann.

Fink, P. (1992). Surgery and medical treatment in persistent somatizing patients. *Journal of Psychosomatic Research, 36,* 439–447.

Gates, J. R., Luciano, D., & Devinsky, O. (1991). The classification and treatment of nonepileptic events. In O. Devinsky & H. Theodore (Eds.), *Epilepsy and behavior* (pp. 251–263). New York: Wiley-Liss.

Gold, M. E., Siegel, J. E., Russell, L. B., & Weinstein, M. C. (1996). *Cost effectiveNEPSs in health and medicine*. Oxford University Press.

Gumnit, R. J. (1993). Psychogenic seizures. In E. Wyllie (Ed.), *The treatment of epilepsy: Principles and practice* (pp. 692–695). Philadelphia: Lea & Febiger.
Hadler, N. M. (1996). If you have to prove you are ill, you can't get well: The object lesson of fibromyalgia. *Spine, 21,* 2397–2400.
Hadler, N. M., Carey, T. S., & Garrett, J. (1995). The influence of indemnification by workers' compensation insurance on recovery from acute backache: North Carolina Back Pain Project. *Spine,* 20, 2710–2715.
Hauser, W. A., & Hesdorffer, D. C. (1990). Epilepsy: Frequency, causes and consequences. Landover, MD: Epilepsy Foundation of America.
Hauser, W. A., Rich, S. S., Lee, J. R. J., Annegers, J. F., & Anderson, V. E. (1998). Risk of recurrent seizures after two unprovoked seizures. *New England Journal of Medicine, 338,* 429–434.
Hellman, C. J., Budd, M., Borysenko, J., McClelland, D. C., & Benson, H. (1990). A study of the effectiveness of two group behavioral medicine interventions for patients with psychosomatic complaints. *Behavioral Medicine, 16,* 165–173.
Henrichs, T. E., Tucker, D. M., Farha, J., & Novelly, R. A. (1988). MMPI indices in the identification of patients evidencing pseudoseizures. *Epilepsia, 29,* 184–187.
Henry, T. R., & Drury, I. (1998). Ictal behaviors during nonepileptic seizures differ in patients with temporal lobe interictal epileptiform EEG activity and patients without interictal epileptiform EEG abnormalities. *Epilepsia, 39,* 175–182.
Hollifield, M., Paine, S., Tuttle, L., & Kellner, R. (1999). Hypochondriasis, somatization and perceived health and utilization of health care services. *Psychosomatics, 40,* 380–386.
Kalogjera-Sackellares, D., & Sackelleres, J. C. (1999). Intellectual and neuropsychological features of patients with psychogenic pseudoseizures. *Psychiatry Research, 86,* 73–84.
Kanner, A. M., Morris, H. H., Luders, H., Dinner, D. S., Wyllie, E., Medendorp, S. V., & Rowan, A. J. (1990). Supplementary motor seizures mimicking pseudoseizures. *Neurology, 40,* 1404–1407.
Kashner, T. M., Rost, K., Cohen, B., Anderson, M., & Smith, G. R. (1995). Enhancing the health of somatization disorder patients: Effectiveness of short-term group therapy. *Psychosomatics, 36,* 462–470.
King, D. W., Gallagher, B. B., Murvin, A. J., Smith, D. B., Marcus, D. J., Hartlage, L. C., & Ward, L. C. (1982). Pseudoseizures: Diagnostic evaluation. *Neurology, 32,* 18–23.
Krahn, L. E., Reese, M. M., Rummans, T. A., Peterson, G. C., Suman, V. J., Sharbrough, F. W., & Cascino, G. D. (1997). Health utilization of patients with psychogenic nonepileptic seizures. *Psychosomatics, 38,* 535–542.
Kristensen, O., & Alving, J., (1992). Pseudoseizures: Risk factors and prognosis. *Acta Neurologia Scandinavica, 85,* 177–180.
Krumholz, A., & Niedermeyer, E. (1983). Psychogenic seizures: A clinical study with follow-up data. *Neurology, 33,* 498–502.
Kuyk, J., Leijten, F., Meinard, H., Spinhoven, P., & Van Dyck, R. (1997). The diagnosis of psychogenic non-epileptic seizures: a review. *Seizure, 6,* 243–253.
Lancman, M. E., Brotherton, T. A., Asconape, J. J., & Penry, J. K. (1993). Psychogenic seizures: A clinical study in 50 patients. *Seizure, 2,* 281–286.
Lepert, L., & Schmitt, D. (1990). Natural history and outcome of psychogenic seizures: A clinical study in 50 patients. *Journal of Neurology, 237,* 35–38.
Lesser, R. P. (1996). Psychogenic seizures. *Neurology, 46,* 1499–1507.
Marks, P. A., & Seeman, W. (1963). *The actuarial description of abnormal personality.* Baltimore: Williams & Wilkins.
Martin, R., Gilliam, F., Kilgore, M., Faught, E., & Kuzniecky, R. (1998). Improved healthcare resource utilization following inpatient video/EEG seizure monitoring confirmed diagnosis of non-epileptic psychogenic seizures. *Seizure, 7,* 385–390.
Matthews, C. G., Shaw, D. J., & Klove, H. (1966). Psychological test performances in neurologic and "pseudoneurologic" subjects. *Cortex, 2,* 244–253.

Mattson, R. H. (1998). Medical management of epilepsy in adults. *Neurology, 51*(Suppl 4), S15–S20.

Meierkord, H., Will, B., Fish, D., & Shorvon, S. (1991). The clinical features and prognosis of pseudoseizures diagnosed using video-EEG telemetry. *Neurology, 41,* 1643–1646.

Mennemeyer, S. T. (1997). Why do health economists not take transfer payments into account? *Journal of Health Services Research and Policy, 2*(3), 195.

Moore, P. M., Baker, G. A., McDade, G., Chadwick, D., & Brown, S. (1994). Epilepsy, pseudoseizures and perceived family characteristics: A controlled study. *Epilepsy Research, 18,* 75–83.

Morris, I., Galezowska, J., Leroy, R., et al. (1994). The results of computer-assisted ambulatory 16-channel EEG. *Electroencephalography and Clinical Neurophysiology, 91,* 229–231.

National Institutes of Health. (1990). National Institutes of Health Consensus Conference: Epilepsy Surgery. *Journal of the American Medical Association, 264,* 729–733.

Nicholl, J. S. (1981). Pseudoseizures: A neuropsychiatric diagnostic dilemma. *Psychosomatics, 22,* 451–454.

Ramani, S. V., & Gumnit, R. (1982). Management of hysterical seizures in epileptic patients. *Archives of Neurology, 39,* 78–81.

Ramani, S. V., Quesney, L. E., Olson, D., & Gumnit, R. J. (1980). Diagnosis of hysterical seizures in epileptic patients. *American Journal of Psychiatry, 137,* 705–709.

Risse, G., Mason, S. L., & Mercer, K. (2000). Neuropsychological performance and cognitive complaints in epileptic and non-epileptic seizure patients. In J. R. Gates & A. J. Rowan (Eds.), *Non-epileptic seizures* (2nd ed., pp. 139–150). Boston: Butterworth-Heinemann.

Rowan, A. J., & Gates, J. (Eds.). (2002). *Nonepileptic seizures: Causation, diagnosis, classification, and treatment.* New York: Demos.

Russell, L. B., Gold, M. R., Siegel, J. E., et al. (1996). The role of cost-effectiveness analysis in health and medicine. *Journal of the American Medical Association, 276,* 1172–1177.

Sackellares, J. C., Giordani, B., Berent, S., Seidenberg, M., Dreifuss, F., Vanderzant, C. W., & Boll, T. J. (1985). Patients with pseudoseizures: Intellectual and cognitive performance. *Neurology, 35,* 116–119.

Sakamoto, A. C., Holthausen, H., & Noachtar, S. (1994). Diagnosis of pseudoepileptic seizures. In P. Wolf (Ed.), *Epileptic seizures and syndromes* (pp. 633–642). London: Libbey & Company.

Saygi, S., Katz, A., Marks, D. A., & Spencer, D. (1992). Frontal lobe partial seizures and psychogenic seizures: Comparisons of clinical and ictal characteristics. *Neurology, 42,* 1274–1277.

Schappert, S. M. (1995). Office visits to neurologists: United States, 1991–1992. *Advanced Data* (267).

Shaw, D. J. (1966). Differential MMPI performance in pseudoseizure, epileptic, and pseudo-neurologic groups. *Journal of Clinical Psychology, 22,* 271–275.

Shaw, D. J., & Matthews, C. G. (1965). Differential MMPI performance of brain-damaged vs. pseudo-neurologic groups. *Journal of Clinical Psychology, 21,* 405–408.

Storzbach, D., Binder, L. M., Salinsky, M. C., Campbell, B. R., & Mueller, R. M. (2000). Improved prediction of nonepileptic seizures with combined MMPI and EEG measures. *Epilepsia, 41,* 332–337.

Strosahl, K. D., & Sobel, D. (1996). Behavioral health and the medical cost offset effect: Current status, key concepts and future applications. *HMO Practice, 10,* 156–162.

Sutula, T. P., Sackellares, J. C., Miller, J. Q., et al. (1981). Intensive monitoring in refractory epilepsy. *Neurology, 31,* 243–247.

Swanson, S., Springer, J., Benbadis, S., & Morris, G. (2000). Cognitive and psychological functioning in patients with non-epileptic seizures. In J. R. Gates & A. J. Rowan (Eds.), *Non-epileptic seizures* (2nd ed., pp. 123–137). Boston: Butterworth-Heinemann.

Synder, S. L., Rosenbaum, D. H., Rowan, A. J., & Strain, J. J. (1994). SCID diagnosis of panic disorder in psychogenic seizure patients. *Journal of Neuropsychiatry, 6,* 261–266.

Thacker, K., Devinsky, O., Perrine, K., Alper, K., & Luciano, D. (1997). Nonepileptic seizures during apparent sleep. *Annals of Neurology, 33,* 414–418.

U.S. Social Security Administration (1999). President Clinton signs the Ticket to Work and Work Incentives Improvement Act of 1999. *Social Security Legislative Bulletin,* 106–115.

Vanderzant, C. W., Giordani, B., Berent, S., Dreifuss, E. E., & Sackellares, J. C. (1986). Personality of patients with pseudoseizures. *Neurology, 36,* 664–668.

Walczak, T. S., Papacosta, S., Williams, D. T., Scheuer, M. L., Lebowitz, N., & Notarfrancesco, A. (1995). Outcome after diagnosis of psychogenic nonepileptic seizures. *Epilepsia, 36,* 1131–1137.

Westbrook, L. E., Devinsky, O., & Geocadin, R. (1998). Nonepileptic seizures after head injury. *Epilepsia, 39,* 978–982.

Wilkus, R. L., & Dodrill, C. B. (1989). Factors affecting the outcome of MMPI and neuropsychological assessments of psychogenic and epileptic seizure patients. *Epilepsia, 30,* 339–347.

Wilkus, R. J., Dodrill, C. B., & Thompson, P. M. (1984). Intensive EEG monitoring and psychological studies of patients with pseudoepileptic seizures. *Epilepsia, 25,* 100–107.

Wurzman, L. P., & Matthews, C. G. (1982). The borderlands of epilepsy: Explorations with the MMPI. Paper presented at the annual meeting of the International Neuropsychological Society, Pittsburgh, February.

PART

VI

LEARNING DISABILITIES

13

CHAPTER

Lorie A. Humphrey
Paul Satz

The Use of Neuropsychological Assessment in Clarifying the Educational Needs of Children with Learning Disabilities

☐ Introduction

Learning disabilities (LDs) are the most frequently diagnosed handicapping condition among school-aged children in America (Culbertson & Edmonds, 1996). They have been cited in the literature for over 100 years, with an early reference by W. Pringle Morgan, who, in 1896, reported on a bright and intelligent young man who was unable to read (Morgan, 1896). "Congenital word blindness" was the term coined by Morgan to describe this disorder, and his observation began a century of study and controversy. For many years after this publication, researchers sought a single deficient process to explain these difficulties. Much of this research stemmed from Orton (1928; 1937), whose theory was that LDs were due to a neurodevelopmental inability to establish cerebral dominance (Culbertson & Edmonds, 1996). In more recent years, these single-factor conceptualizations have given way to more complex conceptualizations of LDs. These more multifaceted theories have emerged in large part from neuropsychological research (Culbertson & Edmonds, 1996).

Estimates of the prevalence of learning disabilities vary, depending on the criterion standard used as well as the population studied. Epidemiologic studies using current IQ discrepancy models with school children suggest reading disorder prevalence estimates of 4% to 9% (American Psychiatric Association, 1994). Rates of up to 20% also have been cited, however (Shaywitz et al., 1990), when absolute (low- achievement model) rather than IQ-relative (discrepancy model) deficits are used. Some epidemiological studies suggest that reading disabilities exist on a continuum with normal reading abilities, which further increases estimated prevalence rates (Shaywitz, Escobar, Shaywitz, Fletcher & Makuch, 1992).

The etiology for LDs is not fully understood, and variability of cause is likely. The frequent observations that learning disabilities run in families and that certain learning problems are more common in male children have encouraged the examination of evidence supporting a genetic/hereditary mechanism of transmission (Pennington, 1995). There is approximately an eightfold risk increase for a child with an affected parent to develop an LD, as compared to a risk factor of 5% in the general population. Specifically, chromosome 6 is a candidate for influencing reading ability (Smith, Brower, Cardon, & DeFries, 1998). Additionally, LDs are more prevalent in children who have suffered known risk factors to the brain, including low birth weight (Hack et al., 1994), brain injury including head injury (Fletcher, Ewing-Cobbs, Miner, Levin, & Eisenberg, 1990), brain tumors (Morris, Krawiecki, Kullgren, Ingram, & Kurczynski, 2000), and brain disease such as bacterial meningitis (Anderson & Taylor, 2000).

Learning disabilities appear to be chronic, with many longitudinal studies supporting the enduring nature of the learning handicap (Satz, Buka, Lipsitt, & Seidman, 1998). Several studies cited in this chapter point to the chronic nature of reading disabilities.

The preponderance of research in the field of LDs has been done with reading disorders, or developmental dyslexia. Studies over the years have supported the hypothesis that core deficits in phonological processing (or the understanding of speech/symbol relationships allowing for words to be correctly decoded) underlie reading disabilities in most people (Wagner & Torgerson, 1987). Additionally, problems with rapid visual processing (Martin & Lovegrove, 1988) have implicated the magnocellular system of the visual system in dyslexia. A causal relationship with poor reading, however, has not been established (Hulme, 1988). More recent fMRI studies continue to find a relationship, however (Eden et al., 1996). A third hypothesis currently receiving a great deal of attention is that of general deficits in rapid temporal (i.e., sequential) processing across sensory modalities (e.g., auditory, visual, tactile) in people with dyslexia (Tallal, Miller, & Fitch, 1993).

Neurobiology of Learning Disabilities

The assumption that LDs are due to anomalies in the central nervous system has been made by neurologists and neuropsychologists for many years and was explicitly stated by the National Joint Committee on Learning Disabilities in 1981. Despite this history, no reference to the possibility of a central nervous system (CNS) basis for these disorders is made in the *DSM-IV* and, until recently, critics emphasized the lack of consensus regarding this neurological basis (Taylor, 1988). Recent advances in neuroimaging, as well as increased information regarding the genetic heritability of LDs, are providing strong support in favor of the CNS assumption. These findings are detailed below.

With the introduction of X-ray computed tomography (CT) scanning in the 1970s, work began on determining how the brains of people with developmental dyslexia might differ from those of normal readers. Early findings indicated, however, that macroscopic lesions that can be imaged with structural approaches such as CT or MRI are not present in developmental dyslexia (Rumsey, 1996). Exploration of microscopic differences, which are more likely to be implicated in developmental dyslexia, required different approaches.

Postmortem neuropathological studies of the brains of known dyslexics were the first attempts at examining possible cellular abnormalities in people with reading disorders. Galaburda and his colleagues reported anomalies in the brains of four people who were diagnosed as dyslexic prior to their deaths (Galaburda, Sherman, Rosen, Aboitiz, & Geschwind, 1985). Symmetry of the planum temporale (which is usually asymmetrical in humans, with increased size in the left hemisphere), as well as neuronal ectopias and dysplasias too small to be seen on structural MRI were reported in the cerebral cortex of the dyslexic subjects. These anomalies appear to be prenatal in origin, and were distributed bilaterally in the brains of the men, with greatest density being noted along the left Sylvian fissure. Additionally, anomalies were noted in the inferior frontal cortex, and some anomalies were noted in the right hemisphere (Galaburda et al, 1985; Humphreys, Kaufmann, & Galaburda, 1990).

The more recent development of functioning techniques of neuroimaging, such as positron emission tomography (PET) and functional MRI (fMRI), has allowed researchers to examine the hypothesis of microscopic lesions even more thoroughly through studying blood flow activation in the brains of normal and dyslexic subjects. These technologies permit the brain's activity to be examined under varied cognitive challenges, with decreased activation suggesting abnormalities in the brain. More understanding of the brain substrates affecting reading disabilities is now available with these functional technologies.

Results of PET studies suggest that reading utilizes posterior pathways that include the striate and visual association cortex in the occipital lobe, the left angular gyrus, and Wernicke's area in the posterior superior temporal gyrus. The angular gyrus is an association area that appears to be involved in converting visual stimuli into phonological representations. This translation of visually perceived letters into speech sounds is then followed by the semantic processing of the sounds, which appears to be the function of Wernicke's area (Henderson, 1986).

The identification of this pathway for reading was first suggested by PET studies done with normal adult readers. Peterson's group demonstrated that single word recognition is a serial (i.e., sequential) process involving elementary operations (Petersen, Fox, Posner, Mintun, & Raichle, 1988), and activation of the left tempoparietal cortex and left posterior superior temporal cortex has been noted (Rumsey, 1996). Although more extensive activation is seen in the left hemisphere in these studies, some activation in right-sided homologous regions are frequently activated in right-handed men who are normal readers (Rumsey, 1996). This finding parallels findings of left-sided activation in normal readers who are matching words by meaning, as compared to bilateral activation on the same task in people who have dyslexia (Bookheimer, personal communication, April, 2001).

Additionally, studies of the corpus callosum—the largest mass of connecting fibers in the brain, which connect the two hemispheres—suggest that right-handed familial dyslexics (e.g., dyslexia runs in the families of these people) typically show a larger splenium (posterior segment of the corpus collosum) than do normal subjects (Duara et al., 1991; Larsen, Hoien, & Odegaard, 1992). Other studies done with children have demonstrated a smaller genu (or anterior fifth) of the corpus collosum (Hynd et al., 1991), although the presence of children with attention deficit disorders confounded these findings.

Connectionist models of reading also have been suggested (Seidenberg & McClelland, 1989; Waters & Seidenberg 1985) and are an alternative to the serial models discussed above. Bookheimer, Zeffiro, Blaxton, Gaillard, and Theodore (1995) found that location of activation differed depending on whether reading was occurring orally or silently, supporting the model of simultaneous but differing processes occurring during reading.

More recently, the work of the Yale Center for the Study of Learning and Attention has applied the technology of functional MRI to the study of the pathways involved in singleword reading. A comparison of normal adult readers to people diagnosed with dyslexia demonstrated the posterior pathway described above in normal readers, but decreased activation at the angular gyrus and increased activation in Broca's area on the left for dyslexic subjects (Shaywitz et al., 1996). These findings represent preliminary support for the theory that, due to microscopic lesions in specific regions of the left hemisphere, intracerebral reorganization may occur to compensate for these lesions.

Thus, results of the most recent neuroimaging studies support the hypothesis of dyslexia resulting from microscopic lesions, located primarily in the left posterior hemisphere, which interrupt the development of normal phonological processing. Ongoing questions include the role of the right hemisphere in reading processes, as well as the study of connectionist models of reading to complement current sequential processing models.

The Role of Neuropsychological Assessment

Neuropsychological assessment has been assuming an increasing role in the diagnosis of LDs. This approach to assessment, which studies the relationship between brain dysfunction and abnormal behavior, offers a thorough and complex understanding of the cognitive delays that may be present in the student with these disabilities (Pennington, 1991). Beyond assessment, neuropsychological research has been at the forefront of work identifying the neural mechanisms underlying these disorders. Neuropsychologists also have become increasingly involved in issues of treatment of LDs through administering standardized testing and neuroimaging studies both before and after intervention trials (Temple et al., 2000).

The involvement of neuropsychology in the study and assessment of LDs is longstanding. Paul Satz was principal investigator on the NIMH-funded Florida Longitudinal Study, which followed a population of boys from the beginning of school entrance (kindergarten) through grade 6 (Fletcher, Satz, & Morris, 1984). In 1979, Homer B. C. Reed was supporting more study of the relationships between biological handicaps and learning ability, arguing that "neuropsychological deficits selectively impair learning, although intelligence quotients may not be demonstrably affected" (Reed, 1979, pp. 29–30). Reed argued even then that a thorough understanding of the relevance of biological factors to special education are important for creating teaching strategies, evaluating program effectiveness, and making long-range plans for placement and management. The emphasis on the use of neuropsychology in assessing LDs has only increased in the literature since that time (Rourke, 1994; Taylor, 1988).

In beginning to examine the cost-effectiveness of neuropsychological assessment in the field of LDs, several issues must be considered. Traditionally, LD assessment has been done by school psychologists and involved primarily the administration of standardized tests of intellectual functioning and academic achievement. Based on the IQ/achievement discrepancy model of learning disabilities (Rutter & Yule, 1975), the school psychologist's task has been to determine if a significant discrepancy between expected and actual academic achievement is present and, if so, to diagnose an LD. Children so categorized can then qualify for a number of educational services under the Individuals with Disabilities Education Act of 1997 (IDEA, 1997).

In contrast to this traditional approach, neuropsychological assessment of students referred with learning delays is based on a brain/behavior paradigm and includes the assessment of a number of domains of neurocognitive functioning and information processing (Lezak, 1995). Although typically including IQ and academic achievement testing, the neuropsychological assessment focuses more on the child's approach to information processing and learning, and is interested in the intraindividual discrepancies occurring between a number of cognitive domains as well as the child's performance relative to standardized normative data. Specifically, the neuropsychologist sees an LD as an ultimate expression of specific neurocognitive deficits. Because these deficits occur in areas that support academic functioning, they interfere with a student's ability to input or output information academically. Treatment of these underlying impairments therefore makes a profound impact on the student's ultimate ability to participate in classroom learning.

Additionally, the neuropsychologist is interested in the neural substrates of the behavioral problems, creating a broader spectrum of diagnostic possibilities for consideration. These possibilities would include a number of etiologies beyond LDs, such as medical or psychological causes.

Given the expense of the neuropsychological assessment relative to that of the traditional school psychology approach, questions of its cost-effectiveness must be considered. Questions to be raised include whether the more comprehensive neuropsychological assessment offers enough additional information to justify its cost and, more importantly, whether this additional information sufficiently improves the accuracy of treatment planning and ultimately treatment outcome to make it worth the additional expense. Cost-efficiency studies examining these questions have not been done, so these questions remain unanswered.

Cost-effectiveness studies ask whether the costs justify the outcomes when the outcomes are not necessarily measured monetarily (Prigatano, 2002). This approach is well suited to cost-effectiveness studies in which two different approaches to assessment (psychoeducational versus neuropsychological) can be done. The outcomes of the two assessments then can be compared in terms of the efficacy of the information gleaned from each report on treatment planning. Currently, however, the field is lacking many of the scientific studies necessary to demonstrate this efficacy. Additionally, a closer examination of the field indicates that there are questions to be answered before these analyses can be fully undertaken.

Four issues in the field of LDs must be addressed before cost-effectiveness studies can be designed and implemented:

1. What criteria best discriminate students with and without learning disabilities?
2. What are the advantages and disadvantages between traditional psychoeducational assessment and neuropsychological assessment in determining whether an LD exists and in developing a treatment plan?
3. What are the benefits of having additional information about a child's cognitive and emotional profile in developing a treatment plan?
4. How is the outcome of "good intervention" in LDs best measured?

This chapter will attempt to address these four issues through examining the current information and controversies regarding them. Additionally, new treatments for students with LDs and their impact on outcome will be presented.

The Scope of the Issue

For the federal fiscal year (FFY) 1999, under the amended IDEA (1997), the federal government apportioned more than $4.3 billion in allocations for state educational agencies to assist in providing a free appropriate public education to all children with disabilities. Nationally, approximately 50% of the students identified with disabilities fall under the category of "specific learning disabled," making the diagnosis and recommendations for treatment of these children a matter of great fiscal and educational importance.

Given the scope of funding and services available for students with LDs their proper diagnosis and formulation of treatment recommendations are of great concern. Yet, the domain of learning disabilities is rife with controversy regarding the identification, diagnosis, and treatment planning of these students.

Question 1: What Criteria Best Discriminate Students With and Without Learning Disabilities?

The definition of LD has been a subject of debate for as long as the concept has been recognized. The definition used by policy makers and most researchers is the discrepancy model, whereby a child is diagnosed with an LD if he or she is not achieving academically at the expected level. Typically, a comparison of IQ score with scores of academic achievement is done; if discrepant, the child is diagnosed as having an LD.

The main controversy about this approach is that, although it does identify many students with LDs, it fails to identify others. Additionally, it is biased toward students with higher IQ's, making it possible to identify students as learning disabled when their academic scores are actually in the high average range or higher. Another criticism is that some children who do not meet the criteria cut-off established by policy demonstrate neurocognitive profiles with significant academic achievement problems or demonstrate impairment in correlated domains. Given the limited testing they usually receive, however, they are not identified.

The following section will describe current policy statements, as well as discussing the criticisms of the discrepancy model. Alternatives to the traditional discrepancy model will then be discussed, including use of a modified discrepancy model (Buka, Satz, Seidman, & Lipsitt, 1999) and other approaches to using neuropsychological assessment in identifying students with less-standard presentations.

Current Policy Regarding the Discrepancy Model

The term *learning disabilities* was defined by the federal government in 1968, and that definition is still the basis for legislation providing for these children. It reads,

> Children with specific learning disabilities exhibit a disorder in one or more of the basic psychological processes involved in understanding or in using spoken or written language. These may be manifested in disorders of listening, thinking, talking, reading, writing, spell-

> ing, or arithmetic. They include conditions that have been referred to as perceptual handicaps, brain injury, minimal brain dysfunction, dyslexia, developmental aphasia, etc. They do not include learning problems which are due primarily to visual, hearing, or motor handicaps, to mental retardation, emotional disturbance, or to environmental disadvantage. (USOE, 1968, p. 34)

Operationalization of this definition occurred in 1977 using the discrepancy model when the *Federal Register* further defined a learning disability as,

> a severe discrepancy between achievement and intellectual ability in one or more of the areas : (1) oral expression; (2) listening comprehension; (3) written expression; (4) basic reading skill; (5) reading comprehension; (6) mathematics calculation; or (7) mathematics reasoning. The child may not be identified as having a specific learning disability if the discrepancy between ability and achievement is primarily the result of: (1) a visual, hearing, or motor handicap; (2) mental retardation; (3) emotional disturbance; or (4) environmental, cultural, or economic disadvantage. (Fletcher, 1998)

Although these policy statements have been in place since the 1970s, pollsters commissioned by Louis Harris and Associates in 1990 to assess the outcome for people receiving services for disability in education reported discouraging results. These pollsters queried people in dozens of settings about being disabled in America today. The specific question asked was the outcome of persons who had received 15 years' of special education services (from 1975 to the 1990 date of the poll). The answers indicated that "far too many" of the students were, as adults, dependent on their parents, living in their parents' homes, and receiving financial aid from them. Skills for independent or semi-independent living had not been developed in many of those polled, and many were unemployed or working part-time and below the minimum wage (Martin, 1998).

In light of these discouraging findings, the IDEA (1997) was amended and signed into law by President Clinton. This act has attempted to remedy the outcomes described above by addressing issues of transition planning, efficacy of the Individualized Education Program (IEP) process, recognition of the fundamental necessity of good and well-communicated evaluations, and by addressing the need to decrease monies currently going into extensive litigation. IDEA (1997) . . . continues to define LDs based on the discrepancy model established by the *Federal Register* in 1977.

Although the specifics of "expected" and "actual" levels of functioning are not specifically described in IDEA, the *DSM-IV* states that standardized tests in reading, mathematics, or written expression should be used and compared to the student's age, schooling, and level of intelligence (APA, p. 46).

The definition of "discrepancy" varies between organizations and states, but 38 states use the discrepancy model and all but 4 administer IQ tests to determine the expected level of functioning. States vary in what statistics are used to define a "significant discrepancy," with some using a 1.5 standard deviation difference and others using a 2.0 standard deviation difference. Some states use a regression model that was designed to correct for overidentification of students with high IQs.

Controversy Regarding the Discrepancy Model

The use of the discrepancy formula has been controversial in the literature. Critics of the discrepancy model point out that it was originally based on the Isle of Wight studies (Rutter & Yule, 1975) that reported a bimodal distribution of students with reading difficulties. This distribution included two groups: those whose low reading scores were discrepant from their IQ scores, and those who demonstrated a consistency between low reading and low intellectual skills ("general reading backwardness"). This study, on which so much policy has been based, did not exclude children with known brain injury or mental deficiency, thereby introducing a bias in the findings (Fletcher, 1998). This bias may be the reason why the Rutter and Yule findings have not been replicated despite several attempts (Rodgers, 1983; Shaywitz et al., 1992; Silva, McGee, & Williams, 1985), most notably two recent, large-scale studies that did not demonstrate the bimodal distribution (Fletcher et al., 1994; Stanovich & Siegel, 1994). Stanovich and Siegel wrote, "neither the phenotypic nor the genotypic indicators of poor reading are correlated in a reliable way with IQ discrepancy. . . . Thus, the basic assumption that underlies decades of classification in research and educational practice regarding reading disabilities is becoming increasingly untenable" (p. 48).

Clinical knowledge about the development of LDs across time and the subsequent impact of this development on test performance helps elucidate the lack of replication of the Isle of Wight study. One reason for false negative findings using the IQ/achievement model is that information gleaned from the IQ test about the child's ability to process information is not independent of results of tests of academic skills. Thus, for some children with specific LDs the same pathology that is affecting the learning may also impact the ability to perform on some aspects of the IQ test, especially verbal processing.

For example, a high correlation between reading disabilities and language disorders often is seen (Pennington, 1991). Given this finding, the Verbal IQ of the Wechsler Intelligence Scale for Children-III also will be affected by the issues driving the reading disability for some children. For these children, the Full Scale IQ (based as it is on a composite of the Verbal and Performance IQ scores) may be unduly impacted by the language processing difficulties, making it an inappropriate comparison measure. Siegel (1998) wrote that most children with LDs "are deficient in one or more of the component skills that are part of these IQ tests; and, therefore, their scores on IQ tests will be an underestimate of their competence."

Another problem with using IQ testing alone to determine expected functioning is that, for children with LDs, IQ scores tend to decrease with age. This phenomenon, termed the Matthew effect by Stanovich (1986), occurs because intellectual and other cognitive functions are adversely affected by the impact of the LD over time. Stanovich described the Matthew effect as "the tendency of reading itself to cause further development in other, related cognitive abilities, such that the rich get richer and the poor get poorer" (p. 9). Given these effects, the student who has less access to information learned from reading will demonstrate a decrease in overall ability. The decline of IQ scores with increasing age in students with LDs has been suggested (Siegel & Himel, 1998), although the need for longitudinal studies examining this concern remains.

Benefits of the Discrepancy Model

Given these many concerns, why does the discrepancy model continue to be the defining approach as outlined by the *Federal Register* and adopted into practice by most state educational departments? One reason is that this model allows for relatively fast and straightforward assessment of students suspected of having an LD. In order to diagnose a child using this approach, only the IQ and achievement testing must be done.

This approach also allows for consistent decision making to occur regarding which students qualify for services. Although this approach may have limited costs in the short-run, critics maintain that the impact of underidentification for students both during their educational careers and in their adaptation to living as adults outweighs the short-term benefits. This belief has not been examined empirically, however.

Alternatives to the Traditional Discrepancy Model

If the discrepancy model is not used, however, what method of identifying students with LDs would replace it? The lack of a viable alternative to this model likely has been the predominant reason for its continued popularity. Several alternatives have been proposed, and will be discussed below.

One alternative is to define a reading disability based solely on signs of low performance on tests of reading achievement, thereby eliminating the requirement of a discrepancy from intelligence scores (Fletcher et al., 1989; Siegel, 1989). This score would identify both groups of reading-impaired students discussed in the original Rutter and Yule (1975) article, and would likely qualify more students for services than the current policy allows. Critics of this approach, however, express concern that this procedure may overlook students who, although reading at grade level, are compensating for compromised abilities (e.g., in phonological processing) due to their high intelligence. These students ("the gifted learning disabled") would not qualify for services, despite their disability. Another problem with this approach as it is currently used (reading disability ≤ 90 SS) is that it identifies 25% of the population. This high prevalence makes research and treatment of these students too costly and therefore not practical (Paul Satz, personal communication, May, 2001).

An alternative approach to diagnosing children with LDs is to identify intraindividual discrepancies. These are described as being differences among skills in different developmental or instructional domains (Keogh, 1988). Chalfant (1989) suggested that students might show intraindividual differences in three ways: (a) among psychological processes or developmental abilities, (b) between intellectual potential and achievement, and (c) within performance on different tasks or among academic areas. This approach would require that a significant difficulty be identified in a specific skill area, and that successful performance in several other skill areas also be identified in the same student (Shaw, Cullen, McGuire, & Brinckerhof, 1995). This focus on identifying an individual student's learning profile would contribute to better understanding of each student's learning processes and factors that affect them. This approach is well suited to the neuropsychological assessment, wherein examination of many cognitive domains allows for comparison both to standardized normative data and to the individual him- or herself. Significant discrepancies between neurocognitive domains suggest the presence of an LD even though there is not an actual IQ/achievement discrepancy.

Variations in how the discrepancy model might be applied also have been proposed. One major criticism of a straightforward comparison of IQ and achievement test scores is that, using this method, students with high IQs are overrepresented in the learning-disabled groups, and students with low IQ scores are underrepresented. That is, it is easier to demonstrate an IQ/achievement discrepancy when the IQ is higher (Sattler, 1992). In order to address this problem, regression formulas have been introduced that attempt to correct for this bias. Even using the regression model, however, students with higher IQs are overrepresented in LD samples.

Buka et al. (1999) proposed an alternative to the three models of identification noted above. They suggested recalculating a "discrepancy ratio," which is the ratio of the standard score on an achievement test to the standard score for intelligence. They then identified as learning disabled those children whose ratio places them in the bottom 1.5 standard deviation of the distribution for discrepancy scores within four FSIQ strata. Their application of this method to data from the National Collaborative Perinatal Project (NCPP), a longitudinal follow-up epidemiologic study of students retrospectively identified as having LDs 25 years ago, has shown that this method far exceeds other methods (e.g., traditional IQ/achievement discrepancy models including regression formulas as well as use of low reading scores alone) on several domains. High-IQ students were not overrepresented using this approach; nor were low-IQ students. Additionally, further analyses indicated that this group (in comparison to the others) exhibited more of the known or suggested correlates of LD, such as being male, having low SES, and having a history of birth complications or grade retention. Groups identified using the other means demonstrated social and economic bias (e.g., traditional discrepancy models had an overrepresentation of White and high-IQ students; reading failure model alone had an overrepresentation of children of poor parents, ethnic minorities, and greater rates of special classroom placement, grade retention, and delinquency). Thus, this approach offers a significant improvement over the traditional IQ/achievement model.

A recently published study that addressed the question of subtypes among children with reading disabilities raised other issues in determining how students should be identified (Morris et al., 1998). In identifying students for this study, *both* the discrepancy model and the low reading rate criteria were used, thereby creating a more heterogeneous sample. A normal control group also was included. Students were administered traditional tests of IQ and achievement and also were given a number of measures of cognitive and language functioning. Reading disability subtypes then were calculated using a cluster analysis. This analysis of eight measures of cognitive and language functions yielded seven reliable subtypes of reading disabilities, only half of which met the IQ/achievement discrepancy requirements. Reading failure was validated with a phoneme deletion task.

Both of these studies demonstrate that the traditional application of the IQ/achievement discrepancy model may underidentify students with LDs. Additionally, the Morris et al. study demonstrated that the use of the traditional discrepancy model alone also underidentifies students, but that the addition of other paradigms–including low reading rate and examination of larger cognitive profiles–identifies many more students who may need services. Current policy statements in many states do not allow for these additional students to be diagnosed as learning disabled if the discrepancy criteria are not met. The point must be made, however, that by relaxing the criteria to include low achievement (reading ≤ 90), a much larger sample of cases is yielded, some of which have no cognitive sequelae.

The neuropsychologist stands in a unique position of being able to identify additional students because they are able to identify intraindividual differences between cognitive domains that are affecting a child's learning and academic success. Taylor (1988) wrote:

> The rationale for comprehensive testing is to investigate the nature and extent of cognitive impairments that accompany learning disabilities. A battery that is comprehensive will make it possible to observe the kinds of skill dissociations that frequently occur in chil-

> dren with brain injuries or learning disabilities. . . . Measures of the skills actually required for academic learning merit special consideration. (p. 797)

Although this approach is viable and would certainly identify more students in need of services, there are no clear guidelines to aid the neuropsychologist in deciding what level of discrepancy constitutes a disorder. Development of such guidelines would create an initial step in creating policy that would allow for the diagnosis of nonspecific LDs acceptable by the states.

☐ Question 2: What Are the Advantages and Disadvantages of Traditional Psychoeducational Assessment and Neuropsychological Assessment in Determining Whether a Learning Disability Exists?

Another question is the degree and type of training necessary to perform a thorough assessment of a child with a suspected LD. Diagnostic assessments of LDs have taken place predominantly in educational domains, under the purview of school psychologists. With the advent of neuropsychological paradigms (Adams & Rourke, 1992, p. 5) as well as the work in further clarifying their neurocognitive origins and subtypes of LDs the role of the neuropsychologist in assessing these children has become increasingly prominent. Given that the neuropsychologist also is trained as a clinical psychologist, the interplay of neurocognitive issues with those of emotion also can be examined. These more expanded examinations of learning issues have raised new questions regarding the definition and diagnosis of LDs. Questions about the use of neuropsychological assessment include whether the neuropsychologist has adequate training in educational interventions to thoroughly assess for an LD whether it is important to understand underlying brain functions in determining if a child has an LD the degree of clinical psychological expertise needed to understand the relationship of cognition and emotion, and how the two professions might work together. These questions will be discussed in the next section.

Psychoeducational Assessment of Learning Disabilities

Division 16 of the American Psychological Association is committed to the area of school psychology. Division 16 "is composed of scientific-practitioner psychologists whose major professional interests lie with children, families, and the schooling process" (APA, Online, Division 16, 2002). One population served by school psychologists is "families who request diagnostic evaluations of learning disabilities," and procedures include "diagnostic assessments to support eligibility for and delivery of services within statutorily regulated contexts that integrate diagnostic information from other professionals to support recommendations for educational modifications and community services" (APA Online, Division 16, Goals and Objective, 2002).

The emphasis of the LD assessment administered by most school psychologists is on whether there is a discrepancy between developmental-cognitive processes (often assessed with an IQ test) and achievement skills. School psychologists are trained to employ the discrepancy model in diagnosing LDs although environmental demands, reactions of others, and interaction effects also are considered (Sattler, 1992). The battery given by a school psychologist is designed to address the discrepancy question and also to assess all seven areas of LD eligibility outlined by the 1997 *Federal Register* (e.g., oral expression, listening comprehension, written expression, basic reading skills, reading comprehension, mathematics calculation, and mathematics reasoning). Sattler recommends administration of a standardized IQ test (such as the Wechsler Scales or the Stanford Binet), or use of specialized measures (such as the Kaufman Assessment Battery for Children, Raven's Progressive Matrices, or the Pictorial Test of Intelligence) to assess developmental-cognitive processes. Additionally, his approach advocates using standardized tests of academic achievement (e.g., Wide Range Achievement Test–Revised, Woodcock Johnson–Revised standardized tests of achievement, or the Illinois Test of Psycholinguistic Abilities) to assess reading, writing, and arithmetic (Sattler, 1992).

The educational battery described above makes several assumptions about LDs. First, it assumes that the discrepancy model is adequate for the identification of students with learning disabilities. Second, assessment typically is isolated to the seven domains described above, so impairment in other neurocognitive domains that might be implicated or even driving the learning delays are not considered. Third, this approach to LD assessment assumes that the standardized instruments used are sufficient to measure the domain indicated. Specific guidelines as to how to assess a given domain are not offered. For example, it might be important to administer a "word attack" test along with a measure of single-word reading and reading rate to be sure that phonological awareness has been adequately assessed in students with suspected reading disabilities.

There are several strengths in the psychoeducational assessment, described in Table 13.1. First, the training of school psychologists emphasizes school and educational issues, with specific training in how to interface with school personnel. This background can improve the integration of testing results into the educational environment. Second, the school psychologist is trained in intervention strategies, allowing for specific application of test results to the child's individual education program. Third, the school psychologist's approach to LD assessment employs the use of standardized instruments whose raw scores have been compared to national normative data, allowing for empirical interpretation of the results. Fourth, this approach answers the questions raised by

TABLE 13.1. Strengths of a Psychoeducational Assessment

- Integration of testing results into the educational environment, given the school psychologist's training in school/educational issues.
- Specific application of testing results to intervention, given school psychologist's training in intervention strategies.
- Use of standardized instruments allowing for empirical interpretation of the results.
- Answers the questions raised by current policy statements and provides a standardized method for deciding who qualifies for services.
- Academic assessment may be more in-depth.
- School psychologist works as part of a larger team of allied professionals who also contribute aspects of assessment to the educational planning phase, thereby creating a thorough approach to treatment planning.

current policy statements. It provides a standardized method for deciding who qualifies for services and placement within the school system. Although concerns remain as to the appropriateness of this classification system, placement can be done relatively quickly, and it provides an apparently impartial decision regarding who will receive services and who will not. A fifth strength is that the approach to academic assessment often is more in-depth than that provided by neuropsychology. School psychologists receive more didactic training in the specifics of school-based learning. Their assessments, therefore, may address academic achievement more comprehensively. Finally, the school psychologist works as part of a larger team, with allied professionals who also contribute aspects of assessment to the educational program-planning phase. Their psychoeducational findings can be combined with testing results from other disciplines (e.g., speech/language and occupational therapy) to create a more thorough approach to treatment planning.

Despite these many strengths, there also are concerns about the psychoeducational approach to LD assessment. The first is that the training of the school psychologist in the assessment of LDs is more limited than that of the neuropsychologist. Some school psychologists have only master's level training, and the training of doctoral-level school psychologists includes considerable emphasis on other aspects of the profession, including school adjustment, treatment of behavior problems, and adverse social conditions that threaten healthy development in school and community (APA, Division 16). This emphasis on other issues may leave gaps in the LD assessment provided by the school psychologist. Additionally, training in how to assess for LD is specifically designed to address the discrepancy question. More complex conceptualizations of LDs, such as those proposed by neuropsychologists, have not been the focus of training for school psychologists, making them less prepared to discuss more subtle interpretations of learning disabilities. Third, given the smaller cognitive test battery used, results of this approach are vulnerable to the impact of extraneous variables such as test error or inattention. For example, if a given domain is measured by only one instrument and the child is hungry or tired at the time it is administered, validity is in jeopardy. Fourth, because it focuses on the academic achievement of the student, training of the school psychologist does not include extensive didactics on the meaning of score patterns as they relate to neurocognitive profiles. This can lead to confusion in understanding the larger patterns suggested by the child's testing profile as well as underidentification of students who do not display the traditional IQ/achievement discrepancy, but who, nonetheless, have CNS-based anomalies that interfere with their ability to learn. Perhaps the greatest risk with this approach is that, given the lack of training in CNS disorders and their behavioral presentations, the school psychologist may not identify which difficulties are primary to the CNS dysfunction and which are secondary to it. For example, it is important to identify whether a psychological depression has led a child to avoid the challenge of reading due to apathy, or whether the reading disability is based on a primary deficit in phonological processing and only secondarily leads to depressive affect about the reading failure. If the primary issue has not been correctly identified, it may not receive the attention it requires for successful treatment of the child's learning problems. Rather, treatment recommendations could be developed which address only the limited information about the final impact of the neurocognitive difficulty on tasks of reading, writing, and arithmetic. These results therefore may lack the specificity that could lead to more successful resolution of the underlying causes of the LD.

Neuropsychological Approach to Assessment

The directory of the Association of Postdoctoral Programs in Clinical Neuropsychology (APPCN) states that neuropsychology is a clinical specialty that has "proceeded at an exponential pace" (*APPCN Directory*, 2000–2002, p. 1) since peer-reviewed journals in the field first appeared in the late 1970s. Division 40 of the American Psychological Association (Division of Clinical Neuropsychology) was recognized in 1983. Division 40 and the International Neuropsychological Society (INS) developed a task force to develop guidelines for training at the doctoral, internship, and postdoctoral levels; and, in February 1992, the inaugural national meeting of postdoctoral clinical neuropsychology training programs was held in San Diego. The APPCN was developed at this meeting and was formally incorporated in 1994 (*APPCN Directory*, 2000–2002, p. 2). The aspirational guidelines for education and training of neuropsychologists were further discussed at the Houston Conference in 1997.

A clinical neuropsychologist is defined as

> a professional psychologist who applies principles of assessment and intervention based upon the scientific study of human behavior as it relates to normal and abnormal functioning of the central nervous system. The clinical neuropsychologist is a doctoral-level psychology provider of diagnostic and intervention services who has demonstrated competence in the application of such principles for human welfare through:
>
> A. Successful completion of systematic didactic and experiential training in neuropsychology and neuroscience at a regionally accredited university,
> B. Two or more years of appropriate supervised training applying neuropsychological services in a clinical setting,
> C. Licensing and certification to provide psychological services to the public by the laws of the state or province in which he or she practices,
> D. Review by one's peers as a test of these competencies (Reports of the INS-Division 40 task force on education, accreditation, and credentialing, pp. 29–34).

Neuropsychological assessment includes the integration of findings from a number of sources. Developmental history–including prenatal and perinatal information, developmental milestones, educational and psychological history, and current developmental levels–is queried. Additionally, medical history–including any complications in birth and delivery, childhood diseases, brain injury, and history of accidents or fractures–is considered. Family history also is obtained, with a thorough investigation of family learning patterns, educational attainment, behavioral or psychological difficulties, and actual diagnosed disorders. Assessment also includes examining the child's current living situation, including primary languages spoken in the home, comorbid sensory–motor issues, means of discipline used in the home, recent losses, and the general level of stress in the family. Consultation with other professionals offering services to the child is important, including pediatricians, educators, and allied professionals. Testing itself is done using standardized neuropsychological instruments administered under the supervision of a trained neuropsychologist.

Most neuropsychologists use the hypothesis-testing model rather than a standardized battery. This model proposes that assessment of brain function should take place using a domain-specific approach whereby several preidentified neurocognitive domains are assessed, but the specific instruments used to assess them are not prescribed. This approach to testing requires extensive training on the part of the neuropsychologist, as in it the specific elements of the battery are chosen *during the course of the assessment*, as more and more details about the behavior and its presentation become known (Lezak, 1995). The hypothesis-testing model is based on the growing knowledge that many brain-based abnormalities may lead to similar broadly defined behavioral presentations, and that it is only in the application of tests assessing very specific aspects of functioning that diagnostic clarity can be reached.

The *process approach* to neuropsychological assessment (Kaplan, 1988) represents an extension of the hypothesis-testing model. This approach emphasizes that the diagnostic information lies, not just in the final score received by the child, but also in his or her approach to the task at hand. For example, although the final score on the Block Design subtest of the WISC-III yields some valuable information, other aspects of the performance–such as the tendency to rotate the blocks, perception of the gestalt of the block design, and organizational efficiency in approaching the task–offer further crucial diagnostic information and must be integrated into the final interpretation of results.

The *brain/behavior paradigm* of neuropsychology contributes to a specific approach to assessment of LDs. The neuropsychologist assesses for the presence of an LD by testing a number of neurocognitive domains derived from research on the brain. These include intelligence, academic achievement, attention, executive functioning, language, visual–perceptual and visual–perceptual–organization skills, memory, motor functioning, and social/emotional functioning (Culbertson & Edmonds, 1996). In the hypothesis-testing model, each of these domains is assessed using a number of instruments, so no cognitive findings are based on the results of one test alone (P. Satz, personal communication, January 12, 1996). Instruments are standardized, with raw scores being compared to standardized normative data, so the child's performance can be compared to that of other children in the same age group as well as to the child's own (through comparison of intraindividual discrepancies between domains).

There are several assumptions inherent in the use of the neuropsychological approach to the assessment of LDs. The first is that understanding the development of the CNS is crucial if one is to correctly identify and understand the nature of a given child's difficulty with learning. Neuropsychologists believe that brain dysfunction interacts with other variables to produce the symptoms of a specific LD (Rourke, 1994). Therefore, it is only through assessing brain/behavior relationships that an LD can be identified. Further, neuropsychologists assume that brain dysfunction can be identified through the use of neuropsychological instruments–validated through research with patient groups with known CNS lesions–and through correlations between neuropsychological testing findings and results of neuroimaging studies. Neuropsychologists also assume that a developmental, brain-based disability may result from microscopic abnormalities in the brain and may affect one or more behavioral domains. These abnormalities may or may not be identifiable. Another assumption of neuropsychology is that psychological factors may exacerbate or even drive the presenting issues and, therefore, must be thoroughly examined. Finally, the neuropsychologist assumes that "primary" deficits in functioning, resulting from CNS anomalies, may lead to "secondary" deficits that further exacerbate the LD and create treatment complications that must be addressed (Pennington, 1991).

There are several strengths of the neuropsychological approach to the assessment of LDs. The neuropsychological assessment, like the psychoeducational evaluation, uses standardized instruments that allow for the application of normative data in evaluating the severity of a student's delays. Additionally, given that the neuropsychological assessment typically includes both intellectual and academic achievement testing, it is able to ascertain whether a child meets criteria for an LD using the traditional discrepancy model. In addition to answering this question, however, the additional information gleaned from the neuropsychological assessment on how a child processes information offers deeper clarity about his or her learning profile. This additional information makes it possible to identify children with LDs who do not meet the traditional discrepancy cut-off model, and also allows for the development of a specific and individualized treatment program based on considerable information about how a given child learns best. Additionally, the neuropsychologist's extensive training in brain/behavior relationships allows him or her to add appropriate measures to the battery as unfolding results implicate other, unhypothesized areas of dysfunction. Because all neurocognitive domains are assessed, no areas of delay will be overlooked, allowing for more comprehensive treatment planning.

The training of the neuropsychologist provides for an integrated interpretation of the data, combining the findings from multiple domains into a meaningful, integrated whole (see Table 13.2). The combined knowledge base of brain functioning, psychological factors, behavioral paradigms, and assessment creates a comprehensive understanding of an individual's neuropsychological presentation. This integrative approach creates a more complete and comprehensive picture of a child's learning profile and informs treatment decisions made pursuant to the examination. Finally, the neuropsychologist's training in CNS functioning allows him or her to identify potentially harmful or treatable medical conditions that may be underlying the LD presenta-

TABLE 13.2. Strengths of a Neuropsychological Assessment

- Use of standardized instruments allows for the application of raw scores to normative data.
- Neuropsychological assessment is able to ascertain whether a child meets criteria for a learning disability using the traditional discrepancy model.
- Due to more accurate assessment of "expected" level of functioning based on measurement of several neurocognitive domains, it is possible to identify children with learning disabilities who do not meet the traditional discrepancy cut-off model.
- Additional neuropsychological information offers deeper clarity about student's learning profile through identification of processing deficits underlying academic difficulties.
- Allows for development of a very specific and individualized treatment program that incorporates an understanding of the student's strengths as well as delays.
- More thorough assessment allows for assessment of additional domains that might otherwise be missed, thereby lessening the risk that an area of delay will be overlooked.
- Clarification of the appropriateness of specific interventions allows for the creation of a more comprehensive treatment plan.
- Identification of primary and secondary symptoms allowing for prioritization of services.
- Training in CNS functioning allows neuropsychologist to identify potentially harmful or treatable medical conditions that may be underlying the learning disability presentation.
- Training in clinical psychology allows for interpretation of emotional issues and their role in exacerbating or ameliorating learning differences.

tion. The first author recalls a case in which a child with chronic headaches and a sudden onset of math difficulties was denied further medical treatment (CT scan) by his HMO in part due to the diagnosis of an uncomplicated LD with psychological issues made by his school psychologist. It was not until 4 months later, when the child lost vision in one eye, that the CT scan was ordered and a benign brain tumor in the right hemisphere was diagnosed. Unfortunately, because of the late diagnosis of the tumor, the optic nerve had been crushed and the monocular blindness and math disability were irreversible.

There also are criticisms of the neuropsychological approach to LD assessment. One concern is related to the diversity of training that neuropsychologists receive. Many lack information about educational processes and interventions that may make their application of findings to treatment planning less thorough or pertinent. Neuropsychologists traditionally do not receive training in academic interventions and so may be at a loss as to how to make specific recommendations following their exam. Additionally, a lack of understanding of educational policy and law on the part of the neuropsychologist may interfere with the ultimate usefulness of the exam. Incorrect terminology or poor understanding of the criteria for service provision may prevent a child from receiving the interventions he or she requires. To address these concerns, certain training guidelines are necessary but not sufficient. More work must be done to outline what a student of neuropsychology must do to prepare for this kind of specialized assessment.

Another complaint about the neuropsychological assessment is the length of the exam. Because so many domains are assessed using multiple instruments, a neuropsychological exam typically requires far more time to administer. This factor can contribute to fatigue for the student, unless the assessment is broken up into at least 2 days. A question that must be addressed by neuropsychologists is how to be comprehensive in the exam without being so extensive as to create a negative effect.

Also, given the extensive training of the neuropsychologist as well as the time required for test administration, scoring, and interpretation of data, the neuropsychological assessment is considerably more expensive than traditional psychoeducational examinations. Means of allaying these costs must be explored if neuropsychological assessment is to remain a viable option for families.

Finally, given the complexity of the neuropsychological results and the specific language used by most neuropsychologists, interpretations can be difficult to understand unless great care is taken to make the neuropsychological report comprehensive and useful to the lay reader. The neuropsychological report written for a student with an LD must be comprehensive to parents (some of whom also may have LDs) and to educators, who may be unfamiliar with these concepts. The use of professional jargon in the report likely will interfere with the readers' comprehension and therefore lessen its impact and usefulness. More straightforward descriptions of the results and their ensuing impressions will be important if the full effectiveness of the assessment is to be reached.

Integration of the Two Models

The comparison of the assessment models for LDs described above illustrates that both approaches bring different strengths to the process. Several options have been generated in how to integrate these two models in order to bring the advantages of each discipline to the LD assessment.

Some school psychologists have proposed that students in this field be offered increased training in neuropsychology, so that their evaluations can reflect the knowledge and insight that the study of brain/behavior relationships brings. Hynd (1989) advocated that school psychologists be trained at the doctoral level and receive training in subspecialties such as neuropsychology. Cecil R. Reynolds described the importance of an understanding of the biological bases of behavior for the school psychologist. He stated that when school psychologists take on the role of diagnosis, treatment planning, treatment delivery, and vocational planning for students with biologically based learning problems in the absence of knowledge in biological bases of behavior, it is, "certainly unethical and probably constitutes malpractice" (Reynolds, 1989, p. 61).

Hesitations about training school psychologists in neuropsychology also have been expressed. Certainly, school psychologists would need to be trained at the doctoral level to qualify for this level of assessment. The most recent aspirational guidelines for training neuropsychologists (Houston Conference, 1997) required a full-time, 2-year postdoctoral fellowship, given the extent of this field of knowledge. If school psychologists seek training in neuropsychology, these aspirational guidelines should be considered.

A second approach to integrating these two fields would be to include more in-depth training in LDs during neuropsychological postdoctoral fellowships. Such training would include study of interventions and treatment programs for LDs, as well as study in the legal aspects of this domain. In a pilot program at UCLA, we are offering a full-year course to the neuropsychology postdoctoral fellows that includes didactics on the conceptualization and assessment of LDs, as well as guest speakers who address intervention and legal issues. Students involved in this program report improved abilities to apply the results of the neuropsychological assessment to the child's learning profile and intervention planning.

A third model that has been used to integrate these two training modalities is a consultative approach. The educational psychologist would complete the first aspect of the assessment, including administration of the IQ test, academic testing, and a thorough intake. A neuropsychologist would then review the results with the educational psychologist to determine if further assessment is indicated. This approach would allow the neuropsychologist to apply his or her expertise regarding medical risk factors and primary neurocognitive delays to the diagnostic and treatment planning process. If further neuropsychological testing is indicated, it could be done in part by a neuropsychology resident, thereby further allaying the cost and making the licensed neuropsychologist more available for consulting about other children's results.

These models represent three different approaches to combining the neuropsychologist's expertise in diagnosing students with the understanding of the educational psychologist. These approaches acknowledge that there are not enough trained neuropsychologists, and addresses this gap as well as the cost of having a neuropsychologist complete the entire assessment. Further dialogue between the two disciplines, as well as pilot programs that model these different approaches, will add more information to this developing collaboration.

Question 3: What Are the Benefits of Having Additional Information About a Child's Cognitive Profile in Developing a Treatment Plan?

The goal of assessment is appropriate treatment that produces the maximum benefit. As was stated earlier, in 1999 the federal government apportioned over $4 billion in allocations for state-level support of the IDEA (1997). This amount does not include state funding for specific LDs, nor the private contributions of parents and schools in treating children with these disorders. Given this level of financial support for the treatment of these disorders, it is imperative that treatment plans be precise and that they accurately reflect the most compelling needs of the student. Unfortunately, the lack of specificity of patterns of impairment and strength afforded by the psychoeducational evaluation limits the amount of information available in designing a treatment plan. Work on the subtyping of LDs is ongoing, and with it comes the increasing knowledge that there are cognitive deficiencies underlying a child's inability to acquire normal reading, writing, or arithmetic skills (see Table 13.3). The neuropsychological assessment individualizes the identification of specific cognitive patterns of deficits. Rourke (1994) wrote:

> The aim of this . . . procedure is to fashion remedial programs tailored to the individual's specific assets and deficits. Indeed, it has been our clinical experience that a remedial management intervention that fails to "fit" the neurocognitive ability makeup of the child can, in effect, be counterproductive in respect to the acquisition of adaptive, academic, and psychosocial skills. (pp. 497–498)

This next section examines two indices to be considered in treating the child with an LD. These indices include (a) identification of primary, correlated, secondary, and artifactual symptoms and (b) the need for a profile of strengths and weaknesses in order to develop treatment, including remediation strategies and development of compensatory strategies.

The first issue is the identification of primary, correlated, secondary, and artifactual

TABLE 13.3. The Clinical Utility of a Neuropsychological Evaluation

- Accurately identifies core problems, producing clarity about the child's learning profile.
- Identifies neurocognitive and psychological strengths that will support compensatory strategies.
- Reduces family frustration by providing more comprehensive information about the child's learning differences.
- Allows for prioritization of intervention based on information that given symptoms are primary or secondary to the core deficits.
- Guides educators and therapists to remediation not obvious without a brain/behavior paradigm.
- Suggests avenues for compensation and appropriateness of accommodation planning.
- Heightens the effectiveness of interventions by specifying more precisely the nature of the core deficits.
- Allows for the interpretation and integration of psychological data with the neuropsychological and academic findings.

symptoms. Primary symptoms are "universal, specific, and persistent in the disorder" (Pennington, 1991, p. 27). Their identification is necessary for subtypes of a given disorder to be identified, as actual subtypes demonstrate the same primary symptoms. Correlated symptoms differ from primary symptoms in that they represent concomitant symptoms that "have the same etiology as primary symptoms, but arise from the involvement of different brain and or organ systems" (Pennington 1991, p. 28). An example would be the correlation of speech and language disorders in many children diagnosed with dyslexia. These two sets of symptoms often are seen together, but neither is universal or specific to the disorder. A third consideration is secondary symptoms, which are consequences of either core or concomitant symptoms. An example would be unusual eye movements in dyslexic children during reading. Pennington (1991) explained that, given faulty phonological processing, these children must scan text in a more exploratory fashion because of their inability to rely on codes. Artifactual symptoms are those that appear to cluster together but are actually not based on an apparent association.

Treatment providers must be clear about the status of the symptoms they are attempting to impact. Logic would suggest that one should address the primary symptoms first, in order to have the most enduring effect. Treatment of primary symptoms also will affect existing secondary symptoms, as well as interfere with the development of additional secondary symptoms.

A second index to consider in evaluating treatment is the role of remediation versus compensatory strategies. These approaches involve teaching to the child's weakness (remediation) and to the child's strength (compensation; Torgerson, 1998). Remediation techniques are designed to address the primary features of the syndrome. Although full remediation of an LD likely is not possible, early interventions aimed at remediating the core deficits have demonstrated significant effectiveness. Torgerson (1998) described a remedial study with 8- to 11-year-old children identified as learning disabled by their school district. Students identified as having phonological processing problems received intensive individual instruction for 8 weeks (80 hours of instruction), followed up by participation in the LD classroom once a week for 8 weeks. The Auditory Discrimination in Depth program by Lindamood-Bell was used to instruct the children in embedded phonics (Lindamood & Lindamood, 1984). This program is designed to fill in the gaps of each child's word-reading systems through presenting phonemes using visual and kinesthetic as well as auditory cues. Results of this study were that the children's alphabetic reading skills and their ability to recognize and comprehend real words both improved significantly. This program demonstrated the need for identification of the specific characteristics of a given child's LD in order to maximize treatment effects.

Another approach to remediation of brain-based cognitive deficits was proposed by Paula Tallal's group. Tallal maintained that, in individuals with dyslexia, there is a general deficit in rapid temporal (i.e., sequential) processing across sensory modalities (e.g., auditory, visual and tactile; Tallal et al., 1993). Her group developed an adaptive training exercise mounted as computer games, designed to drive improvements in temporal processing skills. The authors reported that children undergoing 8 to 16 hours (in a 20-day period) of such training demonstrated a marked improvement in their ability to recognize brief and fast sequences of nonspeech and speech stimuli (Merzenich, Jenkins, Johnson, Schreiner, Miller, & Tallal, 1996). More recent fMRI studies have shown that normal readers demonstrate left prefrontal activity in response to rapidly changing nonlinguistic acoustic stimuli, whereas dyslexic subjects do not demonstrate this activation. Following the computerized remediation program, however, Temple et al. (2000) reported increased left prefrontal cortical activation, similar to what is seen initially in normals. Studdert-Kennedy and Mody (1995) attributed the deficits described by Tallal et al (1993) to difficulty in discriminating highly similar stimuli rapidly, and not to problems with judging the order of these stimuli.

In addition to teaching to a child's weaknesses, however, a comprehensive treatment program also must enhance and develop a child's strengths. Compensation should be implemented either when the child's core deficits are not amenable to treatment or when the core impairment is interfering with the acquisition of knowledge or the development of other skills. Whereas remediation techniques attempt to actually ameliorate the core deficits, compensatory interventions try to circumvent the gaps the LD has created.

Learning-disabled children must become proficient at compensating for their areas of deficit through using intact cognitive abilities (such as verbal memory, visual learning, or application of higher-level thinking to more basic skills). The identification of strengths does not take place in a systematic fashion using a standard psychoeducational battery in which only the IQ and academic domains are assessed. With a neuropsychological battery, specific assets are identified clearly across neurocognitive domains. These can include intact memory systems, social and psychological abilities (making a child more amenable to resource support), visual or verbal strengths (suggesting alternate modalities for presenting information in the classroom), and skills such as attention or executive functioning. Study of individual cases, however, indicates that these assets cannot be assumed. The first author recently assessed a boy whose assets were not entirely consistent with his learning profile. Despite a language-based reading disorder, his verbal memory was stronger than his visual memory, indicating that verbal modalities should continue to be emphasized and only secondarily supported by visual presentations. In a case such as this, when assets are specifically identified they offer a rich source of information as to how the treatment program should proceed.

One avenue for compensatory support in LD children is the use of computer technology. Many technologies exist to support the child with LDs and are very helpful, but their proper application requires a thorough understanding of the child's entire profile. For example, for some children for whom written language is difficult, the use of a word processor and keyboarding are indicated. However, if this same child, has demonstrated difficulties with psychomotor processing and fine motor development yet has well-developed sequencing and organizational skills, he or she would likely benefit more from developing dictation skills that allow him or her to use voice-to-print systems. Without this level of information about the child's strengths and concomitant weaknesses, however, he or she might be prescribed a keyboarding class—and time that could be spent teaching dictation skills would be lost.

A similar situation exists with the use of accommodations for testing. Many students with LDs request extended time on testing, meaning they are given additional time to complete standardized measures (such as the Stanford Achievement Testing). For many students, however, this accommodation is not the most appropriate. An impulsive student with poor reading skills may not use the extended time, and would be better served by the accommodation of having a proctor sit with him or her and read the items aloud. This second intervention strategy will address both the student's impulsivity and his or her weak reading skills, and represents a true individualized accommodation. In order to arrive at such a specific request, however, information about the student's attention and impulsivity as well as about his or her reading is necessary.

Question 4: How Is the Outcome of "Good Intervention" in Learning Disabilities Best Measured?

Although there are many benefits to using a neuropsychological assessment in diagnosing and creating treatment plans for LDs, there also are concerns about this level of assessment. A neuropsychological assessment typically is very costly, given the advanced training of the neuropsychologist and the amount of time required to complete it. The number of tests administered also raises concerns, especially in the case of child assessment, as some may be too long for some children. The question of the length of the exam raises the question of whether the time required justifies the additional information yielded.

We have not located any studies comparing the cost-effectiveness of neuropsychological assessment to a more traditional psychoeducational evaluation. In beginning to approach how one might study such a comparison, we developed a questionnaire that was mailed to parents of children who had received both psychoeducational evaluations and neuropsychological assessments. The purpose of this exercise was to explore the kinds of questions that might be pertinent to such a comparison, the attitudes of the parents queried, the actual costs incurred in each evaluation, and the perceived value of each type of assessment. Value included both actual savings (through a decrease in services or more economical use of services due to more focused interventions) and projected savings (through a discussion of what other services or costs might have been incurred had early identification and treatment not taken place).

These questions were addressed in an 11-page questionnaire that included short-answer items asking for itemized costs of each type of assessment, Yes/No columns querying specific domains assessed by each type of assessment, Likert scales examining specific ways in which the assessment was or was not valuable to the diagnostic and treatment planning process, and open-ended questions about actual savings (a description of services and actual money saved) and projected savings.

This project was done in order to create a beginning point for future studies through gathering information about the areas listed above, and through identifying attitudes of parents about completing such a form. The parents of five children who had been assessed using both approaches were contacted by phone, and all expressed an interest in participating. They then were sent the questionnaire and asked to complete and return it to the examiners. The neuropsychological assessment of all five families had been done by the first author; so, given that the completed forms were not anonymous, there was a clear bias present. Perhaps not surprising given this bias, the results of the questionnaires indicated far more appreciation for the neuropsychological assessment over the psychoeducational assessment. Additionally, for all of the families who were sent forms, the neuropsychological assessment had been specifically sought out because the parents were not satisfied that the information gleaned from the psychoeducational assessment was sufficient. Obviously, future studies should involve families for whom this bias is controlled through random selection of those who receive both types of assessment and are then queried about them.

Despite these biases, some interesting findings were noted. The first was that the parents had a great deal of difficulty completing the questionnaire. Although all were initially open to participating, and some even stated considerable interest in having an opportunity to express themselves in this forum, only two families ultimately completed the questionnaire, despite significant follow-up from the first author. This may have been due, in part, to the length of the questionnaire as well as to the inclusion of open-ended questions regarding the projected savings resulting from the exam. Because the first author had not received responses, despite phone calls several weeks after the questionnaires had been distributed, she offered to change the format to include a phone interview in which parents could discuss the differences orally. None of the families responded to this offer and, in the end, only two families completed the questionnaire (although for one family the mother and father each completed a questionnaire independently).

Thus, one of the findings from this project was that parents, initially eager, were ultimately reticent about participating. When asked about this reticence, the families commented on the amount of time it took to complete the more open-ended questions, as well as on how difficult it was to state how their children's futures may have been changed by the assessment. Unlike situations in adult neuropsychology where specific outcomes (such as time of return to work or savings from being able to pursue specific jobs) can be assessed, the effect of a thorough neuropsychology assessment on the ultimate outcome of a child's life is far less clear and is impacted by many additional variables.

Results of the three questionnaires collected are reported in Table 13.4. Family A completed one questionnaire about their 6-year-old son who had previously been diagnosed with hypotonia and developmental delays. Results of the neuropsychological assessment indicated that he did not present with autism but, rather, struggled with fine motor delays, attention deficit hyperactivity disorder, and early academic problems. Family B completed two questionnaires (one from each parent) regarding their 12-year-old son, who was previously diagnosed with speech and language delays and a specific LD. Results of the neuropsychological assessment indicated ongoing severe difficulties in both of these domains, despite significant classroom-based interventions.

The results shown in Table 13.4 support the impression that the neuropsychological assessment costs the family more, especially if the psychoeducational evaluation is provided free of charge by the school district. Additionally, the neuropsychological assessment does not necessarily save the family money in the short run. For one family it translated into additional private services (increased occupational therapy), thereby increasing the financial output for the family and the insurance company. In the case of the school district approving tuition for attendance at a school for students with special needs, however, there were considerable annual savings for the family ($46,000 annually).

Although more costly, both families stated that the neuropsychological assessment provided more thorough assessment of domains. Interestingly, the families both indicated that a more thorough assessment of academic achievement had been provided by the neuropsychological assessment, despite the assumption that the school psychologist might have received more training in the assessment of academic domains.

Both families indicated that the neuropsychological assessment described their child's

TABLE 13.4 Results of Cost-Efficiency Questionnaire

Cost of Assessment			
Psychoeducational Evaluation		Neuropsychological Assessment	
Family A	Family B	Family A	Family B
Done by school district	Done by school district	$2,135.00	$2,849.00
No cost to family	No cost to family		

Domains Assessed			
Psychoeducational Evaluation		Neuropsychological Assessment	
Family A	Family B	Family A	Family B
Cognitive domains	Memory/language	Cognitive domains	Cognitive domains
Minimal academic	Minimal academic	Full academic	Full academic
Social/emotional	No social/emotional	Social/emotional	Social/emotional

Value of Each Type of Assessment
(Average score for each question is reported, lower score is more favorable.)

Question	Psychoeducational	Neuropsychological
Child's learning difficulties described in detail?	6.33	2.66
Other diagnoses ruled out?	1	5.0
Clear guidance for treatment planning?	6.33	1.66
Specific guidance for MD?	7.33	2.66
Specific guidance for teacher	8.5	3.00
Specific guidance for educational therapist	6.0	2.0**
Specific guidance for language therapist/OT?	7.0**	2.75**

Actual Savings	
Family A	Family B
Cost to family was increased as additional OT was added to treatment plan.	Child was funded by school district for nonpublic school tuition due to increased information provided by neuropsychology exam.
Additional cost: $60.00/week	Actual savings: $46,000/year

learning difficulties in greater detail than did the psychoeducational assessment. Additionally, they stated that more clear guidance for treatment planning both in general and to specific providers was offered by the neuropsychological assessment. The question of which assessment made a more clear differential diagnosis yielded interesting results. Family A indicated that only the psychoeducational evaluation ruled out autism, although the neuropsychologist's report expressed the opinion that the child did not present with autism (contrary to a prior diagnosis of developmental delays made by the school district). Family B indicated that no differential diagnoses were ruled out by either assessment.

The question of projected savings of either assessments yielded qualitative responses by both families. Family A reported that the information gleaned from the neuropsychological assessment, over and above the psychoeducational assessment, helped them make the decision to provide their child with medication for an attention deficit disorder, which they believed was improving his participation in all aspects of his treatment, thereby improving his prognosis. These parents also reported that the additional information provided by the neuropsychological assessment allowed their son to maintain his level of special services provided by the school district, which represented a change from their earlier stance to decrease services.

Family B stated that the neuropsychological assessment played an important role in obtaining funding for special schooling for their son. They stated that the provision of this new learning environment had greatly lessened their son's need for more intensive intervention in the future. They said they believed that, without his transfer to the special school, he would have become increasingly depressed, possibly requiring medication in the future; he would have become increasingly oppositional; and he would not have been able to consider higher levels of education. They also stated that their belief that he would have needed more intensive vocational support in the future without the interventions he was now receiving. They also reported a "happier and more cohesive home environment" as a result of his increased support at school.

Thus, results of the project suggest a few starting points for future research (see Table 13.5). One quasi-experimental approach would be to identify several families who have had a psychoeducational evaluation and another group whose children have undergone a neuropsychological assessment, and give both groups a questionnaire querying the actual costs, the information gleaned, the usefulness of the information for treatment planning, and the actual and projected savings stemming from the assessments. Given the difficulty with completing the lengthy questionnaires, the information should be gathered either through a simpler, more objective instrument or through an interview approach. Another approach would be to identify a small group of students who would receive both types of assessment at different times, and then do a comparison of the perceived value of each approach. A third approach would be identify two groups of children receiving either one type of assessment or the other, and follow them longitudinally for 2 to 3 years to determine the ongoing usefulness of the information for treatment planning.

A second issue that could be addressed using cost-efficiency studies would be the cost or benefit of the discrepancy model in identifying students with LDs. One such study might include having a neuropsychological assessment done on students already identified using the discrepancy model and adapting treatment using the added information, and then compare these students' outcomes with students who do not receive the additional assessment. Such a project would quantify how much added advantage there is in the information offered by the additional neuropsychological testing.

Thus, many approaches to validating the cost-efficiency of neuropsychological assessments are available and could be done to further inform education departments about the advantages of having more rather than less information available on their students' learning profiles.

☐ Conclusion

Outcomes of students with LDs have consistently been found to be poor and include chronic learning problems, difficulties with attaining higher levels of education, and

TABLE 13.5. Areas of Potential Research in Cost-Efficiency of Neuropsychological Assessment for Learning Disabilities

- Query parents of children receiving either psychoeducational or neuropsychological evaluations regarding actual costs, usefulness of the information for treatment planning, and actual and projected savings stemming from the assessments.
- Give both types of assessment to randomly selected children over a 2-year period and then compare perceived value (of parent, child, and school) of the information gleaned from each assessment.
- Administer either psychoeducational or neuropsychological assessment to randomly selected children and then follow their rate of progress over a few years to determine impact of treatment planning.
- Administer additional neuropsychological instruments to students identified as learning disabled using traditional discrepancy model and adapt treatment plan based on additional information learned from neuropsychological testing. Compare these children's progress to children who did not receive additional neuropsychological testing after a 1-year period.

(in some cases) substance abuse and criminal behavior (Satz et al., 1998). Given these data, it is imperative that children with LDs be identified and given the treatment necessary for them to participate in optimal living. This chapter has sought to describe a few of the key issues in the LD field, including use of the discrepancy model in making diagnoses, strengths and weaknesses of psychoeducational versus neuropsychological assessments, and practical application of information gleaned from thorough assessment to treatment decisions. The chapter also described an introductory project about how a cost-efficiency study regarding the neuropsychological assessment of students with suspected LDs might be done. Given the concerns about outcome for these students, studies of how best to arrive at the proper diagnosis and treatment plan are of great importance.

☐ References

APA Online: Division 16-School Psychology. (2002). www.apa.org/about/division/div16.html

APA Online: Division 16-School Psychology: Goals and Objectives. (2002). www.indiana.edu/˜div16/G&O.html

APPCN Association of Postdoctoral Programs in Clinical Neuropsychology, Directory 2000–2002. http://www.appcn.org, (1–2).

Adams, K. M., & Rourke, B. P. (Eds.), (1992). *TCN guide to professional practice in clinical neuropsychology*. Berwyn, PA: Swetz-Zeitlinger.

American Psychiatric Association. (1994). *Diagnostic and statistical manual of mental disorders* (4th ed.). Washington, DC: Author.

Anderson, V. A., & Taylor, H. G. (2000). Meningitis. In K .O. Yeats, M. D. Ris, & H. G. Taylor (Eds.), *Pediatric neuropsychology research, theory, and practice* (pp. 117–148). New York: Guilford Press.

Bookheimer, S. Y., Zeffiro, T. A., Blaxton, T., Gaillard, W., & Theodore, W. (1995). Regional cerebral blood flow during object naming and word reading. *Human Brain Mapping, 3*, 93–106.

Buka, S. L., Satz, P., Seidman, L., & Lipsitt, L (1999). Defining learning disabilities: The role of longitudinal studies. *Thalamus, 16*(2), 14–27.

Chalfant, J. C. (1989). Diagnostic criteria for entry and exit from service: A national problem. In L. B. Silver (Ed.), *The assessment of learning disabilities: Preschool through adulthood* (pp. 1–25). Austin, TX: PRO-ED.67

Culbertson, J. L., & Edmonds, J. E. (1996). Learning disabilities. In R. L. Adams, O. A. Parsons, J. L. Culbertson, & S. J. Nixon (Eds.), *Neuropsychology for clinical practice* (pp. 331–408). Washington, DC: American Psychological Association.

Duara, R., Kushch, A., Gross-Glenn, K., Barker, W. W., Jallad, B., Pascal, S., Loewenstein, D. A., Sheldon, J., Rabin, J., Levin, B., & Lubs, H. (1991). Neuroanatomic differences between dyslexic and normal readers on magnetic resonance imaging scans. *Archives of Neurology, 48,* 410–416.

Eden, G .F, VanMeter, J. W., Rumsey, J. M., Maisog, J. M., Woods, R. P., & Zeffiro, T. A. (1996). Abnormal processing of visual motion in dyslexia revealed by functional brain imaging. *Nature, 382,* 6–69.

Fletcher, J. M. (1998). IQ-discrepancy: An inadequate and iatrogenic conceptual model of learning disabilities. *Perspectives, 24*(1), 10–11.

Fletcher, J. M., Espy, K. A., Francis, D. J., Davidson, K. C., Rourke, B. P., & Shaywitz, S. E. (1989). Comparisons of cutoff and regression-based definitions of reading disabilities. *Journal of Learning Disabilities, 22,* 334–335.

Fletcher, J. M., Ewing-Cobbs, L., Miner, M. E., Levin, H. S., & Eisenberg, H. M. (1990). Behavioral changes after closed head injury in children. *Journal of Consulting and Clinical Psychology, 58,* 93–98.

Fletcher, J. M., Satz, P., & Morris, R. (1984). The Florida Longitudinal Project: A review. In S. Mednick, Harway, & K. M. Finnello (Eds.), *Handbook of longitudinal research* (pp. 233–258). New York: Praeger.

Fletcher, J. M., Shaywitz, S. E., Shankweiler, D. P., Katz, L., Liberman, I. Y., Stuebing, K. K., Francis, D. J., Fowler, A. E., & Shaywitz, B. A. (1994). Cognitive profiles of reading disability: Comparisons of discrepancy and low achievement definitions. *Journal of Educational Psychology, 86,* 6–23.

Galaburda, A. M., Sherman, G. F., Rosen, G. D., Aboitiz, F., & Geschwind, N. (1985). Developmental dyslexia: Four consecutive patients with cortical anomalies. *Annals of Neurology, 18,* 222–233.

Hack, M., Taylor, H. G., Klein, N., Eiben, R., Schatschneider, C., & Mercuri-Minich, N. (1994). School-age outcomes in children with birth weights under 750 g. *New England Journal of Medicine, 331*(12), 753–759.

Henderson, V. W. (1986). Anatomy of posterior pathways in reading: A reassessment. *Brain and Language, 29,* 119–133.

Hulme, C. (1988). The implausibility of low-level visual deficits as a cause of children's reading difficulties. *Cognitive Neuropsychology, 5,* 369–374.

Humphreys, P., Kaufmann, W. E., & Galaburda, A. M. (1990). Developmental dyslexia in women: Neuropathological findings in three patients. *Annals of Neurology, 28,* 727–738.

Hynd, G. W. (1989). Futures in psychology: Commentary. In M.Fine (Ed.), *School psychology: Cutting edges in research and practice* (pp. 63–65). Washington, DC: National Education Association and National Association of School Psychologists.

Hynd, G. W., Semrud-Clikeman, M., Lorys, A. R., Novey, E. S., & Eliopulos, D., (1991). Corpus callosum morphology in developmental dyslexia and attention deficit-hyperactivity disorder (ADHD): Morphometric analysis of MRI. *Journal of Learning Disabilities, 24,* 141–146.

Kaplan, E. (1988). A process approach to neuropsychological assessment. In T. Boll & B. K. Bryant (Eds.), *Clinical neuropsychology and brain function: Research, measurement, and practice* (pp. 125–167). Washington, DC: American Psychological Association..

Keogh, B. (1988). Improving services for problem learners: Rethinking and restructuring. *Journal of Learning Disabilities, 21*(1), 19–22.

Larsen, J. P., Hoien, T., & Odegaard, H. (1992). Magnetic resonance imaging of the corpus callosum in developmental dyslexia. *Cognitive Neuropsychology, 9,* 123–134.

Lezak, M. D. (1995). *Neuropsychological assessment* (3rd ed.). New York: Oxford University Press.

Lindamood C. H., & Lindamood, P. C. (1984). *Auditory discrimination in depth*. Austin, TX: PROED, Inc.

Lovegrove, W, Martin, F., & Slaghuis, W. (1986). A theoretical and experimental case for a visual deficit in specific reading disability. *Cognitive Neuropsychology, 3,* 225–267.

Martin, F., & Lovegrove, W. (1988). Uniform field flicker masking in control and specifically-disabled readers. *Perception, 17,* 203–214.

Martin, J. D. (1998). The individuals with disabilities education act's (IDEA) coming of age in the Congress. *Perspectives of the International Dyslexia Association, 24*(1), 28–29.

Merzenich, M. M., Jenkins, W. M., Johnson, P., Schreiner, C., Miller, S. L., & Tallal, P. (1996). Temporal processing deficits of language-learning impaired children ameliorated by training. *Science, 5*(271), 77–81.

Morgan, W. P. (1896). A case of congenital word blindness. *British Medical Journal, 2,* 1378.

Morris, R. D., Krawiecki, N. S., Kullgren, K. A., Ingram, S. M., & Kurczynski, B. (2000). Brain tumors. In K. O. Yeats, M. D. Ris, & H. G. Taylor (Eds.), *Pediatric neuropsychology research, theory, and practice* (pp. 74–91). New York: Guilford Press.

Morris, R. D., Stubing, K. K., Fletcher, J. M., Shaywitz, S. E., Lyon, G. R, Shankweiler, D. P., Katz, L., Francis, D. J., & Shaywitz, B. A. (1992). Subtypes of reading disability: Variability around a phonological core. *Journal of Educational Psychology, 90*(3), 347–373.

Orton, S. T. (1937). *Reading, writing, and speech problems in children.* New York: W. W. Norton.

Orton S. T. (1928). Specific reading disability-Strephosymbolia. *Journal of the American Medical Association,* 90, 1095–1099.

Pennington, B. F. (1995). Genetics of learning disabilities. *Journal of Child Neurology, 10,* S69–S77.

Pennington, B. F. (1991). *Diagnosing learning disorders: A neuropsychological framework.* New York: Guilford Press.

Petersen, S. E., Fox, P. T., Posner, M. I., Mintun, M., & Raichle, M. E. (1988). Positron emission tomographic studies of the processing of single words. *Journal of Cognitive Neuroscience, 1,* 153–170.

Prigatano, G. (2002). Health care economics and clinical neuropsychology. In G. Prigatano & N. Pliskin (Eds.), *Clinical neuropsychology and cost outcome research: A beginning.* New York: Psychology Press.

Reed, H. B. C. (1979). Biological defects and special education: An issue in personnel preparation. *The Journal in Special Education, 13*(1), 9–33.

Reports of the INS-Division 40 task force on education, accreditation, and credentialing (1987). *The Clinical Neuropsychologist, 1*(1), 29–34.

Reynolds, C. R. (1989). Biological bases of behavior and school psychology: Riches or ruin? In M. Fine (Ed.), *School psychology: Cutting edges in research and practice.* Washington, DC: National Education Association and National Association of School Psychologists.

Rodgers, B. (1983). The identification and prevalence of specific reading retardation. *British Journal of Educational Psychology, 53,* 369–373.

Rourke, B. P. (1994). Neuropsychological assessment of children with learning disabilities: Measurement issues. In G. R. Lyon (Ed.), *Frames of reference for the assessment of learning disabilities.* Baltimore: Brookes.

Rumsey, J. M. (1996). Neuroimaging in developmental dyslexia: A review and conceptualization. In G. R. Lyon & J. M. Rumsey (Eds.), *Neuroimaging: A window to the neurological foundations of learning and behavior in children* (pp. 57–77). Baltimore: Brookes.

Rutter, M., & Yule, W. (1975). The concept of specific reading retardation. *Journal of Child Psychology and Psychiatry, 16,* 181–197.

Sattler, J. M. (1992). *Assessment of children.* San Diego: Jerome M. Sattler.

Satz, P. (Principal Investigator). (1970-1979). *Specific developmental dyslexia: A longitudinal study.* Washington DC: National Institute of Health grant (MH19415).

Satz, P., Taylor, H. G., Friel, J., & Fletcher, J. M. (1978). Some developmental and predictive precursors of reading disabilities: A six-year follow-up. In F. Pirozzolo & J. Wittrock (Eds.), *Dyslexia: A critical appraisal of current theory* (pp. 313–347). New York: Academic Press.

Satz, P., Buka, S., Lipsitt, L, & Seidman, L. (1998). The long-term prognosis of learning disabled children. In B. K. Shapiro, J. A. Pasquale, & A. J. Capute (Eds.), *Specific reading disability: A view of the spectrum* (pp. 223–250). Timonium, MD: York Press.

Seidenberg, M. S., & McClelland, J. L. (1989). Visual word recognition and pronunciation: A computational model of acquisition, skilled performance, and dyslexia. In A. M. Galaburda (Ed.), *From reading to neurons* (pp. 255–303). Cambridge, MA: MIT Press.

Shaw, S. F., Cullen, J. P., McGuire, J. M., & Brinckerhof, L. C. (1995). Operationalizing a definition of learning disabilities. *Journal of Learning Disabilities, 28*(9), 586–597.

Shaywitz, S. E., Escobar, M. D., Shaywitz, B. A., Fletcher, J. M., & Makuch, R. (1992). Evidence that dyslexia may represent the lower tail of a normal distribution of reading ability. *The New England Journal of Medicine, 326*(3), 145–150.

Shaywitz, S. E., Shaywitz, B. A., Fletcher, J.M., & Escobar, M.D. (1990). Prevalence of reading disability in boys and girls. *Journal of the American Medical Association, 264,* 998–1002.

Shaywitz, S. E., Shaywitz, B. A., Pugh, K. R., Skudlarski, P., Fulbright, R. K., Constable, R. T., Bronen, R. A., Fletcher, J. M., Liberman, A. M., Shankweiler, D. P. Katz, L., Lacadie, C., Marchione, K. E., & Gore, J. C. (1996). The neurobiology of developmental dyslexia as viewed through the lens of functional magnetic resonance imaging technology. In G. R. Lyon & J. M. Rumsey (Eds.), *Neuroimaging: A window to the neurological foundations of learning and behavior in children* (pp. 79–94). Baltimore: Brookes.

Siegel, L. (1998). The discrepancy formula: Its use and abuse. In B. K. Shapiro, J. A. Pasquale, & J. Capute (Eds.), *Specific reading disability: A view of the spectrum* (pp. 123-135). Timonium, MD: York Press.

Siegel, L. (1989). The development of working memory in normally achieving and subtypes of learning disabled children. *Child Development, 60,* 973–980.

Siegel, L. S. & Himel, N. (1998). Socioeconomic status, age, and the classification of dyslexia and poor readers: The dangers of using IQ scores in the definition of reading disability. *Dyslexia.*

Silva, P. A., McGee, R., & Williams, S. (1985). Some characteristics of nine year old boys with general reading backwardness or specific reading retardation. *Journal of Child Psychology and Psychiatry, 26,* 407–421.

Smith, S. D., Brower, A. M., Cardon, L. R., & DeFries, J. C. (1998). Genetics of reading disability. Further evidence for a gene on chromosome 6. In B. K. Shapiro, P. J. Accardo, & A. J. Capute (Eds.), *Specific reading disability: A view of the spectrum* (pp. 63–74). Timonium, MD: York Press.

Stanovich, K. E. (1986). Matthew effects in reading: Some consequences of individual differences in the acquisition of literacy. *Reading Research Quarterly, 21,* 7–29.

Stanovich, K. E., & Siegel, L. S. (1994). Phenotypic performance profile of children with reading disabilities: A regression-based test of the phonological-core variable-difference model. *Journal of Educational Psychology, 86,* 24-53.

Studdert-Kennedy, M., & Mody, M. (1995). Auditory temporal perception. Deficits in the reading-impaired: A critical review of the evidence. *Psychonomic Bulletin and Review, 2,* 508–514.

Tallal, P., Miller, S., & Fitch, R. H. (1993). Neurobiological basis of the case for the preeminence of temporal processing. In P. Tallal, A. M. Galaburda, R. R. Linas, & C. von Euler (Eds.), *Temporal information processing in the nervous system: Special reference to dyslexia and dysphasia* (pp. 27–47). New York: New York Academy of Sciences.

Temple, E., Poldrack, R. A., Protopapas, A., Nagarajan, S., Salz, T., Tallal P., Merzenich, M. M., & Gabrieli, J. D. (2000). Disruption of the neural response to rapid acoustic stimuli in dyslexia: Evidence from functional MRI. *Proceedings of the National Academy of Science, USA, 200*(25), 13907–13912.

Taylor, H. G. (1988). Neuropsychological testing: Relevance for assessing children's learning disabilities. *Journal of Consulting and Clinical Psychology, 56*(6), 795–800.

Torgerson, J. K. (1998). Instructional interventions for children with reading disabilities. In B. K. Shapiro, J. A. Pasquale, & A. J. Capute (Eds.), *Specific reading disability: A view of the spectrum* (pp. 197–220). Timonium, MD: York Press.

United States Office of Education. (1968). *First annual report of the national advisory committee on handicapped children.* Washington, DC: U.S. Department of Health, Education, and Welfare.

Wagner, R. K., & Torgerson, J. K. (1987). The nature of phonological processing and its causal role in the acquisition of reading skill. *Psychological Bulletin, 101,* 193–212.

Waters, G. S., & Seidenberg, M. S. (1985). Spelling-sound effects in reading: Time-course and decision criteria. *Memory and Cognition, 13,* 557–572.

PART

VII

REHABILITATION, PSYCHOTHERAPY, AND PATIENT MANAGEMENT

14

CHAPTER

Leonard Diller
Yehuda Ben-Yishay

The Clinical Utility and Cost-Effectiveness of Comprehensive (Holistic) Brain Injury Day-Treatment Programs

Introduction

An understanding of a brain injury day-treatment program (BIDTP), which is comprehensive or holistic in focus, may be approached on four levels: first, by a formal statement defining the major features of a BIDTP; second, by the way patients spend time in treatment; third, by the key process features of a program that define and drive its goals; and fourth, by the insights provided by a case demonstration. In this chapter we first explain the nature of a BIDTP in terms of the different levels and then examine issues of utility–outcomes and costs.

A formal definition helps in setting the unique features and characteristics of a program. Patient time usage is a form of accountability to look at a dimension of program participation. For example, Medicare has a 3-hour rule to provide a standard for the amount of treatment time in a given day for an inpatient stay in a comprehensive medical rehabilitation program. An institution that does not provide 3 hours a day of therapy is not reimbursed for inpatient services. A process approach enables one to go beyond the formal labeling of therapies and defines more precisely what is being treated, specifying the reason for and the underlying logic of the treatment and how treatment is carried out. We consider each of these levels in turn. A case illustration permits a close-up of some of the subtleties that elude conventional outcome assessments.

Definition of a Holistic Program

Comprehensive holistic neuropsychologic rehabilitation programs offer integrated multimodal treatments that emphasize improvement in self-awareness and acceptance of altered life status along with teaching compensatory skills for adequately coping with residual impairments and disabilities (Malec & Basford, 1996). Because many community reentry and remedial programs claim to be holistic and many day-treatment programs offer multiple therapies that are designed to permit people with disabilities to remain out of institutions, the concept of holistic day treatment maybe ambiguous. A consensus conference in 1994 (Malec & Basford, 1996; Trexler et al., 1994) attempted to define the essential elements of holistic day-treatment programs (see Table 14.1).

The elements to look for in deciding whether a program is holistic are the contents of the program; the organization of the team delivering the contents; the emphasis on

TABLE 14.1. Defining Features of Comprehensive Holistic Day-Treatment Programs*

1. Neuropsychological orientation
   A. Cognitive and meta cognitive impairments
   B. Neurobehavioral impairments
   C. Interpersonal and psychosocial issues
   D. Affective issues
2. Integrated treatment
   A. Formal staff meetings
   B. Team leader who manages for each patient
   C. Program or team leader with at least 3 years of experience in traumatic brain injury rehabilitation
   D. Integrated goal setting and monitoring
   E. Transdisciplinary staff roles
3. Group treatment
   A. Awareness
   B. Acceptance
   C. Social pragmatics
4. Dedicated resources
   A. An identified team core
   B. Dedicated space
   C. A patient staff ratio no greater than 2:1
5. Neuropsychologist part of the treatment team, not just a consultant
6. Formal and informal opportunities to involve significant others on a weekly basis
7. Inclusion of a dedicated vocational or independent living trial
8. Multiple outcomes assessed
   A. Productive activity
   B. Independent living
   C. Psychosocial adjustment
   D. Emotional adjustment
9. Include dedicated vocational or independent living trial
10. Multiple outcomes

* The elements comprising a holistic program were aggregated to construct a scale. In a survey of 10 holistic programs and 8 programs delivering services in discipline-specific, traditional ways differences between program styles were noted (Malec and Basford, 1996)

a peer-group approach (and the therapeutic community), which provides the context, or milieu, within which learning takes place; a commitment of resources needed to foster and reinforce therapeutic interventions; a need for systematic and meaningful family or significant other involvement; a deliberate and concerted effort to relate the treatment to the patient's functional (real life) experiences; and a concern with measuring outcomes that span several domains of the individual's life, including the role of the individual in the family and community and the extent of his or her personal and vocational adjustment.

A holistic program is suited to address the specific needs of patients in postacute rehabilitation settings. Some of the central problems accompanying cognitive deficits due to brain damage are the individual's unawareness of problems, failure to acknowledge limitations resulting from the brain damage, and inability to take advantage of the remedial steps toward the correction of functionally incapacitating deficits due to problems in malleability. Unawareness is closely tied to problems in acquiring compensatory skills and learning to live with limitations; to cooperate with a program; and to accept of the premise that rehabilitation is about learning to compensate for deficiencies in functional life, rather than seeking total restitution. Part of the rehabilitation process, therefore, includes education about the nature of the deficits and their impact on the person's functional life. In a holistic program, the problem that may be first brought to the person's attention and singled out for remedial intervention also is given careful consideration. Usually, it is that basic neuropsychologic disorder (e.g., problems in initiation or impulse control, an attentional disorder, or a socially inappropriate behavior) that lends itself most easily to amelioration, so a relatively quick "learning curve" can be achieved and thus demonstrate to the person that problems can be overcome. A second consideration in deciding which of the person's deficits to single out for early remediation is whether successful amelioration of this first problem increases the chances that the person's other, higher-level cognitive and neurobehavioral problems will become accessible to systematic remedial and therapeutic intervention.

Budgeting Treatment Time in Holistic Rehabilitation

How a person budgets available resources is a practical translation of his or her values and priorities in life. In rehabilitation, how time is used (i.e., how time is allocated for specific program elements and the way these elements are coordinated) is a practical expression of the program's philosophy. There are, as yet, no formal data on time usage in comprehensive holistic programs. But a review by Trexler (2000) of a number of programs described by Caetano and Christensen (2000); Christensen (2000); Daniels-Zide and Ben-Yishay (2000); Klonoff et al. (2000); Malec, Smigielski, DePompolo, and Thompson (1993); Prigatano et al. (1984); Trexler (2000); and Wilson et al. (2000) and reveals that a typical holistic program operates 4 to 5 hours a day, 3 to 5 days a week, with durations of a treatment cycle ranging from 4 to 8 months. Some programs have fixed time intervals; others have great individual variability. Malec and Moessner (2000) reported a mean duration of 179.8 days, with a range from 53 to 297 days. On the other hand, the NYU-RUSK (Daniels-Zide & Ben-Yishay, 2000) day program offers a treatment cycle (5 hours a day, 4 days a week) amounting to a minimum of 400 hours of treatment over a 5-month period. The 400 hours of a typical cycle of treatment are broken down as follows:

- Participants spend 40 hours (10%) in daily orientation and systematic training to recognize their deficits, to understand the rationale for the remedial training, and to formulate practical behavioral goals on how to compensate for these problems Trainees spend 120 hours (30%) in small-group cognitive therapeutic exercises designed to foster adequate interpersonal communications skills, and acceptance of their predicament and limitations, and to improve self-esteem.
- They spend 120 hours (30%) on individual cognitive remedial training to help attain mastery, habituation, and transfer of compensatory skills into their functional repertoire.
- They spend 40 hours (10%) in group communal (i.e., all trainees, their significant others, and the staff) reviews of accomplishments and restatements of the philosophy of rehabilitation.
- And 80 hours (20%) are devoted to individual counseling, including family sessions.

These program components are coordinated so as to allow for maximum reinforcement of the remedial-therapeutic activities that take place in any of the formally designated time allocations. The groups (i.e., the larger community or the smaller, ad hoc groupings based on clinical considerations) serve as communities of supporting and validating peers, role models, and constructive critics. When participants complete a cycle, 50% to 60% typically are recommended for a second cycle of remedial training; another 20% advance to a work trial consisting of placement in real work situations with careful monitoring and supervision until they are deemed employable; the remainder may be discharged to continue studies or work in their places of residence.

All programs emphasize significant amounts of time in group along with individual treatment. The variations in time budgets in holistic day-treatment programs depend on local circumstances and the relative emphases placed on different program features. Some programs introduce work trials in the initial intensive remedial phase of treatment, or allocate more time for work trials (Christensen, 2000; Prigatano et al., 1984); some use more discipline-specific skills, such as speech therapy (Klonoff et al., 2000); some devote a major portion of time to motoric components of activities of daily living, aimed at improving home independence (Klonoff, 2000; Trexler, Eberle, & Zappala, 2000); and other programs (Daniels-Zide & Ben-Yishay, 2000) commence the work trials after the program trainee has completed the intensive remedial phase (for one or more cycles) and met the minimum specified requirements.

The Treatment Process

In a holistic program, the goals cannot be separated from the treatment process. Making the trainee aware of the problems that must be compensated for and the rationale for the treatments is an integral part of the process. The treatment process, thus, is designed to explicitly address several important themes, which are essential for its success. These include answering a few key questions: What is being treated at any given time? What problem is being brought to the trainee's awareness, and what must the trainee understand about the nature and functional consequences of the injury? What modalities are used in the treatment, and what is their relevance to the outcomes being sought? How are the cognitive–remedial and psychotherapeutic interventions prioritized and integrated to produce the desired functional improvements?

What Is Being Treated?

Because a major task of cognitive rehabilitation is to make a student out of a patient, it is important that the learner have a clear statement of the problem. In some programs, patients are referred to as trainees or students to identify their roles. Part of the thrust is to optimally engage the trainee in the rehabilitation process and to help him or her become aware of deficits and understand their consequences. Significant effort is exerted to help the trainee explain the problem and provide meaningful instances of its manifestations in his or her functional life. Initially, the trainee may be able to state the problem without fully understanding it or inferring its practical consequences. But acknowledgment of the problem—even though, in the early stages, the trainee's understanding of it may be vague—is necessary. The explicit acknowledgment usually is the first painful step toward its acceptance. The demand that the trainee acknowledge a problem explicitly is accompanied by reassurance from the staff and positive feedback from peers, while making sure the trainee is not being overwhelmed. Making acknowledgment and ownership of the problem possible is thus an important step in the process of neuropsychological rehabilitation. And, to make it possible, it must be one of the priorities in program planning and treatment.

What Theories Guide the Treatment?

A common thrust is a therapeutic approach that attempts to help trainees discover in their personality makeups characteristics (e.g., resilience, persistence, the ability to trust others) they can mobilize to help confront losses and limitations in a palatable way. Drawing on the work of Goldstein (1942, 1959), Ben-Yishay (2000) noted that brain injury affects motivation and emotion as profoundly as cognition. The phenomenology of the person may be altered so that the world is experienced in concrete, stimulus-bound ways, with diminished aspects of higher-level mental life such as abstract and critical evaluative thinking, as well as the ability to empathize or see things from the perspective of others. With altered cognition, a person's coping abilities become tenuous, so that he or she (as an organismic defense) becomes totally oriented to automatically assume a defensive posture aimed at avoiding catastrophic reactions. Failing that, the person often will actually experience a catastrophic reaction, which has all of the characteristics of extreme anxiety. Hence, an integral part of the rehabilitation process (how treatments are delivered and in the way in which they are structured programmatically) is to ensure that trainees do not experience catastrophic responses and (by feeling safe) will gradually relinquish their defensive postures, which impel them to avoid challenges. Other rehabilitation theorists have attempted to elaborate or add to the principles that should guide the processes of a holistic program (Prigatano, 1999).

☐ Presenting the Problem to the Patient

The decision of which problem is first selected for presentation to patients occurs after a complete neuropsychological evaluation, clinical interviews with program candidates and significant others, and in-vivo observations of candidates' behaviors in functional contexts. Since the definition of the problem usually is couched in terms of "the first step toward mastery" and is an integral part of the treatment, the problem must be translated to fit into the trainees' narratives of themselves and their experiences—for who has the problem may be as important as the content of the problem. In most instances there are multiple problems, or some of the problem may be only partially understood, so deciding on which problem to focus the treatment must be weighed carefully. Treatment priorities must be set against the background of the importance and functional relevance of the problem(s), their amenability to treatment, and practical logistics. Problems tend to be formulated to trainees in functional behavioral terms. For example, problems resulting from adynamia or dyscontrol (i.e., dysinhibition) may be respectively characterized as "difficulty initiating thoughts or actions" or "inadequate consideration of how your action may affect others." Similarly, problems resulting from impaired attentional functions may be characterized as "difficulty to focus on the task at hand" or "a difficulty to screen out irrelevant external or internal stimuli/thoughts." And so on.

☐ Major Modalities of Treatment

Therapeutic Milieu

The milieu is perhaps the most critical part of the holistic treatment, in that it creates a safe (i.e., regulated and predictable) environment for the trainees (Ben-Yishay, 2000). The milieu encourages openness and acceptance of limitations, permitting participants to respond nondefensively. It helps to destigmatize ownership and expression of deficits and to assuage the "narcissistic wound" (Klonoff & Lage, 1991) associated with brain injury. It encourages freedom to explore latent skills and supports courageous acts in venturing into activities and experiences that were previously part of the trainee's repertoire or inclinations but have been (defensively) avoided since the brain injury. The milieu provides a dynamic community for people drawn together by the consequences of their respective brain injuries, each with obstacles to be tested and overcome. Both the diversity and the communality of the issues that confront the members enhance the affective reinforcement critical to make the learning experiences significant. A major problem for people who sustain severe disabilities is that of no longer feeling "helpful" (Dembo, Leviton, & Wright, 1956). By concrete demonstration, the milieu provides a platform for people to act helpfully to one another and thus feel helpful. Prigatano (1999) and Christensen (2000) emphasized the value of group attachment and the trust it engenders in the essential contributions of others in a therapeutic milieu in developing effective ways of dealing with complex issues of sorting out hope and reality.

Cognitive Remediation

Cognitive remediation has received a good deal of attention, clinically and scientifically, for the last three decades (Cicerone et al., 2000). The first decision to be made when confronting the issue of whether to treat a cognitive problem is whether a deficit can be remediated, ignored, or compensated for. In holistic rehabilitation, the decision takes place in the context of other treatment considerations: the malleability of the patient; the nature and severity of the cognitive deficit; the patient's understanding of the functional relevance of the treatment; and the patient's capacity as well as tolerance for engaging in intensive and protracted remedial training to produce the necessary habituated compensatory skills—which, alone, can enhance the patient's functional adjustment. Ben-Yishay and Diller (1993) noted that striving for compensatory skills is far more likely to be successful than a direct attack on a deficit. Ben-Yishay, Diller, Gerstman, and Gordon (1970), in line with the more generic philosophy of rehabilitation, presented evidence that "saturated cueing" (i.e., attempts to build skills by minimizing the potential for error) is useful for individuals with severe cognitive deficits. Individuals with severe cognitive deficits may not learn from their mistakes. Similarly, Evans et al. (2000) indicated that error-free learning might be more useful for people with more severe memory deficits and in facilitating retrieval of implicit memory (e.g., names), but may not be the best approach for learning novel associations (e.g., routes or programming a computer). A further important consideration in cognitive remediation is that, for many individuals, the remediation of deficits is not an end in itself. The experience of loss of self-esteem and repeated failure to cope disposes the patient toward restricting, as part of the organismic defense, the full utilization of still-intact abilities; and failing to forestall the occurrence of a catastrophic response will result in the patient feeling overwhelmed. Hence, the guided practice of cognitive remedial tasks, in a small-group format carefully calibrated to optimize information processing, and the gradual build-up the patient's sense of success in engagement in problem-solving tasks, are useful ways of (a) reinforcing the patient's sense of mastery and coping and (b) helping the patient regain the preinjury, (i.e., normal) attitude of welcoming new cognitive and interpersonal challenges, without feeling vulnerable and disposed to automatically assume defensive postures. The dual purposes of cognitive remedial training have been clearly articulated by Ben-Yishay and Prigatano (1990) and Prigatano and Ben-Yishay (1999).

Psychotherapy

Goldstein (1942; 1959) noted the central tasks of psychotherapy with brain-injured persons: making the patient aware of the deficits imposed by the brain injury; helping the person accept the losses, restrictions, and limitations due to diminished capacities; and assisting the patient in finding (new) meaning in life after rehabilitation. Present-day applications of Goldstein's notions in the context of holistic, therapeutic milieu programs have been described by Ben-Yishay & Daniels-Zide (2000) and Prigatano and Ben-Yishay (1999).

Working through the feeling of loss is a familiar theme in psychotherapy. Indeed, some schools of psychotherapy identify the feelings of loss experienced at an early age as being at the core of personality and lifelong adjustment problems. The loss experienced with brain injury, however, poses a somewhat different situation. First, the loss is intrapersonal (i.e., the person experiences it as a shattering blow to his or her sense of self). Second, the loss, although keenly felt, may be hard for the person to grasp because it is filtered through a fragmented cognitive apparatus. Therefore, the patient may be able neither to adequately work through it mentally nor to initiate reparative behavioral steps. Third, the relationship between what is lost (e.g., normalcy of attentional or executive functions, diminished or disrupted skills) and what is experienced by the patient as the loss ("I can't go back to my old job, by which my identity was defined") is hard to reconcile. Hence, mourning the perceived loss (i.e., the loss of the job) blocks the patient's capacity and readiness for seeking or accepting help. In addition, psychotherapy may be difficult because of short attention span or language problems, which may be gross or subtle. With the development and flowering of different schools of psychotherapy (Karasau, 2000), there is recognition that many techniques are common and useful in conducting psychotherapy. There is also recognition that the common desiderata for good candidates to profit from psychotherapy are the experience of a felt need for help, at least some awareness of a problem, and the capacity to develop a trusting relationship. These features apply to individuals with brain damage as well, except for the aforementioned modifications imposed by the sequelae of brain injury. The following case illustrates some of these blends of therapeutic modalities

A Case Illustration: The Usefulness of a Holistic Program

Marge entered our program 4 years after her injury. She was 23 years old at the time. In the setting of our "therapeutic community," Marge underwent two consecutive 20-week cycles of intensive remedial–rehabilitative treatments (September 1993 through July 1994), followed by 12 additional weeks of guided work trials (September through December 1994). Following discharge from active rehabilitation, Marge became competitively employed, earned a college degree (with distinction), established a satisfactory and lasting relationship with a live-in boyfriend, and began pursuing studies toward a graduate degree.

The Injury

On November 16, 1988, at the age of 19, in her freshman year at college, Marge sustained a severe closed head injury in a motor vehicle accident, resulting in left ventricular hemorrhage and punctuate hemorrhages in the frontal and occipital regions of her brain. She was comatose for 9 days, and the duration of the posttraumatic amnesia (PTA) was assessed as 14 days. She emerged with multiple, circumscribed cognitive deficits and with a mild left hemiparesis, indicating that she sustained coup-contrecoup brain injuries in the accident.

Background

Marge was the oldest of three siblings. Her parents had been divorced for years. Marge's father was an active alcoholic; her mother, employed as an office manager, was involved in psychotherapy; and both of Marge's younger siblings were having serious emotional problems, including alcohol and drug abuse. Of all the members of her family, it was Marge who functioned best in all spheres: She excelled academically throughout her primary, high-school, and college years; she abstained totally from alcohol, as well as from other recreational drugs; and she was a star athlete in cross-country (long-distance) running. Marge was socially popular (by virtue of her athletic prowess) but, otherwise, she did not maintain many intimate friendships. She led a disciplined life, dedicated to her studies, to practicing long-distance running, and to helping her working mother care for her siblings and with housekeeping chores.

Conventional Rehabilitation Proves a Failure

Approximately 2 months following her injury, Marge was transferred for inpatient rehabilitation to a well-known rehabilitation center. There, she underwent intensive multimodal rehabilitation for about 7 weeks. After her discharge from inpatient rehabilitation, Marge entered a day program in her state. She attended this day program for nearly 6 months, after which she discharged herself against medical advice, determined to resume her studies at college, where she had been a scholarship student and a star athlete. But, despite her heroic efforts, Marge failed to meet even the minimum requirements of academic life, because of her many cognitive deficits. Greatly discouraged, she was compelled to leave college and return home.

This failure to resume academic life did not persuade Marge to seek further rehabilitation at the day program from which she earlier discharged herself. In the first place, her motivation to leave the program was (as the final report stated) "having difficulty buying into" the notion that rehabilitation was essentially about learning to compensate for rather than achieve a total restitution of, her deficits, and because "she was overwhelmed by everyone telling her what she needs and what to do." Marge, in short, failed to establish the necessary therapeutic alliance with her rehabilitation counselors and rejected, out of hand, their admonition that she apply "the many [compensatory] strategies [she was taught] because she never had to use [such devices] preinjury."

Thus, for 3 years after the failed attempt to resume her academic studies, Marge embarked on a dogged quest to regain both her cognitive competence and her financial independence. She did this on her own, without the help of rehabilitation professionals, because she perceived their "messages" concerning rehabilitation to be a threat to her ego-identity and hence totally unacceptable. Her efforts included spending long hours at the public library, working (part-time) as a cashier at a supermarket, and intermittently auditing some courses at a nearby community college. Her quest, however, proved unrewarding, frustrating, and utterly demoralizing.

Marge Agrees to Enter Our Program

In October of 1992, Marge's attorney, with the active help of her mother, succeeded in persuading Marge to undergo a 2-week evaluation in our program. The hope was that Marge would find the program interesting enough to seek entry. Marge came, observed, and participated in various program activities with a group of peers who were in treatment. She underwent comprehensive testing, which included several remedial probes (designed to assess her ability to benefit from cognitive and interpersonal remedial interventions), and was provided the opportunity to have a series of dialogues with several (articulate and highly motivated) patient–trainees who, prior to their head injuries, were academically trained and highly accomplished professionals in their respective fields. Impressed by what she had seen and heard, Marge agreed to seek entry into our program, if funds for her treatment became available. Nearly 1 year later, her attorney secured a settlement of her legal case, and Marge enrolled promptly into our program.

The Process of Rehabilitation Begins

The scope of this chapter does not permit a detailed account of Marge's ultimate success as a result of her total "immersion" (for a period of 18 months) in our program.

This process involved a series of multifaceted, integrated, mutually reinforcing therapeutic and remedial interventions. These interventions were tailored to Marge's personality and psychological needs, and they were judiciously applied within our holistic, therapeutic-community-type program by exploiting maximally the clinical leverages afforded by it. The following sections selectively summarize the highlights of Marge's gradual transformation, emphasizing those aspects of the process that best illustrate the corrective powers inherent in this approach to neuropsychological rehabilitation.

1. Cognitively, 4 years after her injury, Marge exhibited the following core problems:
   a. She was mildly impulsive, had difficulty modulating her emotional responses, was frequently (organically) irritable, and felt unable to "shake off" her irritability.
   b. She had difficulty concentrating because of her inability to "screen out," at will, irrelevant thoughts.
   c. Her information-processing abilities (speed as well as efficiency) and her communication skills were mildly impaired due to a combination of (mild and subtle) aphasia and her tendency to be a "noisy listener."
   d. Her memory functions were mildly impaired (but only in a circumscribed manner).
   e. Also, her convergent, divergent, and executive higher-level reasoning functions were impaired (mildly and differentially).

These problems were gradually ameliorated by systematic and lengthy cognitive remedial training, once Marge became emotionally committed to the rehabilitation thesis.

2. Interpersonally, Marge initially presented as a somewhat dysphoric, withdrawn, socially uncomfortable person who was extremely self-critical and self-deprecatory. She tended to "bruise" easily when offered constructive criticism, and she found the rehabilitation thesis (i.e., compensation not restitution, with some brain-injury sequelae permanent) difficult to "swallow." She was frightened by and preoccupied with thoughts of "what if" (i.e., questions concerning what her deficits portended for her future).
3. Marge's preinjury ego-identity[1] could be characterized as, "I must keep running and excelling." This image, or "definition," of herself, we surmised, was developed early in her life and served as a bulwark against (what she perceived in her father's and her siblings') loss of self-control, inability to cope, and ultimately failure in life. We felt we understood why Marge—typically a hardworking and persistent person—was earlier unwilling or unable to embrace the rehabilitation thesis: To her, the message of rehabilitation (a process of learning to adjust to misfortune, rather than seeking total restitution) represented an existential threat to her very "existence." Her ego-identity demanded that she return to her previous ability, to be in control, and to excel physically and intellectually. Nothing less was acceptable to her.

Hence, we realized that Marge needed help to achieve a successful transformation from an ego-identity that mandated that she "excel or perish" to a reconstituted ego-identity that would enable her to find satisfaction and meaning in the accomplishments and lifestyle that rehabilitation would make possible.

---

[1]Ego-identity, as conceptualized by Erik Erikson, consists of one's master motive and self-image—the kind of person she felt she *ought* to be.

Emergence of a Reconstituted Ego-Identity

Marge's ultimate success (18 months later) in developing a "new," reconstituted ego-identity was facilitated by a variety of carefully planned, integrated, and timed (a) small-group "exercises," (b) special cognitive interpersonal assignments, and (c) personal counseling. Some key examples of each type of remedial activity are briefly described below:

1. *Group exercises:* In the presence of her peers, significant others, and visiting professionals, Marge participated in several exercises:
   a. *She engaged in special interview exercises.* She was instructed to role-play a psychologist (a member of the program team) and interview "herself," as role-played by a member of the staff. In her interview, Marge, acting as the psychologist, had to follow a carefully scripted and choreographed scenario specifically designed by the staff to confront her (in a carefully "calibrated" fashion, so as not to overwhelm her) with her particular psychological dilemma. In her capacity as "beginning psychologist," Marge had to consult—on camera, in the presence of the entire community—with another member of the staff who was role-playing her senior supervisor. Thus, through the staff person who role-played herself and her intermittent consultations with her supervisor, Marge underwent a step-by-step review, discussion, and working-through of her existential dilemma—as viewed empathetically but objectively by others. At the end of the proceedings, Marge received feedback from all those who attended the sessions on the extent to which she exhibited "grace under fire," her open-mindedness; and her capacity to relate empathetically to her "interviewee" (herself).
   b. *She engaged in guided dialogues with role-model peers.* Such guided dialogues were aimed at providing Marge with opportunities to exchange views with some of her peers, whom she admired for their moral courage, articulateness, and the willingness to examine and ultimately accept their disabilities. Thus, Marge was encouraged to become inspired and to emulate her peers' example.
   c. *She received "oral report cards."* In the presence of the entire community, Marge received interim and final oral report cards from a senior member of the staff. These report cards covered her progress, or the lack of it, in all areas that were critical for her rehabilitation (awareness and understanding, malleability, mastery and application of compensatory strategies, acceptance of her predicament and self, and current competence in managing her affairs and readiness to become productive).
2. *Special cognitive–interpersonal assignments:* As part of her individualized cognitive training, challenged to exercise good membership in the (therapeutic) community, Marge engaged in two more assignments:
   a. *She was assigned to train a particular peer–trainee who needed special coaching in how to conduct himself in various interpersonal situations.* Marge had to exercise in this assignment empathy, sound judgment, exquisite didactic skills, and infinite patience. She was supervised in these activities by a member of the team who provided a critique and a role model, as the occasion warranted.
   b. *She was assigned to act as master of ceremony (MC) during special presentations of her peer group.* Following meticulous preparations and rehearsals, Marge was assigned to act as MC of presentations by her peers and herself to a large audience consisting of members of the trainees' families, friends, and invited professionals.

As the MC, Marge's task was to introduce the speakers and assist those of her peers who forgot their respective assignments or needed assistance in maintaining or regaining their composure. In a word, Marge "ran the show" and had to ensure that everything went smoothly. At a later date, she reviewed during personal counseling her videotaped performance and was impressed by her competence and poise.

3. *Personal counseling functions:* To help her personalize, "work-through," and apply many lessons learned from the group exercises, the cognitive training, and the various special assignments as part of her community membership, Marge and her personal counselor worked assiduously to translate these "lessons" into behavioral templates or resolutions for applying such templates in her daily life away from the program. Included in Marge's regular sessions with her personal counselor were ad-hoc, conjoint sessions with her mother—who, as a result of her own regular participation in the weekly group sessions for the trainees' significant others, had become an ally and enthusiastic endorser of the staff's clinical objectives for Marge.

Outcome

Marge's successful transformation is encapsulated by the following quote from her final program graduation speech, published in a recent article by Ben-Yishay and Daniel-Zide (2000).

> The old me did strive to be successful in what I did. In my preinjury life, I measured [success] on a scale geared for speed and agility. . . . I have had to revise my preinjury "ruler" to a new, more appropriate measurement of success. . . . I will be pleased [making progress] no matter how small [the steps]. . . . I have the hardy strength and strong character of a cross-country runner.

As her statement clearly shows, Marge's struggle to reconstitute her ego identity involved a difficult and painful process: She had, as she put it, to adopt a new yardstick for measuring success in life. This entailed a shift from a competitive view (Was she the best student? The fastest runner?) to a subjective one (i.e., finding meaning and satisfaction in her rehabilitation gains, no matter how small or slow in coming). To make this transformation, Marge invoked two "old" personality attributes ("hardy strength and the strong character of a cross-country runner") which, preinjury, served her competitive drive for excellence and at present help her find meaning in her life. Without the benefit of the holistic therapeutic milieu approach, we submit, Marge would have continued to languish in her former bitter and defeated state.

☐ Is Holistic Rehabilitation Worthwhile?

Holistic rehabilitation emerged during times of great need, such as wartime or with increased civilian auto accidents, when there was great emphasis on fulfilling health needs and attendant social problems created by disease and injury. As multiple needs in health care grew, questions of costs and benefits of all aspects of health care became urgent. Third-party payers imposed cost containment by stipulating limitations on the use of health-care resources and further delimited access to medically necessary treatment. No clear definition was provided for what constituted "medically necessary" treatments, and only minimal provisions were made for catastrophic situations. To accommodate this new development, rehabilitation developed a metric for defining benefit by formulating a vocabulary (impairment, disability, handicap) capable of defining medical necessity in terms of aspects of recovery cast in functional terms. Thus, improvement is indicated by a reduction in dependency (disability) and the facilitation of return to premorbid social roles, or to living with the family, and by returning to work (handicap). Relief of personal burden indicated by reduced disability could be translated into reductions in the costs of the burden (Heinemann et al., 1997), and return to work could be translated into dollars earned and taxes yielded by earnings postrehabilitation. Reports of outcomes of cognitive rehabilitation programs tended to adapt to these dimensions (Wilson, 1997).

We encourage researchers who want to measure the cost-effectiveness of BIDTPs to consider variables listed in Table 14.2.

In addition to the call for limiting the use of health-care resources to medically necessary treatments, there has been a call for evidence-based studies to be used as guides for practice. In order to contain mushrooming federal expenditures on health care, the U.S. government created a special agency within the Public Health Service—the Agency for Healthcare Research and Quality (AHRQ)—to develop guidelines for clinical practice. The guidelines were established by panels of experts who sorted information in terms of (a) levels of scientific evidence derived from published studies demonstrating efficacy of treatments and, where evidence was insufficient, (b) degree of clinical consensus. Evidence-based practice created a paradigm for all professionals who deliver services to support reimbursement when challenged by third-party payers. It has become a driving force in the current health-care marketplace. A number of different models have been advanced to assess the value of the evidence for the benefits of treatment.

Levels of Scientific Evidence for Holistic Rehabilitation

Cicerone et al. (2000) developed a three-tier approach to documenting evidence for cognitive rehabilitation, which was then applied as a guideline for practice in neuropsychological rehabilitation. Level I includes well-designed, clinical prospective trials and prospective quasi-randomized trials. Level II indicates prospective, nonrandomized cohort studies; retrospective, nonrandomized case-controlled studies; and single case designs that permit quantitative comparisons across treatment conditions. Level III includes clinical series without controls or single case design studies with adequate statistical analysis of results. This method of analysis was applied to 15 published stud-

TABLE 14.2. Outcome Measures to Consider When Studying the Cost-Effectiveness of BIDTP Programs Compared to Other Treatment Approaches

- Reduction in dependency (disability)
- Facilitation of return to premorbid social roles or living with the family
- Return to work (handicap) with economic consequences such as dollars earned and taxes paid
- Relief of personal burden indicated by reduced disability

ies of holistic rehabilitation, which were carefully sifted from a large body of literature and evaluated in terms of scientific credibility. One study was Level I, 4 were Level II, and 10 were Level III. All of the studies indicated the usefulness of holistic rehabilitation. After subjecting these published reports to scrutiny with regard to the criteria of evidenced-based practice, it was concluded that the evidence for comprehensive holistic rehabilitation falls short of meeting criteria for a standard of practice (requiring clear evidence from at least two randomized controlled trials), but meets the standard for a recommended practice guideline (positive results from at least one randomized trial). To cite two examples: A Level-I study found that patients receiving either 160 hours of cognitive remediation or merely social support improved their performance on neuropsychological tests and achieved alleviation of their depression, significantly beyond what could be attributed to spontaneous recovery, based on stable, multiple-baseline testing (Ruff & Niemann, 1991). A Level-II study (Rattok et al., 1992) featuring three groups of matched patients with traumatic brain injury who received 400 hours of treatment each found (a) that the group which received more intensive cognitive remediation showed more gains on cognitive tests than the other two groups; (b) that the group which received more intensive training in the area of interpersonal skills showed greater gains in interpersonal areas than the cognitive group; (c) and that the group which received a balance of both trainings (cognitive and interpersonal) showed improvement in both areas. On follow up at 9 months, employment in the open market ranged from 52% (cognitive group) to 78% (social/interpersonal group). Cicerone et al. (2000) recommend that the greatest improvement in overall functioning may occur with combinations of cognitive–remedial and interpersonal therapeutic interventions.

☐ What Kinds of Outcomes Are Assessed in Holistic Rehabilitation?

Holistic programs have reported improvement in a variety of outcome areas, including independent living skills, language, family living, leisure time usage, stable social relationships, mood, quality of life, and living status. Return to work has received the most attention as an outcome measure (Malec & Basford, 1996). In part, this occurs because individuals entering holistic programs generally are seeking solutions for long-term outcomes and behavioral issues that confront families who have lived with patients after discharge from inpatient settings (Evans, 1997). In a sense, these values–shared by families, third-party payers, and trainees–are similar to those of the population at large (Hosack, Malkmus, & Evans, 1991). As a global measure, employment after brain injury has been shown to be strongly associated with a sense of well-being, social integration, and home and leisure activities (O'Neill et al., 1998). Changes on neuropsychological tests, although statistically significant, have yielded only modest results (Rattock et al., 1992; Ruff & Neimann, 1990; Teasdale, Hansen, Gade, & Christensen, 1997). Improvement in neuropsychological test performance does not appear to be the major predictor of gainful employment after BIDTP programs.

It is difficult to assess holistic programs versus other programs regarding outcomes, because patients and services may not be comparable. A review of published literature (Malec & Basford, 1996) compared outcomes of published cases of postacute brain-injury rehabilitation (PABIR; *n* = 856) with non-PABIR (*n* = 796) and found superiority for the PABIR group (71% vs. 53%) regarding employment. A further analysis of the results, comparing 357 patients who received holistic PABIR with 462 who received nonholistic PABIR, found that the largest differences occurred among those who did not return to work (Malec & Basford, 1996). High et al. (1997) reported that patients who were able to participate in an outpatient holistic program or rehabilitation (*n* = 42) showed a higher rate of return to work (65%) than did those who could not participate (*n* =18; 45%)–despite the fact that the two groups were similar on discharge from an inpatient setting. This report is similar to one published a decade earlier (Prigatano et al., 1984).

More recently, Ben-Yishay and Daniels-Zide (2000) pointed to a dimension of outcome that had not been considered previously, but that may lend itself as a way of regarding outcomes from a vantage point that differs from conventional approaches. In addition to traditional indicators of outcome in terms of reductions of disability or handicap, one can look at acceptance of disability as an outcome variable. In a pilot study, graduates of a holistic program who rated highest on acceptance of their disability (i.e., explicitly acknowledging the losses associated with disability with equanimity), while at the same time trying to optimize their functioning, found more meaning in their lives. On follow-up, they felt more productive, reported themselves as more at peace, and had more satisfying social lives and a greater capacity for intimacy. Although there are no data regarding incidence of acceptance following rehabilitation, one might hypothesize that graduates of holistic programs will have a higher acceptance rate than those of other types of interventions. Although the notion of acceptance is presented in a context of the "examined life," it overlaps the idea of quality of life in the sense of subjective reaction to the fit between expectations and achievements (Duggan & Dijkers, 2001).

☐ Cost–Effectiveness

By far the most common concern about the holistic approach is cost (Wilson, 1997), because it is labor-intensive. Some programs operate on a 1:1 staff-to-patient ratio, (Trexler, 2000), some at a 2:1 ratio (Daniels-Zide & Ben-Yishay, 2000), whereas others may have less-intense staff-to-patient ratios. Staff/patient ratios may differ within the same program due to situational fluctuations. For example, a review of staff-to-patient-ratios at the NYU–RUSK program over a 10-cycle period of 5 months per each cycle indicated that, although the number of patients ranged from 8 to 12 per cycle, the number of full-time staff remained the same (5).

A low staff-to-patient-ratio is important, because of the need to devote much time to formulate, implement, and monitor short- and long-term goals in a coordinated fashion. This is necessary to ensure total immersion in the program to magnify the key messages, which the staff conveys to participants, and to deal with resistance and obstacles to their implementation. A parallel concern is how much treatment is needed. This translates into two related questions concerning the intensity and duration of treatment required for optimal outcomes. Although there are no hard and fast rules, most programs offer 4 to 5 hours of treatment, 3 to 5 days a week, for 4 to 6 months. However, in many cases it is difficult to meet such requirements, and treatment is thus offered at less-intense levels, over longer periods of time. For example, at the outpatient department of the Rusk Institute of Rehabilitation Medicine, a less-intensive and modified version of holistic treatment program is offered, ranging from 2 to 8 hours a week. Such a program is delivered to a larger number of participants (120 to 135) and involves 6 months to 2 years in duration, with an average treatment time of 250 hours (Sherr, personal communication, 2000).

Costs and Revenues

Revenues and costs in rehabilitation are considered as proprietary, so comparative information is difficult to obtain. Indeed Cope, Cole, Hall, and Barkan (1991) reported that a large-scale California HMO reneged on an initial agreement to participate in a study comparing persons who received and did not receive postacute care. Insurers are reluctant to come forth with information, saying it is too variable from policy to policy, from case to case, and even from time to time. Gathering cost data is further complicated by the fact that programs typically have multiple payer sources, which negotiate different rates for the same treatments or place different restrictions on treatment, such as the number of treatment sessions they approve. These negotiations are complex and time-consuming. Similarly, collection also is labor- and time-intensive and often does not reflect billings. The calculation of costs also is complicated: direct versus indirect costs; family versus third-party payer costs; long-term versus short-term costs; no wonder, therefore, revenue and cost data lag even further behind outcome data.

The ideal approach, therefore, is to conduct studies that have the capacity to obtain outcomes and costs across subjects. This can generally be obtained where there is a system of care that permits tracking of referrals, services, and follow-up costs. Larsen, Mehlbye, and Gertz (1991) reported on the medical savings following a holistic program in Denmark, in which the program repaid its investment within 3 years after completion. The importance of this issue is seen in an announcement in the *Federal Register* on January 21, 1998. Priority for funding for the 17 programs sponsored by the U.S. Department of Education's National Institute of Disability and Rehabilitation Research (NIDRR) under the Traumatic Brain Injury Model Systems includes the investigation of the efficacy of alternative methods of service delivery interventions after inpatient rehabilitation discharge, and determination of the relationships between cost of care and functional outcomes. Given that there are 17 model system programs in a position to track patients who have completed inpatient rehabilitation, a number of paths of inquiry could be followed. One path would be the formulation of different experimental designs. The second would consist of different ways of measuring costs. A differing design might involve comparing individuals who follow different paths of treatment after discharge from acute rehabilitation based on payer source rather than clinical need. For example, there is a higher probability that patients supported by governmental funds (e.g., Medicaid or Medicare) or by HMOs will be discharged to skilled nursing facilities rather than to holistic rehabilitation programs (Chan et al., in press). High et al. (1997) found that patients attending a holistic outpatient program showed a 65% return-to-work rate, compared with patients who followed alternate path (a 45% return to work). Outcome studies of this type provide golden opportunities to estimate dollars saved as a result of one type of rehabilitation program versus another.

It also should be noted that patients who did not participate in the outpatient program did not differ from those who did clinically; they differed only on the basis of payer source. This type of study—although it involves nonrandom assignment of patients to various types of treatment and is based on retrospective matching of data—yields important findings. Studies of this type also might yield data on vocational and living arrangements, which are the major concerns of publicly funded programs. For holistic programs, it is important to focus on the study of psychological constructs such as acceptance and life satisfaction. Corrigan, Smith-Knapp, and Granger (1998) found that a measure of life satisfaction in a follow-up of persons with traumatic brain injury showed a fluctuation in "life satisfaction" over time. One measure of benefits is an indicator expressed as *years of healthy life*. A year of healthy life is a year of freedom from symptoms or health problems (Kaplan, 1993). Years of healthy life can be used to provide meaningful units of health outcomes, which could, in turn, be translated into costs. Controlled studies with random assignment can provide reliable data on costs. Such studies usually occur within a common payer source and require the ability to randomize treatment and control groups in advance.

Measuring payer costs can be approached in different ways:

1. Programs with large numbers of subjects who are government-funded, can trace outcomes and actual payments for treatments using Medicaid and Medicare databases. The advantage of this approach is that one can measure actual costs. The disadvantage is that this measures only one aspect of costs for a delimited but significant population.
2. Direct costs also can be ascertained by combining information on costs and services received in a given month (McKenzie, Shapiro, & Siegel, 1998). Indirect costs can be approximated by calculating lost wages, lost wages of caregivers and cost of public assistance. This methodology draws on the emerging field of lifetime care planning (Max, Rice, & McKenzie, 1991).

☐ Conclusions

Although definitive data are still lacking, it is possible to draw the following inferences from existing information:

1. Comprehensive holistic neuropsychological rehabilitation programs are empirically supported.
2. Holistic programs are most useful for dealing with behavioral, personal adjustment, and vocational issues, particularly when there is an interaction among multiple cognitive, neurobehavioral and psychosocial factors.
3. Holistic programs are the most likely vehicle for reestablishing a person's ego-identity, including helping the individual find meaning and personal satisfaction in life after rehabilitation.
4. Although the costs of such programs are difficult to determine—hence, their cost-effectiveness is hard to demonstrate—positive evidence is beginning to appear.

Table 14.3 briefly lists the clinical utility of such programs.

TABLE 14.3. Clinical Utility of Holistic BIDTPs

- Provides a therapeutic environment that allows for a clear identification of problems imposed by brain injury.
- Coordinated staff activities help patients improve self-awareness, acceptance, and the use of practical compensation techniques on the effects of brain injury.
- Helps patients reestablish meaning in life with often reported increased percentages of productive lifestyle.
- Often helps patients return to work when traditional rehabilitation programs have failed.
- Allows for families to have a greater appreciation of the affects of brain injury and to deal with the patient in a more effective manner.

References

Ben-Yishay, Y. (2000). Postacute neuropsychological rehabilitation: A holistic perspective. In A. L. Christensen & P. B. Uzzel (Eds.), *International handbook of neuropsychological rehabilitation.* New York: Kluwer Academic/Plenum.

Ben-Yishay, Y., & Daniels-Zide, E. (2000). Examined lives: Outcomes after holistic rehabilitation. *Rehabilitation Psychology, 45,* 112–130.

Ben-Yishay, Y. & Diller, L. (1993). Cognitive remediation in traumatic brain injury: Update and issues. *Archives of Physical Medicine and Rehabilitation, 74,* 203–231.

Ben-Yishay, Y., Diller, L., Gerstman, L. G., & Gordon, W. A. (1970). Relationship between initial competence and ability to profit from cues in brain damaged individuals. *Journal of Abnormal Psychology, 75,* 248–259.

Ben-Yishay, Y., & Prigatano, G. P. (1990). Cognitive remediation. In M. Rosenthal et al. (Eds.), *Rehabilitation of the adult and child with traumatic brain injury* (2nd ed.). Philadelphia: F.A. Davis.

Chan, L., Doctor, J., Temkin, N., MacLehose, R. F., Esselman, P., Bell, K. R., & Dikmen, S. (in press). *Archives of Physical Medicine and Rehabilitation.*

Caetano, C., & Christiansen, A. L. (2000). The CRBI at the University of Copenhagen: A participant-therapist perspective. In A. L. Christensen & B. P. Uzzell (Eds.), *International handbook of neuropsychological rehabilitation.* New York: Kluwer Academic/Plenum.

Christiansen, A. L. (2000). Neuropsychological practice in post-acute rehabilitation. In A. L. Christensen & B. P. Uzzell (Eds.), *International handbook of neuropsychological rehabilitation.* New York: Kluwer Academic/Plenum.

Cicerone, K. D., Dahlberg, C., Kalmar, K., Langenbahn, D. M., Malec, J. F., Berquist, T. F., Felicitti, T., Giacino, J. T., Harley, J. P., Harrington, D. E., Herzog, J., Kneipp, S., Laatsch, L., & Moss, P. A. (2000). Evidenced based cognitive rehabilitation: Recommendations for clinical practice. *Archives of Physical Medicine and Rehabilitation, 81,* 1596–1615.

Cope, D. N., Cole, J. R., Hall, K. M., & Barkan, H. (1991). Brain injury: Analysis of outcome in a post acute rehabilitation system, Part 1; General analysis. *Brain Injury, 5,* 111–125.

Corrigan, J. D., Smith-Knapp, K., & Granger, C. (1998). Outcomes in the first 5 years following traumatic brain injury. *Archives of Physical Medicine and Rehabilitation, 79,* 298–305.

Daniels Zide, E., & Ben-Yishay, Y. (2000). Therapeutic milieu day program. In A. L. Christensen & B. P. Uzzell (Eds.), *International handbook of neuropsychological rehabilitation* (pp. 183–194). New York: Kluwer Academic/Plenum.

Dembo, T., Leviton, G., & Wright, B. (1956). Adjustment to misfortune-a problem of social psychological rehabilitation. *Artificial Limbs, 3,* 4–62.

Duggan, C. H., & Dijkers, M. (2001). Quality of life after spinal cord injury. *Rehabilitation Psychology, 46,* 3–25.

Evans, J. J., Wilson, B. A., Schuri, U., Andrade, J., Baddley, A., Bruni, O., Canavan, T., Sala, S. D., Green, R., Laakksonen, R., Lorenzi, L., & Taussik, I. (2000). A comparison of "errorless" and "trial and error" learning methods for teaching individuals with acquired memory defects. *Neuropsychological Rehabilitation, 10,* 67–101.

Evans, R. W. (1997). Postacute neurorehabilitation: Roles and responsibilities within a national information system. *Archive Physical Medicine and Rehabilitation, S17.*

Goldstein, K. (1959). Notes on the development of my concepts. *Journal of Individual Psychology, 15,* 5–14.

Goldstein, K. (1942). *After effects of brain injuries in war: Their evaluation and treatment.* New York: Grune & Stratton.

Hall, K. M., & Johnston, M. V. (1994). Outcomes evaluation in TBI rehabilitation. Part II, measurement tools for a nationwide data system. *Archives of Physical Medicine and Rehabilitation, 75*(Supp.), SC10–8.

Heinemann, A. W., Kirk, P., Hastie, B. A., Semik, P., Hamilton, B. B., Linacre, J. M., Wright, B. D., & Granger, C. V. (1997). Relationships between disability measures and nursing effort during medical rehabilitation for patients with traumatic brain and spinal cord injury. *Archives of Physical Medicine and Rehabilitation, 74,* 566–573.

High, W. M., Jr., Sherer, M., Boake, C., Gollaher, K., Bergloff, P., Newton, C. N., & Ivanhoe, D. (1997). Effects of postacute rehabilitation on social functioning one to three years following traumatic brain injury. *Journal of International Neuropsychology Society, 3*(abstract), 59.

Hosack, K., Malkmus, D., & Evans, R. W. (1991). *Family priorities in post acute rehabilitation for persons with acquired brain injury.* Londenderry, NH: Learning Services Corp.

Kaplan, R. M. (1993). *The Hippocratic predicament: Affordability, access, and accountability in American medicine.* San Diego: Academic Press.

Karasau, B. (2000). On the road to the millennium: The procession of times and paradigm. *American Journal of Psychotherapy, 54,* 141–148.

Klonoff, P. S., & Lage, G. A. (1991). Narcissistic injury after traumatic brain injury. *Journal of Head Trauma Rehabilitation, 6,* 11–21.

Klonoff, P. S., Lamb, D. G., Henderson, S. W., Reichert, M. V., & Tully, S. L. (2000). Milieu-based neurorehabilitation at the adult day hospital for neurological rehabilitation. In A. L. Christensen & B. P. Uzzel (Eds.), *International handbook of neuropsychological rehabilitation* (pp. 195–214). New York: Kluwer Academic/Plenum.

Larsen, A., Mehlbye, J., & Gertz, M. (1991). *Does rehabilitation pay? An analysis of the social and economic aspects of brain injury rehabilitation.* Copenhagen: AKF Forlaget.

Luria, A. M. (1963). *Restoration of the brain after trauma.* London: Pergammon. (Original work published in 1948)

Malec, J., & Basford, J. S. (1996). Postacute brain injury rehabilitation. Review article. *Archives of Physical Medicine and Rehabilitation, 77,* 198–207.

Malec, J. F., & Moessner, A. M. (2000). Self-awareness, distress, and postacute rehabilitation outcome. *Rehabilitation Psychology, 45,* 227–241.

Malec, J. F., Smigielski, DePompolo, R. W., & Thompson, J. W. (1993). Outcome evaluation and prediction in a comprehensive-integrated post-acute outpatient brain injury rehabilitation program. *Brain Injury, 7,* 15–29.

Max, W., McKenzie, E. J., & Rice, D. P. (1991). Head injury: Costs and consequences. *Journal of Head Trauma Rehabilitation, 6*(2), 76–91.

McKenzie, E., Shapiro, S., & Siegel, J. (1998). The economic impact of traumatic injuries. One year treatment related expenditures. *Journal of American Medical Association, 260,* 3290–3296.

Mehlbye, J., & Larsen, A. (1994). Social and economic consequences of brain damage in Denmark: A case study. In A. L. Christensen & B. P. Uzzell (Eds.), *Brain injury and neuropsychological rehabilitation: International perspectives* (pp. 257–267). Hillsdale, NJ: Lawrence Erlbaum.

New York Times. (2001). Hospitals look abroad for patients paying retail. July 23, 2001; vol. CL, No 51, 833; p 1.

O'Neill, J., Hibbard, M. R., Brown, M., Jaffe, M., Sliwinski, M., Vandergoot, D., & Weiss, M. J.

(1998). The effect of employment on quality of life and community integration after traumatic brain injury. *Journal of Head Trauma Rehabilitation, 13,* 68–79.

Prigatano, G. P (1999). *Principles of neuropsychological rehabilitation.* New York: Oxford University Press.

Prigatano, G. P., & Ben-Yishay, Y. (1999). Psychotherapy and psychotherapeutic interventions in brain injury rehabilitation. In M. Rosenthal et al. (Eds.), *Rehabilitation of the adult and child with traumatic brain injury* (3rd ed.). Philadelphia: F.A. Davis.

Prigatano, G. P., Fordyce, D. M., Zeiner, H. K., Roeuche, J. R., Pepping, M., & Wood, B. C. (1984). Neuropsychological rehabilitation after closed head injury in young adults. *Journal of Neurology Neurosurgery and Psychiatry, 47,* 505–513.

Rattok, J., Ben-Yishay, Y., Ezrachi, O., Lakin, P., Piasetsky, E., Ross, B., Silver, S., Vakil, E., Zide, E., & Diller, L. (1992). Outcome of different treatment mixes in a multidimensional neuropsychological rehabilitation program. *Neuropsychology, 6,* 395–416.

Ruff, R. M., & Niemann, H. (1991). Cognitive rehabilitation versus day treatment in head injured adults: Is there an impact on social and emotional life? *Brain Injury, 4,* 339–347.

Sherr, R. L. (2000). Personal communication.

Teasdale, T. W., Hansen, H. V., Gade, A., & Christensen, A. L. (1997). Neuropsychological test scores before and after brain injury in relation to return to employment. *Neuropsychological Rehabilitation, 7,* 23–42.

Trexler, L. E., Diller, L., Gleuckauf, R., Tomusk, A., Anreiter, B., Ben-Yishay, Y., Buckingham, D. Christensen, A.-L., Grant, M., Klonoff, P., Malec, J., Mauer, B., & Seller, S. (1994). *Consensus conference on the development of a multi-center study on the efficacy of neuropsychological rehabilitation,* Zionsville, IN.

Trexler, L. E. (2000). Empirical support for neuropsychological rehabilitation. In A. L. Christensen & B. P. Uzzell (Eds.), *International handbook of neuropsychological rehabilitation* (pp. 137–150). New York: Kluwer Academic/Plenum.

Trexler, L. E., Eberle, R., & Zappala, G. (2000). Models and programs of the Center for Neuropsychological Rehabilitation: 15 years experience. In A. L. Christensen & B. P. Uzzell (Eds.), *International handbook of neuropsychological rehabilitation* (pp. 215–230). New York: Kluwer Academic/Plenum.

Wilson, B. A. (1997). Cognitive rehabilitation: How it is and how it might be. *Journal of International Neuropsychology Society, 3,* 487–496.

Wilson, B. A., Evans, J., Brentnall, S., Bremner, S. A., Keohane, C., & Williams, H. (1999). The Oliver Zangwill Center for Neuropsychological Rehabilitation: A partnership between health care and rehabilitation research. In A. L. Christensen & B. P. Uzzel (Eds.), *International handbook of neuropsychological rehabilitation* (pp. 231–246). New York: Kluwer Academic/Plenum.

15

CHAPTER

Mary Pepping
George P. Prigatano

Psychotherapy After Brain Injury: Costs and Benefits

Introduction

As the authors of Chapter 14 pointed out, psychotherapy of brain-dysfunctional patients often is a part of holistic brain injury day-treatment programs. This service also can be provided in other settings. Regardless of the setting, individual psychotherapy after brain injury is one of the services most specifically directed at helping patients deal with their fragmented sense of loss and rebuilding meaningful lives. Psychotherapy after brain injury also can be applied to family members who care for brain-injured loved ones, although we will not address this important topic in this chapter (see Prigatano, 1999).

The purpose of this chapter is to discuss how one might measure the costs and benefits of psychotherapy when applied to individuals who have suffered brain injury. In an attempt to do this, we will reapproach the definition of psychotherapy and describe the settings in which psychotherapy typically is conducted with brain-dysfunctional patients. We also will consider the basic question of why psychotherapy should be attempted after brain injury. Research findings and clinical observations regarding the ingredients that make psychotherapy effective are important when planning cost outcome analysis. By focusing on these variables, one can obtain a more reasonable picture of when the benefits of psychotherapy clearly outweigh the costs.

Because many readers may not be familiar with the practical details of attempting psychotherapy with brain-dysfunctional patients, two brief case scenarios are presented. One highlights when psychotherapy was effective; the other demonstrates an instance when it was largely ineffective. We will review these case scenarios in an effort to demonstrate possible cost outcome studies for this patient population.

Definitions and Opinions

Psychotherapy can be defined in several ways (Prigatano, 1999; Prigatano, Fordyce, Zeiner, et al., 1986). When applied to persons who have an acquired brain injury (e.g., traumatic brain injury [TBI], ruptured aneurysm, or brain tumor), it involves, at a minimum, face-to-face dialogue between the patient and a psychologist (neuropsychologist) or qualified mental health provider (e.g., a psychiatrist or social worker) who has a good understanding of the patient's neuropsychologic impairments. The aim of the therapy is to provide an experience that improves the patient's intrapsychic (affective state, characterological factors, self-awareness) and interpersonal (e.g., behavioral tendencies, impact on others, understanding of social situations) adaptations. These adaptations should result in improved ability to work as well as in maintaining or reestablishing a meaningful life after the inevitable sorrows associated with brain injury.

The settings in which psychotherapy are conducted can be quite varied. Individual psychotherapy for a person with acquired brain injury often occurs within the context of a holistic day-treatment program (as noted above). Psychotherapy also may precede the involvement of such programs. In this instance, the goal is to help patients prepare themselves for the rigors of such work. Psychotherapy also can begin on an inpatient neurorehabilitation unit, as the individual is struggling to understand what is wrong and needs the emotional support of a clinical neuropsychologist during the early stages following brain injury.

In other instances, individual psychotherapy may be applied several months or even years after hospitalization and rehabilitation. Brain-dysfunctional patients may require ongoing psychological support when dealing with the effects of the brain injury, particularly when their preinjury personality characteristics were such that they have a difficult time dealing with any major losses.

Also, individual psychotherapy may be a key component to continuing brief but interdisciplinary rehabilitation programs (Kaipio, Sarajuuri, & Koskinen, 2000). For example, Finnish investigators noted that holistic programs may be reduced in length for some individuals if they receive considerable ongoing psychotherapy at the end of such rehabilitation programs (Kaipio et al., 2000). One can see, therefore, that psychotherapy can occur in different settings, at different times during recovery, and in varying degrees of frequency or intensity. The costs involved certainly are dictated, in part, by these factors and the overall setting in which the therapy is administered.

Why Do Psychotherapy After Brain Injury?

Damage to the brain during young adulthood and beyond not only produces cognitive, perceptual, sensory, and motor disturbances, it produces predictable changes and patterns of emotional and motivational responding (Prigatano et al., 1986). In addition, patients have inevitable emotional reactions to their changed abilities and resultant sense of impaired self-value or esteem. Depending on preinjury or premorbid personality characteristics, there may be a reasonable adjustment to these changes that requires minimal or no psychotherapy. In other instances, an individual may be so overwhelmed by the changes that psychotherapeutic interventions are useless in controlling depression and suicidal behavior. Whatever the situation, the experienced clinical neuropsychologist who attempts to do psychotherapy with brain-dysfunctional patients recognizes that there is a need to help patients come to grips with how they have changed. This has been described as dealing with the problem of *lost normality* (Prigatano, 1995).

In addition to this, there is another problem that is somewhat unique to certain patients—particularly those who suffer diffuse TBI to heteromodal cortices (Prigatano, 1999). These individuals may have partial awareness of their disturbances in higher cerebral functioning but not fully appreciate the degree to which their judgment is adversely affected. These two interacting problems (i.e., the problem of impaired awareness after brain injury combined with strong but misguided attempts to assert a sense of normality) can lead to substantially poor judgment and associated poor choices by patients with brain injury. Perhaps the key contribution of working with brain-injured patients from a psychotherapeutic point of view is to help them deal with these two interacting problems.

Poor awareness and poor choices can have profound economic and personal impacts. In some instances, these result in patients quitting jobs impulsively or going through multiple jobs without stopping to ask themselves why they are having difficulties maintaining work. In other instances, it can mean problems with emotional dyscontrol and alienating individuals who are trying to help. The psychotherapist who attempts to work with brain-dysfunctional patients must have a good understanding of the problems of impaired awareness when dealing with lost normality to be of maximum help to these individuals. Although all patients do not suffer from these difficulties, these two dimensions are extremely important, particularly after TBI.

In cases of focal brain injury, other problems may emerge. For example, O'Brien and Prigatano (1991) noted that a patient with alexia without agraphia became depressed when he recognized that his inability to read stopped him from being a business executive. The patient had good insight as to his limitations, but he was overwhelmed by the limitations. Psychotherapy in this case helped him learn to compensate for his reading difficulties and guided him into volunteer work that was truly meaningful for him.

Another patient with a focal lesion in the left temporal lobe was returned to work without appropriate appreciation of his neuropsychological disturbances (Prigatano & Smith, 2000). This patient feared that he was "going crazy" as he experienced problems in reading and spelling and an inability to comprehend materials he could easily comprehend in the past. The neuropsychological evaluation helped him understand the underlying problems. This naturally led into psychotherapeutic sessions in which the patient came to grips with his altered status and restructured his life in light of his previous values and experiences.

These brief case scenarios and numerous clinical and research reports (Anderson, Gundersen, & Finset, 1999; Becker & Vakil, 1993; Bennett & Raymond, 1997; Buskirk, 1992; Cicerone, 1989, 1991; Drubach, McAlaster, & Hartman, 1994; Langer & Padrone, 1992; Miller, 1993; Prigatano & Ben-Yishay. 1999) document that each psychotherapy endeavor and alliance with a brain-injured patient has to be taken on an individual basis. Yet, there are recurring themes that emerge in the psychotherapy of brain-dysfunctional patients. They give us insight as to the potential benefits of psychotherapy after brain injury.

Potential Benefits of Psychotherapy After Brain Injury

Depending on patients' premorbid personality characteristic and their acquired neuropsychological disturbances, the benefits of psychotherapy can be varied. We are impressed, however, that the following five benefits are frequently seen:

1. The reduction of anxiety and depression in the face of altered abilities.
2. A sense of hope that comes from not feeling "alone" with their disturbances in higher cerebral functioning.
3. A meaningful reduction of confusion as to what is "wrong" with their functioning and, therefore, a more reasonable approach to compensating for the disabilities.
4. The appropriate use of guidance in making choices regarding issues of productivity and interpersonal relationships.
5. An experience that is truly "emotionally corrective," in so far as it helps patients understand the fabric of their lives and thereby, either reestablish (or, for the first time, establish) meaning in the face of frustration and suffering.

Some of these benefits have no reasonable economic markers. For example, what does it mean to have a meaningful existence in terms of dollars? However, the making of appropriate choices regarding work can have profound economic impact, as noted above. Researchers in these areas must again look at objective and subjective markers of value when conducting cost outcome research on these various dimensions.

How Does Psychotherapy Work? Considerations for Cost Outcome Studies

Any meaningful analysis of the costs and benefits of psychotherapy must be predicated on some understanding of the essential ingredients for successful psychotherapeutic work, particularly when patients have suffered a catastrophic illness. In an exceptionally thoughtful paper, Frank (1984) discussed therapeutic components shared by all psychotherapists. He pointed out that therapists generally have the capacity to understand what patients are experiencing. They foster reasonable expectations for hope and help. They combat patients' sense of alienation via strengthening their therapeutic relationship or alliance. They provide new learning experiences. They arouse emotions, but help patients better cope with those emotions. They enhance patients' sense of mastery or self-efficiency.

When applied to work with brain-dysfunctional patients, the treating neuropsychologist must have the training to allow him or her to understand what the patient is experiencing (Prigatano, 1999). This requires considerable training in neuropsychology as well as psychodynamic theory, learning theory, and a good appreciation of animal behavior as it reflects the underpinnings of human behavior. This type of training and knowledge is only learned over many years and with a considerable effort. It is costly training in terms of the psychologist's formal education, ongoing supervision, and need for continuing education. These factors have to be reasonably included in any cost outcome analysis.

The psychotherapist must be able to combat a patient's sense of alienation via strengthening the therapeutic alliance. Many individuals have emphasized the importance of the psychotherapeutic alliance in psychotherapy (Klonoff, 1997; Luborsky, 1976). It takes time to develop a therapeutic alliance. One area of very fruitful research is actually looking at the amount of time and costs necessary to establish a therapeutic alliance with different types of brain-dysfunctional patients who have different premorbid characteristics. If one could simply answer that question in terms of dollars, one could then sensibly assess the benefits of such a bond. Repeatedly, we have noted that the establishment of a good alliance with the patient and family members translates into substantially better rehabilitation outcome (Klonoff, Lamb, & Henderson, 2000; 2001; Prigatano et al., 1994).

The psychotherapist must provide a new learning experience for the brain-dysfunctional patient. Many times, this has to be done in the context of a holistic program, but not always. In some instances, the psychotherapist works with patients and their family members as well as with other health-care providers to guide the process. For example, some individuals can be given work trials with the aid of an experienced occupational therapist or vocational rehabilitation counselor, who simultaneously works with the consulting clinical neuropsychologist who is doing psychotherapy with the brain-dysfunctional patient. In this context, the patient may learn how old and new response tendencies are interfering with adjustment to a work setting. This type of ongoing dialogue among all involved parties, rooted in day-to-day work and mediated by the neuropsychologist, is important in helping brain-injured patients obtain real-life learning experiences that help them cope with the problem of lost normality.

As Frank (1984) pointed out, psychotherapy arouses emotions. It arouses emotions in the therapist as well as in the patient. The capacity of the therapist to understand these emotions may be very important in understanding how to approach the patient and maintain a therapeutic alliance during the difficult times. This requires a fair degree of psychological maturity on the therapist's part. Often, therapists have experienced their own individual psychotherapy in order to do their work. The costs of one's own psychotherapy as an aid to doing psychotherapy with brain-dysfunctional patients should further be considered in any cost outcome studies.

Finally, as Frank (1984) noted, psychotherapy must help the patient have a sense of mastery or self-efficacy. This has been discussed in numerous settings (e.g., Ben-Yishay & Prigatano, 1990; Prigatano, 1995). That sense of new mastery is important in helping patients become independent of the psychotherapist. Although some patients clearly need long-term psychotherapy, one of the major goals of psychotherapy should be helping the patient become independent of the psychotherapist.

In this regard, we want to emphasize what we think is the major contribution of learning theory and behavioral modification to the psychotherapeutic work with brain-dysfunctional patients. Behavioral theorists have emphasized the importance of antecedent and consequent conditions in modifying ongoing behavior. They emphasize that clear goals must be established, and one should measure to the degree to which various reinforcers help achieve these goals. We are in support of the notion that psychotherapy with brain-dysfunctional patients should have specific goals in order to determine if it is successful and, for purposes of this chapter, to determine whether it is cost-effective. Without clear outcome goals, one cannot assess the effects of psychotherapy with brain-dysfunctional patients.

In this latter regard, we would suggest three major goals in working with brain-dysfunctional patients (Prigatano, 1999; Prigatano et al., 1986). These three goals are to help the patient return to a productive lifestyle, to maintain mutually satisfying interpersonal relationships, and to develop a unique sense of individuality. It is beyond the scope of this chapter to discuss these topics in detail. But we believe that behavioral markers as to whether these goals are achieved are important in any cost–outcome analysis.

One final point should be made regarding psychotherapy with brain–dysfunctional patients that is important to the study of cost outcome research. Gunther (1971) suggested years ago that a brain or spinal cord injury often produces substantial psychological regression in individuals. This regression may present itself in various ways, but it is often described as seen as "complex states of denial and depression" (p. 574). Therapists and family members often become frustrated when dealing with patients who appear to be denying their disabilities or who are severely depressed and will not participate in rehabilitation programs. Often, such patients can be so overwhelming to therapists (including psychotherapists) that they act punitively toward these patients (see Prigatano, 1999). In some instances, patients are discharged from rehabilitation programs under the guise that they are either not honest in what they are saying or not motivated to work at rehabilitation activities. We would suggest that one go cautiously before assuming that a patient is dishonest or unmotivated to work at rehabilitation. Often, patients are so overwhelmed by what has happened to them and have such complicated neuropsychological disturbances that they cannot adequately engage the psychotherapeutic or rehabilitation process. An area of considerable research interest is the ability and skill of therapists to engage such patients. If one could understand what it takes to actually engage patients at all phases of rehabilitation, this would provide a very important fulcrum for starting to measure the true value of psychotherapy with brain-dysfunctional individuals.

We will now present two case scenarios that provide in more detail what is actually done in psychotherapy. Then we will try to apply some of our thoughts to analyzing the cost and benefits involved in these two cases.

Case Example 1: When Psychotherapy Was Useful

Jeff[1] was a single, right-handed, college educated male, aged 33. He suffered post right arteriovenous malformation rupture at age 7, with only partial clipping possible, and rerupture and complete clipping at age 19.

Residual Symptoms. Jeff exhibited visual perceptual disturbances, left hemiparesis, upper extremity greater than lower extremity, and poorly controlled anger and depression. He had been psychiatrically hospitalized twice in recent years, once with a self-inflicted knife wound to the stomach. He was being tried on a combination of Haldol and a tricycle antidepressant, which seemed to be helping reduce the more extreme moods and outbursts. Prior to this recent change in medications, he had been increasingly verbally abusive, and occasionally physically abusive to his parents, who were in their 60s and with whom he had lived all of his life. His parents were at their emotional and physical limits with Jeff. They wanted to help him live on his own with

[1]Names, biographical data, and other important identifying features in both case examples have been changed to protect confidentiality while remaining true to general issues and thrust of treatment.

their support and occasional supervision. However, they were understandably very concerned about his depression, his suspiciousness, and the possibility that he would hurt himself or someone else if he became too lonely, brooding, or otherwise upset.

Jeff had never successfully held a job and had not looked for work for many years at the time of his admission to the brain-injury program. He spent much of his time reading about politics and history or watching news shows on television. He liked to visit with his parents and two sisters. Other than contact with his immediate and extended family, Jeff had no friends.

Strengths. Jeff had excellent verbal skills and a loyal and supportive family. He excelled at verbal puns, was willing to engage in the process of treatment, and displayed good attendance at treatment and a willingness to discuss and debate issues. He enjoyed writing poetry and was a prodigious reader of political texts.

Treatment. In a full time, milieu-oriented outpatient treatment program, Jeff was able to participate in a wide variety of individual treatments, of which individual psychotherapy was one key component. He also was able to learn the lists of problems and strengths that other people had based on their brain injuries. This shared reality made it easier for Jeff to understand and accept why he might be having some long-standing difficulties in his interactions with others.

He learned in individual therapy about his problems with perception, and how these led to some of his erroneous conclusions about other people's attitudes and behavior toward him. In the individual psychotherapy hour, when Jeff would (typically) make comments that were offensive or "crazy," he had an opportunity to receive feedback. This feedback was from someone who liked him and appreciated his many attributes, but who had no intention of letting him get by without some direct therapeutic confrontation regarding his destructive comments. At times, those individual therapy sessions ended early or shifted to a less in-depth consideration of topics, because Jeff was understandably frightened when considering the fact that what couldn't be trusted were his own unaided perceptions.

By being part of a small group of patients, Jeff was able (with a considerable amount of follow-up and practice in his individual psychotherapy hours) to trust other patients and staff in the groups and to tolerate public discussion of problem behaviors. This first occurred in a very general, education-oriented sense, but, with time, also on a more personal level.

With psychoanalytic appreciation for the defense mechanism of projection and the nature of profound narcissistic wounds to the self, his psychotherapist, with some ongoing good supervision at her disposal, worked first and foremost to help Jeff feel less like "a bad person." This approach involved helping Jeff develop a sense of connection, belonging, and acceptance by his fellow program participants, who also were struggling with brain injury. It was probably the first time since early primary school that Jeff felt he was an integral part of a close circle of peers. In addition, his psychotherapist was a single woman approximately his age, who shared a love of poetry and puns and with whom Jeff was able to form a therapeutic alliance. It was probably the first psychologically intimate relationship Jeff had had with a woman his age and provided an important, corrective emotional experience for him.

No part of the process was easy for Jeff, or for his treating therapists. In spite of the significant challenges facing him, however, he had enjoyed all his life the consistent and unwavering presence of his family, which likely made it easier for him to believe that the treatment staff and patients could function like a good family for him.

As a direct result of psychotherapeutic intervention and approximately 6 months of outpatient treatment, the direct and indirect benefits have been as follows:

1. Jeff has never been psychiatrically hospitalized since his treatment; he is now over 15 years post treatment and doing well.
2. He is no longer in need of psychotherapeutic treatment to maintain adaptive behavior, and is not using outpatient resources, other than very occasional rechecks with his physician to monitor general health and medications.
3. He has been stable for many years on a medication regimen that was effectively monitored during his psychotherapy treatment, when Jeff was observed multiple times each week.
4. He is living independently and contributing to the local economy by his rent payments, grocery shopping, book purchases, and newspaper and cable TV subscriptions.
5. His father's problems with high blood pressure improved, as did his mother's gastric difficulties, following Jeff's treatment and moves toward independence. Their need for outside medical and psychotherapeutic support (and their expenditure of health-care dollars) was reduced.
6. Jeff's interactions with his family improved to the point that he was welcome to visit several times a week and to join the family for dinner or church or outings, while he continuing to live in his own apartment, about two blocks away from his parents. This helped further reduce his risk of depression and isolation, and also helped serve as a reality check on his more outrageous misperceptions and delusions.
7. Jeff has remained in touch with his primary therapist over the years, sending occasional letters or cards (almost always with some kind of pun or political comment). He has established a regular routine of household chores, meal preparation, reading, walking for exercise, visiting his family, enjoying his sisters' children, and attending church.

It was through intensive psychotherapeutic treatment that Jeff was able to learn to keep some of his more provocative statements to himself and to resume his role as a productive member of the community, rather than as an individual draining mental health, medical, and family resources, and giving very little back. He may be an eccentric uncle at this point in his life, but he is not a dangerous one. Instead, he is an excellent example of a brain-injured patient with a very challenging and chronic set of neurologically mediated problems in perception and behavior.

For this man, and for many others like him, practical guidelines and corrective emotional experiences provided via the strong individual psychotherapeutic alliance–in the context of a small, supportive group of patients with similar problem–have contributed significantly to a positive, permanent improvement in behavior. The resulting reduction in economic, emotional, and long-term social costs as a result of comparatively time-limited treatment–for a man who otherwise appeared to be on the path to multiple future psychiatric hospitalizations and probable long-term institutional placement when his parents could no longer care for him–is enormous.

Ideas for Cost Outcome Studies for Jeff (and Patients Like Him). The preceding case clearly demonstrates why individuals attempting to do cost outcome research on psychotherapy have preferred to use the cost-effectiveness model. In fact, Miller and Magruder (1999) edited a text specifically on the cost-effectiveness of psychotherapy. Within this method of analysis, the outcome measures often are thought to be noneconomic in nature, reflecting the degree to which quality of life has been improved, reduction in depression, anxiety, and so on.

In considering the specific outcomes that were accomplished with Jeff, one could use various cost–outcome analyses. One could invoke a willingness-to-pay model (see Chapter 2) and ask Jeff's parents what it would be worth in terms of dollars if they could substantially reduce their son's verbal aggressiveness and angry outbursts. Although most psychotherapists are not trained to think along these lines, it would be interesting to actually have dollars signs attached to, let's say, a 50% reduction in these outbursts, and then determine what the actual costs of psychotherapy were to produce a certain percentage of improvement. Consumers may be surprised to find that they are actually receiving greater value than they literally purchased in this willingness-to-pay model. In this regard, it is interesting to note that a few years ago *Consumer Reports* did a survey as to whether or not consumers were satisfied with their experiences in psychotherapy (Strupp, 1996). Not surprisingly, generally speaking they were satisfied with the outcomes, and people were willing to pay for the service.

In addition to invoking a willingness-to-pay model, one could compare the actual costs of medications for patients like Jeff 5 years prior to the onset of psychotherapy versus the cost of medications 5 years after psychotherapy. By comparing patients who had received psychotherapy versus no psychotherapy, one could determine whether the cost–benefit ratio was favorable after psychotherapeutic work. In this latter design, one is measuring the dollars saved in medication costs as a result of psychotherapy.

One also could measure the actual preprogram costs of Jeff's inpatient and outpatient psychiatric care, including his family's need for outpatient psychiatric consultation related to his care. One could then compare those preprogram costs, extrapolated into his future adult years, compared to the cost of his brain-injury program and subsequent psychiatric follow-up needed by Jeff and his family. The value of the product and actual savings in this case are abundantly clear. Thus, one can see that cost–benefits studies are indeed possible when assessing the value of psychotherapy in the health-care environment.

Finally, an important area to further investigate when considering the cost and benefits of psychotherapy is the indirect impact such treatment may have on family members. In fact, Jeff's father showed improvement in his blood pressure following successful psychotherapeutic treatment of his son, resulting in reduced need for the father's own medical care. This should not be forgotten when conducting such research. We find this an interesting observation and believe this could be replicated in group studies. That is, family members, particularly parents of brain-dysfunctional patients, may well enjoy improved health as a result of successful psychotherapeutic treatment of a brain-injured child. This type of analysis would include measures of both medical outcomes and the person's subjective sense of well-being. Once again, we can envision both objective and subjective markers of the value of psychotherapy after brain injury.

Case Example 2: When Psychotherapy Was Not Useful

Charlie was a single, left-handed 33-year-old with 2 years of college (AA degree). He suffered a severe TBI in a car accident at age 31, with a 3-week coma. He sustained diffuse, global injury, with greater right hemisphere impairment, including evacuation of large right frontal-temporal-parietal subdural hematoma.

Residual Symptoms. Charlie had visual perceptual deficits, along with poor design recall and profoundly reduced awareness of his deficits. Even when difficulties were consistently pointed out, Charlie would simply listen in a pleasant manner, as if the information did not register with him in any real way (e.g., in a manner that might be expected to affect his view of residual abilities and options). There were also rather classic frontal signs, including childlike demeanor and behavior and being somewhat silly or immature in interactions with others. No frank hemiplegia was present, but there were clear reductions in left body side sensory and motor skills, including poor tactile recognition and reductions in fine motor speed. Fairly well-preserved verbal intelligence and a preinjury history as a competitive tennis player were additional areas of strength. Charlie's preinjury adjustment appeared to be a healthy one with respect to his education and work history. In addition, at the time of his accident, he was engaged to be married. He and his fiancée had been involved with each other for several years; there was no actual date set for a wedding. She also had two children from a prior marriage. Charlie was the only child of older parents, and was particularly close to his mother, who did not approve of his fiancée.

Charlie had been returning from a tennis tournament late at night, driving some distance, when he apparently fell asleep at the wheel and crashed head-on into the base of a freeway pylon. His car was demolished, and he spent several months in the hospital and in inpatient rehabilitation with a variety of physical injuries in addition to his severe TBI.

The accident appeared to offer an opportunity for Charlie's mother to bring his relationship with his fiancée to an end by eventually barring her from the hospital, from participation in any treatment as a family member, and from any continued contact with Charlie. The fiancée did call to speak with one of the authors, and informed this psychologist that a variety of issues had been coming to a head in her relationship with Charlie at the time of the accident. One of these issues was his relationship with his mother and her level of influence in his decisions. The fiancée described the mother as intimidating, overbearing, controlling, and unusually intimate with her son, to a degree that made the fiancée uncomfortable. Charlie did not seem to see the problem in the same light.

The fiancée loved him and had wanted to marry him, but she felt now that there was no way for her to make contact with him, as his mother was in full control of the situation. The fiancée reportedly had been asked by Charlie's mother to withdraw from the relationship. With his diminished capacities, reduced drive and awareness, and increased dependence on his mother, Charlie was in no position to contravene his mother's wishes. The fiancée's judgment was that the situation was impossible to rectify, and she withdrew.

When he came for his initial evaluation and subsequent treatment, Charlie indicated that he very much wanted to return to his preinjury life as a professional tennis player. His primary regular employment had been a combination of coaching and ongoing involvement in the semiprofessional tennis circuit. He was performing well enough at the time his accident occurred to be on the brink of breaking into the professional level of tennis.

His mother was understandably concerned about his overall level of functioning, separate from the issue of tennis, and wanted to know what could be done to restore her son to as fully functional a life as possible. Through considerable sacrifice and effort on her part, Charlie was enrolled in a program of treatment. He never spoke of his father, nor did he appear to have much involvement with him. Charlie's mother and Charlie moved into housing together near the program. They occasionally took long weekends to drive home, which was a considerable distance away, during his months in treatment.

Strengths. Charlie was a hard-working, disciplined, and dedicated athlete prior to his injury. He had been trying for a long time to break into the next level of his sport and had not yet made it, but he was persisting in spite of this. He was willing to accept the kind of "coaching" inherent in some aspects of good treatment and willing to use compensatory techniques (e.g., for memory). His basic verbal reasoning was good, and he had well-preserved reading ability and basic academic skills. He was approachable about areas of difficulty. He also was punctual and had perfect attendance in the program.

Treatment. In a full-time, milieu-oriented outpatient treatment program, Charlie (similarly to Jeff) was able to participate in a wide variety of individual and group treatments, with individual psychotherapy as one key component. In some ways, Charlie initially appeared to be a better treatment risk than Jeff. Charlie had had some preinjury success in his adult life, and he was only 2 years postinjury, not 25 years postinjury. Even though there were issues with respect to establishing his own fully independent relationship, he was not paranoid, he was not angry and combative, he had not struck his parents–in general, he had been little trouble to anyone.

Unlike Jeff, Charlie tended to smile vaguely, in a somewhat childlike fashion, at much of the information that was discussed. This was a pattern that persisted throughout the months of treatment. He seemed reasonably interested but generally untouched by almost all that transpired. We initially presumed that his general level of passivity was a direct result of the severity of his TBI. Certainly the brain injury was (and remains) a significant contributing factor.

Initially, we simply redoubled our efforts in treatment to make sure the ideas discussed and feelings potentially generated would be presented and handled in safe and supportive ways. Charlie liked to draw and had been fairly artistic, so we made use of drawings and art to reflect on his current situation and ways to understand and address it. There also was extensive use of humor and feedback in the individual and group treatments, and Charlie appeared to enjoy the program and his contact with both peers and staff.

Charlie also performed very well on a clerical work trial, where his good verbal and numeric abilities were put to use in bookkeeping activities. He seemed to enjoy this aspect of treatment the most (i.e., being back in a regular work environment). We had great hopes for his future promise in a clerical capacity. Although he was not speedy, he was quite accurate, and his supervisor (who was a regular employer within a hospital setting) felt that Charlie would be able to work competitively.

Yet, in spite of all our efforts and our reasonably sophisticated understanding of the various neuropsychological, characterological, and familial issues that might be operating, Charlie seemed to remain outside the gravitational pull of the therapeutic alliance. He did not appear removed or regressed in a psychologically traumatized fashion; nor did he appear resigned to his fate. He also was not so concrete that he couldn't understand some of the finer points of psychological inquiry. He remained hidden in a pleasantness that provided no entry.

In that context, he gave the overall appearance of being a very good little boy, who was perfectly willing to do what was asked and be courteous about it. It was just that the more adult aspect of him was either no longer present or not available for real contact, scrutiny, or influence. Perhaps this aspect of the self was not available for reflective contact with him, even in the privacy of his own mind. He did not appear terribly bothered by his deficits, or concerned about his future in the way that other young men his age would be. He seemed content with his current living situation and content to let his mother hold sway in his life.

The more we got to know his mother, the better we also appreciated the degree to which a pleasant, passive, and hidden way of being might be the only way to remain unscorched when she began her "march to the sea." Although she wanted Charlie to be helped as much as possible with his problems, when the discussions moved to specific goals toward independence or eventually being able to live on his own or return to work, she became less enthusiastic. She had helped him establish Social Security Disability, which was certainly understandable. So, although she wanted to be assured that she and Charlie had done all they could to restore his skills to a functional level, she did not want him to take the next steps to a more competitive and therefore independent level.

In retrospect, it appeared that Charlie, fate, and his mother may all have inadvertently conspired to remove the questions and challenges of an individuated life outside the home. Charlie was never a particularly reflective or psychologically minded man. He had been trying for a long time to break into the big leagues and had not made it. It wasn't clear that he was going to make it. The injury allowed him an unexpected opportunity to escape from the pressures of a future wife and her children, as well as from the potential failure of his career path in the world of professional sports. On another, far more primitive level, it may have allowed him to unconsciously fulfill his mother's need for Charlie to remain her true life partner.

We learned an important lesson from this case, and have had the chance to learn it again and again when all of the family and personal issues are not clear up front. The lesson is this: If your patient's primary and long-standing source of emotional support—be it wife, husband, mother, father, child, or friend—is not in favor of competitive employment, with some of its inherent risks and challenges, it is extremely unlikely that your patient will ever do paid work again, regardless of his or her actual level of talent or potential for employment.

Unfortunately, this can be a difficult fact to elucidate upon initial contact, especially when a family genuinely wants improvement and appears to agree with productivity goals. Perhaps their hope is to see their loved one miraculously restored to all or most of his or her prior self.

When it is clear that this level of recovery or coping is not going to occur, a shift may happen within the family that is not made public to the team. We all think we have the same goals, but family goals have shifted midstream, while ours have not. Families do not want their relative discharged early from good treatment, so there is no incentive to "come clean" with respect to actual goals.

Although therapy did help Charlie improve some of his more childlike social behaviors, gave him an opportunity for realistic feedback regarding his residual strengths and weaknesses, and provided him with a positive and successful work trial experience he likely never would have had on his own, the overall program was a comparative waste of time and money. Charlie was going to remain on disability and likely not be employed in any capacity outside the home. He was not going to live independently, and he had already been at a functional level preprogram so that he could do fairly well at home. For Charlie, some outpatient occupational and speech therapy—time limited in nature and at a much less intense frequency, duration, and cost—may have been enough to help him improve his leisure time and his memory compensatory techniques. He did not need months of intensive individual psychotherapy and group psychotherapy treatment with a strong return-to-work focus in order to return home to live with his parents, with no independent or work life established outside the home.

Ideas for Cost Outcome Studies for Charlie (and Patients Like Him). Charlie's example clearly demonstrates that the therapist was not able to establish a therapeutic alliance with this patient. The case also illustrates that the patient's family members were not supportive of the patient becoming independent. The cost of psychotherapy certainly was not justified by the outcome. This negative finding needs to be squarely assessed when doing outcome studies on the effectiveness of psychotherapy.

We believe that a careful delineation of the variables that put a patient at risk for not benefiting from psychotherapy should be systematically considered when doing cost–outcome research. Although there is not any definitive list, we would suggest that the following patient characteristics should be considered when psychotherapy has been unsuccessful: level of cognitive deficit, history of being able to form a working alliance prior to injury, ability to modify behavior with insight, capacity to establish reasonable goals, capacity to manage anxiety and depression, freedom from psychosis, motivation to become independent, and ability to have "philosophical patience" in the face of personal suffering (Prigatano, 1999). In addition to these patient characteristics, family members also must be willing to see positive change in order for them to make progress. We suggest that analysis of the family's characteristics also provides useful insights into why psychotherapy may fail in some instances.

We also would emphasize that, when psychotherapy is not effective, one should evaluate the therapist's characteristics. What were the goals of psychotherapy as seen through the eyes of the patient and psychotherapist? How much time did the psychotherapist actually spend with the patient? Was the therapist committed to the patient's psychotherapy? Was he or she able to seek out consultative help when having difficulty working with the patient? Was he or she skilled in psychodynamically oriented psychotherapy as well as in other methods of psychological intervention? Did he or she have experience in working in a holistic rehabilitation setting as a necessary background to doing psychotherapy work with these patients?

In short, we are suggesting that a careful analysis of patient and therapist characteristics (as well as family characteristics) will provide insight into why psychotherapy may fail. This information is needed when conducting studies on cost outcomes.

Summary and Conclusions

We have attempted in this chapter to revisit what psychotherapy is and how it can be applied to brain-dysfunctional patients. We have addressed the question of why psychotherapy should be attempted and also tried to illustrate the potential benefits of psychotherapy for various types of brain-dysfunctional patients. Moreover, we have reviewed what appeared to be crucial ingredients to successful psychotherapy and argued that, if those ingredients are studied in cost outcome analyses, one is able to get a better understanding of the true value of psychotherapeutic interventions after brain injury.

Furthermore, we have provided two case scenarios that are common in our experience. They highlight when psychotherapy is effective versus when it is not. Both cases have a lot to teach us about the relative values of different forms of cost outcome studies. Although cost-effectiveness studies seem to be the most prominent method of measuring the usefulness of psychotherapy in health care, other methods (even methods using direct cost–benefits) also could be of some use.

We have attempted to highlight what variables should be considered and provided some rudimentary ideas of what kinds of cost–benefits and cost-effectiveness ratios could be calculated in doing research in this area. Finally, Table 15.1 summarizes in broad terms the clinical utility of psychotherapy with brain-dysfunctional patients

Although not the focus of this chapter, we would like to make one final point: Neuropsychological and psychological assessment of brain-dysfunctional patients is an important component to their psychotherapeutic work (Prigatano, Pepping, & Klonoff, 1986). Such assessments allow clinicians to have a reasonable understanding of whether or not an individual is likely to benefit from psychotherapy, and whether he or she can be meaningfully engaged in rehabilitation programs. Too often, in the context of managed care, clinicians do not perform an adequate preliminary psychological and neuropsychological examination because of the financial strains placed on them. As Finn (1996) so clearly demonstrated, just the review of evaluation results with the patient can function as a form of initial intervention and lay the groundwork for much of what is to come. Future research on outcome and cost-effectiveness should also consider the role of these evaluations and how they may dovetail with formal psychotherapy to produce the best outcome for patients we serve.

In a related line of work, Ciechanowski, Katon, Russo, and Walker (2001) clearly documented that if the clinician knows how to talk to the patient in light of that patient's history of interpersonal relationships using Bowlby's concepts (1973), the patient's

TABLE 15.1. Clinical Utility of Psychotherapy with Brain-Dysfunctional Patients

1. Establish a therapeutic alliance that helps patients engage the rehabilitation process.
2. Clarify for patients (and many times families and rehabilitation staff) the nature of the patients' neuropsychological deficits and how they may be interacting with premorbid personality strengths and weaknesses.
3. Help patients understand (i.e., experience) their neuropsychological strengths and limitations in the hopes that, with this information, they can be guided to make better choices in life, especially regarding issues of productivity.
4. Help patients control negative emotional reactions, which clearly interfere with the ability to maintain work as well as with interpersonal relationships. This type of intervention also may include behavioral modification strategies as well as insight-oriented psychotherapeutic interventions.
5. Help patients come to grips with their existential situation (i.e., improving awareness/acceptance) and, in that context, help them reexperience joy and pleasure in life.

adherence to medical treatment protocols is substantially improved. This can lead not only to greater treatment compliance but to many dollars saved in the health-care arena. Clinical neuropsychologists need to follow these leads and establish their own ongoing, relevant, and measurable outcomes for gauging the cost-effectiveness of their work. They also need to take this information back to their practices and incorporate the findings to appropriately modify clinical interventions.

References

Andersson, S., Gundersen, P. M., & Finset, A. (1999). Emotional activation during therapeutic interaction in TBI: Effect of apathy, self-awareness and implications for rehabilitation. *Brain Injury, 13*(6), 393–404.

Becker, M. E., & Vakil, E. (1993). Behavioral psychotherapy of the frontal-lobe injured patient in an outpatient setting. *Brain Injury, 7*(6), 515–523.

Bennett, T. L., & Raymond, M. T. (1997). Emotional consequences and psychotherapy for individuals with mild brain injury. *Applied Neuropsychology, 4*(1), 55–61.

Ben-Yishay, Y., & Prigatano, G. P. (1990). Cognitive remediation. In E. Griffin, M. Rosenthal, M. R. Bond, & J. D. Miller (Eds.), *Rehabilitation of the adult and child with traumatic brain injury* (pp. 393–409). Philadelphia: F. A. Davis.

Bowlby, J. (1973). *Attachment and loss, volume II: Separation, anxiety and anger.* New York, Basic Books.

Buskirk, J. R. (1992). Headlock: Psychotherapy of a patient with multiple neurological and psychiatric problems. *Bulletin of Menninger Clinic, 56*(3), 361–378.

Cicerone, K. D. (1991). Psychotherapy after MTBI: Relation to the nature and severity of subjective complaints. *Journal of Head Trauma Rehabilitation, 6*(4), 30–43.

Cicerone, K. D. (1989). Psychotherapeutic intervention with TBI patients. *Rehabilitation Psychologist, 34*(2), 105–114.

Ciechanowski, P. S., Katon, W. J., Russo, J. E., & Walker, E. A. (2001). The patient-provider relationship: Attachment theory and adherence to treatment in diabetes. *American Journal of Psychiatry, 158*, 29–35.

Drubach, D., McAlaster, R., & Hartman, P. (1994). The use of a psychoanalytic framework in the rehabilitation of patients with traumatic brain injury. *American Journal of Psychoanalysis, 54*(3), 255–263.

Finn, S. E. (1996). *Using the MMPI-2 as a therapeutic intervention*. Minneapolis: University of Minnesota Press.

Frank, J. D. (1984). Therapeutic components shared by all psychotherapies. In J. H. Harvey & M. M. Parks (Eds.), *The master lecture series, volume 1: Psychotherapy research and behavior change* (pp. 5–37). Washington, DC: American Psychological Association.

Gunther, M. S. (1971). Psychiatric consultation in a rehabilitation hospital: A regression hypothesis. *Comprehensive Psychiatry, 12*(6), 572–585.

Kaipio, M.-L., Sarajuuri, J., & Koskinen, S. (2000). The INSURE program and modifications in Finland. In A.-L. Christensen & B. P. Uzzell (Eds.), *International handbook of neuropsychological rehabilitation* (pp. 247–258). New York: Kluwer Academic.

Klonoff, P. S. (1997). Individual and group psychotherapy in milieu-oriented neurorehabilitation. *Applied Neuropsychology 4*(2), 107-118.

Klonoff, P. S., Lamb, D. G., & Henderson, S. W. (2001). Outcomes from milieu-based neurorehabilitation at up to 11 years post-discharge. *Brain Injury, 15*(5), 413–428.

Klonoff, P. S., Lamb, D. G., & Henderson, S. W. (2000). Milieu-based neuro-rehabilitation in patients with traumatic brain injury: Outcome at up to 11 years post-discharge. *Archives of Physical Medicine and Rehabilitation, 81*(11), 1535–1537.

Langer, K. G., & Padrone, F. J. (1992). Psychotherapeutic treatment of awareness in acute rehabilitation of TBI. *Neuropsychological Rehabilitation, 2*(1), 59–70.

Luborsky, L. (1976). Helping alliances in psychotherapy. In J. L. Cleghorn (Ed.), *Successful psychotherapy* (pp. 92–116). New York: Brunner/Mazel.

Miller, L. (1993). *Psychotherapy of the brain-injured patient: Reclaiming the shattered self.* New York: W.W. Norton.

Miller, N. E., & Macgruder, K.M. (1999). *Cost-effectiveness of psychotherapy: A guide for practitioners, researchers, and policymakers.* New York: Oxford University Press.

O'Brien, K. P., & Prigatano, G. P. (1991). Supportive psychotherapy for a patient exhibiting alexia without agraphia. *Journal of Head Trauma Rehabilitation, 6*(4), 44–55.

Prigatano, G. P. (1999). *Principles of neuropsychological rehabilitation.* New York: Oxford University Press.

Prigatano, G. P. (1995). 1994 Sheldon Berrol, MD, Senior Lectureship: The problem of lost normality after brain injury. *Journal of Head Trauma Rehabilitation, 10*(3), 53–62.

Prigatano, G. P., & Ben-Yishay, Y. (1999). Psychotherapy and psychotherapeutic interventions in brain injury rehabilitation. In M. Rosenthal (Ed.), *Rehabilitation of the adult and child with traumatic brain injury* (3rd ed., pp. 271–283). Philadelphia.: F. A. Davis.

Prigatano, G. P., Fordyce, D. J., Zeiner, H. K., Roueche, J. R., Pepping, M., & Wood, B. C. (1986). *Neuropsychological rehabilitation after brain injury.* Baltimore: The Johns Hopkins University Press.

Prigatano, G. P., Klonoff, P. S., O'Brien, K. P., Altman, I., Amin, K., Chiapello, D. A., Shepherd, J., Cunningham, M., & Mora, M. (1994). Productivity after neuropsychologically oriented, milieu rehabilitation. *Journal of Head Trauma Rehabilitation, 9*(1), 91–102.

Prigatano, G. P., Pepping, M., & Klonoff, P. (1986). Cognitive, personality and psychosocial factors in the neuropsychological assessment of brain-injured patients. In B. Uzzel & Y. Gross (Eds.), *Clinical neuropsychology of intervention* (pp. 135–166). Martinus Nijhoff.

Prigatano, G. P., & Smith, K. A. (2000). The role of psychotherapy in a neurological institute. *BNI Quarterly,* 16(3), 7–11.

Strupp, H. H. (1996). The tripartite model and the *Consumer Reports* study. *American Psychologist, 51*(10), 1017–1024.

16

CHAPTER

Barbara A. Wilson
Jonathan Evans

Does Cognitive Rehabilitation Work? Clinical and Economic Considerations and Outcomes

What Is Cognitive Rehabilitation?

At its basic level, cognitive rehabilitation can be regarded as remediation or reduction of cognitive deficits following insult to the brain. However, a number of alternative definitions can be found in papers published since the term gained popular usage in the 1980s. Many of the existing definitions are imprecise or limiting, such as those proffered by Gianutsos (1980s, p. 37): "a service designed to remediate disorders of perception, memory and language," and by Wood (1990, p. 3): "Cognitive rehabilitation uses an assortment of procedures to improve or restore a diverse collection of abilities and skills." Closer to our own view is a definition by Sohlberg and Mateer (1989), who suggested,

> Cognitive rehabilitation . . . refers to the therapeutic process of increasing or improving an individual's capacity to process and use incoming information so as to allow increased functioning in everyday life. This includes both methods to restore cognitive function and compensatory techniques. (pp. 3–4)

Sohlberg and Mateer continued by stating, "Cognitive rehabilitation applies to therapy methods that actually retrain or alleviate problems caused by deficits in attention, visual processing, language, memory, reasoning/problem solving, and executive functions" (p. 4).

Ben-Yishay and Prigatano (1990) offered a variation on this when they suggested that cognitive rehabilitation is "the amelioration of deficits in problem solving abilities in order to improve functional competence in everyday situations (p. 395).

One factor missing from such definitions is a recognition that any kind of rehabilitation is an interactive process involving the disabled person, therapeutic staff, and probably also relatives and the wider community (McLellan, 1991). Recognizing the fundamental importance of this interactive process, in this chapter we have taken as our basic premise that cognitive rehabilitation is "a process whereby brain injured people work together with health professionals to remediate or alleviate cognitive deficits arising from a neurological insult" (Wilson, 1996, p. 637). Our arguments in this chapter will be supported by an extension of this premise to include any strategy or technique that enables brain-injured people and their families to understand, come to terms with, bypass, or reduce cognitive deficits in order to function as adequately as possible in an environment that is most appropriate to them.

☐ A Brief History of the Development of Cognitive Rehabilitation

Although a relatively new discipline, the origins of rehabilitation go back a long way, as witnessed in the surgical papyrus document acquired by Edwin Smith in 1862 (described by Walsh, 1987), showing that treatment of brain-injured people can be traced back to Ancient Egypt some 2,500 to 3,000 years BC. However, the examples from the Smith papyrus provided by Walsh are more related to medical aspects of treatment rather than rehabilitation in any of the senses described above. Modern-day rehabilitation probably began during World War I as a result of improvements in the survival rates of head-injured soldiers (Goldstein, 1942). As Poser, Kohler, and Schönle (1996) reminded us in their historical review of neuropsychological rehabilitation in Germany: "Many of the rehabilitation procedures developed in special military hospitals during World War I are still in use today in modern rehabilitation—at least to some extent" (p. 259). Poser et al. (1996) suggested that the first important publication recognizing the role of rehabilitation was that by Poppelreuter (1917), which dealt with the treatment of visual impairment in a group of 700 soldiers seen in Germany between 1914 and 1916. Interestingly, as far back as 1917, Poppelreuter argued for an interdisciplinary approach between psychology, neurology, and psychiatry; in a paper published in 1918, he emphasized the importance of the patient's own insight into the effects of disabilities and treatment.

Goldstein (1942), also writing about World War I, stressed the importance of cognitive and personality deficits following brain injury, and touched upon what would be called today cognitive rehabilitation strategies (Prigatano, 1986). In 1918, Goldstein (quoted by Poser et al., 1996) was concerned with decisions about whether to try to restore lost functioning or to compensate for lost or impaired functions—and, as is well-known through recent documentation, this debate is alive and well at the beginning of the twenty-first century. This is true also of Goldstein's interest in work therapy (vocational therapy), which constitutes an important part of modern rehabilitation methodology.

During World War II, Luria (in the [then] Soviet Union) and Zangwill (in the United Kingdom) were both working with brain-injured soldiers. In a paper describing Luria's contributions to neuropsychological rehabilitation, Christensen and Caetano (1996) suggested that World War II was the most significant factor in Luria's development of neuropsychological rehabilitation methods. One important principle stressed by both Luria and Zangwill was that of "functional adaptation," whereby an intact skill is used to compensate for a damaged one; and we have already seen that Goldstein was committed to a similar concept. Luria's publications of 1963 and 1970, and his work with Naydin, Tsvetkova and Vinarskaya (Luria et al., 1969) are well worth reading today for the insights they offer. So too is Zangwill's (1947) paper, in which he discusses, among other things, the principles of reeducation and refers to three main approaches to rehabilitation: compensation, substitution, and direct retraining. In the United States, the most influential people in rehabilitation during World War II were Cranich; (1947) and Wepman (1951), who both worked with people with aphasia, and Aita (1946, 1948), who set up a day-treatment program for men with penetrating injury to the brain.

The next major move forward probably came with the Israeli programs, yet again stimulated by wars, such as those described by Najenson et al. (1974) and Ben-Yishay (1978). Ben-Yishay (1996) described in some detail the origins of his approach, the evolution of the therapeutic milieu concept, and the philosophy behind his thinking. At about the same time that Ben-Yishay was developing his therapeutic milieu program, greater numbers of survivors of road traffic accidents prompted the growth of specialist rehabilitation centers in the United States, such as the Rancho Los Amigos Hospital in California (Malkmus, Booth, & Kodimer, 1980). The first program to call itself a cognitive rehabilitation program appears to be that of Diller in New York (Diller, 1976). Diller and Ben-Yishay have worked closely together for more than 20 years, and the former was one of Ben-Yishay's main supporters in setting up the Israeli program. Prigatano's (1986) program in Oklahoma also was heavily influenced by Ben-Yishay, adopting a holistic approach (described below). Prigatano later moved his program to Phoenix, Arizona. In turn, he influenced Christensen, who opened a similar program in Copenhagen, Denmark, in 1995 (Christensen & Teasdale, 1995); and Wilson and colleagues who opened the Oliver Zangwill Centre in Cambridgeshire, England in 1996 (Wilson et al., 2000).

A more detailed history of neuropsychological and cognitive rehabilitation can be found in Boake (1996).

☐ Underlying Theoretical Bases for Cognitive Rehabilitation

In her foreword to the 1989 Sohlberg and Mateer book *An Introduction to Cognitive Rehabilitation,* Gianutsos suggested that cognitive rehabilitation is born of a mixed parentage, including neuropsychology, occupational therapy, speech and language therapy, and special education. Others draw from different fields: McMillan and Greenwood (1993), for example, believed that rehabilitation should draw on clinical neuropsychology, behavioral analysis, cognitive retraining, and group and individual psychotherapy. Still others believe only one "parent" is necessary, and these tend to be supporters of the use of theories from cognitive neuropsychology to inform treatment. In the first issue of the prestigious journal *Cognitive Neuropsychology,* Coltheart (1984) argued that rehabilitation programs should be based on a theoretical analysis of the nature of the disorder to be treated. Mitchum and Berndt (1995) suggested that the goal of cognitive rehabilitation is "the development of rational therapies that are based upon a theoretical analysis of the nature of the disorder that is targeted for treatment" (p. 13).

Most people working in cognitive rehabilitation argue that theoretical models are necessary for appropriate treatment, although they also may argue that they are not necessarily sufficient on their own. The situation is made more complex because there is disagreement as to what constitutes a theoretical model. Gianutsos (1991), for example, claimed that cognitive rehabilitation is the application of theories of cognitive sciences to traumatic brain injury (TBI) rehabilitation. Apart from the fact that it is not only people with TBI who receive cognitive rehabilitation, Gianutsos's approach does not appear to be influenced by theories from cognitive science, as she favors the repeated practice approach whereby patients or clients engage, for the most part, in computerized, cognitive exercises (Gianutsos, 1981, 1991; Gianutsos, Cochran, & Blouin, 1985; Gianutsos & Matheson, 1987). There is little if any evidence in these papers of theories of cognitive neuroscience. Similarly, the influential Sohlberg and Mateer book, although arguing that rehabilitation should be scientific and grounded in theory, does not follow its authors' own advice, according to Robertson (1991):

> [T]he theories of normal neuropsychological functioning which Sohlberg and Mateer present as underlying their treatment and assessment methods are frankly facile. They are not theoretical models, but collections of headings to guide assessment and treatment. (p. 88)

Robertson conceded that many of the approaches make intuitive sense, but he objected to them being called theoretical models.

The most influential theories are without doubt those from cognitive neuropsychology, particularly from the fields of language and reading (see, for example, Coltheart, 1991; Mitchum & Berndt, 1995; Seron & Deloche, 1989). We have already referred to one of these models. Although it is true that theoretical models from cognitive neuropsychology have been highly influential in helping us to understand and explain related phenomena (Wilson & Patterson, 1990), and in helping us to develop assessment procedures, the trap waiting for them is rehabilitation irrelevance (Robertson, 1991). Wilson (1997a) also argued that models from cognitive neuropsychology tell us what to treat but not how to treat and that they are therefore insufficient on their own to guide us through the many intricate processes involved in the rehabilitation process.

Other theoretical approaches used in rehabilitation since the 1970s (e.g., Ince, 1976; Lincoln, 1978) and in cognitive rehabilitation (for example, Wilson, 1981; 1991a) are those from learning theory and behavioral psychology. Behavioral assessments to (a) identify and measure variables that control behavior, (b) select treatment, and (c) evaluate treatment (Nelson & Hayes, 1979) have been employed in cognitive rehabilitation programs (see, e.g., Wilson, 1987), and numerous approaches from behavior therapy and behavior modification can and have been adopted for helping people with memory, perceptual, reading, and language disorders (Wilson, 1987; 1991a; 1997a; 1999). As one of us (Wilson) said in 1989: "behavior therapy and behavior modification have generated a technology of learning based on careful observation and concerned with the gradual increment of appropriate behaviors or the decrement of inappropriate behaviors" (p. 123). A behavioral approach usually is incorporated into cognitive rehabilitation because it provides a structure, a way of analyzing cognitive problems, a means of assessing everyday manifestations of cognitive problems, and a means of evaluating the efficacy of treatment programs. It also, of course, supplies us with many existing treatment strategies such as shaping, chaining, modeling, desensitization, flooding, extinction, positive reinforcement, response cost, and so forth—all of which can be modified or adapted to suit particular rehabilitation purposes.

There are critics of this approach (see, e.g., Prigatano, 1997), but we suggest that much of the criticism is based on a misunderstanding of the role of behavioral or learning theories in cognitive rehabilitation. In the first place, the majority of psychologists engaged in cognitive rehabilitation do not adhere to rigid behavioral approaches such as those described by Skinner (1953) and Kazdin (1975). Instead, they tend to use elements such as task analysis or anxiety management techniques, modifying these strategies to make them appropriate for the brain-injured client's neurological and neuropsychological status. It is wrong, therefore, to criticize their use in cognitive rehabilitation as though they were simply a mirror image of Skinner's extreme proposals. Second, behavioral techniques are not used in isolation but are supplemented by theories, models, and technologies from a number of other areas. As Lafferty (1997) pointed out in a television interview, we should not be confined by our own theoretical framework. If rehabilitation is to advance, we need to draw from a number of theoretical bases (Diller, 1987; Wilson, 1987a).

Finally in this section we would like to consider the holistic approach as pioneered by Diller (1976), Ben-Yishay (1978), and Prigatano (1986). Proponents of this approach regard it as futile to separate the cognitive sequelae of brain injury from the emotional, social, and functional sequelae. After all, how we think, remember, communicate, and solve problems affects how we feel emotionally and how we behave, and vice versa. Most holistic programs are concerned with increasing a client's awareness, alleviating cognitive deficits, developing compensatory skills, and providing vocational counseling. All such programs provide a mixture of individual and group therapy. "Although there is as yet no irrefutable evidence of the success of the holistic programs, they appear to have been subjected to more research on efficacy than other approaches" (Diller, 1994). Furthermore, Cope (1994) argued that there is reasonably convincing evidence that comprehensive rehabilitation does make a substantial difference in the reduction of handicap for brain-injured patients.

Cognitive rehabilitation, then, is carried out in a number of ways (discussed in more detail by Wilson, 1997a). Combining the strengths of these approaches probably is the best way forward. Clinically, the holistic approach probably is the best for the majority of brain-injured people. However, this approach, as advanced by Prigatano and Ben Yishay, could perhaps be improved by incorporating ideas and practical applications from learning theory, such as task analysis, baseline recording, monitoring, and the implementation of single case experimental designs to individual treatment programs; and by referring to cognitive neuropsychological models in order to identify cognitive strengths and weaknesses in more detail, to explain observed phenomena, and to make predictions about cognitive functioning.

☐ Is Cognitive Rehabilitation Clinically Effective?

General Issues

This is not an easy question to answer, and one could make a positive or negative case according to the evidence one selects, or according to how one chooses to interpret the question. One of the prerequisites when conducting research is to make sure the initial questions one asks are posed in such a way as to make them answerable. Just as we would not undertake research in order to answer a general question such as "Are drugs effective?" so we should not be expected to answer directly the broad question above relating to cognitive rehabilitation. We need to ask more specific questions, so that any examination of evidence we undertake relates to particular areas that can be highlighted and analyzed adequately. As far as our purpose is concerned in this section, we need to find out which programs or techniques work for which people under which circumstances.

Many health economists, managers, scientists, physicians, and others believe there is only one way to evaluate the effectiveness of rehabilitation, and that is through the use of randomized, controlled trials, preferably under double-blind conditions. Yet, as Mai (1992) pointed out, it is hard to see how double-blind conditions can be applied in rehabilitation. Therapists and psychologists cannot be blind to the treatment they are giving and, in most cases, neither can patients be blind to the treatment they are receiving. It is possible in some cases, however, to conduct single-blind trials in which an assessor does not know which treatment has been provided (see, e.g., Wilson, 1997b). The Proceedings of the Aspen Neurobehavioral Conference (1998) go so far as to suggest that evaluation studies of rehabilitation should include only those in which the researchers evaluating programs are not the clinicians carrying them out.

Another important factor making such research very difficult, if not almost impossible, is that it is rarely if ever ethical to randomly allocate patients to treatment or no treatment. For example, in one study (Wilson, Shiel et al., 1994), we found that severely head injured people admitted to general wards without specialist head-injury services were more likely to develop contractures, inhalation pneumonia, and behavior problems than those admitted to specialist wards. Randomly allocating to treatment or no treatment in order to conduct a tighter piece of research in this area would be extremely hard if not impossible to justify.

Even though there is a place for randomized, controlled trials (RTCs) (leaving aside the more controversial decision to make them double-blind), and conceding that certain investigations can only be carried out in this way, we must nevertheless recognize that it is necessary to go beyond the limitations imposed by RCTs in order to evaluate cognitive rehabilitation adequately. As Andrews (1991) reminded us, the RCT "is a tool to be used, not a god to be worshipped" (p. 5). He argued that the RCT is an excellent tool in research where "the design is simple, where marked changes are expected, where the factors involved are relatively specific, and where the number of additional variables likely to affect the outcome is few and can be expected to be balanced out by the randomization procedure" (p. 5). Unfortunately, most investigations into the efficacy of rehabilitation are more complex, and (as already stated), randomization is not possible in most rehabilitation circumstances. It would be hard, for example, to have a control group receiving no rehabilitation or different treatment in a rehabilitation center committed to providing a holistic program for all its clients.

In their review of the literature on postacute brain-injury rehabilitation, Malec and Basford (1996) found that only one study of holistic rehabilitation had used an RCT. This study, reported by Ruff et al. (1989), described how 40 people with brain injury (from 1 to 7 years postinsult) were randomly allocated to an experimental or control group. The experimental group received a structured cognitive rehabilitation program together with psychotherapy. Both groups improved on a set of neuropsychological test measures, with no significant effects of group or interaction. We argue below, however, that standardized tests are not the best outcome measures to use when evaluating cognitive rehabilitation.

There are studies employing RCTs to look at more specific questions. For example, von Cramon, Matthes-von Cramon, and Mai (1991) wanted to discover whether specific problem-solving training benefited patients with brain injury. Patients in the study had difficulty planning, organizing, and problem solving, as measured by tests, observations, and rating scales. They were alternately allocated to specific problem-solving training (PST) or to memory training (MT). The procedures were clearly specified and the patients allocated to PST benefited to a significantly greater extent than those allocated to MT, as measured by posttreatment assessment. The fact that others have also used RCTs to evaluate particular aspects of rehabilitation (e.g., Berg, Koning-Haanstra, & Deelman, 1991) suggests that they have a place in answering certain questions. We must, however, consider other methodologies, such as surveys, direct observations, and single case experimental designs, in order to build up a broader picture of clinical effectiveness (Wilson, 1997b).

Published Findings

In a recently published report by the Agency for Health Care Policy and Research (AHCP&R), Oregon (Chesnut et al., 1999), 2,536 abstracts from articles on rehabilitation were traced to find answers to five specific questions, one of which was concerned with cognitive rehabilitation. The report was based on 363 articles, of which 114 related to cognitive rehabilitation with the specific question: "Does the application of compensatory rehabilitation enhance outcomes for people who sustain TBI?" Of the 114 potential articles, only 32 reached the final selection to evaluate effectiveness, with the remainder being excluded for various reasons such as review articles being purely descriptive, there were fewer than five subjects, and so on. Eleven of the 32 were RCTs, with 5 measuring relevant health outcomes and 6 measuring intermediate outcomes. The authors of the report concluded, that "along with the small size of the studies and the narrow range of interventions studied, the lack of information about the representativeness of the included patients makes it difficult to apply the findings of these studies to cognitive rehabilitation practice generally" (p. 55). In other words, the RCTs did not tell us much about the effectiveness of cognitive rehabilitation in any general sense.

The cognitive rehabilitation section of the report was published separately (Carney et al., 1999). The authors stated that, although the desired outcome of cognitive rehabilitation is improvement in daily function, many of the outcome measures are intermediate measures rather than health outcomes. By "intermediate measures," the authors mean test scores (123 tests of cognition were described in the studies). The question was posed as to whether improvements on test scores predict improvement in real-life function. The authors concluded, whereas there appears to be some relationship between intermediate measures and employment, the association is not strong." We question the wisdom of using test scores at all, irrespective of whether they are intermediate or direct, and recommend instead that rehabilitation therapists should consider the final outcome of their treatment. Scores on cognitive tests are surely not the way to evaluate the efficacy of cognitive rehabilitation. If, as we have argued, the ultimate goal of rehabilitation is to enable people with disabilities to function as adequately as possible in their most appropriate environment, then information on changes in scores on the Wechsler Scales, or any other standardized test, will not give us the information we require. JC, a densely amnesic patient known to us (Wilson, J. C. & Hughes, 1997), has shown no improvement on standardized tests over a 10-year period, yet he now lives on his own, is self-employed, and is completely independent thanks largely to excellent use of compensatory strategies. By most rehabilitationists' standards, these outcomes are very good indeed, yet if standardized tests had been used as measures of success, JC would have failed dismally.

One of our own studies mentioned in the AHCP&R report is an evaluation of NeuroPage, an electronic memory aid (Wilson, Evans et al., 1997). We measured the everyday memory failures of 15 clients during a 6-week baseline and then provided them with a pager to remind them of their target behaviors. Following 12 weeks using NeuroPage, the pager was withdrawn and we then monitored the clients for a further 3 to 4 week period. In the initial baseline period, the mean success rate for the 15 clients was 37%. In the pager phase this increased to over 85%. There was some drop back in the posttreatment (second baseline) phase to 74% but not to baseline levels; in fact, some clients had learned their routines during the 12-week pager phase. Not only was there a significant increase in success rate between the first baseline and treatment for the group as a whole, but every individual showed a statistically significant increase between the two stages. Although the AHCP&R report (Chestnut et al., 1999) acknowledges that this study was useful, it said, "the observational design of this study weakens its value as evidence of effectiveness" (p. 63). However, we would argue that, far from being a weakness, direct measures of real-life behaviors are a very strong way of indicating changes brought about by cognitive rehabilitation strategies. We targeted the real-life problems identified by clients and their families; we measured these for several weeks, thus having a control period (subjects being their own controls); we provided a clearly specified intervention; and we monitored clients once the pager was removed. Furthermore, we showed that the effectiveness of NeuroPage was not dependent on whether clients came from a particular diagnostic group; we showed that NeuroPage could be used once a day or several times during the day; and we saw that it is a flexible tool making a real difference to the quality of the everyday lives of the memory-impaired people in the study. Tackling real-life targets and individualizing programs within a specified framework is the way forward in cognitive rehabilitation. Clare and colleagues (Clare et al., 1999, 2000) also applied this principle to people with Alzheimer's disease. The client and family select the targets and then we find a way, using in this case errorless learning principles, to teach new information.

To return to the question of whether cognitive rehabilitation is clinically effective, we could use the AHCP&R report (Chesnut et al., 1999) to say that there is an "absence of strong and sufficient evidence for a direct effect of cognitive interventions on health and employment . . . and associations between performance on cognitive tests and post-trauma employment and productivity were inconsistent" (pp. 63–64). Alternatively, we could say that the question is too broad to be answerable and we need to look at other ways of asking (and answering) it. We can, for example, evaluate the effectiveness of some treatment procedures. We have already described the Wilson et al. (1997) NeuroPage study and the von Cramon et al. (1991) problem-solving therapy study. There are numerous other examples we could cite: Thoene and Glisky (1995), for example, investigated three methods of teaching names to memory-impaired people and found that face–name associations led to improved learning.

Single Case Experimental Designs and Small Group Studies

There are also numerous single case experimental designs demonstrating that it is possible to remediate or alleviate the cognitive deficits of certain brain-injured people. Wilson (1999), for example, described how a man who was completely unable to read following a gunshot wound was taught to read successfully 5 years later and achieved a reading age of 13 years. The value of single case experimental designs is that they allow us to evaluate an individual's response to treatment, to see if the client is changing over time, and to find out whether any changes are due to natural recovery or to the intervention itself. In other words, we can tease out the effects of treatment from the effects of spontaneous recovery and other nonspecific factors. Given that rehabilitation is planned for individuals, evaluation should take place at the individual as well as the group level, and the choice of individual or group study will again depend on the kind of questions that need answering. For example, if we want to find out whether a head-injured person is benefiting from an attention training program, we need to employ a single case experimental design. If we want to find out how many people appear to be benefiting from a particular procedure, we need to conduct a group study.

A group study would not necessarily inform us as to how any particular client within the group was or was not benefiting from any intervention, because each individual within the group is likely to have a different combination of deficits, be differently motivated, and have a different level of severity of impairment from all others in the group. Group studies average out performances, so individual differences are masked. Single case experimental designs, on the other hand, avoid many of the problems inherent in group designs. They are often chosen specifically for their ability to evaluate an individual's progress through cognitive rehabilitation, and they are, of course, perfectly respectable as far as their scientific methodology is concerned (Gianutsos & Gianutsos, 1987; Hersen & Barlow, 1982; Kazdin, 1982). An individual study can provide information that is complementary to a group study and, indeed, the two approaches should be held in equal regard. Large group studies are required when individual variations need to be shared out; single case (and small group) studies are preferable when each individual is monitored for a period of time, each acting as his or her own control, and when baselines are used instead of control groups.

A criticism often aimed at single case and small group studies points to their inability to generalize, because their findings apply only to the individual subject. Such criticism is not entirely fair and may be used by critics whose preferred methodology (large group studies) may not provide generalization because results are averaged and cannot therefore apply to individuals, most of whom will differ from the mean. We would argue that it is incorrect to assume that we cannot generalize from individual subjects. The whole history of neuropsychology provides examples of such generalization. From Broca's patient "Tan" (Broca, 1861) to H.M. (Scoville & Milner, 1957) to other classic cases in neuropsychology (Code, Wallesch, Joanette, 1996), we have not only learned a great deal from individual patients but also learned how to diagnose particular syndromes based on findings from these single cases.

Hersen and Barlow (1982) pointed out, "To increase the base for generalization from a single case experiment, one simply repeats the same experiment several times on similar patients, thereby providing the clinician with results from a number of patients" (p. 57). Gianutsos and Gianutsos (1987) went even further, arguing that it is only through single case designs that generalizability can be established through systematic replication with controlled changes across variables that might be expected to affect generalization. In light of such historical and contemporary findings, we would argue that single case experimental designs, with their ability to allow us to evaluate generalization systematically, should be embraced by those concerned with the efficacy of cognitive rehabilitation.

Establishing General Principles

We have shown in this chapter that some therapeutic techniques in the field of cognitive rehabilitation are effective; and we have argued that single case experimental designs offer a methodology that can be adapted more widely in the quest for establishing the effectiveness or otherwise of rehabilitation techniques. It also is possible to draw out some general principles that have been established in the field of cognitive rehabilitation. For example, the once widespread technique of trying to restore lost functioning through drills and exercises has been shown to be ineffective, at least in terms of its ability to generalize into real-life tasks (Robertson, 1990; Sloan & Ponsford, 1995; Sturm & Willmes, 1991). Repetition by itself is not an effective learning strategy (Baddeley, 1997). In the field of memory therapy it has been shown that distributed practice in the form of spaced retrieval (also known as expanding rehearsal) is a better method of learning than rote rehearsal (Camp, 1989; Clare & Wilson, 1997; Moffat, 1989). Visual imagery also is more efficacious for name learning than rote rehearsal, and preexposure to the faces to be learned is even more helpful (Downes et al., 1997; Wilson, 1987). A strategy known as PQRST (Preview, Question, Read, State, & Test) is better at enhancing recall of written material than straightforward repetition (Wilson, 1987a).

Perhaps the most exciting recent work in new learning has been in the area of errorless learning, a teaching technique whereby people are prevented (as far as possible) from making mistakes during the learning process. The effectiveness of this method has been convincingly demonstrated with memory impaired people (Baddeley & Wilson, 1994; Squires, Hunkin, & Parkin, 1997; Wilson, Baddeley, Evans, & Shiel, 1994; Wilson & Evans, 1996). Trial-and-error learning, or learning from our mistakes, is all very well when one has a reasonable episodic memory, but for those without adequate memory functioning, making a mistake can lead to the strengthening of an incorrect response.

Table 16.1 provides some examples of different research designs used to evaluate the effectiveness of cognitive rehabilitation.

☐ Summary of the Clinical Effectiveness of Cognitive Rehabilitation

There is increasing evidence to support the view that rehabilitation can improve cognitive functioning (Robertson, 1999). Rehabilitation programs may work through teaching people to compensate for their difficulties (Wilson & Watson, 1996), through helping them to learn more efficiently (Baddeley & Wilson, 1994; Downes et al., 1997; Wilson, Baddeley, et al., 1994), or through achieving restoration (or partial restoration) of functioning resulting from plasticity and exercising (Robertson & Murre, 1999; Robertson, Tegnér, Tham, Lo, & Nimmo-Smith, 1995; Sturm, Willmes, Orgass & Hartje, 1997). Robertson (1999) argued that restoration may be possible after relatively small lesions, whereas compensatory processes are more likely to underlie recovery from larger lesions. Although this idea is similar to that offered by Poppelreuter in 1917, Robertson based his views on connectionist models aimed at predicting recovery. Plaut (1996) also used a connectionist model to predict recovery, and argued that the degree of relearning and generalization varies considerably depending on the lesion location—

TABLE 16.1. Examples of Different Research Designs Used to Evaluate the Clinical Efficacy of Some Aspects of Cognitive Rehabilitation

Research Design	Example	Result	Comments
Randomized control trial	Berg et al. (1991) randomly allocated TBI patients to memory strategy training, drill and repetitive practice or control group.	Both memory strategy and drill/repetitive practice, groups subjectively rated their memory as better, but only the strategy group scored significantly better on objective tests of memory.	Not clear how well results generalized to real–life tasks.
Randomized control trial/crossover design	Wilson et al. (2001): People with memory or planning problems randomly allocated to treatment (pager) for 7 weeks or waiting list. After 7 weeks people on waiting list received pager.	Significant effects of pager, which reduced everyday problems.	Target behaviors were selected by clients, families, and therapists. So real-life tasks were selected for treatment.
Three group design—two approaches to learning compared	Baddeley and Wilson (1994) compared 16 amnesic people with 16 young control participants and 16 older control participants on learning a stem completion task using errorless and errorful learning.	Errorless learning was significantly better than errorful learning, particularly for the people with amnesia.	Although these results were potentially important clinically, the experiment did not address real-life problems.
Three group design—two groups with brain injury and a control group compared on various tasks	Alderman (1996) looked at brain-injured people who did not respond to a token economy program and compared this group with brain-injured responders and controls on divided attention tasks.	With exaggerated verbal feedback, the brain-injured nonresponders were able to achieve the level of the other groups.	Not clear whether these results would apply to everyday life.

TABLE 16.1. Continued

Research Design	Example	Result	Comments
Two group design (alternate allocation to treatment or control group)	Von Cramon et al. (1991): Brain-injured people alternatively allocated to problem solving training (PST) or control group.	People in PST group improved on some objective tests and on behavioral ratings by ward staff.	Appeared to be generalization for some people in PST group.
One group design baseline-treatment-postbaseline monitoring	Wilson et al. (1997): 15 people with memory or planning problems monitored for 6 weeks, given a pager for 12 weeks and monitored for 4 weeks, after return of the pager.	Significant improvement for group and for each individual between baseline and treatment. For most, improvement was maintained when pager returned.	Real-life tasks targeted.
Single case experimental designs	Wilson et al. (1994): A series of single case designs to compare errorful and errorless learning for real life tasks.	In each case errorless learning was superior to errorful learning.	Errorless learning is better than trial-and-error learning for people with severe memory problems; not clear if this is true for other cognitive problems.

and this, in turn, has implications for understanding the nature and variability of improvement following brain injury. Plaut's model appears to address retraining rather than compensation, although, as both Zangwill and Luria believed during World War II, both are important aspects of rehabilitation.

Is Rehabilitation Cost Effective?

Despite differences in the provision of rehabilitation in the United Kingdom, the United States, Australia, and so forth, all countries are interested in whether results justify costs. For a discussion on how rehabilitation is purchased in the United Kingdom, see McCarthy (1999); and for an interesting account of the industrialization of rehabilitation, particularly as it relates to the United States, see Diller (2000).

Wood, McCrea, Wood, and Merriman (1999) said that international opinion about the clinical and cost-effectiveness of neurorehabilitation is divided, with considerable skepticism seen among neurologists, neurosurgeons, and others, but with enthusiasm among some staff providing such rehabilitation. Wood et al. discussed two types of costs, direct and indirect. Direct costs refer to the provision of treatment, and indirect costs refer to social burdens such as time off work and sickness benefits. So is rehabilitation cost-effective?

In one American study of 145 brain-injured patients (Cope, Cole, Hall, & Barkan, 1991), the estimated savings in care costs following rehabilitation for people with severe brain injury was over £27,000 ($40,500) per year. The number of people requiring 24-hours-per-day care dropped from 23% to 4% after rehabilitation. A Danish study (Mehlbye & Larsen, 1994) reported that spendings in health and social care for patients attending a nonresidential program were recouped in 3 years. The costs of not rehabilitating people with brain injury are also considerable, given the fact that many are young, with a relatively normal life expectancy (Greenwood & McMillan, 1993). Cope (1994) suggested that postacute rehabilitation programs can produce sufficient savings to justify their support on a cost–benefit basis. On a slightly different theme, a study by West et al. (1991) claimed that people with TBI who had attended a supported work program earned more than the program cost after 58 weeks of supported employment. Furthermore, after 2.5 years, there was a net gain to the taxpayers who had ultimately funded the service. This did not include the indirect costs, such as savings from family members who were able to return to work. Three case studies reported by Bistany (1988) estimated annual and lifetime costs with and without a specialized rehabilitation program. The estimated lifetime saving was over $1 million (U.S.) dollars for each of the three individuals.

Wood et al. (1999) were interested in the clinical and cost-effectiveness of a postacute neurobehavioral community rehabilitation program. They looked at 76 people surviving severe brain injury who attended the program. The majority had sustained their injuries more than 2 years prior to admission, and all had spent at least 6 months in rehabilitation. In terms of improved social outcomes and savings in care hours, it was found that the most cost-effective provision was to provide rehabilitation within 2 years of head injury. Nevertheless, it was still worthwhile in terms of clinical and cost-effectiveness to offer rehabilitation to those who were more than 2 years postinsult.

It also is possible to estimate the costs of separate components of a rehabilitation service. For example, the NeuroPage® project (referred to earlier) was shown to save money for the British Health Service and Social Services. Prior to the program, one client (described originally by Evans, Emslie, & Wilson, 1998) had a week's respite care every 3 months to give her family a break. Her local health authority paid for this, at a cost of $2,000 for 1 week's care (i.e., $8,000 per annum). Since having the pager, she has never needed respite care, so over a 5-year period her health authority has saved $40,000. Another client on the same system who was seen 7 years post head injury learned to live independently with the pager (Wilson, Emslie, Quirk et al., 1999). After being involved in a 16-week research project (baseline for 2 weeks, pager for 7 weeks, and postbaseline monitoring for 7 weeks), the young man moved into his own apartment, with 24-hour care provided by Social Services. An estimate of the costs for the carers (based on Wood et al., 1999) was $11 per hour (i.e., $264.24 per day, $1,849.68 per week, and $96,183.36 per year). Within 3 months, the man was able to manage with one carer for 12 hours rather than two carers over 24 hours, thus halving the costs to Social Services.

The research on NeuroPage is now complete, and a commercial service is available. The cost of providing this is $90 per client per month. This covers the hire of a pager, air time, a contribution to the salary of the staff member running the program, overheads, and a royalty to the developer of NeuroPage. Although this is a considerable amount of money to find for some families, most of the clients are funded by Health or Social Services. In the long term, money is likely to be saved in a number of ways, not only through reduced stays in hospitals and a reduction in the number of carers, but also because medication is taken reliably, hospital visits are missed less often, and family members can return to work.

Although much needs to be done, there is growing evidence that neuropsychological rehabilitation programs are effective clinically and economically and contribute toward improving quality of life. We end with a case study of one young man who illustrated each of these points.

☐ Case Example

The following case study provides a good example of the clinical and cost-effectiveness of neuropsychological rehabilitation. Although it does not represent a controlled, empirical test of the effectiveness of rehabilitation, the case strongly suggests that, without the opportunity to engage in a postacute neuropsychological rehabilitation program, the outcome would have been much worse.

At the time of his injury, Mark was an international property underwriter for a large insurance company, working in the city of London. His hobby was mountain biking, and while on a holiday in Switzerland 2.5 years ago, he fell 1,000 feet down a mountain. He had stopped on his bike to take some photographs and fell while remounting his bike. He suffered three broken ribs, a broken finger, multiple lacerations to his legs, and a very severe head injury. He was airlifted to a specialist hospital in Switzerland. He was in coma for 1 week. An acute CT scan revealed diffuse axonal injury; edema; small, deep mid-line hemorrhages; and a subdural hematoma, which was evacuated via a burr hole. He required a tracheostomy for 11 days. He also contracted meningitis, pneumonia, and septicemia. He was transferred to the National Hospital in London and then to an acute rehabilitation center, also in London.

At that time, Mark was ataxic and sometimes agitated. He needed two people to help him stand from sitting. His posttraumatic amnesia was 6 weeks in length. He made good progress in acute rehabilitation, particularly in terms of physical functioning. However, 9 months postinjury, when he began an intensive neuropsychological rehabilitation program at the Oliver Zangwill Centre (see Wilson et al., 2000), he continued to experience significant cognitive difficulties. The most significant impairment was in memory (particularly delayed recall), affecting both visual and verbal memory. He also had some attention problems, particularly with sustained attention. His general intellectual, perception, and language skills were intact. He had some mild problems with planning tasks and was described by relatives as lacking initiative in comparison to his premorbid personality. He had some insight into his difficulties, but initially did not appreciate the nature and extent of his memory difficulties and the potential impact of such impairments on his work.

With the rehabilitation team, Mark set some specific goals for his program, which lasted 20 weeks—the first 10 weeks being intensive (i.e., 5 days per week) and the second 10 weeks being divided between home, work, and the rehabilitation center. There were five goals for his program:

1. to develop an awareness of his strengths and weaknesses in a written form consistent with his neuropsychological profile, and to describe how any problems would affect on domestic, social, and work situations;
2. to identify whether he could return to his previous employment;
3. to manage his financial affairs independently;
4. to demonstrate competence in negotiation skills as rated by a work colleague;
5. to develop a range of leisure interests.

To achieve these goals Mark engaged in a program that consisted of both group work (e.g., understanding brain injury group, memory group, planning/problem-solving group) and work with individual team members.

There were many elements to Mark's program, but one of the most critical was helping him cope with memory difficulties. His insight into these problems was achieved by education about the nature of memory and the problems that may exist after brain injury (through understanding brain injury group and memory group). He was given feedback from the results of standardized assessments. He was asked (prompted and monitored) to keep a diary of memory errors. He was asked to consider his work role and to identify the demands on memory that were made as part of his work. He developed better insight into his difficulties, which had a "down side" in that he began to feel low as he became less confident that he would be able to return to work. However, the rehabilitation team supported him in developing a set of strategies to compensate for the problems. He adopted these strategies successfully, using a large diary for appointments and "things to do." He began to use a computer contacts card system for recording relevant information about brokers who came to him with business. He also learned to use mnemonic strategies for remembering people's names and other information. Mark recognized that the ability to judge risk effectively was the essence of his premorbid success as an underwriter, and that his ability to do this depended on picking up on and remembering pieces of information about locations (e.g., earthquake zones), companies, and situations that might present a risk. To compensate for his memory in relation to this issue, he developed a database of information about insurance risks (i.e., details of major losses and disasters compiled from the Lloyds list), in order to keep up to date with information, and to which he could refer when assessing risk associated with new business. Many of these strategies might be used by nonmemory-impaired underwriters, but Mark had previously been successful without any of them. For this reason he had to go through the process of appreciating the nature of his difficulties, accepting the need for memory aids, implementing strategies, and evaluating their value.

Critical to Mark's successful return to work was a program of step-wise increases in the level of work responsibilities. Initially he shadowed other underwriters, who asked him for his views on business offered to them by brokers. Next he undertook "minimal risk" business, such as insurance renewals. Then he was able to make underwriting decisions, but these had to be checked by his manager. Finally, he was given full underwriting authority. This staged approach was necessary for a variety of reasons. It allowed his manager to develop confidence in Mark's judgment in a high-risk business; it enabled Mark to develop his confidence; and it allowed time for Mark to learn to apply the strategies he had developed to compensate for memory problems.

At a time in his recovery when the rate of biological, spontaneous recovery might be expected to be slowing, Mark continued to experience considerable cognitive problems. It is difficult to be certain what would have happened to Mark had he not had the opportunity to undertake a postacute rehabilitation program, but it seems reasonable to speculate that he would have tried to return to work (if given the opportunity by his employers) and almost certainly would have failed. More likely, perhaps, particularly given the financial risks attached to the business in which he works, he would not have been given the opportunity to return to work by his employers, who needed the reassurance of the clinical team that it was appropriate for Mark to commence work. His program consisted of a combination of education and practical work to help him develop the necessary insight and strategies to compensate for problems. The group-based nature of the rehabilitation appeared to facilitate the development of insights, and also provided Mark with a supportive environment at a time when he was feeling low as a result of increased insight. Close working with supportive employers was critical.

Seven months after beginning his rehabilitation program, Mark was reinstated on the company payroll, and after another 12 months he remained employed. He continues to use the strategies he learned, which he reports are absolutely necessary to his success at work. By being in work he contributes to the cost of his rehabilitation through the tax he pays on his salary and the tax his company pays as a result of Mark's success. By being in work, welfare costs also are saved. Although it is true that not all patients undertaking rehabilitation are in a position to make such clinical or financial gains, cases such as Mark's illustrate that rehabilitation can be both clinically and cost-effective.

Summary and Conclusions

This chapter considers several definitions of cognitive rehabilitation, preferring the one proposed by Wilson (1996), that "Cognitive rehabilitation is . . . a process whereby brain injured people work together with health professionals to remediate or alleviate cognitive deficits arising from a neurological insult" (p. 637). A short history of cognitive rehabilitation is presented, focusing on progress made during World Wars I and II, the 6-day war in Israel, and the beginning of holistic programs. The following section discusses the underlying theoretical bases for cognitive rehabilitation and reaches the conclusion that we should combine the strengths of several theoretical approaches, particularily the holistic approach, theories of cognitive functioning, and theories of learning.

The next point addressed is whether cognitive rehabilitation is clinically effective. Questions regarding effectiveness should be posed so they can be answered rather than posed in a general way, such as "does rehabilitation work?"—which is essentially unanswerable. Research designs are considered, published findings reported and critically evaluated, and some general rehabilitation principles described. The conclusion to this section is that there is increasing evidence to support the view that rehabilitation can improve cognitive functioning.

The final section is concerned with the cost-effectiveness of rehabilitation. Despite scepticism in some quarters, there is evidence from several studies that cognitive rehabilitation is cost-effective. A case study of one man who sustained a severe traumatic brain injury illustrates how rehabilitation for this person was both clinically and cost-effective.

References

Aita, J. A. (1948). Follow-up study of men with penetrating injury to the brain. *Archives of Neurological Psychiatry, 59,* 511–516.

Aita, J. A. (1946). Men with brain damage. *American Journal of Psychiatry, 103,* 205–213.

Alderman, N. (1996). Central Executive Deficit and Response to Operant Conditioning Methods. *Neuropsychological Rehabilitation, 6*(3), 161–186.

Andrews, K. (1991). The limitations of randomized controlled trials in rehabilitation research. *Clinical Rehabilitation, 5,* 5–8.

Baddeley, A. D. (1997). *Human memory: Theory and practice* (Rev. Ed.). Hove, UK: Psychology Press.

Baddeley, A. D., & Wilson, B. A. (1994). When implicit learning fails: Amnesia and the problem of error elimination. *Neuropsychologia, 32,* 53–68.

Ben-Yishay, Y. (1996). Reflections on the evolution of the therapeutic milieu concept. *Neuropsychological Rehabilitation, 6,* 327–343.

Ben-Yishay, Y. (Ed.). (1978). *Working approaches to remediation of cognitive deficits in brain damaged persons: Rehabilitation monograph.* New York: New York University Medical Center.

Ben-Yishay, Y., & Prigatano, G. P. (1990). Cognitive remediation. In M. Rosenthal, E. R. Griffith, M. R. Bond, & J. D. Miller (Eds.), *Rehabilitation of the adult and child with traumatic brain injury* (2nd ed., pp. 393–409). Philadelphia: F.A. Davis.

Berg, I. J., Koning-Haanstra, M., & Deelman, B. G. (1991). Long term effects of memory rehabilitation: A controlled study. *Neuropsychological Rehabilitation, 1,* 97–111.

Bistany, D. V. (1988). Cost benefits of rehabilitation programs. In A.-L. Christensen & B. P. Uzzell (Eds.), *Neuropsychological rehabilitation* (pp. 87–101). Boston: Kluwer Academic Publishers.

Boake, C. (1996). Editorial: Historical aspects of neuropsychological rehabilitation. *Neuropsychological Rehabilitation, 6,* 241–243.

Broca, P. (1981). Nouvelle observation d'aphémie produite par une lésion de la moité postérieur des deuxième et troisième circonvolutions frontales. *Bulletin de la Sociéte Anatomique de Paris, 36,* 398–407.

Camp, C. J. (1989). Facilitation of new learning in Alzheimer's disease. In G. Gilmore, P. Whitehouse, & M. Wykle (Eds.), *Memory and aging: Theory, research and practice* (pp. 212–225). New York: Springer.

Carney, N., Chesnut, R. M., Maynard, H., Mann, N. C., Patterson, P., & Helfand, M. (1999). Effect of cognitive rehabilitation on outcomes for persons with traumatic brain injury: A systematic review. *Journal of Head Trauma Rehabilitation, 14,* 277–307.

Chesnut, R. M., Carney, N., Maynard, H., Patterson, P., Mann, N. C., & Helfand, M. (1999). Rehabilitation for traumatic brain injury. *AHCPR Publ.* (no. 99-EOO6).

Christensen, A.-L., & Caetano, C. (1996). Romanovich Luria: (1902–1977). Contributions to neuropsychological rehabilitation. *Neuropsychological Rehabilitation, 6,* 279–303.

Christensen, A.-L., & Teasdale, T. (1995). A clinical and neuropsychological led post-acute rehabilitation programme. In M. A. Chamberlain, V. C. Neuman, & A. Tennant (Eds.), *Traumatic brain injury rehabilitation: Initiatives in service delivery, treatment and measuring outcome* (pp. 88–98). New York: Chapman & Hall.

Clare, L., & Wilson, B. A. (1997). *Coping with memory problems: A practical guide for people with memory impairments, relatives, friends and carers.* Bury St Edmunds, UK: Thames Valley Test Company.

Clare, L., Wilson, B. A., Breen, E. K., & Hodges, J. R. (1999). Learning face-name associations in early Alzheimer's disease. *Neurocase, 5,* 37–46.

Clare, L., Wilson, B. A., Carter, G., Breen, K., Gosses, A., & Hodges, J. R. (2000). Intervening with everyday memory problems in dementia of Alzheimer type: An errorless learning approach. *Journal of Clinical and Experimental Neuropsychology, 22,* 132–146.

Code, C., Wallesch, C.-W., Joanette, Y., Lecours, A. R. (Eds.). (1996). *Classic cases in neuropsychology.* Hove: Psychology Press.

Coltheart, M. (1991). Cognitive psychology applied to the treatment of acquired language disorders. In P. Martin (Ed.), *Handbook of behavior therapy and psychological science: An integrative approach* (pp. 216–226). New York: Pergamon Press.

Coltheart, M. (984). Editorial. *Cognitive Neuropsychology, 1,* 1–8.

Cope, D. N., Cole, J. R., Hall, K. M., & Barkan, H. (1991). Brain injury: Analysis of outcome in a post-acute rehabilitation system. *Brain Injury, 5,* 111–139.

Cope, N. (1994). Traumatic brain injury rehabilitation outcome studies in the United States. In A.-L., Christensen & B. P. Uzzell (Eds.), *Brain injury and neuropsychological rehabilitation: International perspectives* (pp. 201–220). Hillsdale, NJ: Lawrence Erlbaum.

Cranich, L. (1947). *Aphasia: A guide to retraining.* New York: Grune & Stratton.

Diller, L. (2000). Cognitive rehabilitation during the industrialization of rehabilitation. In A.-L. Christensen & B. P. Uzzell (Eds.), *International handbook of neuropsychological rehabilitation* (pp. 315–325). New York: Kluwer Academic/Plenum.

Diller, L. L. (1994). Changes in rehabilitation over the past 5 years. In In A.-L., Christensen, B. P. Uzzell (Eds.), *Brain injury and neuropsychological rehabilitation: International perspectives* (pp. 1–15). Hillsdale, NJ: Lawrence Erlbaum.

Diller, L. L. (1987). Neuropsychological rehabilitation. In M. J. Meier, A. L. Benton, & L. Diller (Eds.), *Neuropsychological rehabilitation* (pp. 3–17). Edinburgh: Churchill Livingstone.

Diller, L. L. (1976). A model for cognitive retraining in rehabilitation. *The Clinical Psychologist, 29,* 13–15, 1976.

Downes, J. J., Kalla, T., Davies, A. D. M., Flynn, A. F., Ali, H., & Mayes, A. R. (1997). The pre-exposure technique: A novel method for enhancing the effects of imagery in face-name association learning. *Neuropsychological Rehabilitation, 7,* 195–214.

Evans, J. J., Emslie, H. C., & Wilson, B. A. (1998). External cueing systems in the rehbilitation of executive impairments of action. *Journal of the International Neuropsychological Society, 4,* 399–408.

Gianutsos, R. (1991). Cognitive rehabilitation: A neuropsychological specialty comes of age. *Brain Injury, 5,* 363–368.

Gianutsos, R. (1981). Training the short- and long-term verbal recall of a post-encephalitis amnesic. *Journal of Clinical Neuropsychology, 3,* 143–153.

Gianutsos, R. (1980). What is cognitive rehabilitation? *Journal of Rehabilitation, 1,* 37–40.

Gianutsos, R., Cochran, E. E., & Blouin, M. (1985). *Computer programs for cognitive rehabilitation, vol. 3: Therapeutic memory exercises for independent use.* Bayport, NY: Life Science Associates.

Gianutsos, R., & Gianutsos, J. (1987). Single case experimental approaches to the assessment of interventions in rehabilitation psychology. In B. Caplan (Ed.), *Rehabilitation psychology* (pp. 453–470). Rockville, MD: Aspen Corp.

Gianutsos, R., & Matheson, P. (1987). The rehabilitation of visual perceptual disorders attributable to brain injury. In M. Meier, A. Benton, & L. Diller (Eds.), *Neuropsychological rehabilitation* (pp. 303–241). London: Churchill Livingstone.

Goldstein, K. (1942). *Aftereffects of brain injury in war.* New York: Grune & Stratton.

Greenwood, R. J., & McMillan, T. M. (1993). Models of rehabilitation programmes for the brain-injured adult–I: Current provision, efficacy and good practice. *Clinical Rehabilitation, 7,* 248–255.

Hersen, M., & Barlow, D. H. (1982). *Single case experimental designs.* Oxford: Pergamon Press.

Ince, L. P. (1976). *Behavior modification in rehabilitation medicine.* Baltimore: Williams & Wilkins.

Kazdin, A. E. (1982). *Single case research designs.* New York: Oxford University Press.

Kazdin, A. E. (1975). *Behavior modification in applied settings.* Chicago: Dorsey Press.

Lafferty, A. (1997). Quote from a BBC Television programme on genetics.

Lincoln, N. B. (1978). Behaviour modification in physiotherapy. *Physiotherapy, 64,* 265–267.

Luria, A. R. (1970). *Traumatic aphasia.* The Hague: Mouton.

Luria, A. R. (1963). *Recovery of function after brain injury.* New York: Macmillan.

Luria, A. R., Naydin, V. L.,Tsvetkova, L. S., & Vinarskaya, E. N. (1969). Restoration of higher cortical functions following local brain damage. In V. Vinken & G. W. Bruyn (Eds.), *Handbook of clinical neurology: Volume 3* (pp. 368–433). New York: Elsevier.

Mai, N. (1992). Discussion: Evaluation in constructing neuropsychological treatments. In N. Von Steinbüchel, D. Y. von Cramon, & E. Pöppel E (Eds.), *Neuropsychological rehabilitation* (pp. 96–99). Berlin: Springer-Verlag.

Malec, J. F., & Basford, J. S. (1996). Post acute brain injury rehabilitation. *Archives of Physical Medicine and Rehabilitation, 77,* 198–207.

Malkmus, D., Booth, B. J., & Kodimer, C. (1980). *Rehabilitation of the head injured adult: Comprehensive cognitive management.* Downey, CA: Professional Staff Association of Rancho Los Amigos Hospital.

McCarthy, M. (1999). Purchasing neurorehabilitation in the UK National Health Service. *Neuropsychological Rehabilitation, 9,* 295–303.

McLellan, D. L. (1991). Functional recovery and the principles of disability medicine. In M. Swash & J. Oxbury (Eds.), *Clinical neurology* (pp. 768–790). Edinburgh: Churchill Livingstone.

McMillan, T. M., & Greenwood, R. J. (1993). Model of rehabilitation programmes for the brain-injured adult–II: Model services and suggestions for change in the UK. *Clinical Rehabilitation, 7,* 346–355.

Mehlbye, J., & Larsen, A. (1994). Social and economic consequences of brain damage in Denmark. In A.-L. Christensen, & B. P. Uzzell (Eds.), *Brain injury and neuropsychological rehabilitation: International perspectives* (pp. 257–267). Hillsdale, NJ: Lawrence Erlbaum.

Mitchum, C. C., & Berndt, R. S. (1995). The cognitive neuropsychological approach to treatment of language disorders. *Neuropsychological Rehabilitation, 5,* 1–16.

Moffat, N. (1989). Home based cognitive rehabilitation with the elderly. In L. W. Poon, D. C. Rubin, & B. A. Wilson (Eds.), *Everyday cognition in adulthood and late life* (pp. 659–680). Cambridge: Cambridge University Press.

Najenson, T., Mendelson, I., Schechter, I., David, C., Mintz, N., & Groswasser, Z. (1974). Rehabilitation after severe head injury. *Scandinavian Journal of Rehabilitation Medicine, 6,* 5–14.

Nelson, R. O., & Hayes, S. C. (1979). Some current dimensions of behavioral assessment. *Behavioral Assessment, 1,* 1–16.

Plaut, D. (1996). Relearning after damage in connectionist networks: Towards a theory of rehabilitation. *Brain and Language, 52,* 25–82.

Poppelreuter, W. (1917). *Die psychischen Schädigungen durch Kopfschuß im Kriege 1914/1916, Vol. 1: Die Störungen der niederen und höheren Sehleistungen durch Verletzungen des Okzipitalhirns.* Leipzig: Voss.

Poser, U., Kohler, J. A., & Schönle, P. W. (1996). Historical review of neuropsychological rehabilitation in Germany. *Neuropsychological Rehabilitation, 6,* 257–278.

Prigatano, G. P. (1997). Learning from our successes and failures: Reflections and comments on "Cognitive rehabilitation: How it is and how it might be." *Journal of the International Neuropsychological Society, 3,* 497–499.

Prigatano, G. P. (1986). Personality and psychosocial consequences of brain injury. In G. P. Prigatano, D. J. Fordyce, H. K. Zeiner, J. R. Roueche, M. Pepping, & B. C. Wood (Eds.), *Neuropsychological rehabilitation after brain injury* (pp. 29–50). Baltimore: The John Hopkins University Press.

Proceedings of the Subcommittee on TBI Rehabilitation at the Fourth Annual Aspen Neurobehavioral Conference. Aspen, CO, April 1998.

Robertson, I. (1990). Does computerised cognitive rehabilitation work? A review. *Aphasiology, 4,* 381–405.

Robertson, I. H. (1991). Review of M. M. Sohlberg & C. A. Mateer (1989) and X. Seron & G. Deloche (Eds.) (1989). *Neuropsychological rehabilitation, 1,* 87–90.

Robertson, I. H. (1999). Theory-driven neuropsychological rehabilitation: The role of attention and competition in recovery of function after brain damage. In D. Gopher & A. Koriat (Eds.), *Attention and performance XVII: Cognitive regulation of performance: Interaction of theory and application* (pp. 677–696). Cambridge, MA: The MIT Press.

Robertson, I. H., & Murre, J. M. J. (1999). Rehabilitation after brain damage: Brain plasticity and principles of guided recovery. *Psychological Bulletin, 125,* 544–575.

Robertson, I. H., Tegnér, R., Tham, K., Lo, A., & Nimmo-Smith, I. (1995). Sustained attention training for unilateral neglect: Theoretical and rehabilitation implications. *Journal of Clinical and Experimental Neuropsychology, 17,* 416–430.

Ruff, R. M., Baser, C. A., Johnston, J. W., Marshall, L. F., Klauber, S. K., Klauber, M. R., & Minteer, M. (1989). Neuropsychological rehabilitation: An experimental study with head-injured patients. *Journal of Head Trauma Rehabilitation, 4,* 20–36.

Scoville, W. B., & Milner, B. (1957). Loss of recent memory after bilateral hippocampal lesions. *Journal of Neurology, Neurosurgery, and Psychiatry, 20,* 11–21.

Seron, X., & G. Deloche (Eds.). (1989). *Cognitive approaches in neuropsychological rehabilitation.* Hillsdale, NJ: Lawrence Erlbaum.

Skinner, B. F. (1953). *Science and human behaviour.* New York: The Free Press.

Sloan, S., & Ponsford, J. (1995). Managing cognitive problems. In J. Ponsford, S. Sloan, & P. Snow (Eds.), *Traumatic brain injury: Rehabilitation for everyday adaptive living* (pp. 33–64). Hove, UK: Lawrence Erlbaum.

Sohlberg, M., & Mateer, C. (1989). *Introduction to cognitive rehabilitation.* New York: Guilford Press.

Squires, E. J., Hunkin, N. M., & Parkin, A. J. (1997). Errorless learning of novel associations in amnesia. *Neuropsychologia, 35,* 1103–1111.

Sturm, W., & Willmes, K. (1991). Efficacy of a reaction training on various attentional and cognitive functions in stroke patients. *Neuropsychological Rehabilitation, 1,* 259–280.

Sturm, W., Willmes, K., Orgass, B., & Hartje, W. (1997). Do specific attention deficits need specific training? *Neuropsychological Rehabilitation, 7,* 81–103.

Thoene, A. I. T., & Glisky, E. L. (1995). Learning of name-face associations in memory impaired patients: A comparison of different training procedures. *Journal of the International Neuropsychological Society, 1,* 29–38.

von Cramon, D. Y., Matthes-von Cramon, G., & Mai, N. (1991). Problem solving deficits in brain injured patients: A therapeutic approach. *Neuropsychological Rehabilitation, 1,* 45–64.

Walsh, K. (1987). *Neuropsychology: A clinical approach* (2nd ed.). Edinburgh: Churchill Livingstone.

Wepman, J. M. (1951). *Recovery from Aphasia.* New York: Ranald Press.

West, M., Wehman, P., Kregel, J., Kreutzer, J., Sherron, P., & Zasler, N. (1991). Costs of operating a supported work program for traumatically brain-injured individuals. *Archives of Physical Medicine and Rehabilitation, 72,* 127–131.

Wilson, B. A. (1999). *Case studies in neuropsychological rehabilitation.* New York: Oxford University Press.

Wilson, B. A. (1989). Models of cognitive rehabilitation. In R. L. L. Woods & P. Evans (Eds.), *Models of brain injury rehabiliation* (pp. 117–141). London: Chapman & Hall.

Wilson, B. A. (1997a). Cognitive rehabilitation: How it is and how it might be. *Journal of the International Neuropsychological Society, 3,* 487–496.

Wilson, B. A. (1997b). Research and evaluation in rehabilitation. In B. A. Wilson, D. L. McLellan (Eds.), *Rehabilitation studies handbook* (pp. 161–187). Cambridge: Cambridge University Press.

Wilson, B. A. (1996). *La réadaptation cognitive chez les cérébro-lésés.* In M. I. Botez (Ed.), *Neuropsychologie clinique et neurologie du comportement* (2nd ed., pp. 637–652). Montreal: Les Presses de l'Université de Montreal.

Wilson, B. A. (1991a). Behaviour therapy in the treatment of neurologically impaired adults. In P. R. Martin (Ed.), *Handbook of behavior therapy and psychological science: An integrative approach* (pp. 227–252). New York: Pergamon Press.

Wilson, B. A. (1991b). Theory, assessment and treatment in neuropsychological rehabilitation. *Neuropsychology, 5,* 281–291.

Wilson, B. A. (1987a). *Rehabilitation of memory.* New York: Guilford Press.

Wilson, B. A. (1987b). Single case experimental designs in neuropsychological rehabilitation. *Journal of Clinical and Experimental Neuropsychology, 9,* 527–544.

Wilson, B. A. (1981). Teaching a man to remember names after removal of a left temporal lobe tumour. *Behavioural Psychotherapy, 9,* 338–344.

Wilson, B. A., Baddeley, A. D., Evans, J. J., & Shiel, A. (1994). Errorless learning in the rehabilitation of memory impaired people. *Neuropsychological Rehabilitation, 4,* 307–326.

Wilson, B. A., Emslie, H. C., Quirk, K., & Evans, J. J. (1999). George: Learning to live independently with NeuroPage. *Rehabilitation Psychology, 44,* 282–296.

Wilson, B. A., & Evans, J. J. (1996). Error free learning in the rehabilitation of individuals with memory impairments. *Journal of Head Trauma Rehabilitation, 11,* 54–64.

Wilson, B. A., Evans, J. J., Brentnall, S., Bremner, S., Keohane, C., & Williams, H. (2000). The Oliver Zangwill Centre for Neuropsychological Rehabilitation: A partnership between health care and rehabilitation research. In A.-L. Christensen & B. P. Uzzell (Eds.), *International handbook of neuropsychological rehabilitation* (pp. 231–246). New York: Kluwer Academic/Plenum.

Wilson, B. A., Evans, J. J., Emslie, H., & Malinek, V. (1997). Evaluation of NeuroPage: A new memory aid. *Journal of Neurology, Neurosurgery, and Psychiatry, 63,* 113–115.

Wilson, B. A., J. C., & Hughes, E. (1997). Coping with amnesia: The natural history of a compensatory memory system. *Neuropsychological Rehabilitation, 7,* 43–56.

Wilson, B. A., & Patterson, K. E. (1990). Rehabilitation and cognitive neuropsychology: Does cognitive psychology apply? *Journal of Applied Cognitive Psychology, 4,* 247–260.

Wilson, B. A., Shiel, A., Watson, M., Horn, S., & McLellan, D. L. (1994). Monitoring behaviour during coma and post traumatic amnesia. In A.-L. Christensen & B. Uzzell (Eds.), *Progress in the rehabilitation of brain-injured people* (pp. 85–98). Hillsdale, NJ: Lawrence Erlbaum.

Wilson, B. A., & Watson, P. C. (1996). A practical framework for understanding compensatory behaviour in people with organic memory impairment. *Memory, 4,* 465–486.

Wood, R. L. (1990). Towards a model of cognitive rehabilitation. In R. L. Wood & I. Fussey (Eds.), *Cognitive rehabilitation in perspective* (pp. 3–25). London: Taylor & Francis.

Wood, R. L., McCrea, J. D., Wood, L. M., & Merriman, R. N. (1999). Clinical and cost effectiveness of post-acute neurobehavioural rehabilitation. *Brain Injury, 13,* 69–88.

Zangwill, O. L. (1947). Psychological aspects of rehabilitation in cases of brain injury. *British Journal of Psychology, 37,* 60–69.

17
CHAPTER

Ruben J. Echemendia
Mark Lovell
Jeffrey Barth

Neuropsychological Assessment of Sport-Related Mild Traumatic Brain Injury

☐ Introduction

The inclusion of sport neuropsychology in a volume on the economics of clinical neuropsychology is fitting because the development of sport neuropsychology was driven by market forces. Mild traumatic brain injuries (MTBIs), or concussions, have been an area of concern in contact sports for a long time. Until the introduction of neuropsychological instruments and approaches, sport medicine was unable to reliably quantify the presence or severity of a concussion. Neuropsychology had much to offer sports medicine, but traditional neuropsychological batteries lasting 6 to 10 hours were not feasible with athletic teams, because of the multiple demands on an athlete's time. In many cases, the athlete's schedule is so structured that it is difficult to find even 1 hour of free time. Therefore, sport neuropsychology developed as a means of quickly and efficiently assessing the neurocognitive sequelae of MTBI. In this sense, sport neuropsychology displays true cost-effectiveness, as relatively little money is being spent to identify athletes at risk for injury due to an injury sustained because of premature return to play.

In the pages that follow, the history of sport neuropsychology will be outlined, followed by a discussion of the epidemiology of sport-related MTBI, a review of empirical studies on MTBI, and a discussion of the clinical and methodological considerations that are integral to sport neuropsychology. Finally, a discussion will be presented regarding the financial issues in this area.

A Historical Perspective

Almost three decades ago, Symonds (1962) speculated that the effects of even the mildest concussions may include permanent neurocognitive impairment. Ten years later, in landmark clinical research, Gronwall and Wrightson (1974) noted that return to work was slow and attention and rapid mental processing were deficient in some New Zealand factory workers who suffered MTBIs. These positions and contributions to the scientific literature were the precursors to the burgeoning efforts in the 1980s and 1990s to define and understand mild head injury and postconcussion syndrome.

Although there is no universally accepted definition of concussion, it is a term that is used widely within the medical community to describe a "trauma induced alteration in mental status that may or may not be accompanied by a loss of consciousness" (Quality Standards Subcommittee, American Academy of Neurology, 1997). Within neuropsychology, the terms mild brain injury and MTBI have been used interchangeably with the term concussion. Because concussion is widely used in the medical literature, this chapter will use the term interchangeably with MTBI, although we believe that MTBI is a more accurate descriptor of the phenomenon.

A large epidemiological study of more than 1,200 head-injured patients (55% of which were categorized as mild trauma) by Rimel, Giordani, Barth, Boll, and Jane (1981) at the University of Virginia revealed poor return to previous employment rates (34%) for mild head injuries at a 6-month follow-up visit. Subsequent neuropsychological assessment of a subset of these mildly injured patients (Glasgow Coma Scale >12; loss of consciousness < 20 minutes; and < 48 hour hospitalization with no significant collateral trauma) documented significant neurocognitive impairment in almost a quarter of these patients (Barth et al., 1989). Although this research appeared to further substantiate the Gronwall and Wrightson findings, it was appropriately criticized for its lack of a comparison group and the fact that, in epidemiological studies, factors such as premorbid cognitive functioning, substance use and abuse, and litigation are uncontrolled. Factors such as these may be critical when analyzing the mechanisms of mild head injury and risk for poor outcome.

In order to address these clinical research issues and control for the above-mentioned factors, investigators at the University of Virginia pioneered a unique line of scientific inquiry that avoided the pitfalls of engaging a matched control group and, instead, used subjects as their own controls. To investigate mild acceleration-deceleration head injury (similar to that found in automobile accidents, which were the primary mechanism of injury in their previous epidemiological research), they studied football players in a Sports as a Laboratory Assessment Model (SLAM; Barth et al., 1989; Barth et al., in press;). In this study, more than 2,300 college football players from 10 universities underwent brief neurocognitive testing at preseason and at postseason. Those players who suffered mild concussions (change in consciousness, but not necessarily loss of consciousness) were reassessed, along with matched, red-shirted control (non-playing) subjects, at 24 hours, 5 days, and 10 days postinjury, in order to document neurocognitive deficits and recovery curves in young, healthy, motivated athletes, for whom preseason baseline abilities had been established. Findings indicated decreased neurocognitive efficiency and lack of ability to take advantage of the practice or learning effects (which were evident in the control group) by the mildly concussed group at 24 hours and 5 days postinjury. No statistical differences were found between the injured players and the controls by 10 days posttrauma, suggesting a short and likely complete recovery curve in this population, with few complicating risk factors.

There has, of course, been interest in sports medicine for many years; however, the SLAM approach to the assessment of concussion has helped to focus attention on an important public health issue and provided a method for studying this mild head injury phenomenon. Neurocognitive assessments are being applied in a variety of sports and across high school, college, and professional venues in this country and abroad using the preseason baseline and serial follow-up model.

☐ Epidemiology of Sport-Related MTBI

Traumatic brain injury is a serious health concern, with an estimated 1.5 to 2 million such injuries occurring each year in this country (NIH Consensus Panel, 1999). The overall head-injury prevalence rate ranges from 2.5 to 6.5 million, with many MTBIs going undiagnosed and untreated. The NIH Consensus Panel (1999) reported that because mild head injury is so frequently underdiagnosed, it is likely the societal burden is significant. Their report also stated that only 3% of patients admitted to the hospital are sports-recreation-induced MTBIs. However, the vast majority of sport-related head injuries are quite mild and unreported, making accurate incidence estimates difficult. Mild head injuries may go undiagnosed as loss of consciousness often is considered necessary for such reporting. Importantly, most mild concussions do not involve loss of consciousness (Cantu, 1998).

Sport-related MTBI is a major public health concern because the majority of these injuries occur among children and young adults (ages 5 to 24 years), and multiple injuries can result in significant disability and, in rare cases, death (e.g., second impact syndrome). More frequently, difficulties in cognitive functioning are noticed in educational and vocational settings (NIH Consensus Panel, 1999). Approximately 300,000 people each year sustain a sport-related traumatic brain injury (with many more suffering mild concussions), and this problem is compounded by the fact that athletes are at risk for multiple head injuries and possibly more serious, permanent disability (Thurman, Branche, & Sniezek, 1998). At all age groups, males have approximately twice the risk of females for sustaining a TBI (National Center for Injury Prevention and Control, 2000). In contrast, data from the NCAA Injury Surveillance System indicate that women in soccer, basketball, and lacrosse have higher injury rates than men.

In one of the largest epidemiological studies of its kind, Powell and Barber-Foss (1999) investigated the incidence of MTBI in varsity athletes at 235 high schools. They documented 1,219 MTBIs, which constituted 5.5% of the total injuries, with football accounting for the largest number of concussions (63.4%), followed by wrestling (10.5%), female soccer (6.2%), male soccer (5.7%), and female basketball (5.2%). Other sports accounted for less than 5% of injuries, including male basketball (4.2%), female softball (2.1%), baseball (1.2%), female field hockey (1.1%), and female volleyball (0.5%). The majority of injuries resulted from tackles, takedowns, or collisions. In soccer, the majority of MTBIs occurred during heading, yet the data reported do not indicate whether the injuries were sustained during head-to-ball, head-to-head, or head-to-ground contact (or jarring body-to-body collisions while heading). Based on their large sample, Powell and Barber-Foss (1999) estimated that the national incidence of MTBI across 10 sports is 62,816 cases per year, with the majority of injuries occurring in football. Importantly, these estimates do not include sports such as ice hockey, rugby, or lacrosse, which are at high risk for MTBI.

Contemporary Models in Sports Neuropsychology

The clinical use of neuropsychological assessment in sports has developed only recently. Although both the National Football League (NFL) and the National Hockey League (NHL) have adopted neuropsychological testing as a standard procedure prior to and following concussion, the clinical application of neuropsychological assessment procedures in college and high school athletics has been limited to research programs and is not yet in widespread use at the clinical level. One notable exception at the college level is the Penn State Concussion Program, which has been using neuropsychological test data clinically with a broad range of sports since 1995. The clinical models that have been employed in the NFL and NHL have emphasized the preseason baseline evaluation of the athlete. This model also has become the predominant model in programs that have been established at both the high school and university levels.

Baseline or preparticipation neuropsychological assessment is important because of the significant individual differences among athletes (Echemendia & Julian, 2001; Lovell & Collins, 1998). Following injury, an athlete's performance is compared to his or her baseline level of performance, rather than to group normative data. The postinjury neuropsychological evaluation of the athlete generally should take place within 24 to 48 hours of the suspected MTBI. A follow-up neuropsychological evaluation is recommended within 5 to 7 days after injury, prior to return to competition to assure that the athlete has returned to preinjury baseline levels of functioning. This time interval represents a useful and practical time span and appears to be consistent with animal brain metabolism studies that have demonstrated metabolic changes in the brain that persist for several days following injury (Hovda et al., 1999). Sport-specific neuropsychological protocols are briefly reviewed below.

Football

Following the model initially developed by Barth and his colleagues (Barth et al., 1989; Macciochi, Barth, Alves, Rimel, & Jane, 1997) and based on the need for more sensitive MTBI evaluation procedures in professional football players, a neuropsychological evaluation program was instituted with the Pittsburgh Steelers in 1993 (Lovell & Collins, 1998). This represented the first clinically oriented project designed to help team physicians make return-to-play decisions following a suspected MTBI. This approach involved the preseason baseline assessment of each Steeler player as well as follow-up testing in the event of injury during the season. Post-MTBI assessments were repeated within 24 hours after a suspected MTBI, and again approximately 5 days postinjury.

Table 17.1 provides a listing of the neuropsychological instruments that were originally used with the Pittsburgh Steelers and which have now been adopted by the NFL Subcommittee on MTBI. This test battery has been revised recently with the addition of the several tests from the Wechsler Adult Intelligence Scale-III (WAIS-III; Symbol Search, Digit Symbol and Digit Span; Wechsler, 1997).

As can be seen in Table 17.1, the NFL test battery was constructed to evaluate multiple aspects of cognitive functioning but primarily focused on the assessment of atten-

TABLE 17.1. Pittsburgh Steelers Neuropsychological Test Battery

- Post-Concussion Symptoms Scale
- Orientation Test
- Stroop Test
- COWAT
- Digit Span (WMS-R)
- Hopkins Verbal Learning Test
- Symbol Digits Modalites (written)
- Trail Making Test
- Grooved Pegboard Test

tion processes, information processing speed, and memory. This test battery recently was subjected to an initial factor analysis and yielded four general factors: (a) verbal memory, (b) visual memory, (c) verbal processing/attention, and (d) visual attention (Woodard et. al., 1999). The total time for administration of the test battery is approximately 30 minutes.

Ice Hockey

As a result of heightened awareness and concern about brain injury in professional hockey, the NHL formally instituted a league-wide neuropsychological assessment program for the 1997 season. Preseason neuropsychological testing was mandated for all players, and baseline testing became a routine part of each team's preseason training camp.

The NHL neuropsychology program was designed to yield meaningful clinical information regarding the postinjury status of athletes, and neuropsychological test results have become a valued component of care following concussion. Return-to-play decisions are made based on neuropsychological test results; additional neurodiagnostic studies, such as MRI; and the players' self-report of postconcussion symptoms.

The design of the NHL neuropsychology program is somewhat more complicated than the NFL program, due to several factors. First, the multiple languages spoken within the professional hockey ranks (e.g., French, English, Russian, Czechoslovakian, Swedish, Finnish, and German) created a challenge with regard to construction of a standardized test battery. Two test batteries were constructed. Table 17.2 presents the tests that are used with native and nonnative English-speakers. As can be seen, the general battery is weighted toward nonverbal tasks, and the non-English version eliminates all frankly verbal tasks.

In addition to the issue of evaluating athletes from different cultural and language backgrounds, the logistics of a typical hockey schedule differ significantly from football and complicate the assessment model. In professional football, games typically are played on weekends, and the teams return home, often immediately after the game. This allows for the neuropsychological assessment of injured athletes in the home city within 24 to 48 hours of injury. In professional hockey, however, teams often embark on long (2 to 3 week) road trips and typically receive medical treatment outside their home city. Therefore, any league-wide program aimed at the systematic evaluation of MTBI needed to be structured so that all athletes have access to neuropsychological

TABLE 17.2. NHL Neuropsychological Test Battery for Native and Nonnative English Speakers

English Battery	*ESL Battery*
Symptoms Inventory	Symptom Inventory
Orientation Test	Orientation Test
Penn State Cancellation Test	Penn State Cancellation Test
Symbol Digit Modalities	Symbol Digit Modalities
Color Trailmaking	Color Trailmaking
Brief Visuospatial Memory Test–Revised	Brief Visuospatial Memory Test–Revised
Controlled Oral Word Association Test	
Hopkins Verbal Learning Test	

testing, wherever they are injured. This required the establishment of a league-wide network of neuropsychologists throughout the United States and Canada.

The NHL battery was constructed to evaluate athletes' functioning in the areas of attention, information processing speed, verbal fluency, and memory. Whenever possible, multiple forms of tests are used for baseline and follow-up assessments. Tests were selected by the NHL Neuropsychology Advisory Board, which is currently composed of Drs. Mark Lovell, Ruben Echemendia (program codirectors), William Barr, Elizabeth Kozora, and Don Gerber. The NHL test battery is administered in standard order and can be completed in approximately 30 minutes. In keeping with our previous experience with amateur and professional athletics, we recommend preseason baseline testing, follow-up testing within 24 to 48 hours of a suspected MTBI, and a 5-day follow-up evaluation.

☐ Neuropsychological Studies of Sport-Related MTBI

Although a fair amount of research has been conducted into the epidemiology of sport-related MTBI, relatively few studies have examined the neurocognitive functioning of athletes post-MTBI. A brief review of the studies that have been published will be grouped by sport for ease of presentation.

Football

As we stated earlier, the first study to examine the effects of MTBI in football players was conducted by Barth and his colleagues (1989), who first made use of a preseason neuropsychological baseline, which allowed for the comparison of preinjury scores with post-MTBI scores. Using the Trail Making Test (TMT), Symbol Digits Modalities Test (SDMT), and Paced Auditory Serial Addition Task (PASAT), these authors found that cognitive and information processing deficits were apparent within 24 hours of injury in the MTBI group when compared to their noninjured controls. A rapid, although incomplete recovery was demonstrated over the 5 to 10 days following MTBI. It was reported that the TMT resulted in pronounced practice effects that reduced its efficiency in differentiating between the injured and control groups. Olesniewicz, Sallis, Jones, and Copp (1997) examined NCAA division III athletes and found deficits in memory, visual scanning, attention, word fluency, and mental flexibility in athletes who sustained moderate to severe MTBI. Collins et al. (1999) reported neurocognitive deficits in NCAA division I football players at 24 hours, 3 days, and 5 days after mild concussion. Lovell and Collins (1998) examined 63 members of a varsity college football team at preseason and at the conclusion of the season. The difference in test scores between preseason and postseason was minimal for noninjured players, although practice effects were found for the TMT, Digit Span, and Grooved Pegboard. Four players who sustained MTBIs during the season were examined 24 hours following injury, and their postinjury scores were below their preseason baseline scores. The scores of the injured players returned to or exceeded baseline at the postseason evaluation.

Collins et al. (1999) found significant baseline differences in college football players who reported a history of concussion, when compared to those with no history of concussion. Players with a history of two or more concussions had significantly lower scores on TMT and SDMT than those with only one concussion. An interesting, although preliminary finding emerged whereby those players with multiple concussions and a diagnosis of learning disabilities (LD) had significantly lower scores than those with no history of LD and two or more concussions. Collins and colleagues (1999) also reported data on 16 athletes who sustained concussions during the study period. When compared to noninjured controls, the concussed athletes scored significantly worse than controls at 24 hours, and these differences persisted until "at least" 5 days after injury.

Soccer

Not only can soccer players sustain a MTBI through player contact (e.g., head to head, foot to head), equipment contact (e.g., goalpost), and contact with the ground, it has been speculated that they may experience neurocognitive changes because of "heading" the ball. For example, Schneider and Liche (1975) estimated that a kicked ball with half power may travel at 82.3 kilometers per hour and impact the head with a force of 116 kp. At full power, the impact was estimated at 200 kp. Given the number of heading contacts per game, significant concern has arisen regarding the cumulative neurocognitive effects of heading over the many years of a soccer player's career. Several studies have reported increases in symptoms (e.g., headache, dizziness, decreased memory, decreased concentration) and EEG changes following heading (Barnes et al., 1998; Kross, Ohler, & Barolin, 1983; Tsvaer & Storli, 1981). Abreau, Templer, Schuyler, and Hutchinson (1990) reported an increase in headaches among players who headed the ball frequently, but they did not detect any neuropsychological impairment. In a pilot study, Putukian, Echemendia, and Mackin (2000) did not find any significant differences in neurocognitive functioning among college male and female soccer players after 20 minutes of heading practice.

Few neuropsychological studies have been conducted on the effects of MTBI on soccer players. Abreau et al. (1990) compared soccer and tennis players on the Raven Progressive Matrices, SDMT, Perceptual Speeded Test, and the PASAT. Noninjured soccer players reported more symptoms characteristic of MTBI than did the tennis players, but there were no differences between the groups in neuropsychological test performance. In contrast, Matser, Kessels, Lezak, Jordan, and Troost (1999) found significant differences between amateur soccer players and controls (swimmers and distance runners) on the Complex Figure Test, the Wisconsin Card Sorting Test, and the Wechsler

Memory Scales. Those players with a greater number of concussions had the poorest test scores. The conclusions of this study must be tempered by the fact that the soccer players consumed alcohol at a rate significantly greater than the control group athletes.

Boxing

Many studies have reported abnormal radiologic findings among boxers (Casson et al., 1984; Casson, Sham, Campbell, Tarlau, & DiDomenico, 1982; Kaste et al., 1982; Ross, Cole, Thompson, & Kim, 1983; Sironi, Scotti, Ravagnati, Franzini, & Marossero, 1982). EEG abnormalities also have been detected (Busse & Silverman, 1952; Kaplan & Browder, 1954). McLatchie et al. (1987) found abnormalities in 1 of 20 CT scans of amateur Scottish boxers. They also found abnormalities in 8 of 20 EEG recordings, and abnormal neuropsychological test scores in 9 of 20 boxers. These findings led the authors to suggest that neuropsychological techniques were more sensitive than traditional neurophysiological techniques in detecting abnormalities among boxers. Brooks, Kupshik, Wilson, Galbraith, and Ward (1987) found no evidence of impaired neuropsychological functioning among active amateur boxers when compared to nonboxing controls. Differences were found, however, between the boxing and nonboxing groups (e.g., Raven's mean IQ of 106.8 for the controls, mean IQ of 82.7 for boxers), which call into question the results of the study. Thomassen, Juul-Jensen, de Fine Olivarius, Braemer, and Christensen (1979) found that former amateur boxers performed significantly worse than soccer players on the vocabulary subtest of the WAIS, measures of motor functions with the left hand, visuospatial operations, some language operations, and memory. Kaste et al. (1982) discovered minimal differences between amateur boxers and population means on a wide range of neuropsychological measures. Roberts (1969) found a significant relationship between deficits in memory and verbal skills and career length among professional boxers. Casson et al. (1984) examined professional boxers and noted abnormal performance on several neuropsychological instruments (TMT, SDMT, Wechsler Memory Test, Bender-Gestalt). These neuropsychological test scores were highly correlated with CT and EEG abnormalities. Murelius and Haglund (1991) found no differences in neuropsychological performance between Swedish amateur boxers, soccer players, and track and field athletes. They did find that boxers with a greater number of matches scored more poorly than those with fewer matches.

Multisport Studies

Guskiewicz, Riemann, Perrin, and Nashner (1997) examined a group of mixed-sport NCAA division I athletes and found no differences on neuropsychological measures (TMT, Digit Span, Stroop), Hopkins Verbal Learning Test (HVLT) between concussed athletes and noninjured controls at 1, 3, 5, and 10 days post-MTBI. Echemendia, Putukian, Mackin, Julian, & Shoss (2001) presented the initial findings of a multisport collegiate program at Penn State University. Baseline data were collected on more than 900 athletes from football, men's and women's soccer, men's ice hockey, men's and women's basketball, wrestling, and women's lacrosse. The assessment battery included the HVLT, SDMT, TMT, Controlled Oral Word Association Test (COWAT), Stroop, Vigil Continuous Performance Task, a five-word list learning task, and a Post-Concussion Symptoms checklist. Data from the first 29 concussed athletes were reported for 2 hours, 48 hours, 1 week, and 1 month post-MTBI. Significant differences were found between the concussed players and their controls at 2 hours and 48 hours postinjury. A pattern of scores was detected in which the injured players performed worse at 48 hours postinjury than they did at 2 hours postinjury. Also of interest was the finding that self-reported symptoms after MTBI differentiated injured from noninjured players at the 2-hour evaluation but failed to differentiate the groups at 48 hours postinjury. This finding calls into question the current practice of returning an athlete to sport solely on the self-report that their symptoms have cleared. No significant multivariate group differences were found at 1 week postinjury, but univariate analyses did suggest group differences on some of the neuropsychological measures.

Other Sports

Although ice hockey has one of the highest prevalence rates for concussion (see Echemendia & Julian, 2001), it has received little attention in the literature thus far. Data from the NHL Neuropsychological Testing Program will soon shed light on this issue. In Australian professional rugby players, Hinton-Bayre, Geffen, and McFarland (1997) found that measures of information processing speed (Speed and Capacity of Language Processing Test) were sensitive to the effects of MTBI. Cremona-Meteyard and Geffen (1994) studied Australian Rules Football players and found that a long-term consequence of MTBI may be a diminished ability to respond quickly to expected events.

Taken together, these studies suggest that neuropsychological instruments reliably differentiate between athletes who have sustained an MTBI and those who have not. The data also suggest that neuropsychological tests may be useful information in the return-to-play decision.

☐ Methodological Considerations

Selecting an appropriate test battery for assessing MTBI in athletes can be a challenging task because of the unique demands of the sports environment. Athletes, particularly at the college and professional levels, have very hectic schedules and their time is at a premium. Team functions often are tightly scheduled, with little time for "extraneous" activity. The neuropsychologist generally has little time to spend with an athlete, and test batteries rarely exceed 30 minutes in length. This time limitation contrasts with the extended batteries that are customarily administered in typical clinical neuropsychological practices. Similarly, testing conditions in sports are sometimes less than ideal, because tests may need to be administered in locker rooms, hallways, or even on airplanes and buses. Because of the volume of testing that must be conducted (e.g., a college football team may have 120 athletes) as well as the travel schedules of many teams, psychometricians, athletic trainers, or team physicians often perform testing in addition to the neuropsychologist. As these individuals do not have neuropsychological training, tests must be selected that can be administered without extensive training.

Because most sport neuropsychology testing programs examine an athlete serially after a concussion, it is important that the test–retest characteristics of a test are known. Whenever possible, tests should be included that have multiple alternate forms, so that practice effects may be minimized.

Taken together, these issues suggest that, in order to develop an efficient battery that is sensitive to the effects of MTBI, tests must be selected based on their ease of administration, length, availability of alternate forms, sound psychometric properties, previous use with athletes, and the amount of frustration they generate. For example, although the PASAT has been used extensively with the MTBI populations, the level of frustration it generates often creates a negative set with athletes, which then leads to decreased motivation and cooperation.

The vast majority of athletes have never encountered a neuropsychologist and know little about neuropsychological testing. In some cases, athletes may be suspicious of our motivation and have concerns about how the test data will be used. They may be concerned that the test data will be given to coaches or management or used for selection purposes. They may be unsure of the role of the baseline testing in relation to the postinjury testing. Many of these issues are easily alleviated by a thorough discussion of the role of the neuropsychologist with the team and of the ways the data will, and will not, be used.

Even though athletes may understand the purpose of the program and how the data will be used, their level of motivation may wax and wane. Some players may be unmotivated to perform well during baseline testing because they may feel threatened by the tests, are bored, or feel they have better things to do with their time. They may feel that there is no clear benefit to them for good performance. In contrast, athletes usually are highly motivated following an injury to perform at their best, because return to play may be contingent on good performance. These fluctuating levels of motivation may cause difficulty for the neuropsychologist who is faced with making a return-to-play recommendation. Increased motivation may be interpreted as "recovery" from baseline levels. In light of this, neuropsychologists must be vigilant to signs that a player is unmotivated at baseline and take steps to increase his or her motivation. For example, apparently unmotivated players may be told that, because the baseline data are so important to accurate decision making, if their baseline data are considered suspect they may have to retake the battery. It also may be suggested to them that an inaccurate baseline may actually lead to a longer time away from sport following an injury, because of the need to take a more conservative approach.

Some researchers (Hinton-Bayre et al., 1997) have advocated the use of multiple baselines in order to negate practice effects. In this approach the athlete is administered a baseline battery on two occasions, and the higher of the two scores is used as the player's baseline. It is believed that the readministration of the battery within a short time period will maximize the practice effects, thereby reducing their impact on subsequent assessment. However, because the magnitude of practice effects is a function of the time delay between testing sessions, and the time between baseline assessment and postinjury evaluations is highly variable, it is unlikely that multiple baselines will have a significant impact on practice effects in clinical applications. Additionally, multiple baselines require more time with athletes, and many teams will not allow the extra time.

☐ Clinical Considerations

Relationship with Teams/Players

The role of consultant to sports organizations is a relatively new one for neuropsychologists. Many neuropsychologists have had only limited interactions with athletes, particularly at the professional level. Furthermore, neuropsychologists traditionally have had only limited interactions with other sport-related professionals such as coaches, athletic trainers, and agents. To interact effectively both with the athletes and with other support personnel, it is imperative that the neuropsychologist clearly identifies who he or she is and what his or her role is with the team. As noted earlier, athletes initially may be skeptical about why they are being evaluated and how the neuropsychological test data will be used. For example, during the initial establishment of the program in professional football, there was concern on the part of the athletes that the information would be used to determine their intellectual status or as additional performance criteria, such as time in the 40-yard sprint. This misunderstanding was easily corrected by providing the athletes with a brief written summary of the program. This summary explained the potential importance of the evaluation program and outlined the psychologist/client relationship with regard to release of test data. A clear description of roles as well as the use of test data will help minimize possible ethical dilemmas, such as dual relationships and violations of confidentiality. (For a discussion of the ethical issues involved in sport consultation, see Echemendia and Parker, 1998).

Establishing Rapport

Although the establishment of good rapport with clients is generally regarded as an essential component of the neuropsychological evaluation, establishing good rapport is particularly important when working with athletes. At the college and professional levels, athletes who are undergoing neuropsychological evaluation are well aware of the potential financial and personal impact of test performance on their return to the playing field. Therefore, there often is a keen awareness of the test performance with regard to career status and, ultimately, their ability to earn a living. This overall backdrop, coupled with clients who are by nature highly competitive, may create a pressure-filled environment that does not lead to optimal test performance. For this reason, we often suggest that evaluations be completed outside of the traditional neuropsychological laboratory, in an environment where the athletes feel comfortable. This often involves finding a quiet room within the arena or stadium where the team practices.

Important Factors in the Interpretation of Test Results

MTBI History. In interpreting neuropsychological test data following a suspected MTBI in an athlete, it is particularly important for the neuropsychological consultant to understand the athlete's neurological history. First, given the proposed link between multiple concussions and level of impairment (Collins et al., 1999), it is best to obtain a thorough history of head injuries that may have resulted in MTBIs. In gathering this information it is important to query the athlete with regard to (a) loss or alteration of consciousness, (b) retrograde and anterograde amnesia following each injury, (c) period of posttraumatic confusion, (d) neurologic symptoms, and (e) loss of practice or playing time. If a parent, friend, or spouse accompanies the athlete, it is useful to seek collateral information from these sources.

Educational History. As is the case in general neuropsychological practice, the educational background of the athletes may have a significant effect on how their postinjury test data are interpreted. Not only is an understanding of the players' educational backgrounds necessary to establish expectations for performance on the particular neuropsychological test instrument or test battery, LDs also have recently been linked to poorer neuropsychological test performance, particularly when these athletes have a prior history of MTBIs (Collins et al. 1999). Although this potential relationship awaits further study, it has been suggested that LD athletes may be more vulnerable to the effects of concussion than non-LD athletes.

Return-to-Play Decision Making

As mentioned previously, the clinical implementation of neuropsychological assessment in sports has evolved primarily to aid in return-to-play decision making. At the current time, neuropsychological assessment generally is regarded as the most sensitive method of evaluating the injured athlete following a suspected MTBI (Echemendia & Julian, 2001; Lovell & Collins, 1998). We actively support the use of neuropsychological assessment as an important component in making return-to play decisions. However, we also feel an obligation to emphasize that neuropsychological assessment procedures represent only one component of the return-to-play decision-making process (see Echemendia & Cantu, in press). Return-to-play decisions rarely should be made based solely on neuropsychological test results, but should include an assessment of the athlete's postconcussive symptoms, neurodiagnostic information (such as MRI when available), and psychological characteristics. For example, if a player has returned to baseline on neurocognitive measures and is symptom-free yet reports that he or she is frightened to return to play because of concerns about being reinjured, it may be wise to hold the player out until the fear can be adequately addressed.

Reaction of Players to Injury

There is tremendous variability in how athletes react to their injuries. Reactions may vary from complete denial of difficulty to catastrophic overreaction to mild postinjury difficulties. At all levels of competition, there often is pressure to perform, which that may lead athletes to minimize or deny their injuries. This represents a component of the expectations that athletes must "play hurt" and not "let the team down." Whereas this expectation represents an important aspect of athletic culture and is based on the ability of athletes to continue to perform when suffering from minor orthopaedic injuries (e.g., sprains or muscle pulls), this approach can have devastating consequences when applied to brain injury. A major part of our efforts in educating athletes over the past 10 years has been directed toward improving their understanding that the brain is not "just another muscle" and requires special care. Although largely successful thus far, there is an ongoing need for player education.

End-of-Career Decision Making

Assisting the injured athlete in making end-of-career decisions represents one of the most complex processes that the sport neuropsychologist will face. This decision does not hinge solely on neuropsychological test scores but also involves the athlete's history of injury, estimated risk of reinjury, financial status, and other, less tangible issues. The decision process usually involves the athlete, his or her family, several physicians, an athletic trainer, and (at the professional level) sports agents. This often is a traumatic time in the athlete's life and he or she may require a referral for supportive or family psychotherapy. At the current time, there are no clear criteria for retirement. However, retirement decisions should not be based solely on how many MTBIs the athlete has suffered, but should instead focus on the athlete's level of functioning. As a general rule, we counsel athletes to consider retirement when (a) there are sustained deficits documented by neuropsychological testing; (b) the athlete has nonremitting symptoms such as headaches, balance difficulties, or photosensitivity and; (c) the athlete appears to develop symptoms with less provocation. If any of these criteria are met, we would suggest consideration of retirement.

Rehabilitation Issues

Current efforts aimed at rehabilitating brain-injured athletes have focused primarily on palliative rather than curative treatments. At the current time, there are no validated rehabilitation procedures that lead to recovery of brain function following a sports-related MTBI. The most important component of treating athletic MTBI is to prevent additional injury. The sport neuropsychologist also can play an important role in steering the athlete away from unproven and often expensive therapies such as neurobiofeedback and vitamin therapy.

Although there currently are no treatments that have been found to reverse the effects of an MTBI, treatment of symptoms often is useful and may minimize the suffering of the injured athlete. Treatment should be targeted to the particular symptoms that are most prominent in a given athlete. For instance, if headaches are a major problem, the athlete should be evaluated and treated for headaches. Because athletes usually are acutely aware of their bodies, relaxation and EMG biofeedback training may be useful in alleviating targeted symptoms and in creating a generalized relaxation regimen. If an athlete displays postinjury emotional changes such as depression, antidepressant medication and psychotherapy may be indicated.

Financial Considerations in the Neuropsychological Assessment of Sport-Related Concussion

As we discussed earlier, concussions are frequent occurrences in the world of sports. Athletes are sidelined by concussions on a regular basis, and many have had to end their sporting careers due to repeated concussions. We are not aware of any published studies to date that examine the economic impact of sport-related concussion. In the pages that follow, we will discuss the various financial forces that exist in sport neuropsychology and the extent to which neuropsychology provides a cost-effective approach to injury management. For ease of presentation, we will focus primarily on professional sports. However, parallel costs and benefits can be drawn to amateur sports as well.

Costs associated with sport-related concussion must be broken down into several categories: direct costs of treatment, financial cost of time lost due to injury (to player, agents, endorsements, future contracts, insurance companies, and team), and the emotional costs of being sidelined (to player, family, and team).

Direct Costs of Treatment

The direct costs of treating concussion are relatively minor when compared to the other costs associated with this injury. With very serious concussion, it is possible that a hospital stay of 1 or 2 days will be required. Generally, a CT scan of the brain and an MRI may be ordered. The more typical concussion will require a sideline evaluation by an athletic trainer and a follow-up visit to the team physician.

The most significant financial cost associated with brain concussions at the professional level is time lost from playing. For example, with the average yearly NHL salary at $1.2 million and approximately 80 regular season games, each game is worth approximately $15,000. A recent report on concussions in the NHL indicated that, as of January 11, 2001, 43 concussions were reported by NHL teams, during the 2000–2001 season with head injuries accounting for 9% of all injuries. The January 11, 2001, NHL injury list indicated that 10 players were sidelined due to concussions, with 127 games missed. These 127 games represent $1,905,000 (using the average salary per game), not including other players who missed games due to concussion prior to this date.

The role of neuropsychological testing in sports is to identify the presence and, more importantly, the absence of neurocognitive dysfunction following MTBI. Identifying return to neurocognitive and neurobehavioral baselines following injury enhances player safety by minimizing the risk of premature return to play. These factors have a direct impact on loss of playing time. For example, a professional hockey player reports that he is symptom-free at rest and during exertion 2 days following MTBI. However, his neuropsychological testing shows that he has not returned to baseline levels neurocognitively. In this hypothetical example, the player is returned to play and he sustains a second concussion. Recovery from the second concussion is likely more protracted than the first, and the player is held out of play for 2 to 3 weeks. This player has probably lost 10 games. In contrast, if the player had been held out until the neuropsychological test scores had returned to baseline (usually within 1 week), the second concussion might have been avoided and only 3 games would have been missed. More extreme examples could be presented that would lead to a career-ending injury or even a catastrophic fatal injury (second impact syndrome) as a result of premature return to play.

Additional costs are associated with reduced playing time. Bonuses may not be met because of lost playing time, endorsements may be lost or minimized due to injury status, and future contracts may be compromised. Not only do the players and the teams lose money, the players' agents and the team's insurance companies also lose money. The more games that are missed due to a concussion, the more money is lost.

Indirect Costs

At an indirect level, there are the psychological costs associated with concussion. For players, there often is apprehension and fear because of the unseen nature of the injury and the mystery surrounding brain function. Most athletes are well aware of high-profile players who have been forced to retire because of concussions and fear that this may happen to them. There also are the direct psychological sequelae of the concussion. Confusion, disorientation, feeling like they are in a fog, lethargy, and personality changes are some of the symptoms reported. Athletes frequently become irritable and depressed following concussion. These symptoms also take their toll on family members, who are not accustomed to watching their loved ones in a debilitated state.

Prior to the use of neuropsychological tests, physicians had little to offer players and their families. As traditional radiologic techniques are largely ineffective in detecting abnormalities in concussed athletes, injuries could not be quantified, and the best that could be offered was a "wait-and-see" approach until the symptoms abated. Neuropsychology has provided the sports medicine team with a new tool that has both direct and indirect value in any cost comparisons used with concussions.

Physicians and athletic trainers alike report that neuropsychological testing is highly valuable because, for the first time, test results can quantify the extent of a concussion. These "hard numbers" are very helpful in talking with coaches, general managers, players, and families about the effects of the concussion. Neuropsychological data provide objective evidence that a player should not play. This information is quite useful to a team physician when he or she is telling a coach or general manager that a player cannot play, particularly a star player. We have often been told that the data provide a significant "comfort level" for the team physician and athletic trainer when making return-to-play decisions. This comfort level is shared by the players, who understand the concept that it is risky to return to play prematurely. They also understand the notion that test scores must (at least) reach baseline levels before return to play is recommended.

Following Prigatano's discussion (Chapter 2) of health-care economics, there is considerable "cost–utility" in neuropsychological assessment (see Table 17.3). The value of neuropsychological services has been discussed from the physician's and athletic trainer's standpoint. In addition to providing data on the neurocognitive effects of concussion, the neuropsychologist also is useful in reducing the concerns and anxiety that arise for the players and their families. For example, in the NHL Neuropsychological Testing Program, the neuropsychologist is viewed as an agent of both the NHL and the NHL Players' Association (NHLPA). In this sense the neuropsychologist's role is to provide services independent of the team structure. At times, team physicians are viewed by players as agents of the team (or of the general manager), and their decisions may not be independent of the best interests of the team. The players often view the neuropsychologist as a neutral outsider who is there to provide information. Often, the neuropsychologist spends time discussing the players' concerns about concussions and attempts to reduce fears by providing information to the players and their families.

What are the costs associated with neuropsychological testing? Because sports neuropsychology generally makes use of an abbreviated battery of tests that is administered at baseline and following injury, the usual multihour neuropsychological assessment is largely eliminated. Instead, a 30- to 45-minute battery is used, with a direct cost of approximately $100 per evaluation at present. There often is additional consultation with the team physicians, athletic trainers, families, and players, which is generally not charged but does reflect a nonreimbursed cost borne by the neuropsychologist.

The role of neuropsychological testing programs in sports is not to prevent concussions. Concussions are inherent in many sports, because of their very nature. Neuropsychology is useful to the athlete and the sport medicine team in that it provides valuable information that can be used to improve return-to-play decisions and thus minimize the risk of a second concussion prior to the resolution of the first. This approach likely will reduce complications from concussion that can lead to chronic symptoms, extended periods of time without playing, or even premature career termination. Given the costs of neuropsychological testing in relation to the direct and indirect costs of not playing, neuropsychology seems like a bargain.

TABLE 17.3. Cost-Effectiveness Variables in Sport Neuropsychology

Costs

Neuropsychological
- Baseline Testing
- Postinjury Testing
- Consultation with physicians, players, trainers, and families

Loss of Playing Time
- Direct costs to player
- Direct cost to team
- Direct cost to Worker's Compensation Insurance
- Psychological costs to players
- Psychological costs to families

Indirect Costs/Impact
- Diminished bonuses
- Diminished endorsement deals
- Diminished ability to negotiate for contracts

Outcomes/Benefits

Neuropsychological Evaluation
- Quantifiable marker of concussion
- Early identification of concussion sequelae
- More informed return to play decision thereby minimizing loss of playing time
- Reduced risk of premature career ending injury
- Reduced risk of chronic neurocognitive dysfunction
- Increased physician confidence in return to play decision
- Tangible data to present to players, coaches, and families regarding the extent of injury

Neuropsychologist as Consultant
- Provides added input/information to the team physician
- Uniquely trained to educate the players, families, and teams about the nature and effects of concussions
- Responds to players' apprehension, depression, anxiety, and other psychological symptoms
- Responds to the concerns and fears of players' families

Conclusions and Recommendations for Further Study

Sport-related MTBIs are common throughout contact sports at all levels of play. The frequency of occurrence coupled with the possible negative consequences of MTBI have led many to categorize sport-related MTBI as a significant public health concern. With the advent of sport neuropsychology, the sports medicine team has a reliable, efficient, and cost-effective method for quantifying the severity and duration of neurocognitive changes following an MTBI. Neuropsychology has been thrown into the limelight, and the data published to date suggest that it has a promising future. However, sport neuropsychology is in its infancy, and there are many studies that must be conducted. The following examples of studies merely scratch the surface of a field that is rich in possibilities:

- What is the relative value of intraindividual baseline testing versus the use of interindividual normative data?
- Is there differential predictive ability between neurocognitive findings and neurobehavioral symptoms?
- What is the differential predictive ability of computerized testing versus standard neuropsychological testing?
- What is the cost-effectiveness of computerized testing?
- What is the optimum number of testing periods needed post-MTBI?
- How many concussions are too many?
- Can the use of general return-to-play guidelines be substantiated through neuropsychological testing?

In addition to these questions, sports provide a unique laboratory in which to learn about the course, effects, and phenomenology of MTBI. The ability to obtain baseline data prior to injury is unparalleled in other populations. These baseline data not only provide information regarding return-to-play decisions, they provide a foundation for understanding the natural course of MTBI. The knowledge obtained from these studies will have clear and significant implications for clinical neuropsychology more generally.

In sum, sports have issued a significant challenge to neuropsychology. Although only in its infancy, the field of sport neuropsychology has emerged as a result of this challenge as an economically feasible and cost-effective approach to the problem of sport-related MTBI. As more data are gathered and new approaches developed, sport neuropsychology will continue to expand our knowledge base regarding MTBI in general and to enhance the safety of children, adolescents, and adults who choose to engage in athletic competition.

References

Abreau, F., Templer, D., Schuyler, B., & Hutchison, H. (1990). Neuropsychological assessment of soccer players. *Neuropsychology, 4,* 175–181.

Barnes, B. C., Cooper, L., Kirkendall, D. T., McDermott, T. P., Jordan, B. D., & Garrett, W. E. (1998). Concussion history in elite male and female soccer players. *American Journal of Sports Medicine, 26*(3), 433–438.

Barth, J. T., Alves., W. M., Ryan, T. V., Macciocchi, S. N., Rimel, R. W., Jane, J. A., & Nelson, W. E. (1989). Mild head injury in sports: Neuropsychological sequelae and recovery of function. In H. S. Levin, Eisenberg, H. M., & Benton, A. L. (Eds.), *Mild head injury* (pp. 257–275). New York: Oxford University Press.

Barth, J. T., Freeman, J., & Broshek, D. K. (in press). Mild Head Injury. *Encyclopedia of the brain.* New York: Academic Press.

Brooks, N., Kupshik, G., Wilson, L., Galbraith, S., & Ward, R. (1987). A neuropsychological study of active amateur boxers. *Journal of Neurology, Neurosurgery, and Psychiatry, 50,* 997–1000.

Busse, E. W., & Silverman, A. J. (1952). Electroencephalographic changes in professional boxers. *Journal of the American Medical Association, 149,* 1522–1525.

Cantu, R. C. (1998). Return to play guidelines after head injury. *Clinical Sports Medicine, 17,* 45–60.

Casson, I. R., Sham, R., Campbell, E. R., Tarlau, M., & DiDomenico, A. (1982). Neurological and

CT evaluation of knocked out boxers. *Journal of Neurology, Neurosurgery, and Psychiatry, 45*(2), 170–174.

Casson, I. R., Siegel., O., Sham, R., Campbell., E. A., Tarlau, M., & DiDomenico, A. (1984). Brain damage in modern boxers. *Journal of the American Medical Association, 251,* 2663–2667.

Collins, M., Grindel, S., Lovell, M., Dede, D., Moser, D., Phalin, B., Nogle, S., Wasik, M., Cordry, D., Daugherty, M., Sears, S., Nicolette, G., Indelicato, P., & McKeag, D. (1999). Relationship between concussion and neuropsychological performance in college football players. *Journal of the American Medical Association, 282,* 964–970.

Cremona-Meteyard, S. L., & Geffen, G. M. (1994). Persistent visuospatial attention deficits following mild head injury in Australian rules football players. *Neuropsychologia, 32*(6), 649–662.

Echemendia, R. J., & Cantu, R. (in press). Return to play following cerebral concussion. In M. Lovell, R. Echemendia, J. Barth, & M. Collins (Eds.), *Sports neuropsychology.* Swets & Zeitlinger.

Echemendia, R. J., Putukian, M., Mackin, S., Julian, L., & Shoss, N. (2001) Neuropsychological test performance prior to and following sports-related mild traumatic brain injury. *Clinical Journal of Sport Medicine, 11,* 23–31.

Echemendia, R. J., & Julian, L. (2001). Mild traumatic brain injury in sports: Neuropsychology's contribution to a developing field. *Neuropsychology Review, 11*(2), 69–88.

Echemendia, R. J., & Parker, E. (1998). Ethical issues in the neuropsychological assessment of athletes. In J. E. Bailes, M. R. Lovell, & J. C. Maroon (Eds.), *Sports related concussion and nervous system injuries.* St. Louis: Quality Medical Publishers.

Gronwall, D., & Wrightson, P. (1974). Delayed recovery of intellectual function after mild head injury. *The Lancet, 14,* 605–609.

Guskiewicz, K. M., Riemann, D., Perrin, D. H., & Nashner, L. M. (1997). Alternative approaches to the assessment of mild head injury in athletes. *Medicine & Science in Sports & Exercise, 29,* 213–221.

Hinton-Bayre, A. D., Geffen, G., & McFarland, K. (1997). Mild head injury and speed of information processing: A prospective study of professional rugby league players. *Journal of Clinical and Experimental Neuropsychology, 19*(2), 275–289.

Hovda, D. A., Prins, M., Becker, D. P., Lee, S., Bergsneider, M., & Martin, N. A. (1999). Neurobiology of Concussion. In J. E. Bailes, M. R. Lovell, J. C. Maroon (Eds.), *Sports-related concussion* (pp. 12–51). St. Louis: Quality Medical Publishers.

Kaplan, H. A., & Browder, J. (1954). Observations on the clinical and brain wave patterns of professional boxers. *Journal of the American Medical Association, 156,* 1138–1144.

Kaste, M., Kuurne, T., Vilkki, J., Katevuo, K., Sainio, K., & Meurala, H. (1982). Is chronic brain damage in boxing a hazard of the past? *The Lancet, 2,* 1186–1188.

Kross, R., Ohler, K., & Barolin, G. S. (1983). Effect of heading in soccer on the head—A quantifying EEG study of soccer players [German]. *EEG-EMG Zetschrift fur Elektroenzephalographi Electromyographie und Verwandte Gebiete, 14*(4), 209–212.

Lovell, M. R., & Collins, M. W. (1998). Neuropsychological assessment of the college football player. *Journal of Head Trauma Rehabilitation, 13*(2), 9–26.

Macciocchi, S. N., Barth, J. T., Alves, W., Rimel, R. W., & Jane, J. A. (1996). Neuropsychological functioning and recovery after mild head injury in collegiate athletes. *Neurosurgery, 39*(3), 510–514.

McLatchie, G., Brooks, N., Galbraith, S., Hutchison, J. S. F., Wilson, L., Melville, I., & Teasdale, E. (1987). Clinical neurological examination, neuropsychology, electroencephalography and computed tomographic head scanning in active amateur boxers. *Journal of Neurology, Neurosurgery, and Psychiatry, 50,* 96–99.

Matser, E., Kessels, A., Lezak, M., Jordan, B., & Troost, J. (1999). Neuropsychological impairment in amateur soccer players. *Journal of the American Medical Association, 282,* 971–973.

Murelius, O., & Haglund Y. (1991). Does Swedish amateur boxing lead to chronic brain damage? A retrospective neuropsychological study. *Acta Neurologica Scandanavia, 83,* 9–13.

National Center for Injury Prevention and Control. (2000). Epidemiology of traumatic brain injury in the United States. www.cdc.gov/ncipe/dacrrdp/tbi.htm

NIH Consensus Panel. (1999). Rehabilitation of persons with traumatic brain injury. *Journal of the American Medical Association, 282*(10), 974–983.

Olesniewicz, M. H., Sallis, R. E., Jones, K., & Copp, N. (1997). *The neuropsychological changes that occur from head concussions in football at the National Collegiate American Association Division Three level.* Paper presented at the Sports-Related Concussion and Nervous System Injuries Conference, Orlando, FL.

Powell, J. W., & Barber-Foss, K. (1999). Traumatic brain injury in high school athletes. *Journal of the American Medical Association, 282,* 958–963.

Putukian, M., Echemendia, R. J., & Mackin, R. S. (2000). Acute effects of heading in soccer: A prospective neuropsychological evaluation. *Clinical Journal of Sport Medicine, 10,* 104–109.

Quality Standards Subcommittee, American Academy of Neurology. (1997). Practice parameter: The management of concussion in sports (summary statement). *Neurology, 48,* 581–585.

Rimel, R. W., Giordani, B., Barth, J. T., Boll, J. T., & Jane, J. A. (1981). Disability caused by minor head injury. *Neurosurgery, 9,* 221–228.

Roberts, A. H. (1969). *Brain damage in boxers.* London: Pitman Medical Scientific Publishing.

Ross, R. J., Cole, M., Thompson, J. S., & Kim, K. H. (1983). Boxers—Computed tomography, EEG, and neurological evaluation. *Journal of the American Medical Association, 249,* 211–213.

Schneider, P. G., & Lichte, H. (1975). Untersuchungen zur groesse der krafteinwirkung beim kopfballspiel des fussballers. *Sportarzut un sprtmedizin, 26,* 10.

Sironi, V. A., Scotti, G., Ravagnati, L., Franzini, A., & Marossero, F. (1982). CT scan and EEG findings in professional pugilists: Early detection of cerebral atrophy in young boxers. *Journal of Neurosurgery, 26,* 165–168.

Symonds, C. (1962). Concussion and its sequelae. *The Lancet, 1,* 1–5.

Thomassen, A., Juul-Jensen, P., de Fine Olivarius, B., Braemer, J., & Christensen, A. L. (1979). Neurological, electroencephalographic, & neuropsychological examination of 53 former amateur boxers. *Acta Neurologica Scandinavica, 60*(6), 352–362.

Thurman, D. J., Branche, C. M., & Sniezek, J. E. (1998). The epidemiology of sports-related traumatic brain injuries in the United States: Recent developments. *Journal of Head Trauma Rehabilitation, 13*(2), 1–8.

Tysvaer, A., & Storli, O. (1981). Association football injuries to the brain: A preliminary report. *British Journal of Sports Medicine, 15*(3), 163–166.

Wechsler, D. (1997). *The Wechsler Adult Intelligence Scale–third revision.* San Antonio, TX.: The Psychological Corporation.

Woodward, J. L., Cronic, R., & Medlin, R. (2000). Psychometric characteristics of a brief neuropsychological battery used with professional football players. *Journal of the Interational Neuropsychological Society, 6,* 139.

PART

VIII

SPECIAL TOPICS

18

CHAPTER

Laetitia L. Thompson

Neuropsychological Assessment of Physicians Whose Competency to Practice Medicine Is Being Questioned

☐ Introduction

The utility of neuropsychological assessment of physicians, particularly when there are questions about competency to practice medicine, has been the subject of very little research and, to my knowledge, cost-effectiveness has not been systematically studied. Because this is an area that has only recently received interest from the medical and neuropsychological communities, writing a chapter on this topic presents quite a challenge. The paucity of research precludes a traditional focus on "What does the research tell us?" and leads to a chapter that asks as many questions as it answers.

This chapter explores what neuropsychological assessment services can provide to physicians and the benefits that may accrue to the physician and to the public. The chapter will review data regarding the "impaired" physician and research studies that examine physician competency in relation to cognitive functioning. Several physician-evaluation programs that include some type of neuropsychological assessment will be described. Two programs incorporate a neuropsychological "screen," and the third includes a more comprehensive neuropsychological evaluation. This provides an opportunity to compare the advantages and disadvantages of brief versus more inclusive assessments. In addition, very preliminary data are presented regarding the neuropsy-

---

I wish to thank Michael Gendel, M.D., Stephen Hjelt, J.D., Jane Kennedy, D.O., Elizabeth Korinek, M.P.H., Susan Miller, William Norcross, M.D., William Perry, Ph.D., Sue Radcliffe, and George Thomasson, M.D., for giving me their time and for graciously providing their perceptions and opinions about the neuropsychological contribution of assessment of physician competency.

chological component of one program, mostly to provide a launch point for discussion of important research questions and topics.

A number of professionals involved with the assessment of physician competency were interviewed regarding their perceptions of the utility and cost-effectiveness of neuropsychological evaluation. Informal interviews were conducted with physicians who evaluate and treat other physicians who may be impaired, neuropsychologists who evaluate physicians, administrators of physician-assessment programs, a program administrator of a state medical board, an administrative law judge, and a physician associated with a medical malpractice insurance carrier. Comments from these individuals about their perceptions and ideas for research are incorporated into the discussion. Case vignettes are interspersed throughout the chapter to provide information about the range of issues and various approaches that may be used. Issues related to costs and benefits of neuropsychological evaluation in this context are discussed and, finally, suggested research topics and ideas that might provide empirical information about this important clinical area are presented.

□ Cognitive Capacity to Practice Medicine

The practice of medicine is a highly regarded and responsible profession in our society. As such, the practice of medicine is regulated by state licensing boards, because our society places a priority on the safety of its citizens. Physicians work with citizens in ways that can have great benefit, but their interventions (or lack thereof) also can cause great harm. Therefore, physicians are licensed to practice based on achieving certain levels of training and demonstration of knowledge and proficiency in the practice of medicine.

Because the practice of medicine requires very high levels of cognitive performance, even subtle changes in functioning that might not be noticed in some individuals can affect physician competency. Therefore, it is generally accepted that physicians need to have relatively intact neurocognitive functioning in order to competently and safely practice in their profession (Parker & Coiera, 2000). Trunkey and Botney (2001) recently compared the ongoing evaluation of competency in two professions and noted that assessment of airline pilots is far more rigorous and frequent than are any requirements for physicians.

Physician impairment is defined as the inability to practice medicine with reasonable skill and safety because of physical or mental illness, and it has been estimated that 7% to 10% of the physicians in the United States are impaired sufficiently that their condition affects their work and practice (Van Komen, 2000). The most common diagnoses causing impairment relate to alcohol and drug abuse, emotional disorders, illness due to aging and loss, and physical conditions (Robinowitz, 1983). The prevalence of physical disabilities among physicians is not known, although estimates ranging from 2.5% to 4% have been put forth, albeit without much empirical support (Strax, Wainapel, & Welner, 2000). Recent information from the Federation of State Medical Boards indicated that, of all serious board disciplinary actions against physicians, 28.4% were because of substandard quality of care and 18.1% were because of physician substance abuse. Other major reasons for sanctions concerned unprofessional conduct (14%) and prescribing violations (14.8%; Prager, 2000). Unfortunately, these statistics do not tell us how often impaired cognitive functioning caused or contributed to the problem resulting in disciplinary action.

As noted, many of the problems causing impairment in physicians are psychiatric in nature and include drugs and alcohol (Langsley, 1983). Statistics vary somewhat from report to report, but the data suggest that substance use disorders are not an infrequent problem among physicians. The American Medical Association (AMA) and others have estimated that 7% to 8% of doctors are or will become alcoholics (Steindler, 1975; Webster, 1983). More recent data suggest that physicians have higher rates of alcohol use than the general population, but their rates may be similar to those of similar socioeconomic groups (Dilts & Gendel, 2000). Data from a U.S. community sample of adults in 1990–1991 using *DSM-IIIR* criteria indicated that approximately 14% had alcohol dependence at some time in their lives, with about 7% having had dependence in the past year (American Psychiatric Association, 1994).

Early reports suggested that about 1.5% of practicing physicians had a drug addiction (Modlin & Montes, 1964). This appears to be consistent with more recent information that physicians are similar to the general population in terms of previous experimentation with illicit drugs but were less likely to be current users (Dilts & Gendel, 2000). The major exception to this may involve a greater propensity for physicians to develop dependence on opioids, because medical personnel have ready access to certain opioids compared to the general population (American Psychiatric Association, 1994).

These data suggest that a significant number of physicians are "impaired," and cognitive dysfunction is an important factor in some cases. Concerns about how to detect and manage impaired physicians are not new. In an article in 1969, White cogently discussed the medical profession's responsibility to and for the "senile" physician. He criticized what he saw as attempts to "cover for" physicians who were no longer able to practice, because they had been held in high esteem in the past. His position was that this ultimately did nothing for the physician and certainly did not contribute to public safety. During the past several years, interest has grown in how to develop systematic mechanisms to detect and rehabilitate or remove impaired physicians from practice (e.g., Trunkey & Botney, 2001).

Although one might assume that physicians would be the first to seek information about their symptoms, this is not necessarily the case. Physicians often deny or minimize the import of their own symptoms much more than they would if their patients reported the same information. This may stem from a number of factors (fear of what the symptoms mean, overconfidence in self-diagnosis, concerns about reactions from others, worries about confidentiality, personal economic concerns), but it suggests that physicians cannot always be relied upon to independently seek out diagnosis and treatment (Goldman, 2000).

Role of Neuropsychology

Like everyone else, physicians are subject to illnesses and injuries that may specifically affect their cognitive functioning and their ability to apply their training and knowledge to their work. In these cases, informed decisions should be made on the basis of "hard evidence." Kapur (1997) called for the early involvement of a clinical neuropsychologist when a physician has suspected or established brain pathology. Kapur offered a cogent rationale for seeking early neuropsychological evaluation and consultation:

> Evidence from a clinical neuropsychologist will help to substantiate any observations in work settings related to functional competence, will help to provide an objective and impartial view with regard to cognitive symptoms, and will provide an opportunity for therapy/counseling to be offered at a stage where it may relieve some of the symptoms of brain pathology and prevent coping difficulties in work settings. These types of measures will help to ensure that the self-respect and mental well being of the patient are maintained, and that matters such as career development, financial affairs, etc. can be discussed on a rational basis. (1997, p. 402)

Physicians also are subject to changes in cognitive functioning that occur as a result of "normal aging." This introduces a particularly difficult and perplexing issue in the assessment of physicians with regard to competency to practice medicine. Is it possible that older physicians could be functioning "normally" for their age, but not be doing at all well compared to a reference group of practicing physicians? Could such physicians be considered not competent to practice or not competent to engage in certain activities such as surgery, even though there is no physical or mental illness in question? Or should we assume, if there is no illness present, that prior experience and "wisdom" will compensate for the cognitive decline occurring as a part of aging. These questions correspond to the differences discussed by Heaton, Chelune, Talley, Kay, and Curtiss (1993) between evaluating scores for the purpose of diagnosing disease or injury and evaluating scores in relation to the adequacy of abilities for everyday functioning. Very little empirical data are available to help sort out the cognitive effects of normal aging on the ability to practice medicine, but increasingly physicians are speaking out about the need to be aware of and to accept the changes that aging may produce (Hopkins, 1999).

Research Relating Cognitive Task Performance to Physician Job Performance

Relatively little research has addressed the ecological validity of neuropsychological tests for physician practice. Some physicians have assumed that neuropsychological assessment would not be "sensitive" enough to detect changes or decline in cognitive functioning in highly functioning individual such as medical doctors. For example, in *Injured Brains of Medical Minds*, a neurosurgeon who suffered a mild traumatic brain injury in a skiing accident while attending a conference in Vail, Colorado, wrote an essay about his recovery (Marshall & Ruff, 1997). He noted that he had "respectfully" declined to undergo neuropsychological testing, although it was recommended at the meeting in Vail by the neuropsychologists in attendance. The neurosurgeon perceived himself to have some cognitive difficulties for a number of months following the ski accident, but said, "The neurosurgeon in question here is certain . . . that had he been tested within one week of his injury, performance would have exceeded at least the average of national controls" (Marshall & Ruff, 1997, p. 313). As the testing never took place, this remains an empirical question. Advances in education-adjusted norms and an emphasis on use of "high-level" tests likely increase the sensitivity of neurocognitive tests to subtle deficits in high functioning individuals, but if Dr. Marshall was correct, he makes a good argument for research to develop physician-specific norms.

A few research studies have been conducted to examine performance on neuropsychological tests in relation to performance in specialty residency programs. This research is important because it studies the relationships of neuropsychological performance and clinical proficiency within groups of physicians in training who are not necessarily having difficulty performing their work. Demonstrating significant relationships between variables in groups with a restricted range is a demanding and difficult task. If significant associations are found between psychometric test performance and competency or skill in this type of setting, it bodes well for the utility of neuropsychological testing of physicians who may be having performance difficulties. In a study examining surgery residents' skills, Schueneman, Pickleman, Hesslein, and Freeark (1984) found a significant multiple correlation between neuropsychological test scores and attending ratings of surgical skill ($r = .68$), accounting for 46% of the variance. A subsequent analysis, regressing surgical skill ratings on neuropsychological test performances and Medical College Admission Test (MCAT) scores, revealed a multiple correlation of .80, accounting for 63% of the variance. Measures of nonverbal, visuospatial problem-solving ability were most related to better surgical technique; the Minnesota Paper Form Board Test alone correlated .58 ($p < .001$) with surgical skill rating.

At the end of the Schueneman et al. (1984) paper, three physicians provided discussion, and one of them, Dr. Robert E. Condon, speculated that visual–spatial organizational ability might not only be an important component of surgical skill, but might also be an important element of that "nebulous quality we call surgical judgment, the essence of which is the ability to act on and to pick out from a complex mix those elements that are important, to do so on the basis of incomplete data, and to organize them in such a way that therapy is successful" (Schueneman et al., 1984, p. 294). This is an intriguing hypothesis that has not yet been empirically tested.

A much more recent study examined the relationship of anesthesia knowledge and cognitive and personality measures to anesthesiology resident clinical performance (Reich et al., 1999). The authors employed two cognitive measures that focused on vigilance, divided attention, and speed of information processing (Paced Auditory Serial Addition Test [PASAT] and a visual continuous performance test [Vigil] modified to include an auditory signal detection task). Low scores on the PASAT and high numbers of commission errors on the Vigil predicted poor clinical performance ratings in the residency, independent of personality and academic measures. The measures of anesthesia knowledge also predicted poor clinical performance, but did not do so independently of neuropsychological test performance.

Another line of research related to resident performance investigated the effects of acute sleep deprivation on cognitive functioning. Because of controversy surrounding the required long work hours for medical personnel, especially residents in training, and subsequent effects on patient care, several articles appeared discussing the pros and cons of how resident training is structured and the hours worked (e.g., Condon, 1989a; 1989b). In addition, a few studies attempted to assess the effects of night call and the resulting acute sleep deprivation on cognitive functioning. Bartle et al. (1988) investigated the effects of acute sleep deprivation on surgical residents with a battery of tests focused on attention, speed of information processing, nonverbal problem solving, and fine motor coordination. They evaluated 42 surgical residents on two occasions, one time after a night on call (average of 2 hours of sleep) and the other time after no call (average of 6.5 hours of sleep). Half of the subjects were initially assessed in the sleep-deprived state, and half were initially assessed in the rested state. No significant differences were found between sleep-deprived and rested states on any neuropsychological measure (WAIS-R Digit Symbol, Digit Vigilance, Trail Making, PASAT, Raven's Matrices, Story Memory Test, or Grooved Pegboard). A mood questionnaire revealed, however, that the residents reported being significantly less vigorous and more fatigued, more depressed, more tense, more confused, and more angry when sleep deprived.

Browne and associates (1994) addressed ability to learn and remember in relation to acute sleep deprivation. They had surgical residents and medical students read journal articles either when sleep deprived or when rested and later answer questions about the content. Recall was assessed at 1 week and at 3 months. Although sleep deprived subjects reported increased fatigue and decreased motivation, no difference among sleep groups was found for recall at either 1 week or 3 months.

Lichtor, Zacny, Lane, and Good (1996) reported on two studies regarding how loss of sleep affected performance in anesthesiologists, surgeons, and nurses. They found that after a night on call, medical personnel showed impairment on a coordination task and a vision task, similar in extent to impairment seen after low-dose alcohol ingestion. Further resident performance decrements were seen the next day after a night of sleep at home that had been preceded by a night on call, suggesting that chronic sleep deprivation may be an issue or that there may be delayed effects of acute sleep deprivation. In the second study, the authors found a negative relationship between physician's ability to retain narrative information and sleep, although performance on a simulated, complex medical task was not associated with sleep status.

Taken together, these research studies suggest that only mild, if any, changes in performance occur in young, highly functioning physicians in training as a result of the typical acute sleep deprivation that occurs with residents' schedules. However, the issue of chronic sleep deprivation is more difficult to study and may partly confound the results from the investigations. Furthermore, these studies were done with residents, who are typically young and healthy. It is unclear whether results would be different in older physicians who practice long hours, with periods of significant sleep deprivation.

These studies suggest that at least some neuropsychological results are importantly related to the competent practice of medicine, and that neuropsychological evaluation is relevant to the assessment of physician functioning when there are concerns about cognition. Of course, more research is needed. Such research could specify which tests best predict physician competency, determine the need for physician-specific norms versus the utility of existing norms, explore the relationship between absolute level of functioning and competency in the aging physician, and develop "thresholds" of test performance for clinical concern.

Given our current state of knowledge, neuropsychological evaluation appears to be useful in the evaluation of physicians whose competency to practice is being questioned. As suggested by Dilts and Gendel (2000) in their article on substance use disorders in physicians, clinical assessment is required to determine the degree to which an illness affects ability to practice medicine, and specialized neuropsychological testing often is helpful in this clinical process. Situations in which neuropsychological assessment appears to be most relevant are listed in Table 18.1.

☐ Existing Procedures for Physicians to Undergo Neuropsychological Assessment

In my experience, physicians come to the attention of neuropsychologists via one of three routes: traditional referral, referral via a physician health program, or as part of a physician-competency evaluation.

TABLE 18.1. Major Contributions of Neuropsychological Testing in the Evaluation of Physicians

- Detection of subtle (but professionally significant) impairments in highly functioning professionals that are not picked up by other evaluation methods
- Evaluation of behavioral manifestations of neurological disease (e.g., Parkinson's disease), systemic illness (e.g., chronic obstructive pulmonary disease), or substance abuse/dependence for the purpose of determining safety to practice medicine
- Monitoring of mental functioning in the presence of expected recovery from illness (e.g., stroke) or injury (traumatic brain injury) to help determine whether and when return to practice is safe and appropriate
- Monitoring of progression of cognitive impairment in physicians with chronic illnesses (e.g., multiple sclerosis) to determine whether and when the physician becomes unsafe to practice medicine
- Differentiating depression from dementia in older physicians

Traditional Referral to Neuropsychologist in Clinical Practice

The first route is a traditional referral from a physician whom the physician patient is seeing for a known medical problem or an array of symptoms that are being evaluated for diagnosis. The symptoms or diagnosis lead the physician patient or the referring physician to question whether cognitive impairment is present as part of the disorder. In this scenario, the neuropsychological evaluation often is requested primarily to help with the diagnosis or treatment of the physician patient. Frequently in these cases, the question of ability to practice is secondary, but often it *is* present in the background. Vignette 1 provides an example of this type of clinical referral.

Vignette 1: Physician with Multiple Sclerosis. Dr. J was a 45-year-old physician specializing in internal medicine who was diagnosed with multiple sclerosis (MS) approximately 2 years before undergoing neuropsychological evaluation. He became concerned that he might be experiencing problems with concentration and short-term memory sufficient to affect his medical practice. He consulted with his neurologist, and they decided to pursue a neuropsychological evaluation to obtain objective data about the nature and degree of any cognitive decline. Dr. J's symptoms of MS to date were parasthesias and lower extremity weakness. His course was of a relapsing–remitting nature, and his last exacerbation had occurred about 1 year before the neuropsychological evaluation.

This physician seemed very interested in the testing. He was cooperative and appeared to put forth his best effort. He completed a comprehensive neuropsychological evaluation, including the WAIS–R, the expanded Halstead–Reitan Battery described in Heaton, Grant, and Matthews (1991), California Verbal Learning Test, verbal fluency, and PASAT.

Results of the evaluation were generally within normal limits and suggested only the possibility of minimal cerebral dysfunction. General intellectual functioning was in the superior range, and summary scores were within normal limits. Impaired test results included sustained attention and concentration, letter and category fluency, and unexpected errors on aphasia screening. Efficiency in visual scanning and in following sequential procedures was borderline normal. Clinical interview and psychological screening suggested the presence of at least mild depression.

Recommendations were made for this doctor to seek treatment for his depression. He was given feedback about the areas of impairment on testing and information that the impaired results could be a result of minimal neurocognitive decline, effects of his depression, or a normal variant. Suggestions for possible compensation strategies were provided, but the main conclusion was that his difficulties on testing did not rise to the level likely to significantly impair his ability to practice medicine.

Dr. J expressed considerable relief about the test findings. Obtaining information that he was still functioning well reduced his level of worry and the sense of hypervigilance he had developed about his cognitive functioning. He and his neurologist also thought that the neuropsychological results would provide a useful baseline should he or others around him become concerned about his cognitive functioning at a later point in time.

Referral via Physician Health Program

Many states have an organization that plays a special role in working with physicians who may have psychiatric or medical problems, difficulties with stress or burnout, or questions about practice competency. These programs offer a confidential place for the physician to turn (in some cases, instead of being reported to the Medical Board) for help in diagnosis, evaluation, and appropriate treatment. The evaluation and treatment remain confidential unless the physician is perceived as being dangerous to patients. The second vignette illustrates this type of referral.

Vignette #2: Physician with Report of Memory Problems. Dr. S called the physician's health organization in his state with concerns that Dr. C seemed to be having considerable memory difficulty. Dr. S said he was so concerned that, if Dr. C did not consult with the physician's health organization, Dr. S would report him to the state medical board. After several requests from the physician health organization, Dr. C met with one of the physicians there for an initial interview. At that time, Dr. C denied any cognitive or memory problems, said that his practice was going well, and attributed Dr. S's report to a professional disagreement about a patient's treatment.

There were no obvious memory problems in the interview, but Dr. C's conversational speech was circumstantial, perseverative, and tangential. He scored 28/30 on the Folstein Mini-Mental Status Exam (Folstein, Folstein, & McHugh, 1975). He missed an orientation item and a memory item. Because of the allegation of memory difficulty and the problems in the interview, he was referred for a neuropsychological evaluation and a physical exam. He agreed to the plan, but procrastinated in scheduling appointments, saying that his medical practice was too busy. Only at the strong urging of the doctor at the physician's health program did he actually schedule an appointment for neuropsychological assessment.

At the time of neuropsychological evaluation, the physician was 58 years old. He had a solo medical practice in plastic surgery. He denied any difficulty with his medical practice. At the same time, he had difficulty providing his home address, and he tended to answer questions about his medical history tangentially by telling unrelated or peripherally related stories. His speech was fluent although tangential, and he presented in a distinguished, erudite manner.

Dr. C was generally cooperative with testing procedures, but he worked slowly and had trouble understanding and remembering more complex test instructions. Reminders and extra clarification were provided when possible.

Dr. C's overall performance on the neuropsychological testing was significantly impaired; in fact, the battery was truncated because of his obvious difficulty on many tests. His general intelligence on the WAIS–R was in the low/average range, and his reading comprehension was at the sixth grade level. He was severely impaired in learning new information; even after multiple exposures to the same material, he recalled only a few bits of information. Even his recognition memory on this test was severely impaired; he tended to endorse all items, both those that were correct and other items presented as "foils." He became very confused on problem-solving and complex attentional tasks and could not complete some of them. He was impaired on several tests of visual/spatial and visuoconstructional ability.

This level of performance was much lower than expected from someone of his age and general educational achievement level—and this was a physician who was regularly performing intricate surgery on patients! Specific norms were not available for physicians, but his performance was compared to others with graduate-level academic degrees. Based on the quantitative test data and behavioral observations, the neuropsychologist strongly encouraged a neurological work-up and suggested that Dr. C not perform any surgery or other interventions until he met with the referring doctor from the physician's health program.

Per the physicians' health program, Dr. C was not allowed to continue his surgical practice until further work-up. A neurological evaluation, including lab tests and an MRI of the brain, resulted in a provisional diagnosis of Alzheimer's disease. Dr. C. took a disability retirement.

This vignette highlights the utility of neuropsychological assessment in detecting early dementia before it is obvious from clinical interview and mental status exam, but at a point where it is likely to be significantly affecting job performance. Evaluation was useful to the patient in terms of diagnosis, treatment, and disability status. Evaluation also was useful from a public safety perspective. Dr. C. showed significant cognitive deficits in memory, reasoning, and spatial analysis, and he was apparently quite unaware of his difficulties. He was in a solo practice in which there was little interaction with other physicians. He had an active surgical practice, which, in light of his deficits, seemed to place patients at risk. As far as is known, no adverse effects occurred to his patients prior to his discontinuing his practice, but he likely was at much greater risk of making a serious error than a normally functioning physician would be.

Neuropsychological Assessment as Part of a Physician-Competency Evaluation

Physicians who "get into trouble" with their patients, colleagues, hospitals, or medical boards because of some mistake or unusual behavior may be required to undergo evaluation of competency to practice. Specialized programs have been developed in the United States and Canada to address these issues of physician competency that may arise separately from any known medical condition. A number of these programs now include neuropsychological assessment as part of the evaluation.

Vignette 3: Physician Undergoing Evaluation Because of Concerns About Prescription Practices. Dr. H was a 60-year-old general practitioner referred for a comprehensive evaluation of his competency to practice by his state medical board because of questions about the appropriateness of his prescribing practices. He completed a 3-day evaluation of his knowledge base, interpersonal skills, diagnostic and treatment skills, and cognitive functioning. Cognition was assessed via a screening battery administered to all physicians completing the evaluation. This physician performed poorly on several components of the screening, including verbal memory, cognitive flexibility, and conceptual reasoning. He worked very quickly, but this was often at the expense of accuracy. His level of difficulty on the cognitive screen was sufficient that the neuropsychologist recommended further evaluation.

A comprehensive neuropsychological evaluation revealed mild weaknesses in visual attention and flexibility in problem solving, but his other performances were good, and the more detailed assessment did not suggest difficulties that would preclude the physician from practicing competently. He was provided feedback about his cognitive strengths and weakness and given recommendations for possible compensatory strategies.

This vignette highlights the increased interest in incorporating neuropsychological assessment in the evaluation of the physician in trouble. A number of programs have been developed specifically to evaluate and then, if appropriate, provide education and remediation plans for physicians whose competency to practice is being questioned. Many, but not all, of these programs now include some type of neuropsychological assessment as part of the overall evaluation. The following section describes different programs to illustrate the different ways that neuropsychological assessment is being incorporated into formal physician assessment.

☐ Physician-Assessment Programs: Three Examples

Three physician-assessment and education programs are described for illustrative purposes. The first is a program in Canada that has incorporated brief neuropsychological testing into the protocol. The other two are in the United States: One incorporates a computerized cognitive screen in the standard physician evaluation of competency, and one incorporates a lengthier battery of neuropsychological and psychological tests in the physician evaluation. Description of the Canadian program is based on a published report, whereas description of the two U.S. programs is based on the author's personal knowledge and interviews with professionals working in each.

Physician Review Program (PREP) was developed at McMaster University in Ontario, Canada, under the sponsorship of the College of Physicians and Surgeons of Ontario, the province's medical licensing authority. Turnbull and associates (2000) recently published an intriguing report on a detailed neuropsychological screening battery given to all of the participants in PREP during a 1-year period, 1996–1997. During that year, 27 actively practicing physicians were evaluated through the program. At the end of the intensive 1-day PREP evaluation, the neuropsychological battery was administered (see Table 18.2.)

Physicians were assigned clinical ratings of no, minimal, mild, moderate, or severe difficulty for each of several neuropsychological domains (verbal and visual–spatial problem solving; memory; tracking, concentration, and fluency; and mood), and then given

TABLE 18.2. PREP Neuropsychological Screening Battery

WAIS-R subtests
Wisconsin Card Sorting Test
Rey Osterreith Complex Figure–Copy
Wechsler Memory Scale–Revised Logical Memory–Immediate and Delayed Recall
California Verbal Learning Test (CVLT)
Trail Making Test
Stroop Color Word Test
PASAT
FAS and Animal Naming
Profile of Mood States

a final clinical rating regarding likelihood and severity of general cognitive deficit. Eight physicians scored well on the basic PREP evaluation, and 7 of these were rated as having no, minimal, or mild cognitive impairment on the neuropsychological battery. The 8th physician was not cooperative with the neuropsychological portion of the assessment. The remaining 19 physicians scored poorly on the basic PREP evaluation and, of these, 6 (32%) had moderate or severe cognitive impairment. Therefore, of the 27 physicians referred to the program, 22% evidenced significant impairment on neuropsychological testing. The authors noted that the testing was done "at the end of an already busy day," but they argued that it would be "overly protective" to test under less stressful and fatiguing circumstances, because physicians must work long hours (Turnbull et al., 2000, p. 180). Therefore, rather than concluding that the testing overestimated impairment, the authors concluded that a more detailed neuropsychological evaluation might have revealed an even higher proportion of cognitively impaired physicians. Further, they noted that they had adjusted neuropsychological scores for normal aging. They discussed the (aforementioned) issue that some of the older physicians may have been performing satisfactorily compared to age peers, but not doing well compared to most practicing physicians. Therefore, Turnbull et al. concluded that their results might have *underestimated* the actual number of physicians having significant cognitive difficulty. The authors concluded that the addition of at least a neuropsychological screen had utility, and they cited two specific reasons to support its use: (a) detection of unrecognized yet treatable conditions and (b) prevention of educational interventions in physicians unlikely to benefit.

Colorado Personalized Education for Physicians (CPEP) has provided evaluation and remediation programs for physicians throughout the United States who have either self-referred or been referred by organizations such as state medical licensing boards or hospital credentialing committees because of questions about practice competency. The program started about 10 years ago, and 7 years ago it began using a computerized cognitive screening assessment on a very limited basis (i.e., when there was a known reason why there might be significant cognitive impairment). Three years later, the program added the neuropsychological screen as part of the standard evaluation. The CPEP evaluation now consists of 2 to 3 days of assessment. Before the evaluation, the physician is asked to submit the results of a recent general physical exam and to provide information about the nature and scope of practice along with a history of professional and continuing medical education, licensure, and any malpractice cases or disciplinary proceedings.

The physician completes an in-depth interview and undergoes structured clinical interviews conducted by at least two specialist peers regarding hypothetical cases or the physician's charts (or both) in order to assess knowledge, decision making, and documentation. Interactions with three simulated patients are videotaped to provide information about diagnostic and communication skills, and written tests examine knowledge base in the physician's specialty area. The physician also completes a standardized neuropsychological screen, consisting of the MicroCog Assessment of Cognitive Functioning (Powell et al., 1993). At the discretion of the medical education director, other assessments–such as computer-based clinical simulations or EKG interpretations–may be added.

A recent agreement was reached among the National Board of Medical Examiners, the Federation of State Medical Boards, and Colorado Personalized Education for Physicians to establish the Institute for Physician Evaluation–Colorado. This is the first in a series of planned assessment centers designed to identify and address possible subpar medical practice through an assessment of strengths and deficits and development of a remediation plan when necessary and appropriate. James R. Winn, M.D., executive director of the Federation of State Medical Boards, stated,

> Broader use of clinical assessments could greatly benefit the public, boards, and medicine overall. Boards should be able to intervene earlier, when a couple of complaints suggest that care patterns could be problematic, rather than after patients have been harmed. If the assessment is utilized early on, when a pattern of problematic care is first suspected, physicians may be able to avoid protracted and costly challenges to their licenses. Board investigations could be cut short if doctors demonstrate that their practice is indeed up to snuff. (Prager, 2000)

The neuropsychological screening instrument used at CPEP and interpreted by a clinical neuropsychologist is the MicroCog Assessment of Cognitive Functioning (Powell

TABLE 18.3. MicroCog Assessment of Cognitive Functioning Domains and Subtests

1) Attention/Mental Control
   a) Numbers Forward and Backward
   b) Alphabet
   c) Wordlist 1 and 2
2) Memory
   a) Address-Delayed Recall
   b) Stories 1 and 2-Immediate and Delayed Recall
3) Reasoning/Calculation
   a) Analogies
   b) Object Match
   c) Math Calculations
4) Spatial Processing
   a) Tic Tac
   b) Clocks
5) Reaction Time
   a) Timers 1 and 2 (Auditory and Visual Reaction Time)

et al., 1993). MicroCog cognitive domains and subtests are listed in Table 18.3. The original version of this screening assessment was developed by a group of experts in neuropsychology, neurology, research design, quantitative methods, and computer technology at the encouragement of the board of directors of the Controlled Risk Management Insurance Company, Ltd., and the Risk Management Foundation of the Harvard teaching hospitals. The original normal samples consisted of more than 1,000 physicians and 581 nonphysicians between the ages of 25 and 92 (Powell, 1994). Physicians were tested to examine how MicroCog worked as a test instrument with a well-educated population. The published version of the test is the result of collaboration among the original test developers and the Psychological Corporation. The published test is a modified version of the test given to the original sample, so a new normative sample was collected for the published version, consisting of 810 adults chosen to be representative of the US population of adults. Therefore, although there are physician-normative data for an earlier version of the MicroCog, these data cannot be directly applied to the published version.

As a neuropsychological screening test that is computer administered and scored, Microcog has both the advantages and the disadvantages inherent in computerized testing. Among the advantages are standardization of administration, speed of scoring, precise quantification of reaction and performance times, ease of data handling and computation of scores, and easy implementation of basal and ceiling rules to ensure administration at an appropriate level (Powell et al., 1993). Disadvantages include the fact that some examinees may be unfamiliar with computers or "computer phobic," limitations in the way stimuli can be presented and responses recorded, and the potential effects on motivation of interacting with a computer instead of a human examiner (Powell et al., 1993).

Elizabeth Korinek, M.P.H., executive director of CPEP, said that from her perspective, the addition of the MicroCog neuropsychological screening has been quite beneficial. She indicated that frequently the neuropsychological results are consistent with observations in other aspects of the CPEP evaluation, and the results often provide information about the *nature* of the physician's problem. Given that a goal of the program is to develop education plans, it is her perception that it is very helpful to have information about a physician's ability to learn and remember (Korinek, personal communication, August 29, 2000). Trunkey and Botney (2001) recently endorsed the use of a screening instrument such as MicroCog in evaluating physicians after they reach the age of 50 to help monitor cognitive status as they age.

No formal research has been conducted on the use of this instrument in the CPEP evaluation process, but a limited amount of information has been gathered informally. Of 124 physicians evaluated at CPEP between January 1997 and March 2000, 112 completed the MicroCog. Two of these physicians had completed neuropsychological evaluations before coming to CPEP because of known neurological illness, and they are not included in these data. Of the remaining 110, 82 (75%) were judged to perform within normal limits on the MicroCog or showed only "spotty" difficulties on the test; without additional evidence from other portions of the evaluation, these were not of significant concern. The remaining 28 (25%) physicians performed poorly enough on the MicroCog to raise concerns about significant cognitive impairment, and these physicians were strongly encouraged to undergo more comprehensive neuropsychological evaluation to clarify their cognitive status.

Table 18.4 contains MicroCog summary scores of the 28 physicians who were recom-

TABLE 18.4. MicroCog Summary Percentile Ranks for Referred vs. Nonreferred Physicians

Measure		Group	
		Referred (n = 28)	Not Referred (n = 82)
Age	mean	56.64	49.44
	standard dev.	7.69	8.17
	median	54.5	49
	range	42–77	31–71
Foreign-born	(%)	32.14	13.41
Age-corrected norms for MicroCog			
Speed			
	mean	18.61	51.37
	standard dev.	26.73	29.76
	median	5	54
	range	1–85	1–96
Accuracy			
	mean	18.79	48.56
	standard dev.	16.31	19.43
	median	14	47
	range	1–53	5–95
Proficiency			
	mean	11.04	45.90
	standard dev.	12.24	22.98
	median	7	42
	range	1–58	3–91
Reference group norms for MicroCog			
Speed			
	mean	12.43	41.13
	standard dev.	21.22	27.30
	median	1.5	42
	range	1–86	1–88
Accuracy			
	mean	19.75	59.71
	standard dev.	20.78	20.81
	median	16	63
	range	1–73	6–91
Proficiency			
	mean	7.89	41.83
	standard dev.	9.69	23.98
	median	4.5	38
	range	1–47	4–92

mended to pursue additional evaluation (labeled the *referred group*) and the 82 physicians who did not receive a recommendation to pursue additional neuropsychological evaluation (labeled the *not referred group*). Two types of summary scores are presented; the first percentile summary scores are age corrected (and education corrected to the extent that these physicians are compared to others who have more than a high school education). The second set of percentile summary scores is based on a reference group consisting of 180 participants in the standardization sample between the ages of 18 and 34. According to the MicroCog manual, individuals in this age range generally achieve the highest scores (Powell et al., 1993). The manual indicates that the reference group norms are appropriate when interpretations must address questions about performance relative to optimal adult performance.

Within each normative set, three summary scores are presented. The first is a percentile score based on speed of performance, and the second is based on accuracy. The third, the Cognitive Proficiency Index, is a summary of proficiency (speed and accuracy) across individual subtests. Unfortunately, not all subtests yield a proficiency score, and a few do not contribute to any summary score. Therefore, for individual interpretation it is not sufficient to rely on summary scores alone; they are presented here as preliminary information.

In examining Table 18.4, several points are evident. First, the physicians referred for further neuropsychological evaluation were a little older than those who were not, and a higher percentage of the referred physicians were foreign born and educated (32% vs. 13%). Second, the range of percentile scores across the samples of physicians is broad, regardless of whether you examine scores for the physicians who were referred for further evaluation or the larger group that was not felt to show significant impairment. Third, the means for the referred group appear to be substantially lower than for the other group, but the differences are even more apparent when examining the median scores. For example, the median Cognitive Proficiency for the referred group was at the 7th percentile compared to age peers and at the 4.5th percentile compared to the reference group of young adults. In contrast, the median cognitive proficiency for the nonreferred physician group was at the 42nd percentile compared to age peers with more than a high school education and at the 38th percentile compared to the reference group. The finding that the "better-performing" physicians referred to CPEP were still below the 50th percentile is surprising; it may suggest that as a group physicians referred to these evaluation programs are not functioning as well cognitively as the general group of practicing physicians.

The CPEP staff attempted to learn how many of the 28 physicians obtained the recommended comprehensive neuropsychological evaluations and what the outcomes of the evaluations were. Only 13 of the 28 physicians who were recommended to seek additional evaluation responded to the inquiry from CPEP about this. Twelve reported obtaining follow-up, and 1 reported not obtaining follow-up. Of the 12 who reported undergoing further evaluation, 5 reported that the additional evaluation did not reveal significant deficits; 5 reported that some impairment was found, but not enough to render them incapable of practicing medicine; 1 voluntarily quit practice rather than have his or her license revoked; and 1 physician was found to have a treatable dementia. Unfortunately, we do not know whether the physicians who responded are different from those who did not. A number of those who did not respond may not have followed CPEP's recommendation to obtain further evaluation and did not want to acknowledge this.

The Physician Assessment and Clinical Education (PACE) program at the University of California, San Diego (UCSD), is the final program to be described. Although most of the referrals for evaluation and education come from the California State Board of Medical Examiners, the PACE program is designed to be independent and neutral. Unless a physician is determined to be dangerous to the public, the results of the evaluation and education plan remain confidential. The evaluation takes 2 days. One day involves (a) the doctor undergoing a history and physical exam; (b) the doctor performing a history and physical exam on a mock patient; and (c) the doctor taking a clinical competency assessment in his or her area of specialty, given by faculty in that specialty area at UCSD. Faculty in the physician's specialty area design this competency assessment, and it may consist of written questions, an oral exam relating to patient vignettes, and actual observation of procedures in a simulated context. The second day involves a fairly comprehensive neuropsychological battery that requires 5 to 6 hours for the physician to complete. See Table 18.5 for the tests in the PACE neuropsychological battery.

The neuropsychological evaluation in the PACE program comprises a significant portion of the overall assessment, in terms of both time and significance placed on the results. Dr. William Norcross, Director of the PACE program, expressed the opinion that the neuropsychological evaluation was an important component in the overall assessment. He admitted to being "skeptical" about the need for such a comprehensive psychometric evaluation when the program was first developed, but said he had become convinced that the information from the psychometric testing has significant utility. He said that, although he is not usually "surprised" by the neuropsychological findings, they are useful in documenting specific aspects of the physician's functioning that are contributing to the problems in medical practice and in determining what specific recommendations to make for education, remediation or both (William Norcross, personal communication, September 8, 2000).

Cost–Benefit Analysis

There is no simple answer to the question of costs versus benefits at this time, but there are a number of issues to consider. The professionals interviewed for this chapter provided several salient perceptions.

TABLE 18.5. PACE Neuropsychological Test Battery

WAIS–R Subtests
Information
Digit Span
Vocabulary
Similarities
Picture Arrangement
Block Design
Trail Making Test
Halstead Category Test
Symbol Digit Modalities Test
Numerical Attention Test
Selected tests from the Benton Multilingual Aphasia Exam
Story Memory Test
Modified Complex Figure Test
California Verbal Learning Test
Wide Range Achievement Test–3rd Ed.
Rorschach (as a cognitive assessment tool)
MMPI–2 (as a psychological screening test)

- Neuropsychological assessment is seen as relatively expensive and time consuming.
- The cost is perceived to be a deterrent to voluntary testing.
- Cognitive impairment is a contributing factor to poor medical practice in a small percentage of cases.
- Neuropsychological assessment provides unique objective and defensible information about cognitive functioning.
- Neuropsychological assessment results can provide important diagnostic and practice information.
- The potential cost to the public from cognitively impaired physicians may be very high.
- Neuropsychological screening may provide a potential compromise between the high cost of a comprehensive neuropsychological battery and the limited information obtained from interviews and mental status exams.

The cost of a neuropsychological evaluation (estimated to be $1,500 to $2,500) may seem like a lot of money, but it pales in comparison to harming a patient or facing a malpractice suit. As an example, say a medical malpractice case is settled out of court for $500,000 because of the errors made by a doctor with early dementia. Assume that a neuropsychological evaluation would have identified the dementia and the subsequent risk for the doctor and his or her patients. That $500,000 would pay for 200 to 333 neuropsychological evaluations. This, of course, does not figure in the intangible costs to both the physician and the patient.

Using the costs–benefits equation developed by Drummond, O'Brien, Stoddart, and Torrance (1997), which was explained in Chapter 2 of this volume, one could estimate the costs–benefits in the evaluation of an individual physician. A useful example might be an ophthalmologist who sustains a traumatic brain injury in a motor vehicle accident. He is unconscious for approximately 12 hours and hospitalized for 2 weeks, followed by rehabilitation for about 6 weeks. About 4 months after the accident, he returns to office practice, but is not permitted to perform surgery. He is referred for a neuropsychological evaluation 6 months after the accident, when he wants to resume his surgery practice. He is motivated to undergo the evaluation and pay whatever is necessary. The physician performed well on the neuropsychological evaluation, and his behavior and comportment are appropriate. Based on the neuropsychological evaluation (and positive reports from colleagues and office staff), this physician is allowed to resume his practice without restrictions.

Using the Drummond et al. (1997) equation $\{[(W + V + S_1 + S_2 + S_3) - (C_1 + C_2 + C_3)]\}$–where W = willingness to pay, V = value measured in dollars, S_1 = health-care savings, S_2 = savings in patient/family resources, S_3 = savings in "other resources," C_1 = health-care costs, C_2 = patient/family resources used (costs), and C_3 = costs in other "sectors"–the following costs–benefits analysis can be computed. Willingness to pay (W) was estimated at $3,000 as the top of the range for neuropsychological assessment. The value, in monetary terms, was estimated to be $150,000 per year (60% of his income as an ophthalmologist is based on surgery practice), for 18 years of future practice. Therefore, V = $2.7 million in today's dollars. Savings were difficult to estimate, so 0 was entered for each S value. The cost of the evaluation (C_1) was $1,500 (9 hours of evaluation time and 1 hour of consultation at $150 per hour). Patient resources (C_2) were estimated to be $50 for travel, parking, and lunch on the day of the examination. One day of office practice time was needed for the physician to complete the evaluation, so

C_3 was estimated to be $1,000. The cost–benefit was as follows: [($3000 + $2,700,000 + 0 + 0 + 0) – ($1,500 + $50 + $1000)] = $2,700,450.

Similarly, when a physician is facing an inquiry because of errors or alleged errors, and is placed in the position of documenting ability to practice (and earn a living), the cost of a neuropsychological evaluation seems small. Of course, if the same objectives could be obtained with the use of neuropsychological screening at a cost of only a few hundred dollars, this would be desirable and more cost-effective. The cost-effectiveness of neuropsychological screening is unknown at this time. Screening would be useful and cost-effective only if it were sensitive enough to detect cognitive problems in high-functioning individuals. A useful screen would be designed to detect possible problems that could lead to further, more comprehensive evaluation if the physician had difficulty.

Issues for Research

Little research has been done in this field, so the area is ripe for a wide range of studies addressing a myriad of issues. Among the most basic issues is the lack of normative data for physicians in general or for specialty-practice physicians. Currently, normative data are available (for some tests) for individuals with high levels of education. These normative data appear to be the most relevant for use with this population, and tests with these normative data are the most appropriate for assessment of physicians at this time. This does not obviate the need for research to determine whether physician-specific norms are needed.

How to interpret neuropsychological data in the context of physician practice in general and specialty practice is of great concern. The "ecological validity" of specific neuropsychological tests for the practice of medicine has received limited attention. The studies cited above correlating resident performance with neurocognitive performance provide a start for this type of research, but more data are needed to know what cognitive domains (and what tests) predict physician competency.

Currently, there are no empirical data indicating the average level and range of neuropsychological performance in practicing physicians, or a threshold for concern that could be applied to different specialty areas (e.g., surgery, radiology, or pediatrics). It seems intuitive that a mild decline in visuospatial analysis skill may have different import for a surgeon than for a psychiatrist, but analysis of this currently relies entirely on "clinical" judgment rather than empirical data. Other cognitive abilities (such as memory) may be more universal in their importance for competent practice (Parker & Coiera, 2000).

The issue of how normal aging affects ability to practice medicine was raised at the beginning of this chapter. The competency of older physicians is a concern to many working in this field, and the lack of empirical knowledge makes clinical evaluation and treatment difficult. Research is needed to determine if there are minimal levels of absolute cognitive ability that are necessary to safely practice medicine, regardless of age (or other demographic variables).

Part of the goal of this volume is to consider the cost of neuropsychological evaluation in relation to outcome and benefit. In the case of physician assessment, the monetary cost of the evaluation is likely to be borne by the physician or the health-care system, whereas the benefit may accrue to the physician and to his or her patients. When this type of analysis is conducted, the "cost" of neuropsychological evaluation often no longer seems significant. Future studies examining costs and benefits may be particularly helpful in this area, where the potential stakes to the physician and to public safety are high.

Neuropsychological screening instruments have been presented several times as potentially practical and cost-effective means of evaluating a large number of physicians. The data presented regarding the use of the MicroCog Assessment of Cognitive Functioning in the CPEP program highlights several important research questions. Research is needed to investigate the sensitivity and specificity of screening instruments. It would be useful to investigate the neuropsychological screening performance of physicians referred for physician-competency evaluations compared to a reference group of physicians who are practicing without difficulty. It would be instructive to compare performances on neuropsychological screening with a comprehensive battery of neuropsychological tests to determine what impairments the screen is sensitive to and what impairments are likely to be missed.

Until more research is conducted, neuropsychologists are left with the burden of relying on their clinical judgment. This is similar to the situation neuropsychologists faced 20 years ago with regard to the effects of age and educational achievement on expected neuropsychological test performance. We knew that age and education were important, but had few quantitative guidelines to indicate how to configure them into interpretation. I hope that research will be pursued in the assessment of physician competency that will be as clinically beneficial as the development of demographic-specific norms has been.

In the meantime, this chapter ends with several practical questions that clinicians engaging in this type of practice are encouraged to keep in mind:

- When does a physician need a formal assessment of cognitive functioning?
- What are the purposes of such an assessment? What are the important cognitive domains for this physician's practice?
- What is the scope of the assessment? How will the results be used?
- Who is the assessment for? Who is the client?
- Who has access to the results?
- What is the justifiable cost to determine that a physician has the requisite cognitive abilities to practice medicine? Is a comprehensive battery of tests necessary?

References

American Psychiatric Association. (1994). *Diagnostic and statistical manual of mental disorders* (4th ed.). Washington, DC: Author.

Bartle, E. J., Sun, J. H., Thompson, L., Light, A. I., McCool, S., & Heaton, S. (1988). The effects of acute sleep deprivation during residency training. *Surgery, 104*, 311–316.

Browne, B. J., Van Susteren, T., Onsager, D. R., Simpson, D., Salaymeh, B., & Condon, R. E. (1994). Influence of sleep deprivation on learning among surgical house staff and medical students. *Surgery, 115*, 604–610.

Condon, R. E. (1989a). Resident hours: Only work? *Archives of Surgery, 124*, 1121–1122.

Condon, R. E. (1989b). Sleep deprivation and resident call schedules. *Current Surgery, 46*, 361–364.

Dilts, S. J., & Gendel, M. H. (2000). Substance use disorders. In L. S. Goldman, M. Myers, & L. J. Dickstein (Eds.), *The handbook of physician health: The essential guide to understanding the health care needs of physicians* (pp. 118–137). Chicago: American Medical Association.

Drummond, M. F., O'Brien, B. J., Stoddart, G. L., & Torrance, G. W. (1997). *Methods for the economic evaluation of health care programmes* (2nd ed.). Oxford: Oxford University Press.

Folstein, M. F., Fostein, S. E., & McHugh, P. R. (1975). "Mini-Mental State": A practical method for grading the cognitive state of patients for the clinician. *Journal of Psychological Research, 12,* 189–198.

Goldman, L. S. (2000). When physicians become ill. In L. S. Goldman, M. Myers, & L. J. Dickstein (Eds.), *The handbook of physician health: The essential guide to understanding the health care needs of physicians* (pp. 193–204). Chicago: American Medical Association.

Heaton, R. K., Chelune, G. J., Talley, J. L., Kay, G. G., & Curtiss, G. (1993). *Wisconsin Card Sorting Manual: Revised and expanded.* Odessa, FL: Psychological Assessment Resources.

Heaton, R. K., Grant, I., & Matthews, C. G. (1991). *Comprehensive Norms for an Expanded Halstead-Reitan Battery.* Odessa, FL: Psychological Assessment Resources.

Hopkins, R. (1999). Doctors must accept inevitable consequences of aging (Letter). *British Medical Journal, 318,* 871.

Kapur, N. (1997). *Injured brains of medical minds.* Oxford: Oxford University Press.

Langsley, D. (1983). Foreword. In S. C. Scheiber & B. B. Doyle (Eds.), *The impaired physician.* (pp. ix–x). New York: Plenum Medical Book Co.

Lichtor, J. L., Zacny, J., Lane, B. S., & Good, M. L. (1996). Research grant report: How does night call affect next-day performance in anesthesia? *Journal of Clinical Monitoring, 12,* 277–278.

Marshall L. F., & Ruff, R. R. (1997). Neurosurgeon as victim. In N. Kapur (Ed.), *Injured brains of medical minds* (pp. 313–316). Oxford: Oxford University Press.

Modlin, H. C., & Montes, A. (1964). Narcotics addiction in physicians. *American Journal of Psychiatry, 121,* 358–363.

Parker, J., & Coiera, E. (2000). Improving clinical communication: A view from psychology. *Journal of the American Medical Informatics Association, 7,* 453–461.

Powell, D. H. (1994). *Profiles in cognitive aging.* Cambridge, MA: Harvard University Press.

Powell, D. H., Kaplan, E. F., Whitla, D., Weintraub, S., Catlin, R., & Funkenstein, H. H. (1993). *MicroCog assessment of cognitive functioning manual.* San Antonio, TX: Psychological Corporation.

Prager, L. O. (2000). Doctor sanctions level off; boards try preventive tack. *American Medical News* [Online]. Available: http://www.ama-assn.org/sci-Pubs/amnews/pick_00/prsa0501.html

Reich, D. L., Uysal, S., Bodian, C. A., Gabriele, S., Hibbard, M., Gordon, W., Sliwinki, M., & Kayne, R. D. (1999). The relationship of cognitive, personality, and academic measures to anesthesiology resident clinical performance. *Anesthesia and Analgesia,* 88, 1092–1100.

Robinowitz, C. B. (1983). The impaired physician and organized medicine. In S. C. Scheiber & B. B. Doyle (Eds.), *The impaired physician* (pp. 147–156). New York: Plenum Medical Book Co.

Schueneman, A. L., Pickleman, J., Hesslein, R., & Freeark, R. J. (1984). Neuropsychologic predictors of operative skill among general surgery residents. *Surgery, 96,* 288–295.

Steindler, E. M. (1975). *The impaired physician.* Chicago: American Medical Association.

Strax, T. E., Wainapel, S. F., & Welner, S. (2000). In L. S. Goldman, M. Myers, & L. J. Dickstein (Eds.), *The handbook of physician health: The essential guide to understanding the health care needs of physicians* (pp. 17–38). Chicago: American Medical Association.

Trunkey, D. D., & Botney, R. (2001). Assessing competency: A tale of two professions. *Journal of the American College of Surgeons, 192,* 385–395.

Turnbull, J., Carbotte, R., Hanna, E., Norman, G., Cunnington, J., Ferguson, B., & Kaigas, T. (2000). Cognitive difficulty in physicians. *Academic Medicine, 75,* 177–181.

Van Komen, G. J. (2000). Troubled or troubling physicians: Administrative responses. In L. S. Goldman, M. Myers, & L. J. Dickstein (Eds.), *The handbook of physician health: The essential guide to understanding the health care needs of physicians* (pp. 205–226). American Medical Association.

Webster, T. G. (1983). Problems of drug addiction and alcoholism among physicians. In S. C. Scheiber & B. B. Doyle (Eds.), *The impaired physician* (pp. 27–38). New York: Plenum Medical Book Co.

White, F. P.(1969). Why don't we put senile MDs out of practice? *Medical Economics, 46,* 77–81.

19

CHAPTER

Robert L. Heilbronner
Neil H. Pliskin

Clinical Neuropsychology in the Forensic Arena

> The value of neuropsychological evidence lies in its ability to provide the trier-of-fact with objective data that illuminates the substantive questions that underlie the ultimate issues. (Martell, 1992a)

Introduction

The field of clinical neuropsychology has experienced tremendous growth over the past 60 years, becoming one of the most rapidly expanding divisions in the American Psychological Association. Alongside this growth has been its rapid expansion into the forensic area, which itself is among the fastest growing subdisciplines within clinical neuropsychology (Martell, 1992a; Putnam & DeLuca, 1990, 1991; Sweet, Moberg, & Suchy, 2000). Taylor (1999) documented that neuropsychologists had almost no impact on decisions of the courts prior to 1980, but the situation has changed dramatically since the early 1990s. Clinical neuropsychologists now are called upon routinely to assist the triers of fact (e.g., judges and juries) in understanding the behavioral, emotional, motivational, and cognitive sequelae following insults to the brain as well as to delineate the importance of biopsychosocial variables in modulating brain function and dysfunction (Martell, 1992a; McCaffrey, Williams, Fisher, & Laing, 1997). This chapter focuses on the role, utility, and value of neuropsychological services in the forensic arena. The specific contribution neuropsychologists have in the detection of malingering in forensic settings will be considered separately in Chapter 20.

Forensic neuropsychology, as a subspecialty of clinical neuropsychology, has expanded beyond the domain of the courtroom, and its utility and value must be assessed beyond the world of attorneys and judges. Indeed, neuropsychologists are also used in cases involving worker's compensation, disability determination, educational due process within public school systems, personal injury, criminal, child custody, impaired professional and "fitness for duty," competency, and other cases in which adversarial administrative and judicial determinations are involved. Why are clinical neuropsychologists being called upon more frequently to consult and testify in adversarial proceedings? Sweet (1999) believed this to be a natural outcome of the success of a strong scientist–practitioner orientation. As scientist–practitioners, clinical neuropsychologists are familiar with disciplined scrutiny (i.e., peer review), clinical procedures emphasizing data-based decision making (i.e., accountability), and a hypothesis testing approach (i.e., objective differential diagnosis) to answer questions. Thus, neuropsychologists are especially qualified to operate in the forensic arena. Neuropsychologists also have become prominent figures in the American legal system because state legislatures and courts appreciate the evidence that competent clinical neuropsychologists are able to provide during litigation (Taylor, 1999).

The reader may be interested to find a chapter on forensic neuropsychology in a text largely devoted to cost–outcome research, because what is meant to be proven to health insurance companies is not the same as what has already been proven to attorneys. Indeed, no cost–outcome research or empirical data are being demanded by judges or attorneys, because they are not needed. Neuropsychology as a field, or at least many of its competent constituents, have demonstrated how our expertise is relevant to decisions being made by judges, juries, and other arbiters. The increase in the number of neuropsychologists being asked to provide input in adversarial situations is the very evidence, already proven, that our expertise is valued. Also, the fact that our fees are not customarily discounted, and often are even higher than clinical rates, also is strong testimony that we have already proven our value and worth in the forensic arena.

☐ Professional Issues in Forensic Neuropsychology

The value of what neuropsychologists do is closely related to the quality of their work, which intimately ties into the competency of the person who is writing the neuropsychological report, consulting with the attorney, testifying in court, and so on. The majority of neuropsychologists who work in the forensic arena are historically trained as clinical neuropsychologists. They typically did not choose to develop a forensic practice, or at least they did not decide to do so, until they established their clinical competency and practice. Their forensic experience often began as treating clinical neuropsychologists, when they were asked to testify about patients they had evaluated or treated. After a number of years, they may decide to expand their practice because they enjoy the challenge of forensic work or, more likely, because of the fiscal benefits.

It is important, however, to note that a neuropsychologist who has years of experience consulting and testifying in civil cases involving traumatic brain injury (TBI) may not be well prepared for the rigors and requirements associated with evaluating a criminal defendant. Likewise, a criminal forensic neuropsychologist may not be well skilled in the evaluation of competency to consent to medical treatment in older adults. It is no longer sufficient for neuropsychologists to proclaim that they are proficient in the general practice of forensic neuropsychology, just as it is not good practice (and even potentially unethical: see APA, 1997; Ethics Standard 1.04: Boundaries of Competence) for a neuropsychologist who works almost exclusively with geriatric patients to do an evaluation on a young child. Indeed, there are dramatic theoretical and practical differences between civil and criminal evaluations. There also are critical issues within different types of civil (e.g., competency vs. medical malpractice) and criminal (e.g., competency to stand trial vs. mitigation in capital cases) litigation. Thus, it is critical to obtain appropriate training, supervision, and experience in civil and criminal litigation, and to become familiar with the relevant jurisdictional case law and literature in order to establish competency in the forensic arena.

☐ Practical Issues in Forensic Neuropsychology

One thing that complicates the practice of forensic neuropsychology is a clear understanding of who the client is, or if, in fact, there are responsibilities to multiple parties. APA ethics require psychologists to abide by certain laws and standards when providing psychological services to individuals. This typically includes the maintaining of confidentiality (APA, 1997). When neuropsychologists become involved in doing examinations in the forensic arena, they also have a responsibility to the attorney or judge requesting their professional opinions. It requires considerable clinical skill, knowledge of neuropsychology, and appreciation of the ethics that guide the profession when conducting such examinations and preparing reports.

Unlike traditional clinical neuropsychological evaluations, the results of a forensic evaluation often are not shared with the examinee. In fact, the provision of informed consent at the outset of a forensic evaluation mandates that the examinee be informed of multiple things (e.g., who the referral source is, the limits of confidentiality, that no treatment will be provided), not the least of which is the fact that the neuropsychologist will likely not be the one to provide the results to him or her directly. That is one reason why many neuropsychologists who do extensive forensic work utilize a separate informed consent form designed especially for forensic cases.

How does an attorney or judge evaluate the value and importance of a forensic neuropsychological examination? Ethical guidelines and relevant state mental health laws prohibit them from directly observing the testing process. Consequently, many attorneys do not know what the tests are, how they are scored, what they are measuring, and so on. Moreover, many attorneys do not understand how test scores translate into opinions about brain function and dysfunction, or how a history of multiple head trauma secondary to physical abuse may play a role in a defendant's behavior over a lifetime and in the extant case for which they are being tried. Ultimately, the value of the forensic neuropsychological evaluation is judged by the extent to which the information and opinions assist the attorney in a particular case, whether by gaining a better understanding of complicated neurocognitive issues to aid the attorney in developing or defending a case or through the actual opinions themselves supporting the case.

It is crucial to be vigilant regarding the multiple legal, social, and financial pressures which can influence the objectivity of neuropsychologists' work. Failure to be thorough or objective in the evaluation or presentation of information or testimony could subject the professional to discomforting cross-examination by a well-prepared lawyer. It also might diminish the perceived value of neuropsychological services by the public

TABLE 19.1. Markers of Value of Neuropsychological Assessment for Attorneys in the Forensic Setting

1. There is a viable professional making statements about brain functioning based on normative data.
2. The credibility of a client's testimony can be reinforced by neuropsychological examination findings.
3. Determination of the gravity of reported claims is greatly enhanced by having an objective evaluation conducted by an individual bound by the *Ethical Principles of Psychologists and Code of Conduct* of the American Psychological Association.

(i.e., juries) and legal community (i.e., judges and attorneys) as a whole. Table 19.1 briefly summarizes three major markers of value of neuropsychological assessment for attorneys in the forensic arena.

Like any professional, forensic neuropsychologists need to know the territory in which they work. The world of forensics is very different from the neuropsychology laboratory in a university medical center, hospital, or outpatient clinic, where many neuropsychologists receive their training. It is, by its very nature, adversarial and antagonistic. Moreover, the personalities of the people who work within it often are very different from the people with whom we customarily interact in the clinical setting. The courtroom is a unique environment without equal. Those who consciously choose to become active participants in the forensic arena also must choose to devote the necessary time and effort to understand the rules of the justice system. It means knowing more than the science and practice of clinical neuropsychology—it means knowing how to interact with attorneys and how to behave during a deposition or at trial. This type of learning usually is obtained via direct experience or, at a less experiential level, obtained by reading practical texts devoted toward "mastering" the role of an expert (Brodsky, 1999; Lubet, 1998). Understanding the pertinent civil and criminal statutes, being familiar with relevant jurisdictional case law, and knowing the standards of admissibility (e.g., *Frye v. Daubert*) and *The Federal Rules of Evidence* (especially FRE 401-403 and 702-704) are just a few of the things with which forensic neuropsychologists should be familiar if they are going to provide the triers of fact with well-informed opinions.

Clinical Neuropsychology in Civil Litigation

The most common role for neuropsychologists since they became participants in adversarial legal proceedings has been in civil litigation cases. Neuropsychologists now regularly enter the courts by providing neurocognitive data and inferences regarding brain–behavior relationships in personal injury suits, worker's compensation claims, fitness-for-duty claims, and disability determinations. Most often, neuropsychologists have been retained to assist the triers of fact in the determination of damages following TBI in personal injury litigation. Personal injury litigation extends beyond TBI to include other types of injury as well: for example, toxic torts (e.g., lead poisoning, occupational environmental exposures, electrical injury), and medical malpractice. Regardless of whether the professional initially becomes involved as a health-care provider (i.e., treater) or is retained as an expert witness or consultant on behalf of either the plaintiff or defendant, that person has essentially the same ethical duties and obligations (Heilbronner & Karavidas, 1997). These include conducting a thorough and objective evaluation of the injured person as well as presenting the results of the evaluation in an unbiased and nonargumentative manner. Regardless of whose "side" they are retained by, neuropsychologists rely on their data, clinical interview(s), and record review to arrive at their opinions and conclusions, which must be expressed in terms of a reasonable degree of neuropsychological certainty (probability).

Neuropsychologists also are commonly asked by the court, attorneys, and physicians to perform evaluations designed to address issues related to patient competency in a broad number of situations. One common reason for evaluation relates to matters of competency and guardianship. In such scenarios, the neuropsychologist may be asked to render opinions based on his or her evaluation about the capacity of (for example) an older adult, or a brain-injured, mentally ill, or developmentally disabled adult to manage finances and make independent decisions. Neuropsychologists also are called upon to assess the capacity of individuals to understand and consent to medical treatment. Table 19.2 lists several domains we have found helpful in conducting competency evaluations.

Numerous assessment procedures can be administered to assess these dimensions, and the reader is referred to Lezak (1995) for a comprehensive listing of neuropsychological tests. But, it is important to note that the assessment of different kind of competencies should not depend on any one neuropsychological test, nor should it rely exclusively on the opinion of the neuropsychologist. Multiple cognitive factors–including executive functions, semantic memory, verbal abstraction, attention, and receptive language–have all shown a relationship to functional measures specifically designed to assess competency in older adults (Marson, Cody, Ingram, & Harrell, 1995). Moreover, physicians and family members also provide relevant information that should be used when making a decision about civil competencies.

In civil litigation, the value of neuropsychology is most often judged in monetary terms. That is, how much money the plaintiff will gain through a demonstration of neuropsychological impairment versus how much the insurance company will save by demonstrating that the plaintiff is not as functionally disabled as he or she claims to be.

TABLE 19.2. Domains Commonly Assessed in a Competency Evaluation

1. Level of intelligence
2. New learning and memory capacity
3. Reading comprehension
4. Receptive and expressive language
5. Calculation abilities
6. Abstract reasoning
7. Problem-solving capacity
8. Insight and judgment

However, when issues of guardianship, financial decision-making capacity, competency, and ability to understand medical treatment options are involved, the work of the neuropsychologist has broad implications for quality of life, safety, and independence.

Clinical Neuropsychology in Criminal Litigation

Historically speaking, clinical neuropsychologists practicing in the forensic arena have focused on civil litigation, most often when TBIs are at issue (Heilbronner & Karavidas, 1997; Laing & Fisher, 1997). More recently, however, neuropsychologists have become involved in providing services to the criminal courts (Martell, 1992a; Rehkopf & Fisher, 1997), an area where other mental health professionals (e.g., clinical psychologists, psychiatrists, and social workers) have played a role for many years (Melton, Petrila, Poythress, & Slobogin, 1997). Criminal law is concerned with criminal behavior, acts, or omissions that violate the established norms of society as set forth in its penal laws. The defense attorney who argues that a defendant's brain damage is a mitigating factor to explain his or her criminal actions must establish, by reliable evidence, the link between brain damage and the subsequent alterations in behavior that led to the alleged criminal behavior. The legal "burden of proof" (e.g., preponderence of evidence or beyond a reasonable doubt) and which side has this burden depend on the substantive law of the jurisdiction (Rehkopf & Fisher, 1997).

Martell (1992a) noted that the traditional function of clinical psychology in criminal settings has been to address issues of major mental illness and the impact of such illness on a defendant's behavior relative to requirements of the law. Consequently, the focus has largely been on psychosis or psychiatric disturbance, and not so much on the potential sequelae from brain dysfunction. Given the high rate of brain injuries, seizure disorders, and other central nervous system disorders (e.g., ADHD and LD) among criminal defendants (Blake, Pincus, & Buckner, 1995; Martell, 1992b), it is understandable that there would be a need for neuropsychological expertise in criminal proceedings. Yet, often neuropsychologists are not brought into cases, either because the brain damage is not obvious or because the personnel working on the case (e.g., mitigation specialists and paralegals) do not know what a neuropsychological evaluation is and the value it can offer in these kinds of cases. In fact, when speaking to criminal defense attorneys, public defenders, or prosecuting attorneys, neuropsychologists must spend considerable time explaining how the activities of a neuropsychologist are different from those of a clinical or forensic psychologist. On more than one occasion, attorneys have expected statements about whether or not someone is "insane," or that the Rorschach would have been used during the course of a forensic neuropsychological examination.

As a rule, we recommend that attorneys consider bringing in a clinical psychologist or psychiatrist when the results of the neuropsychological examination suggest the presence of psychosis or a major psychiatric disturbance. Keeping the neuropsychological evaluation directed exclusively toward neuropsychological activities will help to ensure that one is practicing within the boundaries of one's competence. It also will help to minimize the stress and discomfort that can come from effective cross-examination about a subject or issue that the neuropsychologist has not addressed or an area that the expert may not be comfortable opining about. On the other hand, some neuropsychologists are experienced in traditional psychodiagnostics, and they are able to render opinions about the defendant's personality make up, reality testing, or mental state at the time of the offense. These are the persons who usually are the most experienced working in a criminal forensic setting, and they are very familiar with the requisite definitions of terms (competency, diminished capacity, etc.) and the associated laws and statutes of the state or province in which they work.

According to Martell (1992a), the particular appeal of neuropsychological evidence in the criminal context is the expert's ability to bring quantified, normative data on brain–behavior relationships to bear in support of what have traditionally been professional opinions based on mental status exams and clinical interviews. The ability to provide the triers of fact with a normative description of a defendant's neurobehavioral strengths and weaknesses can bring important new information to the criminal decision-making process. Moreover, the capability to relate a known (or suspected) brain lesion to the capacities of the defendant relevant to several legal standards of behavior sets clinical neuropsychology apart from medical/neurological testimony, and ultimately makes it of direct relevance to the issues facing the triers of fact. Consequently, forensic neuropsychology has gained increasing prominence in the criminal arena largely for the purposes of determining the competency of defendants to stand trial and in determining criminal responsibility. Each of these requires an assessment of a defendant's mental state, with specific attention toward orientation and memory and a capacity to "understand" the charges, court principals, nature of the courtroom, and potential pleas and outcomes (Larrabee, 2000).

Neuropsychologists also are involved in other criminal areas. According to Rehkopf and Fisher (1997), there are seven critical junctures in a criminal proceeding at which the defense should be concerned about the mental health and competence of the accused. These include:

1. competence or fitness to proceed with the criminal trial,
2. the advisement of any legal "rights" to the accused and the validity of any statements and confessions (e.g., Miranda warning),
3. the entry of a plea,
4. determination of criminal responsibility,
5. the advisability of having the defendant testify,
6. sentencing or disposition, and
7. imposition of the death penalty and subsequent competence for execution.

Denny and Wynkoop (2000) described a model that helps neuropsychologists identify the mental (cognitive) status of the defendant at three critical periods: (a) before the offense, (b) at the time of the offense, and (c) at the present time (during incarceration while awaiting trial). The goal is to examine the continuity or discontinuity in mental status across time via consistencies or inconsistencies between time and data sources (e.g., subjective and objective). Consistency between past mental status and present mental status helps establish a context in which to place potential neuropsychological functioning at a particular point in time, such as time of the offense. This model is a useful approach for those who are comfortable addressing issues of mental state at the time of the offense, competency to stand trial, future danger, and so on. Our experience is that defense attorneys most often consult with neuropsychologists after another professional has already addressed these issues. Or, they would like to use neuropsychological evidence as a part of the overall psychological work-up of the defendant when issues of brain dysfunction have significance. In mitigation, the neuropsychological evidence usually is reserved for the sentencing phase of the trial, after a defendant has already been found guilty and the judge or jury is asked to consider the role of brain dysfunction and other mitigating factors when deciding on an appropriate sentence for the crime. As noted earlier, the value of neuropsychology is most often judged in monetary terms. In criminal proceedings, wherein deprivation of liberty is an issue, the consequences are more severe. Indeed, the value of what clinical neuropsychology can do is judged in terms of human life, years of imprisonment, emotional suffering of the victim's and the defendant's families, and so on. Following are examples of the value forensic neuropsychological activities can bring to different aspects of a criminal case.

Competency to Stand Trial

The behavioral standards underlying the findings of competency to stand trial arise primarily from the legal language of two cases: *Dusky v. United States* (1960) and *Weiter v. Settle* (1961). Both of these cases set forth legal standards that require a defendant to be oriented to the world around him or her (i.e., have the "mental capacity to appreciate his presence in relation to time, place, and things") and have "memory sufficient to relate (the facts surrounding him [or her] at the time of the offense at the time and place where the law violation is alleged to have been committed) in his [or her] own personal manner" (Weiter, 1961). Per Dusky, competence to stand trial requires a two-pronged test (Melton et al., 1997): a cognitive prong and a cooperation prong. The cognitive prong (Does the defendant, as a result of mental disease or defect, lack the capacity to understand the proceedings against him or her?) concerns orientation and memory, a capacity to understand the charges, court principals, adversarial nature of the courtroom, and potential pleas and outcomes. These requirements are very similar to the mental functions assessed in a standard neuropsychological evaluation (Martell, 1992a). The cooperation prong (Does the defendant lack the capacity to consult with his or her attorney and meaningfully assist in his or her own defense?) requires an evaluation of the defendant's capacity to communicate and actively participate in the litigation process. This involves both speaking and listening. As an example, a defendant with severe attention deficit hyperactivity disorder (ADHD) may be able to speak to and understand his attorney, but be unable to pay attention to lengthy courtroom testimony. The argument could be made that this defendant is unable to assist meaningfully in his or her own defense (Rehkopf & Fisher, 1997).

The literature on the psychological evaluation of competency to stand trial has not addressed neuropsychological assessment in any depth. Indeed, competency is most often assessed via other psychological tests and inventories designed specifically for this purpose (see Grisso, 1986; Melton et al., 1997). But, none of the available instruments includes measures of cognitive ability beyond legal knowledge and decision-making capacity. Thus, determinations of competency to stand trial likely would benefit from neuropsychological assessment, particularly in cases in which the reason for a defendant's apparent incompetency is unclear. A referral for a neuropsychological evaluation could be indicated when a gross mental status exam suggests memory impairment, attention deficits, mental retardation, some other organic basis for incompetency, or malingering. Martell (1992a) maintained that the role of forensic neuropsychology is likely to become even more important *after* a finding of incompetency. In such cases, neuropsychologists can perform serial testing to document any changes in neurobehavioral status over time and to actively evaluate an incompetent defendant's potential for restoration to competency.

Insanity, Diminished Capacity, and Diminished Responsibility

According to Martell (1992a), the forensic neuropsychological issues in this area are less clear than those of competency to stand trial. Nonetheless, there may be an increasingly viable role for neuropsychology in this area. Brain dysfunction is now being viewed as a potential risk factor for violent behavior in combination with other personal, environmental, and situational risk factors (Martell, 1992b). Whereas neuroimaging techniques can provide evidence of the presence, type, location, and size of brain lesions, a neuropsychological evaluation can provide the trier of fact with important information about the behavioral sequelae of a given lesion.

Two standards have been applied to regulate insanity determinations in the United States: the McNaughten standard and the American Law Institute (ALI) standard. Briefly, the McNaughten standard essentially establishes a largely cognitive test for insanity, being concerned primarily with the extent to which the defendant did nor did not *know* what he or she was doing. The ALI standard includes cognitive, affective/emotional, and volitional factors in that the defendant must lack substantial capacity either to appreciate the wrongfulness of his or her conduct or to conform his or her conduct to the requirements of the law. The reader is referred to the relevant literature for a more in-depth discussion of the psychological issues raised by these standards (e.g., Melton et al., 1997; Monahan & Walker, 1990).

According to Martell (1992a), the term "appreciate" implies higher-order cognitive abilities that might range from simple awareness or recognition to a fairly sophisticated ability to note distinctions or to be conscious of the significance, desirability, or impact of behavior. No doubt, this is an area in which forensic neuropsychology can offer valuable information. A number of brain disorders, especially those involving bilateral frontal lobe damage, can effectively impair a person's capacity to accurately perceive or reflect on his or her behavior. The forensic neuropsychologist possesses the skills and abilities to quantify and characterize the nature and degree of impairment exhibited by a defendant, and to aid the fact-finder in determining whether such impairment constitutes a "substantial" lack of capacity. As an example, the neuropsychologist could present data documenting the fact that a defendant falls three standard deviations below the population mean on tests measuring social judgment and certain executive functions (e.g., planning and organization). The trier of fact could then rely on that evidence in determining whether that degree of impairment in those important aspects of behavior constitutes a substantial lack of capacity.

Conceptually distinct from insanity determinations is the evaluation of diminished capacities, which refers to a decreased level of culpability as a result of lesser intent (Clark, 1987). In essence, a diminished capacity defense attempts to reduce the severity of the charge by challenging the mental element of the prosecution's prima facie case (Monahan & Walker, 1990). This is important, because distinctions between murder, manslaughter, and nonnegligent homicide often hinge on whether the prosecution can demonstrate that the crime was committed intentionally, knowingly, recklessly, or negligently (Martell, 1992a). Without invoking the insanity defense (which admits the criminal act, but asserts no criminal intent), defendants can bring into play their mental state by claiming less than the criminal intent required by the charge as a result of factors such as alcohol or drug intoxication, medication use, and neurological conditions (Melton et al., 1997). Most often, forensic neuropsychological evidence is used to establish the cognitive abilities or disabilities of the defendant relevant to the legal definitions of the state of mind required to constitute the defense (Martell, 1992a). For example, a defendant with Alzheimer's disease may lack the ability to organize and plan his or her behavior adequately to form the legal intent required to commit murder, and hence may only be found guilty of a lesser charge.

Often confused with diminished capacity is diminished responsibility. This refers to mitigating circumstances of the crime that warrant a lesser punishment, and it usually is brought before the court during sentencing (Denny & Wynkoop, 2000). Diminished responsibility is common in jurisdictions that no longer have the volitional prong in their insanity standard. It is commonly used in cases of defendants with frontal lobe damage who have impulse control problems that affect their ability to refrain from performing certain criminal acts, or who are unable to appreciate the consequences of the act to any significant degree. In fact, neuropsychological evaluations have proven to be especially useful in this regard, as they can help explain to the trier of fact how the defendant's deficits in cognitive, emotional, and behavioral controls secondary to brain injury are relevant to understanding why the person may have acted in the way he or she did during the criminal act.

Other Competencies in the Criminal Process

Neuropsychological evidence has become increasingly important in a range of other criminal competency issues, including predictions of dangerousness; waiver of *Miranda* rights; and competency to confess, to make a plea, to be sentenced, and to be executed (cf., Heilbrun & McClaren, 1988; Melton et al., 1997). This is especially relevant given the apparent prevalence of brain damage attributed to death-row inmates (Lewis et al., 1988) and the relevance of mental retardation in declaring a defendant incompetent to be executed. Simply stated, being brain damaged (or mentally retarded) in and of itself is not sufficient to declare a defendant incompetent to be executed. Indeed, the neuropsychological evidence must show the degree of brain dysfunction (or mental retardation), and it must help to explain the nature, extent, and course of the brain dysfunction and its consequences in terms of the behavior of the defendant relative to the psycholegal issue at hand.

☐ Conclusions and Future Directions

Current research suggests that standardized neuropsychological test results meet the *Frye Test* (*Frye v. U.S.*, 1923) of "general acceptance," as exemplified by the fact that they are established and recognized in the field of neuropsychology. But, rules governing the admissibility of expert evidence vary by jurisdiction and often by the judge who must determine the admissibility of evidence in a given case. Also, recent court rulings have raised the bar on the admissibility of expert evidence and testimony, requiring not only that they meet the general acceptance standard but that they are scientifically valid (*Daubert v. Merrell Dow*, 1993). Although neuropsychological tests have to undergo and satisfy certain rules of reliability and validity, their validity as it relates to the forensic arena remains to be demonstrated in the real world. Further research is necessary to address the relationship between violence and brain function or dysfunction, between violence and neuropsychological test results, and to establish base rates of brain damage in forensic populations. This may help to ensure the value that clinical neuropsychology can bring to the forensic arena.

References

American Psychological Association. (1997). *Ethical principles of psychologists and code of conduct.* Washington, DC: Author.

Blake, P. Y., Pincus, J. H., & Buckner, C. (1995). Neurologic abnormalities in murderers. *Neurology, 45*, 1641–1647.

Brodsky, S. L. (1999). *Expert, expert witness: More maxims and guidelines for testifying in court.* Washington, DC: American Psychological Association.

Clark, C. R. (1987). Specific intent and diminished capacity. In I. B. Weiner & A. K. Hess (Eds.), *Handbook of forensic psychology*. New York: Wiley & Sons.

Daubert v. Merrell Dow Pharmaceuticals, Inc. (1993). 113 S. Ct. 2786.

Denny, R. L., & Wynkoop, T. F. (2000). Clinical neuropsychology in the criminal forensic setting. *Journal of Head Trauma Rehabilitation, 15*(2), 804–828.

Dusky v. United States. (1960). 362 U.S. 402, 80 S. Ct. 788, 4 L.Ed.2d, 824.

Frye v. United States. (1923). 293 Fed 1013 (D.C. Cir. 1923).

Grisso, T. (1986). *Evaluating competencies*. New York: Plenum Press.

Heilbronner, R. L., & Karavidas, T. (1997). Presenting neuropsychological evidence in traumatic brain injury litigation. *The Clinical Neuropsychologist, 11*(4), 445–453.

Heilbrun, K. S., & McClaren, H. A. (1988). Assessment of competency for execution? A guide for mental health professionals. *Bulletin of the American Academy of Psychiatry and Law, 16*, 892–900.

Laing, L. C., & Fisher, J. M. (1997). Neuropsychology in civil proceedings. In R. J. McCaffrey, A. D. Williams, J. M. Fisher, & L. C. Laing (Eds.), *The practice of forensic neuropsychology* (pp. 117–133). New York: Plenum Press.

Larrabee, G. J. (2000). Forensic neuropsychological assessment. In R. Vanderploeg (Ed.), *Clinician's guide to neuropsychological assessment* (2nd ed., pp. 301–335). Mahwah, NJ: Lawrence Erlbaum.

Lewis, D. O., Pincus, J. H., Bard, B., Richardson, E., Prichep, L. S., Feldman, M., & Yeager, C. (1988). Neuropsychiatric, psychoeducational, and family characteristics of 14 juveniles condemned to death in the United States. *American Journal of Psychiatry, 145*, 584–589.

Lezak, M. (1995). *Neuropsychological assessment*. New York. Oxford University Press.

Lubet, S. (1998). *Expert testimony: A guide for expert witnesses and the lawyers who examine them.* Boston: National Institute for Trial Advocacy..

Marson, D. C., Cody, H. A., Ingram, K. K., & Harrell, L. E. (1995). Neuropsychologic predictors of competency in Alzheimer's disease using a rational legal standard. *Archives of Neurology, 52*, 955–959.

Martell, D. A. (1992a). Forensic neuropsychology and the criminal law. *Law and Human Behavior, 16*, 313–336.

Martell, D. A. (1992b). Estimating the prevalence of organic brain dysfunction in maximum-security forensic patients. *Journal of Forensic Sciences*, 37(3), 878–893.

McCaffrey, R. J., Williams, A. D., Fisher, J. M., & Laing, L. C. (1997). *The practice of forensic neuropsychology*. New York: Plenum Press.

Melton, G. B., Petrila, J., Poythress, N. G., & Slobogin, C. (1997). *Psychological evaluations for the courts: A handbook for mental health professionals and lawyers* (2nd ed.). New York: Guilford Press.

Monahan, J., & Walker, L. (1990). *Social science in law: Cases and materials* (2nd ed.). New York: The Foundation Press.

Putnam, S. H., & DeLuca, J. W. (1991). The TCN professional practice survey: Part 2: An analysis of the fess of neuropsychologists by practice demographics. *The Clinical Neuropsychologist, 5,* 103–124.

Putnam, S. H., & DeLuca, J. W. (1990). The TCN professional practice survey, Part 1: General practices of neuropsychologists in primary employment and private practice settings. *The Clinical Neuropsychologist, 4,* 199–243.

Rehkopf, D. G., & Fisher, J. M. (1997). Neuropsychology in criminal proceedings. In R. J. McCaffrey, A. D. Williams, J. M. Fisher, & L. C. Laing (Eds.), *The practice of forensic neuropsychology* (pp. 135–151). New York: Plenum Press.

Sweet, J. J. (1999). *Forensic neuropsychology.* Lisse, The Netherlands: Swets & Zeitlinger.

Sweet, J. J., Moberg, P. J., & Suchy, Y. (2000). Ten-year follow-up survey of clinical neuropsychologists. *The Clinical Neuropsychologist, 4*(4), 479–495.

Taylor, J. S. (1999). The legal environment pertaining to clinical neuropsychology. In J. J. Sweet (Ed.). *Forensic neuropsychology.* Lisse, The Netherlands: Swets & Zeitlinger.

Weiter v. Settle. (1961). 193 F. Supp. 318 (W.D. Mo.).

20

CHAPTER

William D. Gouvier
Paul R. Lees-Haley
Jill Hayes Hammer

The Neuropsychological Examination in the Detection of Malingering in the Forensic Arena: Costs and Benefits

Introduction

As discussed in the preceding chapter, there are numerous roles neuropsychologists play in the medical–legal arena, and in many of these roles an argument for the cost-effectiveness of neuropsychological services can be made. This chapter will focus on the importance and cost-effectiveness of neuropsychological services specifically in the domain of malingering detection.

Malingering defined is the "intentional production of false or grossly exaggerated physical or psychological symptoms, motivated by external incentives" (APA, 1994). Although the term malingering carries generally negative connotations, we recognize that in certain contexts, such as a prisoner of war feigning illness, malingering behavior can be prosocially adaptive (APA, 1994; Rogers, 1997). Malingering behavior can be categorized by its intent (Price, 1995), differentiating between "simulators" who intentionally fabricate symptoms of illness against a background of normalcy, and "dissimulators," who attempt to portray a picture of normalcy despite a background of illness or deviancy. This chapter will deal exclusively with the simulating type, patients who present most frequently in the context of personal injury litigation.

Malingering behavior also can be classified according to the type(s) of illness or disorder that is simulated. Individuals can feign psychiatric difficulties (Beaber, Marston, Michelli, & Mills, 1985; Rogers, 1997); neurological problems, often including memory and cognitive sequelae typical of closed head injury (Reynolds, 1998; Sweet, 1999); or somatic problems such as chronic back pain or other physical disorders (Larrabee, 1998).

A variety of strategies for identifying these different types of malingering have been extensively reviewed elsewhere (e.g., Hayes, Hilsabeck, & Gouvier, 1999; Reynolds, 1998; Sweet, 1999).

Malingering is not always a simple yes or no distinction. Malingering behavior can range from poor effort during an examination to outright lying and fabrication of symptoms to feign illness or injury.

There is little knowledge of the actual prevalence of malingering, or even how it is to be most appropriately defined. The most conservative might reserve this term solely for persons who fabricate bogus disabilities, whereas others might gladly apply to people with bona fide disabilities who embellish their complaints to ensure the evaluator notices. A key problem is the difficulty in gathering a group of unequivocal malingerers for study; most individuals would be understandably reluctant to self-select themselves into the malingering group, and any who did would arguably be different from most other members of the population. Thus, we are forced to rely on estimates—estimates based analogue research and differential prevalence designs.

Malingering detection strategies vary in their sensitivity, and there has been a trend for increasingly sensitive measures to be introduced as the technology for malingering detection improves (Gervais, Green, & Allen, 1999). Thus, older research using less-sensitive measures such as the Memory for 15 Items or one of the various digit recognition procedures would be likely to generate lower base rate estimates than research using newly introduced measures with higher sensitivity. The estimates for malingering base rates also will vary with the nature of the referral population. One can easily envision a hierarchical taxonomy of situations in which malingering becomes progressively more likely; this is the core assumption of the differential prevalence research designs for studying malingering.

Many patients undergoing evaluation have some incentive to feign or exaggerate their dysfunctions in order to obtain desired ends. Vocational rehabilitation referrals hope to receive services for job training and placement, Social Security applicants hope to obtain financial assistance, workers compensation referrals have financial compensation at issue as well. Most experts would agree that the highest stakes, however, are in the domain of personal injury litigation. Within this domain, estimates range from less than 5% to over 60% of personal injury patients referred for neuropsychological evaluation (Hayes, Hilsabeck, & Gouvier, 1999), but a general trend is noted for the estimates to hover around or above 30% as a reasonable base rate among an outpatient population referred for evaluation in the context of compensation seeking (Allen, Conder, Green, & Cox, 1997; Binder, 1997; Binder, Rohling, & Larrabee, 1997; Gervais, Allen, Green, & Cunningham, 1998; Gervais et al., 1999; Greiffenstein, Baker, & Gola, 1994; Larrabee, 2000; Millis, 1992; Trueblood & Schmidt, 1993).

Regardless of the actual base rate, one fact remains true: The likelihood of false positive misclassification increases as the base rate for malingering goes down. This is a particular source of concern, given that the most commonly used tests of neuropsychological malingering fall short of objective criteria for test effectiveness when the estimated base rate of malingering is 15% or lower (Hayes et al., 1999), and many fall short of the effectiveness criterion even when the estimated base rate for malingering is above 30%. Readers are referred elsewhere (Gouvier, 1999; Gouvier Hayes, & Smiroldo, et al., 1998) for a more detailed discussion of the interrelationships among test sensitivity, test specificity, and population base rates in determining diagnostic accuracy. With the likelihood of misclassification great, the costs of misclassification so high, and the opportunities for successful redress diminished, neuropsychologists need to tread these grounds very carefully.

But tread these grounds we must; despite our limitations and shortcomings, no other professional groups have a technology for malingering detection as well developed as ours. This is important, because the potential societal costs of malingering are huge. In addition to tying up the medical service system and the judicial system with frivolous cases, malingering has a direct monetary cost to society in terms of dollars spent for needless medical care, dollar awards negotiated as part of litigated settlements, and dollar awards granted by judges or juries as part of courtroom litigation. Generally, the stakes climb as we ascend through these cost wasters; however, the number of cases simply receiving medical care is far greater than those involved in settlement negotiation, and settlement cases far outnumber those cases that proceed on to actual courtroom litigation. Therefore, clear reasons exist to focus on malingering detection, regardless of where on the treatment/litigation spectrum the patient lies. Successful detection might catch numerous low-expense cases at the medical care level, and numerically fewer but pricier cases when litigation is involved. It is recognized that malingering detection in the context of routine medical care may offer real and potentially large cost savings, but we will further restrict the focus of this chapter primarily to those persons seen in the forensic context of civil litigation. In such a context, malingered symptoms might appear in any of the three domains; somatic, neurologic, or psychologic, either singly or in combination.

☐ Estimated Costs to Society of Malingering in Civil Litigation

As an example of the costs involved, consider the following statistics extracted from *Eason's Louisiana Quantum Study and Personal Injury Law* (Eason & Eason, 2000). This volume presents an 11-year compilation offering a complete statewide summary of judge and jury awards in personal injury cases by injury type. Of the 54 brain-injury cases reviewed, the awards ranged from $15,000 to $20 million with a mean award value over $1.3 million. Average payouts to brain-injury plaintiffs over the reporting period were approximately $6.5 million per year.

Lawsuits involving physical injuries proved less lucrative for the plaintiffs, but they were vastly more numerous. Drawing again from Eason and Eason—and restricting the physical injury sample to lawsuits involving injuries to the back, neck, and spine—over 10 times as many lawsuits were reviewed (n = 581). Awards ranged from nothing to $875,000, with a mean award value of $97,442. Although the dollar amounts of these awards averaged less than one-tenth of those for brain-injury cases, the tenfold numerical increase in cases brings the costs of back and neck cases only slightly below the costs associated with brain-injury cases. Annually, Louisiana judges and juries awarded $5.15 million in awards for back, neck, and spine injuries over the reporting period. Slightly less costly to society, but no less lucrative for individual plaintiffs and their attorneys, are the cases presenting with purely psychological damages of the sort that might result from a traumatic accident (n = 53). With awards ranging from nothing to $1.5 million, and a mean award value of $103,924, Louisiana judges and juries awarded plaintiffs nearly $16 million dollars over the reporting period, representing a $1.46 million average yearly payout to successful plaintiffs. Taken together, trial awards for brain injuries; back, neck, and spine injuries; and psychological damages resulting from traumatic personal injury lawsuits totaled approximately $13 million per year. Using the 30% base rate estimate, nearly $4 million per year is paid out by judges and juries to malingerers and their lawyers in Louisiana.

The actual costs are far greater than this, however, as the majority of such cases reach settlement before going to trial. Unfortunately, no similar comprehensive compilation of settlement awards was available to provide precise dollar estimates of the cost of awards in litigation proceedings that settle before trial. The U.S. Department of Justice, Bureau of Justice Statistics (2000), has reported that, for every 33 civil lawsuits filed, only 1 ever goes to trial. For purposes of estimating costs, let us accept the 33-to-1 ratio of suits filed to suits tried, and assume that the average settlement dollar award is 50% of mean trial award. By this figuring, the overall expenses for negotiated awards associated with settlement litigation are over 16 times higher than the award costs among cases that go to trial. In Louisiana, estimated negotiated settlements for brain; back, neck, and spine; and psychological accidental damages are $204 million per year, of which an estimated $61 million would go to malingerers and their attorneys distributed across an average of 72 cases per year.

In addition to trial awards and settlements paid, other costs are involved as well. Bogus patients can wrack up sizeable medical bills, and substantial legal expenses are involved in defending personal injury cases as well. The National Insurance Crime Bureau (2000b) has estimated that billions of dollars are spent annually in medical payments for false claims, and that fraudulent claims for workers' compensation are the number one growth area of insurance fraud. Interview data collected with Ms. Jackie Egan–the managing claims attorney with Louisiana Workers Compensation Corporation (LWCC), the largest worker's compensation carrier in Louisiana–can be used to generate estimates of some of these additional costs (personal communication, December 19, 2000). LWCC received approximately 9,500 claims in 2000, of which, historically, 22% go to litigation, and about 125 to 150 per year go to trial. They open about 1,500 legal files a year and, at the end of 2000, approximately one-third of all open files were subrogation cases and approximately 60% were defense files. LWCC supports an in-house legal staff of 19 attorneys and support staff, with an annual legal office budget of $3 million to pay the salaries and rent. Assuming that costs for subrogation and defense cases are comparable, 60% of the budget is spent on defense activities, and fully $1.8 million of the office budget is used for defending claims in litigation. An additional $1.5 million is budgeted annually for other expenses associated with the cases that are in litigation, such as IMEs (independent medical examinations), travel, and depositions. This totals $3.3 million for handling the approximately 1,100 litigation files opened annually, or about $3,000 per file, and includes all litigation cases combined, regardless of whether they proceed to trial. Using the 30% estimate for malingering, LWCC alone spends $990,000 in additional expenses annually in dealing with malingers and their fraudulent or abusive claims. We can apply these numbers to generate estimates of the legal costs of defending malingering claims, and the estimates generated will be conservative ones, based on the greater cost-efficiency of LWCC's in-house legal staff (J. Egan, personal communication, December 19, 2000), as opposed to contracting the defense work to outside law firms.

Applying these defense cost-estimates to the Eason and Eason (2000) data previously described, cost-estimates can be generated as follows: Given an annual average of 72 personal injury cases described by Eason and Eason (2000), plus an additional

2,376 (72 × 33) cases that settle before trial, and an average defense cost of $3,000 per case, total trial defense costs in Louisiana are conservatively estimated at $7.35 million, of which $2.2 million is spent annually defending against the bogus claims of malingerers.

To estimate the medical costs associated with treating malingerers, one can go backward from the NICB (2000) statistics that "billions" of dollars are spent yearly on false medical claims. Conservatively taking that to be $2 billion exactly, and dividing by 50, Louisiana's share of payouts in false medical claims is $40 million.

Overall costs in Louisiana for personal injury awards by settlements plus trial verdicts are on the order of $218 million per year, of which $65 million likely is awarded to persons who malinger for personal gain. Add to that the $40 million paid for unnecessary medical treatment, and the $2.2 million spent defending against malingerers' claims, and the total costs of malingering in Louisiana run about $107.2 million a year. Obviously, huge cost savings can be gained by reducing or eliminating settlement and award payouts to malingerers and their attorneys. To realize these potential savings, without making a high number of false positive misclassifications, we need to be able to detect malingerers with a high degree of sensitivity and specificity.

☐ Strategic Considerations in Malingering Detection

To stem this floodtide of unwarranted payments to malingerers and their attorneys, a decision-making system or judgment algorithm considering factors such as the relative risk or likelihood of malingering, the time available for malingering assessment, the sensitivity and specificity of the test instruments used to detect malingering, and the vulnerability of the instruments to coached evasion of detection is needed. For example, let us examine the relative risk of malingering within the referral population. With all other factors equal, among nonforensic patients receiving health-care services, a relatively low likelihood value might be assigned to referral from the G.I. floor to evaluate the role of stress in chronic ulcer disease, whereas a relatively higher value would be assigned to a referral from the pulmonary floor to evaluate complaints of brain dysfunction stemming from an occupational exposure incident. Whereas the former would be an indication for brief screening only (unless certain other pathognomonic markers were noted), individuals with higher likelihood values (e.g., coming from a higher base rate population) should be assessed via a more in-depth evaluation. As the patient proceeds closer and closer to litigation and trial, the indications for a more comprehensive assessment of malingering increase.

Tables 20.1 and 20.2 present data on several common neuropsychological tests used for malingering detection (Table 20.1) and specific malingering detection tests (Table 20.2). These tables present reported cut-off scores, sensitivity, specificity, false positive error rates, false negative error rates, validity, effectiveness, validity/effectiveness range, time to administer, and rated vulnerability to coaching for these measures. Each of these variables should be considered in the clinician's algorithm for test selection.

- *Sensitivity* refers to the proportion of diagnostic calls that correctly identify true malingerers.
- *Specificity* refers to the proportion of diagnostic calls that correctly identify nonmalingerers.

TABLE 20.1 Characteristics of Neuropsychological Measures in the Detection of Malingering

Authors	Population	Measures	Cut-Off Scores	Sensitivity	Specificity	False Positive Error Rate	False Negative Error Rate	Valid?	Effective at 30% base rate?	Validity Effective Range?	Admin Time	Vulnerability to Coaching
Coleman et al. (1998)	Undergraduate naïve & coached malingerers & controls (n = 90)	CVLT-RD									23.57	Mod-Diff
Iverson & Franzen (1998)	Consecutive patients undergoing neuropsch eval (n = 20 with memory impairment and 20 without memory impairment) and undergraduate simulators (n = 20)	RMT-W RMT-F	<39 <27	95% 65%	100% 100%	0% 0%	5% 35%	Yes Yes	Yes No	6-94 36-64		Unknown Unknown
Prigatano et al. (1997)	Neuropsycholgoical patients (n = 21; 15 not suspected of malingering, 6 suspected of malingering); cognitively impaired patients (n = 25)	DMT & BNI Screen	BNI Screen Total 30 and DMT Total 95%	97%	95%	5%	3%	Yes	Yes	9-91		Unknown
Tenhula & Sweet (1996)	Normal controls (n = 3), simulators (n = 33), TBI pts with neurological sequelae (n = 29)	CT-Total errs	Ask authors	51.1	97.2	2.8	48.9	Yes	No	None	26.43	Mod-Diff
		CT-Errs I & II	Ask authors	75.6	98.1	1.9	24.4	Yes	Yes	27.3–72.7	26.43	Mod
		CT-Errs VII	Ask authors	66.7	91.7	8.3	33.3	Yes	No	42.6–57.4	26.43	Mod
		Bolter	Ask authors	51.1	98.1	1.9	49.9	Yes	No	None	26.43	Mod

		Easy Missed	Ask authors	55.6	98.1	1.9	44.4	Yes	No	47.3–52.7	26.43	Mod
		Difficult Missed	Ask authors	24.4	80.6	19.4	75.6	Yes	No	None	26.43	Mod
Trueblood (1994)	Consecutive out-patients with potential secondary gain, n = 22 probable malingerers, n = 22 matched controls	DS-ACSS	< 7	77%	86%	14%	23%	Yes	No	38–62	6.25	Moderate
		Voc-ACSS	< 7	36%	95%	5%	64%	Yes	No	None	10.0	Moderate
		PC-ACSS	< 7	41%	95%	5%	59%	Yes	No	None	7.25	Easy
		Dsy-ACSS	< 5	27%	100%	0%	73%	Yes	No	None	4.00	Moderate
		Barona-IQ	> 18	45%	100%	0%	55%	Yes	No	None	N/A	Unknown
		Wais-R Indic	> 1	64%	95%	5%	36%	Yes	No	42–58	N/A	Unknown
		CVLT-TWR	< 48	80%	95%	5%	20%	Yes	Yes	26–74	23.57	Mod-Diff
		CVLT-RM	<13	75%	91%	9%	25%	Yes	No	35–65	23.57	Mod-Diff
		CVLT Indic	> 0	90%	91%	9%	10%	Yes	Yes	20–80	23.57	Mod-Diff
Trueblood & Schmidt (1993)	Consecutive out-patients with potential secondary gain, n = 16, probable malingerers, n = 16 matched controls	SPSS Errors	> 17	63%	94%	6%	37%	Yes	No	44-56	15.00	Mod-Diff
		GNDS	> 44	63%	100%	0%	37%	Yes	No	38-62	90.00	Difficult
		DS-ACSS	< 7	69%	94%	6%	31%	Yes	No	38–62	6.25	Moderate
		FTNB Ttl errs	> 5	63%	94%	6%	37%	Yes	No	44–56	6.71	Moderate
		FA Ttl errs	> 3	63%	94%	6%	37%	Yes	No	44–56	6.00	Difficult
		SRT errors	> 8	56%	100%	0%	44%	Yes	No	45–55	11.67	Difficult
		CVLT-RM	< 13	56%	100%	0%	44%	Yes	No	45–55	23.57	Mod-Diff
		Total indicators	> 2	81%	100%	0%	19%	Yes	Yes	20-80	N/A	Unknown

Note. Validity and effectiveness was calculated given a .15 base rate for malingering. CVLT-RD = California Verbal Learning Test Recognition Discriminability; RMT-W=Recognition Memory Test – Words; RMT-F = Recognition Memory Test – Faces; DMT = Digit Memory Test; BNI = BNI Screen for Higher Cerebral Functions; CT-Total Errs = Booklet Category Test Total Number of Errors; CT-Errs I & II = Booklet Category Test Number of Errors on Subtests I and II; CT- Errs VII = Booklet Category Test Number of Errors on Subtest VII; Bolter = Booklet Category Test Number of Bolter et al. items missed; Easy Missed = Booklet Category Test Number of "Easy" Items Missed; Difficult Missed = Booklet Category Test Number of "Difficult" Items Missed; SSP Errors = Speech Sounds Perception Test Errors; GNDS = General Neuropsychological Deficits Scale; DS-ACSS = Digit Span Age-Corrected Scaled Score; FTNB Ttl errs = Finger Tip Number Writing Total Errors; FA Ttl errs = Finger Agnosia Total errors; SRT errors = Seashore Rhythm Test Errors; CVLT-RM = California Verbal Learning Test Recognition Memory; Total Indicators = number of tests in the simulation range; Voc-ACSS = Vocabulary Age-Corrected Scaled Score; PC-ACSS = Picture Completion Age-Corrected Scaled Score; Dsy = Digit Symbol Age-Corrected Scaled Score; Barona-IQ = Barona Index minus obtained WAIS-R IQ; WAIS-R Indic. = number of WAIS-R subtests in the simulation range; CVLT-TWR = California Verbal learning Test Total Words Recalled; CVLT Indic = number of California Verbal learning Test indicators in the simulation range.

TABLE 20.2. Characteristics of Measures Specifically Designed to Detect Malingering

Authors	Population	Measures	Cut-Off Scores	Sensitivity	Specificity	False Positive Error Rate	False Negative Error Rate	Valid?	Effective at 30% base rate?	Validity Effective Range?	Admin Time	Vulnerability to Coaching
Allen, Green, & Rohling (2001)	Patients with poor effort as measured effort as measured by performing worse than chance on the WMT, RMT Words or CVLT Recognition hits (n = 27); Patients with cerebral impairment (n = 56 with moderate to severe TBI, n = 38 with neurological disease; n = 94)	Computerized Assessment of Response Bias	CARB Total Test Score—for test security purposes, this cutoff is held in publications	70	99	1	30	Yes	No	32–68	6-18 Minutes Depending on Effort According to the Authors	Unknown
Arnett, Hammeke, & Schwartz (1995)	Study One: Undergraduate simulators (n = 49), neurologically impaired patients (n = 34)	Memory for 15 Items Test	<3 rows correct	63	74	26	37	Yes	No	None	4.57	Easy
			<9 items correct	61	76	24	39	Yes	No	None	4.57	Easy
			<8 items correct	59	82	18	41	Yes	No	None	4.57	Easy
			<2 rows correct	47	97	3	53	Yes	No	None	4.57	Easy
	Study Two: Simulating medical students (n = 25), neurologically impaired patients (n = 25)		<3 rows correct	76	80	20	24	Yes	No	45–55	4.57	Easy
			<9 items correct	72	84	16	28	Yes	No	45–55	4.57	Easy
			<8 items correct	68	84	16	32	Yes	No	49–51	4.57	Easy
			<2 rows correct	64	96	4	36	Yes	No	41–59	4.57	Easy

Green & Allen (unpublished manuscript)	Normal controls (n = 65), heumatoid rarthritis patients (n = 16), fibromyalgia patients with no disability (n = 50), neurological patients (n = 40), moderate to severe brain injury patients (n = 57), simulated malingerers (n = 25), severe brain injury or neurological disease patients with probable invalid effort (n = 10); therefore, 228 presumed honest responders and 35 presumed invalid responders.	Word Memory Test **In the early trials, this measure is used to measure effort; however, in later trials it is used as a measure of verbal learning and memory. Therefore, it is both a memory and a malingering measure.	<cutoff correct on WMT-IR and <cutoff correct on WMT-DR for test security purposes, this cutoff is held in publications	97	99	1	3	Yes	Yes	5–95	12–18 minutes with 30 minute and 20 minute delays according to test authors	Unknown
Green, Berendt, Allen, & Mandel (unpublished manuscript); Lyle Allen (personal communication January 23, 2001); Gervais, Green, & Allen (1999)	Compensation seeking patients failing the WMT (n =? ?), Compensation seeking patients passing the WMT (n = ??)	Test of Memory Malingering	<45 on Trial 2	38%	99%	1%	62%	Yes	No	None	15 minutes without retention trial according to authors	Unknown

TABLE 20.2. Continued

Authors	Population	Measures	Cut-Off Scores	Sensitivity	Specificity	False Positive Error Rate	False Negative Error Rate	Valid?	Effective at 30% base rate?	Validity Effective Range?	Admin Time	Vulnerability to Coaching
Grieffenstein, Baker, & Gola (1996)	Severe TBI patients (*n* = 55), probable malingerers (*n* = 90)	Memory for 15 Items Test	<10	64	78	22	36	Yes	No	None	4.57	Easy
		Rey Word Recognition List	<6 Correct	80	93	7	20	Yes	Yes	28–72	5.33	Easy
			<5 (total correct minus false positives)	72	84	16	28	Yes	No	45–55	5.33	Easy
Grieffenstein, Baker, & Gola (1994)	Traumatic brain injury patients (*n* = 33), patients with persistent postconcussive syndrome (*n* = 30), probable malingerers (*n* = 43) the data from individuals with TBI and persistent PCS were averaged.	Portland Digit Recognition Test	<59 correct <64 correct	65 75	91 79	9 21	35 25	Yes Yes	No No	45–55 47–53	35.71 35.71	Easy-Mod Easy-Mod
		Rey Word Recognition List	<7 correct <5 correct	80 72	93 84	7 16	20 28	Yes Yes	Yes No	28–72 45–55	5.33 5.33	Easy Easy
Guilmette, Hart, Giuliano, & Leininger (1994)	Brain-damaged subjects (*n* = 20), psychiatric inpatients (*n* = 20), undergraduate simulators (*n* = 20)	Abbreviated Hiscock Forced Choice Procedures (36 total points)	<33 items correct (more than four errors)	85	97.5	2.5	15	Yes	No	38.5–61.5		Unknown

Guilmette, Hart, Giuliano (1993)	Brain-damaged subjects (n = 18), undergraduate simulators (n = 29), undergraduate controls (n = 20)	Hiscock Forced Choice Procedure (72 total points)	<66 (more than six errors)	90	100	0	10	Yes	Yes	11–89	25.00	Easy
Hilsabeck, LeCompte, Zuppardo, & Mitchell (1997)	Undergraduate controls (n = 72), undergraduate simulators (n = 58), severe TBI memory-impaired patients (n = 2)	Word Completion Memory Test	R<9 or Inclusion <15	93	100	0	7	Yes	Yes	8–92	16.67	Moderate
Iverson & Franzen (1996)	Undergraduates (n = 20), psychiatric inpatients (n = 20), memory-disordered	Wiggins & Brandt Autobiographical Interview (total missed of 17)	>3	77.5	100	0	22.5	Yes	Yes	23.5–76.5	6.00	Easy
	patients (n = 20); within subjects analogue design with undergraduates and psychiatric inpatients	Memory for 16 Items Test	>8 Omissions	23	100	0	77	Yes	No	None	4.25	Easy
			>6 Omissions	33	98	2	67	Yes	No	None	4.25	Easy
			<6 Total Correct	40	100	0	60	Yes	No	None	4.25	Easy

TABLE 20.2. Continued

Authors	Population	Measures	Cut-Off Scores	Sensitivity	Specificity	False Positive Error Rate	False Negative Error Rate	Valid?	Effective at 30% base rate?	Validity Effective Range?	Admin Time	Vulnerability to Coaching
Iverson, Franzen, & McCracken (1994)	Psychiatric inpatients (*n* = 60), community volunteer controls (*n* = 60), memory-impaired patients (*n* = 60)	21-Item Test	<9	38	100	0	62	Yes	No	None	15.00	Easy-Mod
			<12	70	96	4	30	Yes	No	35–65	15.00	Easy-Mod
Iverson, Franzen, & McCracken (1991)	Undergraduate controls (*n* = 20), undergraduate simulators (*n* = 20), memory-impaired patients (*n* = 20)	21-Item Test	<5 on free recall	75	72.5	27.5	25	Yes	No	None	15.00	Easy-Mod
			<3 on free recall	35	92.5	7.5	65	Yes	No	None	15.00	Easy-Mod
			<13 on recognition	100	97.5	2.5	0	Yes	Yes	3.5–96.5	15.00	Easy-Mod
			<9 on recognition	65	100	0	35	Yes	No	36–64	15.00	Easy-Mod
Iverson, Green, & Gervais (1999)	Community volunteers (*n* = 38), sophisticated simulators, mainly psychologists (*n* = 15)	Word Memory Test **It was learned on follow-up that the one malingerer classified as honest did not follow the instructions to feign. Therefore, the sensitivity rates may be higher.	<82.5% correct on IR	93	100	0	7	Yes	Yes	8–92	12–18 minutes with 30 minute and 20 minute delays	Unknown
			<82.5% correct on DR	93	100	0	7	Yes	Yes	8-92		

Rose, Hall, & Szalda-Petree (1995)	Uncoached undergraduate simulators (n = 30), coached undergraduate simulators (n = 30), CHI patients (n = 30), community control subjects (n = 30)	Portland Digit Recognition Test—computerized version sensitivity and specificity rates not reported for community control subjects	<40 correct	64	89	11	36	Yes	No	48–52	35.71	Easy-Mod
Slick, Hopp, Strauss, & Spellacy (1996)	Undergraduate controls (n = 95), undergraduate simulators (n = 43), compensation-seeking patients (n = 206), non-compensation seeking patients (n = 32)	Victoria Symptom Validity Test (48 items)—compensation seeking patients were omitted because their simulation status was unknown	Scores of less than 16 on the easy and/or hard items. Questionable and malingering classifications were collapsed to calculate the following data	81	100	0	29	Yes	No	30–70	27.50	Mod-Diff

Note. WMT=Word Memory Test; IR=Immediate Recognition Trial; DR=Delayed Recognition Procedure; Easy = Easy to coach a malingerer to produce an unidentified malingering performance; Moderate = Of moderate difficulty to coach a malingerer to produce an unidentified malingering performance; Difficult = Difficulty to coach a malingerer to produce an unidentified malingering performance. When the median was calculated between two dimensions, mod-diff, or easy-mod was reported.

- *False positive* error rates refer to nonmalingerers who are wrongly labeled as malingerers.
- *False negative* error rates refer to malingerers who escape detection using the particular strategy of interest.
- *Validity* refers to the relatedness of the detection measure to the construct being measured.
- *Effectiveness* refers to whether the overall rate of accurate classifications based on the measure surpasses the classification rate based on base rate predictions alone.
- The *validity effectiveness range* refers to the range of base rates for malingering within which any given test meets criteria for effectiveness.
- *Time to administer* refers to the time commitment needed to administer the measure.
- V*ulnerability to coaching* reflects experts' ratings of how easily the malingering detection strategy can be thwarted or defeated by coaching.

For a more thorough review of these concepts, refer to Rogers (1997) and Hayes and colleagues (1999).

Sensitivity and specificity of the malingering tests are important considerations. Higher levels of sensitivity increase the probability of diagnostic "hits," whereas high specificity guards against false positive accusations. These considerations have been reviewed elsewhere (Gouvier, et al., 1998); and, despite current widespread practices to the contrary, they are no less important in the selection of tests for malingering detection as they are in the selection of tests for other psychodiagnostic purposes (APA, 1985). Should the clinician want a screening tool that would identify almost all potential malingerers (but also risk a high number of false positive identifications), he or she would select an instrument with high sensitivity. Catching most malingerers, but many nonmalingerers, these patients could be followed up using another (perhaps lengthier) measure selected on a basis of its high specificity. This would effectively separate the true malingerers from the false positive nonmalingerers, and serve the dual purpose of catching the suspicious presentations while protecting the honest patients. Validity is computed based solely on a measure's sensitivity, specificity, Type I, and Type II error rates. A test is a valid indicator of malingering when sensitivity/false positive error rate is greater than false negative error rate/specificity (Faust & Nurcombe, 1989). All identified measures were valid; that is, all produced results that were associated with higher-than-chance levels of malingering detection. Effectiveness varies as a function of the base rate for the condition being identified. A measure is regarded as effective when the overall classification accuracy using the measure is better than the overall accuracy of classification when using base rates alone. Therefore, in order for a measure to be effective, the base rate must be greater than the measure's combined false positive and negative error rates (cf. Faust & Nurcombe, 1989; Gouvier et al., 1998). Thus, for any given measure of malingering, there is one base rate cutoff below which the measure is not effective, and another cutoff above which the measure is not effective. Using the aforementioned example, the measure with a 20% overall error rate would be useful to improve classification accuracy when the base rate for malingering is greater than 20% and less than 80%. This measure would not be effective when there is a 15% base rate for malingering, as 80% of the diagnostic judgments from using the test would be right, whereas 85% of the judgments from base rate information only would be right. Of course, in the latter circumstance no malingerers would ever be identified, as all patients would be classified as nonmalingerers.

Similarly, malingering detection strategies can be classified along the dimension of time necessary to complete them. Briefer evaluations, mandated by limited insurance reimbursement for many neuropsychological services, may be all that is feasible at the medical care level, but when these screens indicate the need for further evaluation, most insurance adjustors would be expected to respond favorably to a request for additional hours to rule out suspected malingering. The time measures suggested in the table were compiled from a brief survey of practicing neuropsychologists conducted by the authors.

Tables 20.1 and 20.2 present further survey results for those tests for which sensitivity and specificity data were available; the tests in Table 20.1 are traditional neuropsychological measures sometimes recruited for use as malingering measures, whereas those in Table 20.2 are measures developed for the express purpose of malingering detection. The information depicted in these tables represents a mere sampling of the sort of taxonomy of malingering detection strategies that our profession needs. Although some of the measures appear to be effective across a broad range of malingering base rates, others are not, and more tests become effective the closer the base rate for malingering approaches 50%. The Validity Effectiveness Range column of both tables outlines the base rate range within which each test is effective.

With the introduction of increasingly sensitive and specific tests, our science is advancing to the point where we can identify malingerers with a higher level of confidence than even a few years ago; and we have seen how our contribution in doing so lends support to nationwide efforts to reduce lawsuit abuse, possibly helping to limit ever-rising insurance rates. Table 20.3 briefly summarizes three major markers of value of detecting malingerers using neuropsychological assessment in the forensic arena.

☐ Evidence for Attorney Coaching

A number of investigators have provided evidence suggesting that some attorneys have influenced the data relied upon by forensic neuropsychological experts (e.g., see Baer, Wetter, & Berry, 1995; Dolan, 1994; Legate, 1996; Platt & Husband, 1986; Rosen, 1995; Taylor, Harp, & Elliott, 1992; Wetter & Corrigan, 1995; Youngjohn, 1995). Such influence can present a serious challenge to the validity of malingering detection. Martin, Gouvier, Todd, Bolter, and Niccolls (1992) found that subjects coached on how to malinger performed more like brain-injured examinees than those who were not coached. Attorneys are advocates engaged in an adversarial process, so their possible manipulation of the data on which neuropsychologists rely is not random; on the contrary, it presents a response bias, or systematic error.

TABLE 20.3. Markers of Value of Neuropsychological Services in Malingering Detection

1. Reduce dollar awards for feigned cognitive deficits
2. Reduce unwarranted workman's compensation benefits
3. Document apparent motivated test-taking behaviors that add credence to patients' legitimate claims of cognitive deficits

In some jurisdictions the courts have taken steps to control these influences. For example, in California the Code of Civil Procedure specifically protects mental examinations by prohibiting third parties from participating in independent examinations (Butterworth, 1999). Similarly, in *Ragge v. MCA/Universal Studios* a federal judge held that a third party would not be allowed to sit in on the evaluation (*Ragge v. MCA/Universal Studios,* 165 F.R.D. 605).

Informal personal communications with litigating attorneys suggest that some attorneys feel that it is improper *not* to advise a client prior to a neuropsychological evaluation. Recent literature has elaborated on this finding (Youngjohn, 1995), and Baer and associates (1995) referred to "the increasing likelihood that coaching of test-takers may be occurring in a variety of settings," adding that "it is important for clinicians to understand its impact" (p. 198). Lees-Haley (1997) warned that "if psychologists are not alerted to these influences, their opinions may not be independent and objective; on the contrary, their conclusions may be shaped by an attorney to conform to a litigation strategy" (p. 321). Wetter and Corrigan (1995) reported that 63% of attorneys they surveyed felt they should provide clients with information about psychological test validity measures. Yale law professor and legal ethics teacher Geoffrey Hazard opined that lawyers are supposed to learn facts from their clients, not invent stories for clients, "But the fact of the matter is, lawyers do tell their clients what to do, indirectly. . . . How artificial they are, how artful, varies" (Dolan, 1994, p. A17).

One pernicious effect of outside influence is seen in those cases in which blatant malingering is apparent but the patient passes malingering tests with flying colors. In these cases the neuropsychologists' own tests appear to argue against their conclusions. Innovative research is needed to increase the complexity of malingering testing to the point that coaching becomes ineffective.

Report Writing and Expert Witness Testifying: Some Suggestions

Although report writing and testimony styles are as diverse as the professionals who practice in this domain, with none being "right" or "wrong," a few comments can be made about writing the malingering report. First, given that lawyers are becoming more knowledgable about neuropsychological measures, it is suggested that report authors be wary of releasing too much information about neuropsychological measures in their reports. The authors have seen neuropsychological reports in which the writers had (a) explained the test, (b) described the protocol for test taking, (c) expressed the underlying assumption of the test, (d) portrayed how the client performed on the test, and (e) described how this performance was suggestive of malingering. If this client is subsequently referred for another neuropsychological evaluation, given this information, the attorney and client will have all the data needed for the client to perform as a truly impaired patient, thus possibly fooling the second neuropsychologist. It is suggested that the report author simply state that on several measures specifically designed to detect malingering, as well as on standard neuropsychological testing, the client's performance indicated malingering, response bias, or exaggeration. If further details are needed, the discovery deposition provides an opportunity for the neuropsychologist to provide this additional information.

A second caution centers around expert witness testifying. Anything the expert witness has written (a journal article, report, etc.) or has said (at a workshop, in a trial, or during an television interview) can be brought up in court or during a deposition, and the expert witness can be questioned about these previous statements. Although one may think this would require a rather industrious and rare attorney, technology is aiding attorneys in this regard. For example, several Web sites (e.g., www.idex.com, www.evansreporting.com, www.malpracticedepositions.com, www.mdxintl.com, www.triodyne.com) offer services to insurance companies, lawyers, and corporations, including case details, transcripts, article searches, and more to learn of the writing and speaking record of expert witnesses nationwide. As of this writing, more than 584,213 individuals have "hit" www.idex.com, attesting to the popularity of this type of service. Therefore, when testifying as an expert witness, one should tell the truth and provide only necessary information–and resist the urge to embark on a verbal tirade. This is applicable elsewhere as well; we have noted that presenters on forensic topics at neuropsychology workshops often are reluctant to permit their presentations to be taped, and this is recognized as an exercise in judicial caution.

Final Considerations and Directions for Future Research

In closing, if the Louisiana statistics ($107.2 million annual direct statewide costs of malingering) are taken as typical or average for each of the 50 states, then needless medical claims, defense costs, and cash payouts to malingerers by negotiated settlements or courtroom awards represent a $5.36 billion-a-year industry in the United States. This is a conservative estimate as well, which does not take into account the costs to society of missed work and hiring replacement workers to make up for the absent malingerer in the workplace.

Neuropsychological services have been designed to identify malingerers in the tort system, and their results often are used to hurry malingerers out of the system, many times with greatly reduced or totally denied rewards. Clinical neuropsychologists have developed a technology for detecting malingerers using traditional measures and measures specifically designed to detect malingered cognitive or memory dysfunction. Unfortunately, we are not as far developed in our ability to identify somatic or psychologic malingering, and we still have no good estimates of how good our technology in any of the three domains really is. Although there are no clear estimates of how many malingerers actually get caught and how many slip through, given the potential cost savings of identifying a single malingerer, the actual added costs of evaluating for malingering (estimated at 1 to 2 hours or $200 to $400) seem small. With $1 million average brain-injury awards in Louisiana, malingering evaluations could be added to 5,000 neuropsychological evaluations for the cost savings from a single identified malingerer. For brain-injury assessments, we need only need one additional "hit" for cost-effectiveness to be demonstrated. Given the sensitivity rates cited in Tables 20.1 and 20.2, it is a safe bet that we do a good bit better than a 1-in-5000 hit rate. Perhaps we do substantially better, and it is important that we do so, for every malingerer who slips through the cracks represents an injustice against some defendant, and exorbitant expenses as well.

There is a flip side to this coin, however. As more and more individuals are labeled and identified as malingerers, there is a concomitant risk of increasing numbers of nonmalingering individuals who will be incorrectly labeled. This topic warrants further attention, as many individuals undoubtedly are mislabeled unjustly as malingerers.

Lastly, the four factors discussed in this chapter and three testing factors of sensitivity/specificity, administration time, and vulnerability to coaching all need to be considered in choosing a strategy for evaluating for potential malingering. These considerations should guide the selection of instruments in evaluating any single client, and also contribute toward the development of malingering batteries to be included in neuropsychological assessments of different classes of clients presenting for evaluation. This development will necessarily be a work in evolution, as coaching strategies produce ever-more-sophisticated malingerers. Ultimately, we can look forward to further development and validation of noncoachable approaches to malingering detection, such as the psychophysiological techniques introduced by Rosenfield and Ellwanger (1999), which rely on evoked potential data to provide confirmatory or discomfirmatory evidence of neurocognitive deficits demonstrated by the patient under evaluation.

☐ References

Allen, L., Conder, R. L., Green , P., & Cox, D. R. (1997). *CARB'97 manual for the Computerized Assessment of Response Bias*. Durham, NC: CogniSyst.

Allen, L., Green, P., & Rohling, M. (2001). *A known groups validation study of the Computerized Assessment of Response Bias*. Unpublished manuscript.

American Psychiatric Association. (1994). *Diagnostic and statistical manual of mental disorders* (4th. ed.). Washington, DC: Author.

American Psychological Association. (1985). *Standards of educational and psychological testing*. Washington, DC: Author.

Arnett, P. A., Hammeke, T. A., & Schwartz, L. (1995). Quantitative and qualitative performance on Rey's 15-Item Test in neurologic patients and dissimulators. *The Clinical Neuropsychologist, 9*, 17–26.

Baer, R., Wetter, M., & Berry, D. (1995). Effects of information about validity scales on underreporting of symptoms on the MMPI-2: An analogue investigation. *Assessment, 2*, 189–200.

Beaber, R. J., Marston, A., Michelli, J., & Mills, M. J. (1985). A brief test for measuring malingering in schizophrenic individuals. *American Journal of Psychiatry, 142*, 1478–1481.

Binder, L. (1997). A review of mild head trauma. Part II. Clinical implications. *Journal of Clinical and Experimental Neuropsychology, 19*, 432–457.

Binder, L., Rohling, M., & Larrabee, G. (1997). A review of mild head trauma. Part I: Meta-analytic review of neuropsychological studies. *Journal of Clinical and Experimental Neuropsychology, 19*, 421–431.

Butterworth Legal Publishers. (1999). *1999 California code of civil procedure*. Carlsbad, CA: Author.

Coleman, R. D., Rapport, L. J., Millis, S. R., Ricker, J. H., Farchione, T. (1998). Effects of coaching on detection of malingering on the California Verbal Learning Test. *Journal of Clinical and Experimental Neuropsychology, 20*, 201–210.

Dolan, M. (1994). Defense seldom rests on issues of ethics and duty. *Los Angeles Times*, Wednesday, June 1, p. A17.

Eason, T. J., & Eason, J. H. (2000). *Eason's Louisiana quantum study and personal injury law*. Mandeville, LA: Lawyers Research Publishing.

Faust, D., & Nurcombe, B. (1989). Improving the accuracy of clinical judgment. *Psychiatry, 52*, 197–208.

Gervais, R. O., Allen, L. M., Green, P., & Cunningham, S. (1998). The effects of coaching DSM-IV pain disordered patients on the Computerized Assessment of Response Bias: *Archives of Clinical Neuropsychology, 14*, 97–98.

Gervais, R. O., Green, P., & Allen, L. M. (1999). Differential sensitivity to symptom exaggeration of verbal, visual, and numerical symptom validity tests. *Archives of Clinical Neuropsychology, 14*, 746–747 (abstract).

Gouvier, W. D. (1999). Base rates and clinical decision making in neuropsychology. In J. J. Sweet (Ed.), *Forensic neuropsychology: Fundamentals and practice* (pp. 27–37). Lisse, The Netherlands: Swets & Zeitlinger.

Gouvier, W. D., Hayes, J. S., & Smiroldo, B. B. (1998). The significance of base rates, test sensitivity, test specificity, and subjects knowledge in assessing TBI sequelae and malingering. In C. Reynolds (Ed.), *Detection of malingering in head injury litigation*. New York: Plenum.

Green, P., & Allen, L. (2001). *A multi-group validation study of the Word Memory Test measures of subject effort*. Unpublished manuscript.

Green, P., Behrent, J., Allen, L., & Mandel, A. (2001). *Comparison of the Test of Memory Malingering and the Word Memory Test for identifying response bias in a series of compensation cases*. Unpublished manuscript.

Greiffenstein, M. F., Baker, W. J., & Gola, T. (1996). Comparison of multiple scoring methods for Rey's malingered amnesia measures. *Archives of Clinical Neuropsychology, 11*, 283–293.

Greiffenstein, M. F., Baker, W. J., & Gola, T. (1994) Validation of malingered amnesia measures with a large clinical sample. *Psychological Assessment, 6*, 218–224.

Guilmette, T. J., Hart, K. J., Giuliano, A. J., & Leininger, B. E. (1993). Malingering detection: The use of a forced-choice method in identifying organic versus simulated memory impairment. *The Clinical Neuropsychologist, 7*, 59–69.

Guilmette, T. J., Hart, K. J., Giuliano, A. J., & Leininger, B. E. (1994). Detecting simulated memory impairment: Comparison of the Rey Fifteen-Item Test and the Hiscock Forced-Choice Procedure. *The Clinical Neuropsychologist, 8*, 283–294.

Hayes, J. S., Hilsabeck, R., & Gouvier, W. D. (1999). Assessment of malingering among personal injury litigants. In N. Varney and R. Roberts (Eds.), *Neurobehavioral dysfunction following mild head injury* (pp. 249–290). Mahwah, NJ: Lawrence Erlbaum Associates.

Hilsabeck, R. C., LeCompte, D. C., Zuppardo, M. C., & Mitchell, M. M. (1997). The Word Completion Memory Test (WCMT): A test to detect sophisticated malingerers. Poster presented at the 17th Annual Meeting of the National Academy of Neuropsychology, Las Vegas, N.V. *Archives of Clinical Neuropsychology, 13*, 28.

Iverson, G. L., & Franzen, M. D. (1998). Detecting malingered memory deficits with the Recognition Memory Test. *Brain Injury, 12*, 275–282.

Iverson, G. L., Franzen, M. D., & McCracken, L. M. (1991). Evaluation of an objective assessment technique for the detection of malingered memory deficits. *Law and Human Behavior, 15*, 667–676.

Iverson, G. L., Franzen, M. D., & McCracken, L. M. (1994). Application of a forced choice memory procedure designed to detect experimental malingering. *Archives of Clinical Neuropsychology, 9*, 437–450.

Larrabee, G. J. (2000). *Assessing malingering*. Presented at the American Academy of Clinical Neuropsychology, Chicago.

Larrabee G. J. (1998). Somatic malingering on the MMPI and MMPI-2 in personal injury litigants. *The Clinical Neuropsychologist, 12*, 179–188.

Lee-Haley, P. R. (1997). Attorneys influence expert evidence in forensic psychological and neuropsychological cases. *Assessment, 4*, 321–324.

Legate, B. L. (1996). *Presenting a tort claim in a first party system-strategies for recovery of a loss of earning capacity benefit*. Presented to Canadian Bar Association–Ontario, Continuing Legal Education, June 22, Ontario.

Martin, R. C., Gouvier, W. D., Todd, M. E., Bolter, J. F., & Niccolls, R. (1992). Effects of task instruction on malingered memory performance. *Forensic Reports, 5*, 393–397.

Millis, S. (1992) The Recognition Memory Test in the detection of malingered and exaggerated memory deficits. *The Clinical Neuropsychologist, 6*, 406–414.

National Insurance Crime Bureau (2000a). www.NICB.com.

National Insurance Crime Bureau/Chartered Property and Casualty Underwriters Society (2000). www.stopinsurancecheats.com

Platt, J. J., & Husband, S. D. (1986). Post-traumatic stress disorder in forensic practice. *American Journal of Forensic Psychology, 4,* 29–56.

Price, J. R. (1995). *Identification of malingering and symptom exaggeration.* Workshop presented at the 15th annual conference of the National Academy of Neuropsychology, San Francisco.

Prigatano, G. P., Smason, I., Lamb, D. G., & Bortz, J. J. (1997). Suspected malingering and the Digit Memory Test: A replication and extension. *Archives of Clinical Neuropsychology, 12,* 609–617.

Ragge v. MCA/Universal Studios, 165 F. R. D. 605(C.D. Cal. 1995)

Reynolds, C. (Ed.). (1998). *Detection of malingering in head injury litigation.* New York: Plenum Press.

Rogers R. (Ed.) (1997). *Clinical assessment of malingering and deception.* New York: Guilford Press.

Rose, F. E., Hall, S., & Szalda-Petree, A. D. (1995). Portland Digit Recognition Test–Computerized: Measuring response latency improves the detection of malingering. *The Clinical Neuropsychologist, 9,* 124–134.

Rosen, G. M. (1995). The *Aleutian Enterprise* sinking and posttraumatic stress disorder: Misdiagnosis in clinical and forensic settings. *Professional Psychology: Research and Practice, 26,* 82–87.

Rosenfield, J. P., & Ellwanger, J. W. (1999). Cognitive psychophysiology in detection of malingered cognitive deficit. In J. J. Sweet (Ed.), *Forensic neuropsychology: Fundamentals and practice* (pp. 287–311). Lisse, The Netherlands: Swets & Zeitlinger.

Slick, D. J., Hopp, G., Strauss, E., & Spellacy, F. J. (1996). Victoria Symptom Validity Test: Efficiency for detecting feigned memory impairment and relationship to neuropsychological tests and MMPI-2 validity scales. *Journal of Clinical and Experimental Neuropsychology, 18,* 911–922.

Sweet, J. J. (1999). Malingering: Differential diagnosis. In J. J. Sweet (Ed.), *Forensic Neuropsychology: Fundamentals and practice* (pp. 255–285). Lisse, The Netherlands: Swets & Zeitlinger.

Taylor, J. S., Harp, J. H. & Elliott, T. (1992). Preparing the plaintiff in the mild brain injury case. *Trial Diplomacy Journal, 15,* 65–72.

Tenhula, W. N., & Sweet, J. J. (1996). Double cross validation of the Booklet Category Test in detecting malingered traumatic brain injury. *The Clinical Neuropsychologist, 10,* 104–116.

Trueblood, W. (1994). Qualitative and quantitative characteristics of malingered and other invalid WAIS-R and clinical memory data. *Journal of Clinical and Experimental Neuropsychology, 16,* 597–607.

Trueblood, W., & Schmidt, M. (1993). Malingering and other validity considerations in the neuropsychological evaluation of mild head injury. *Journal of Clinical and Experimental Neuropsychology, 15,* 578–590.

U.S. Department of Justice, Bureau of Justice Statistics. (2000). Civil justice statistics. *www.ojp.usdoj.gov/bjs/civil.htm*

Wetter, M. W., & Corrigan, S. K. (1995). Providing information to clients about psychological tests: A survey of attorneys' and law students' attitudes. *Professional Psychology: Research and Practice, 26,* 474–477.

Youngjohn, J. R. (1995). Confirmed attorney coaching prior to neuropsychological evaluation. *Assessment, 2,* 279–283.

21

CHAPTER

T. Michael Kashner
C. Munro Cullum
Richard I. Naugle

Measuring the Economics of Neuropsychology

☐ Why Economics of Neuropsychology?

The controversy surrounding managed care balancing profits against human suffering–heard echoing in legislative chambers, the news media, and civil courts–is not without precedent. In a letter to Queen Victoria's confidant John Brown, the art critic John Ruskin, appalled that the "immoral" pursuit of wealth was being taught at Cambridge University, referred to the science of political economy as "the most cretinous, speechless, paralyzing plague that has yet touched the brains of mankind." Imminently more concise, Thomas Carlyle in his *Latter-Day Pamphlets* described economics as the "dismal science" when nineteenth-century economists began to espouse poverty as a natural consequence whenever human reproduction outpaced the food supply.

However, economics is not about profits or wealth, it is about scarcity, and in no other industry is scarcity more of an issue than health care. For instance, in 1925, 4% of all goods and services produced in the United States went for health care. By the mid-1960s, the figure had risen to nearly 6%, when *Harper's* magazine first declared that the U.S. health-care industry was "in crisis" (Battistella & Southby, 1968). During the first decade in the new millennium, we can anticipate spending around 18% of our gross domestic product on health care (Burner & Waldo, 1995), with no end to increases in sight. More than ever, it is important that professionals take responsibility to use health-care resources efficiently for patients with medical needs. If the total resources that society allocates for health care cannot be further expanded, it is important to allocate existing resources wisely to ensure we attain the largest "bang for the buck." As with other areas of medicine, cost outcome and clinical efficacy information as it pertains to neuropsychological services is essential. As reflected throughout this text, it is incumbent upon neuropsychologists to make a concerted effort to provide these data and to design appropriate efficacy and cost outcome studies to address these issues.

Health Care as a Market

Traditional economists preach that informed consumers with explicit demands will meet in the marketplace with producers seeking profits. Following their negotiations, suppliers will produce, at the least, technically feasible cost-goods that consumers will be willing and able to purchase from the fruits of their labor. For many industries, these negotiations are regulated by the invisible hand of competitive markets that balance consumer wants with producer capacity to supply.

As an economic market, the healing arts pose some additional challenges to the theory of the invisible hand (Gaynor, Haas-Wilson, & Vogt, 2000). The challenges take the following forms:

1. *Technical:* Health care is a highly technical commodity constantly changing, making it difficult for even professionals, let alone consumers, to be fully up-to-date to understand the benefits and costs of services, information necessary to make informed choices.
2. *Multidisciplinary:* Health care is a product of many people and institutions composed of diverse disciplines and professional associations, making continuity of care difficult.
3. *Life threatening:* Health professionals sometimes make split-second decisions with potentially irreversible and life-threatening consequences at times when patients and their families are shaken with the burden of illness.
4. *Inexact science:* The complexity and diversity of the human organism often makes it difficult to determine if and how health care can influence health, which, in some cases, may not be fully realized until many years after the service is provided.
5. *Uncertainty:* Despite best intentions, health status may change unexpectedly, requiring extensive services that may leave the patient and the patient's family financially challenged or destitute. Health insurance is designed to provide a remedy for such losses.
6. *Moral hazard:* With third-party payers underwriting part of the cost of care, consumers as decision makers will theoretically reap the benefits from care, while being responsible for only part of its costs. Most experts believe that this moral hazard leads to greater utilization of care, and thus *higher* costs, than would have happened under a competitive market (Feldstein, 1979).
7. *Nonprofit status:* Unlike other markets, health care includes a significant share of "not-for-profit" producers, in both private (e.g., voluntary hospitals) and public (Department of Veterans Affairs medical facilities) sectors. These institutions exist in part, according to some, because competitive markets alone may be too slow to provide for the health needs of patients.
8. *Externalities:* The benefits from health services may flow well beyond the patient and the patient's family, as society in general benefits from a healthier workforce. This suggests that investments in health care would be less than that achieved in competitive markets.
9. *Need versus demand:* Some argue that health care serves a higher purpose, that it should be elevated to a "right," and thus should be allocated on basis of medical "need" defined clinically, rather than on "demand" based on patients' willingness and ability to pay.

☐ Can Government Contain Costs?

The lay press generally discusses medical costs in terms of whether it can be *contained.* To contain costs, the federal government has focused on both providers and consumers of health. The 1940s, 1950s, and 1960s gave rise to programs that helped (a) *expand the supply of health-care providers* by financing schools to produce more doctors and nurses (Health Professions Education Assistance Acts of 1963 and 1976; Nurse Training Act of 1964) and institutions to build more hospitals (Hill–Burton Act of 1946). The theory was that increasing supply would induce competition and mitigate costs. Although supplies increased, so did patient use of services, and thus costs. As a result, the federal government forged a partnership with the states and health-care industry to (b) *voluntarily plan* for care that would spread resources geographically and across specialties based on need (Public Health Service Act of 1965 and 1966). During the 1970s, Congress used its spending powers through the newly legislated Medicare program to require hospitals to provide (c) *certification* justifying capital expansion (Social Security Act Amendments; National Health Planning and Resources Development Act of 1974). The federal government also explored (d) *regulating utilization* directly through the first "managed care" programs, known as professional standards review organizations and later as peer review organizations (Social Security Act of 1965; Tax Equity and Fiscal Responsibility Act of 1982). Attacking the issue of moral hazard, federal financing programs such as Medicare included (e) *cost-sharing* arrangements in which consumers paid a share of their health-care bill in the form of a lump-sum payment (deductible), a fixed percentage of the allowable charges (coinsurance), a fixed fee per unit of service (copayment), and a total cap on covered services. The federal government also (f) *regulated fees* of professionals and hospitals, either directly (as in the 1971–1973 Economic Stabilization Program under the Nixon administration, in which all provider fees were fixed) or through prospectively determined pay schedules covering federally financed patients. Finally, the federal government fostered the development of (g) *alternative health-care organizations,* including health maintenance organizations, believed by some to contain costs by emphasizing outpatient over inpatient care, negotiating provider fees, and encouraging the use of preventive care (Kashner, Rush, & Altshuler, 1997).

Although such systems were designed to control costs, concerns about this health-care movement have focused on problems of access to specialty services, including neuropsychological evaluations and treatment. Here, barriers to care are exacerbated by (a) primary care physicians who, as the industry's gatekeeper, often must first refer a patient before beginning neuropsychological care; (b) organized health plans that, as the industry's payer, may exclude neuropsychologists from their lists of preferred providers or neuropsychological services from their lists of covered services; and (c) administrative agencies that, as sources of industry information, mistakenly classify neuropsychological services under "mental health" rather than neurology using current procedural terminology (CPT). To overcome these barriers, the profession must take an active role to collect and analyze scientific data describing clinical outcomes and cost-effectiveness of neuropsychological services, a point made throughout this text, and ultimately to disseminate such findings to increase public and professional awareness.

Algorithm-Based Practices

A practical solution may be through the development of algorithm-based practices. In the absence of expanding its budget for mental health care, the state of Texas fostered a program that brought together leading experts in severe mental illness, explored the latest clinical literature, and developed clinical algorithms by consensus to describe a "best practice" (Gilbert et al., 1998; Rush et al., 1999). These algorithms were designed to help guide clinicians by organizing strategic (what treatments) and tactical (how to treat) decisions into sequential stages that prioritize medication options (Rush & Prien, 1995). This framework permits clinical experts, working with economists, to design recommendations for health care that balance scientifically determined health outcomes of selected treatments with the cost of those treatments (Kashner, Rush, & Altshuler, 1999). Algorithm-based approaches can be used in neuropsychology from diagnostic as well as treatment perspectives. As many disorders have qualitative and quantitative neuropsychological features that aid in differential diagnosis (Naugle, Cullum, & Bigler, 1998), the development of diagnostic algorithms carries promise as a means of objectifying and quantifying aspects of clinical decision making. As we learn more about the sensitivity and specificity of our neurocognitive tests in different populations, we come to better understand which test characteristics best identify and discriminate disorders, and what aspects of the neuropsychological record should be given the most weight by the neuropsychologist interpreting the profile. The distinction between cortical versus subcortical dementia, the presence of lateralized cognitive impairment, and psychiatric versus neurologic disease are but a few examples wherein neuropsychological patterns or "cognitive signatures" (Cullum, 1999) of disorders can be useful and have implications for early/differential diagnosis as well as treatment. The extent to which clinical algorithms can be developed to aid in this process remains to be seen, although early steps in this direction appear promising (Cullum, 1999; Zakzanis, Leach & Kaplan, 1999).

Although only recommendations, clinical algorithms potentially can serve as appropriate guidelines to clinicians, patients, and third-party payers as to what and how services should be produced. This is particularly relevant because market imperfections discussed earlier leave some experts mistrustful that competition, and the invisible hand, alone will solve the balancing problem between "costs" and "outcomes of care."

Cost Outcome Studies

Evaluating the costs and outcomes of health care generally—and algorithms, innovative programs, and professional services in particular—is the business of cost–outcome studies. In the course of developing and testing health-care innovations, medical research can be divided into (a) the basic sciences, both theoretical (Does it work in theory?) and applied (Does it work in a laboratory?); (b) the clinical sciences exploring efficacy (Does it work in controlled settings?); and (c) services research that includes, among other subjects, outcomes research (Does it work in practice?), cost analyses (At what costs for resources required?), and cost outcomes studies that compare costs and outcomes of care (At what value?).

The three components of cost outcome studies are costs, outcomes, and comparing costs with outcomes.

□ Cost Studies

Although frequently confused, there are two different types of cost studies: *Cost of illness studies* (CIS) measure the societal value of resources expended, lost, or otherwise unavailable for other uses, as a consequence of a given health problem. The intent is to predict how the world would improve economically if the prevalence of a given disease dropped from its actual level to zero. The estimation of such costs includes lost wages and productivity (by the patient as well as caregivers). CIS help policy makers understand the economic seriousness of a condition to society at large. As one of several sources of information, CIS cost estimates help policy makers decide how to allocate scarce resources to education, research, and clinical care programs that target different disease areas. In contrast, *cost outcome studies* (COS) focus on evaluating interventions designed to improve health. These studies compare input costs with the change in health outcomes due to a given treatment. COS studies help determine the value of an intervention to deal with a given health problem. CIS studies help policy makers determine if the "economic" seriousness of a health problem warrants further attention in terms of research studies, education programs, and clinical care. COS studies help clinicians and administrators evaluate how best to allocate those resources once a need has been established.

The components comprising costs in CIS studies have been well discussed in the literature (Rice, Hodgson, & Kpstein, 1985):

1. *Direct* health-care cost includes: professional diagnostic, assessment, treatment, and custodial care; the means for the patient to access care, including transportation and child care; support services such as research, and clinical training; and net cost of third party financing. The net costs of third-party financing are administrative costs incurred by third-party payers to enroll patients, manage the program, and pay health care provider. Actual payments for health services usually are not classified as an administrative cost.
2. *Indirect* costs include production loss that results when persons with illness suffer a reduction in work time or a reduction in productivity for time worked. Here, work includes the labor market (self-employed for pay, employed for pay) and household production (household tasks, raising children); administrative costs for criminal justice system (e.g., police, the courts and criminal justice system, and prisons and jails for incarceration); caregiving involving activities of daily living (eating, dressing, purchasing food, personal hygiene, managing finances) provided by both paid persons and unpaid household members; and administration of welfare programs. The latter includes the cost of administering welfare benefits, but does not include actual payments of welfare benefits. Economists consider the latter as a transfer of wealth from one person to another, not representing a net loss to society as a whole (which includes both beneficiary and provider). Indirect costs also include damages caused by illness-related behavioral problems that result in property loss, injuries sustained by victims, and time spent by the patient in jail or prison (whose time would have otherwise been spent productively employed in either the household or

employment). Injuries sustained by victims include both the cost of medical attention and costs due to production loss.

3. Finally, *intangible* costs include an estimate of the cost of pain and suffering experienced internally by the patient and the patient's family and friends, and externally by the wider community.

The components comprising estimates of costs for COS studies have varied across studies. All investigators include some measure of *direct* cost for diagnosing, treating, and assessing patients, and the cost the patient incurs to access those services. During the 1970s and 1980s, COS costs were viewed as a "net" economic change in the cost of illness. Thus, costs were computed as direct costs "minus" the change in indirect costs that were averted due to improved health status and longer life expectancy. Indirect costs are "averted" when patients in better health could earn wages or engage in household activities they would have otherwise been unable to perform, but for their improved health status. Borrowing from the "cost of illness" literature, the purpose was to compare treatment-induced changes in clinical outcomes with changes in economic outcomes (Weinstein & Stason, 1977). Although criticized by economists (Kashner, 1990), subtracting a change in indirect costs on the cost side of the cost-effectiveness equation, in fact, double-counted the health outcomes that were summed on the outcomes side of the equation. The confusion over estimating COS costs was resolved in the medical literature by the U.S. Public Health Service (PHS) Panel on Cost-Effectiveness in Health and Medicine (Gold, Siegel, Russell, & Weinstein, 1996). Begun in 1993, the purpose of the PHS Panel was to standardize methods and reporting procedures to enable policymakers to compare results across studies and for different diagnoses. COS costs were limited to the cost of care, and did not include economic consequences of patient morbidity or mortality, or intangible pain and suffering due to illness. Thus, double-counting morbidity information on both the cost and outcome sides was avoided.

When evaluating the cost of a neuropsychologist's time for an evaluation or intervention for patients with a given disorder, COS costs should include direct health costs of care for all of the patients' health-care providers. The casual observer may ponder why it is important to obtain all health-care costs when the focus should be on the cost of neuropsychologists following relatively limited clinical protocols. Consistent with PHS Panel recommendations, this is necessary to distinguish between real cost changes and mere shifts in costs between patients, other providers, and other payers. Ultimately, the concern for the policymaker is not explicitly the cost of the neuropsychologist but, rather, the bottom-line costs payers must pay to finance the patient's total health-care package, which includes the cost of the neuropsychologist. Both the cost of the neuropsychologist and the bottom-line costs across all services are important.

Cost estimates can be calculated separately by (a) *provider specialty* (neuropsychologist, other psychologists, neurologists, psychiatrists, and general medical care providers), (b) *protocol-related* (protocol providers, other neuropsychologists, and clinicians outside the protocol), (c) *payer source* (paid directly by the patient, through a third-party payer, or incurred by the provider of service), and (d) *disorder* (pertaining to the particular disorder or other medical conditions).

Elements that are contained in cost estimates include these:

1. *labor*, including the salaries, fees, and payments for the time of professional staff (e.g., psychometrists or technician assistants), other support staff, and administrative personnel;

2. *equipment and supplies,* including expendable materials for both clinical and business office-related (e.g., tests and test forms);
3. *building maintenance,* including paid utilities and physical maintenance of premises;
4. *depreciation* for building and equipment, to reflect wear and tear, and to spread out the purchase price over its useful life; and
5. *land* needed for the buildings to house the care providers.

Depreciation and land costs can be calculated in terms of "rent" paid by the provider, or opportunity rent that could have been received had the owner-provider rented the property to someone else. The cost of durable goods also can be calculated by spreading out the cost of its initial purchase price plus the cost of maintenance agreements over the useful life of the durable good. Professional time should include hours spent directly with *or on behalf of* the patient, and on administrative matters. The axiom, "He also serves who only stands and waits" is applicable here. Thus, resources spent on continuing education and training and on standing ready to serve when needed (sometimes referred to as latent service reserve; Donabedian, 1973) should be added to the time spent in patient care for purposes of computing costs.

Others may argue that the cost of neuropsychological services should be assessed as an "add on" to the patient's total health-care costs. The validity of this assumption poses an empirical question: Is it possible that the impact of neuropsychology services on the "bottom line" may be less than what would have been calculated if only the cost of the service alone was considered? This occurs when neuropsychological services offset the need for patients to use other services, so that the impact of using neuropsychologists on the bottom-line costs is less than the actual cost of the neuropsychological services alone. Although some evidence that offsets exist in mental health services generally (Kashner & Rush, 1999), the issue of offsets for neuropsychology has not been researched. Based on the work of Donabedian (1973), there are several reasons why the total cost of care may fall (or rise) for patients seeking care from neuropsychologists (see Table 21.1).

Estimating Direct Costs of Care

Economists typically measure health-care costs by multiplying the quantity of services consumed for each type of service by the cost per unit for that service, and summing the cost for each service over all services. The challenge to investigators are (a) how to classify services, (b) how to measure a "unit cost" for each service type, and (c) how to determine how much of each service the consumer has used over a given time period.

Classification. Services should be classified into clinically meaningful categories, exhausting all care the patient is likely to receive, and should be reasonably specific describing what was actually done for the patient and the level of skills required from the professional, so that the cost to produce the service is likely to remain the same across different health-care providers and over patients who receive the care. Another important characteristic is that data must be available to permit investigators to calculate a "cost per unit of service" and to measure the quantity that patients consumed from each defined service. We recommend (Kashner, Rush, & Altshuler, 1999) counting the number of outpatient procedures as defined by physicians' CPT codes (American Medical Association, 1998), inpatient days by diagnosis-related groupings (*St.*

TABLE 21.1. Changes in Health-Care Cost That Might Be Associated with Neuropsychology

(A1) *Substitution*: Patients may rely on neurologists, psychiatrists, or general medical physicians for cognitive evaluation and treatment procedures that might not be necessary were the patient to access these services through a neuropsychologist.

(A2) *Improved health*: Patients in better mental status are frequently observed physiologically to have better physical status. Cost of care may fall as patients, achieving improved cognitive status and mental health from therapies prescribed following a neuropsychological examination, also see improvement in physical status that, in turn, require fewer medical services.

(A3) *Treatment productivity*: Referring physicians, better informed about the status of their patients through neuropsychological examinations, may be more efficient in achieving the patient's health goals with fewer resources.

(A4) *Adherence*: Physicians, armed with a better understanding of patients' conditions, may be able to better intervene to help patients comply with medical advice and, thus, improve health outcomes of existing services.

On the other hand, medical costs may go up.

(B1) *Discovery*: When examining the patent, the neuropsychologist may discover illnesses and refer patients to seek health-care providers who otherwise they might not have sought.

(B2) *Complementary:* Patients who experience improved cognitive and mental status may begin to place greater importance on their health and, by gaining a "will to live," seek medical care to protect other aspects of their health.

(B3) *Longevity and wealth*: Patients who recover from neurologic illnesses or undergo cognitive rehabilitation and reenter the workforce may have the paradoxical effect of living longer and gaining the financial resources to consume more services.

(B4) *System effect*: Patients with improved neurologic functioning may have better mental capacity to work the system and advocate providers to furnish more health care and third-party payers to underwrite its cost.

Anthony's DRG Guidebook, 1998); and prescription fills by national drug code. Other services are measured in terms of number of days or visits by facility type (e.g., emergency room, long-term psychiatric care, nursing home, addiction rehabilitation, domiciliary care, transitional residence), day-treatment days, family doctor appointments, and home health-care visits. These aggregated measures are not all-encompassing, however, and do not reflect differences in the intensity of care within each service type. These strategies are recommended because such information generally is available on uniform patient billing records maintained by providers for reimbursement purposes, including public facilities such as the Department of Veterans Affairs and state Medicaid programs. When investigating specific protocols, such as evaluations and interventions conducted by neuropsychologists, the specific services pertaining to the protocol could be defined and separately counted from similar services produced outside the protocol. For instance, one could distinguish a service provided by a neuropsychologist from those provided by a neurologist or psychiatrist.

Unit Costs. Consistent with the recommendations from the Pubic Health Service Panel on Cost-Effectiveness Analyses (Gold et al., 1996), unit costs are intended to reflect the lost opportunity, or "opportunity costs," representing societal value placed on the best alternative use for resources allocated to provide care. There are four ways to estimate these costs. First, unit costs can be computed from *microcosting* studies. Here, the investigator traces all inputs used to actually produce a defined service. In some cases, only one resource is actually followed (such as the neuropsychologist's time). The total cost to produce the service is determined by assuming that all costs associated with the neuropsychologist's practice are distributed as the traced resource. These methods have good internal validity in that the investigators understand well how specific services in the protocol were produced, but they may have poor external validity to judge how much similar services would cost had those services been produced using other service providers and in other settings. A second method is to base unit costs on *actual neuropsychologist charges* for each service, adjusted by cost-to-charge ratios. These estimates can come from actual third-party payments to providers that reflect negotiated rates in presumably price-competitive markets. Official estimates of cost to charge ratios are available in the *Federal Register* as applied to the Medicare program. Although having poor internal validity to reflect the actual costs incurred by professionals providing services to study patients, these methods permit investigators to determine how costs may vary if estimates were based on different markets, encompassing a range of third-party payers, managed care plans, and other aspects of economic cost environments across different regions, facilities, and time periods. That is, costs are computed as a range representing "what if" the care were provided under Medicare fees, various state Medicaid fees, third-party payment schedules, or by patients out-of-pocket in affluent markets. Third, unit costs can be computed based on *cost-accounting databases* (Drummond, O'Brien, Stoddard & Torrance, 1997). Here, unit costs are computed by determining the annual total expenditures and imputed rents for equipment and buildings and grounds for a clinician's practice where the service is provided, and dividing by the total number of services that the practice produced over the same accounting period. Finally, *econometric* methods are used to infer unit costs by examining how total costs by facility, or across time, vary with the number of services the facility produced (Barnett, 1997).

Use of Care. Use of care can be computed by (a) administering standardized or structured questionnaires to patients and collateral sources; (b) abstracting medical records maintained by the patient's health-care providers, or (c) extracting administrative or computerized databases from health-care providers, third-party payers, and managed care and utilization review organizations. Advantages and disadvantages of each are reviewed elsewhere (Kashner, 1998; Kashner, Rush & Altshuler, 1999; Kashner, Suppes, Rush & Altshuler, 1999). Briefly, medical charts are considered by many to be a gold standard, although their completeness and accuracy have not gone unquestioned. Computerized administrative files are inexpensive to access, but there have been reported problems with (a) incomplete data; (b) nonreporting of patient "out-of-plan" use; (c) nonstandardized definitions and collection procedures, making interfile merges difficult; and (d) licensing laws and rules of patient confidentiality that complicate file transfers. On the positive side, the billing function and performance evaluation purposes of many administrative files may lead some systems to include checks and balances that ensure data accuracy and completeness (Fowles et al., 1995). Finally, consumer surveys are well known among epidemiologists to measure national use rates. In some cases, surveys are the only method available when provider and administrative files are unattainable. However, the accuracy of self-reports will vary with (a) the saliency of the medical event (interferes with lifestyle, life-threatening situation, impacts vocation or education, recent, more frequent); (b) intensity of care, such as those involving long hospital stays or invasive surgeries; (c) characteristics of the patient, including premorbid factors as well as acquired cognitive impairment; (d) interviewer characteristics, including respondent's expectations and interviewer attitudes and styles; and (e) presence of collateral family members or friends. The presence of cognitive abnormalities among respondents (i.e., errors in comprehension, recall, decreased motivation, and ability to respond) can create special problems when surveying patients with neurological disorders or mental illness. To account for some of these potential confounds, we recommend utilization information be obtained from various, or hybrid sources (Clark, Ricketts, & McHugo, 1996; Dresser, Feingold, Rosencranz, & Coltin, 1997; Kashner, Rush, & Altshuler, 1999) that rely on medical records when available, validated by comparing entries to administrative files and patient self reports, and replaced when unreliable or otherwise unavailable.

☐ Outcomes of Care

Cost–Benefit

Each year hundreds of cost outcome studies are published (Elixhauser, Halpern, Schmier, & Luce, 1998), with most differing in terms of how "outcomes" are defined and measured. As mentioned earlier, outcomes measured in terms of dollar benefits, or so-called *cost–benefit studies,* focus on the economic consequences of a change in health status that has been translated into dollars. Comparing a common dollar benefit with dollar input costs, cost–benefit analyses appeal to policymakers wishing to make results simple to voters and to compare findings across programs competing for legislative appropriations in both health- and nonhealth-related areas. Although the results are simple, its methods are complex and controversial. Foremost, one must (a) assign dollar values to human life and to human suffering, (b) estimate external effects when health benefits spill over to other persons besides the patient (e.g., family, friends, and employers), (c) calculate dollar benefits when health outcomes are uncertain, and (d) determine the "present value" for dollar benefits that accrue over a long time period (compare patients who obtain only temporary relief from symptoms versus a cure leading to long-lasting symptom relief).

Of special interest are methods to estimate dollar values to human life. The two most common approaches are based on human capital (Rice et al., 1985) and willingness-to-pay (Mishan, 1971) theories. Human capital theory measures economic loses by valuing human life with respect to the production potential of the patient in the home, called *household production,* and in the labor market, or *paid employment.* Some have argued these values can be inferred from legislative hearings and court awards for compensatory damages in wrongful death and personal injury actions (Kashner, 1990). However, these methods usually undervalue the very young, who will not be working for a long time, and the old, whose remaining productive life is short. In contrast, willingness-to-pay approaches measure the amount of money patients are willing and able to spend to avoid the effects of symptoms or a disorder. This approach introduces a "wealth bias" that places greater value on the health status of persons with more means to pay for services.

Cost–Utility

Cost–utility analyses (Patrick & Erickson, 1993) are based on measuring health states in terms of a common value, or utility. Borrowed from Jerry Bentham and eighteenth-century utilitarians, utility is a subjective measure of how consumers value different health states. The higher the measured utility, the greater the value and (presumably) the greater the sacrifice consumers would be willing to make to achieve the given health condition.

Utility often is measured using *standard gambles,* in which patients are asked how much risk they would be willing to take to become cured rather than remain in a given health state. The more risk they are willing to take, the less desirable is the given health state. For example, patients willing to risk a 10% chance of death to undergo an operation for chest pains would thus be considered as assigning a value of 10% to reflect the difference in life with chest pains to a life without chest pains. Conversely, patients willing to risk 30% to relieve blindness would have a utility loss of 30%. Here, by comparing a willingness-to-risk example of 30% for blindness and 10% for chest pains, one can determine the extent to which blindness is perceived as a worse condition in the minds of patients. Rather than risking death, one can alternatively examine *time trade-off.* Here, subjects are asked how much life expectancy in a given health state they would be willing to sacrifice in order to live life in a healthy state. The more life expectancy the patient is willing to sacrifice, the less desirable is the given health state (Drummond et al., 1997). In other methods, such as scaling and visual analogue procedures, patients are asked to rank various health states and assign numbers to reflect preferences, or to space each state along a scale so that the intervals between states reflect differences in desirability between outcomes.

Expressing outcomes in terms of measured utility as a *willingness to risk* permits comparisons of health outcomes across diseases, but without introducing the wealth bias found in willingness-to-pay approaches. The enthusiasm for such approaches is understandable, as policy makers can now turn to scientists to help render tough policy decisions regarding "who shall live" (Fuchs, 1974). Scientifically speaking, the enthusiasm for utility analyses in health care (Weinstein, Siegel, Gold, Kamlet & Russell, 1996) has likely outpaced the development of validated instruments to measure utility and the economic theory needed to interpret its findings (Starmer, 2000). Specifically, researchers should consider "whose" utility is being measured, survey techniques depend on respondents with spatial and quantitative skills, and there is evidence that consumer preferences concerning risk and uncertainty are more complex than what these survey tools were designed to take into account. However, the strength of these procedures is that they permit investigators to combine morbidity and mortality information into a single measure. Such tools are helpful to assess how clinical innovations will not only improve life expectancy but improve the *quality* of those years of life that are extended–an area of particular relevance to neuropsychology.

Cost-Effectiveness

Outcome measures based on effectiveness have varied, but generally may be classified by the following:

1. *Use of care:* Health services generally are thought to be "inputs" rather than "outcomes" of clinical care. Yet, certain patterns of health-care utilization can provide some insight into how health outcomes have progressed for some patients. For example, patients with severe mental illness may be viewed as having a bad outcome whenever there is an acute psychiatric readmission, crisis ER visit, or hotline crisis call. On the other hand, favorable outcomes would suggest patient compliance with medication follow-up visits, proper use of prescription drugs, and self-admission into substance abuse rehabilitation programs. Admission to long-term care is of direct interest when the clinical goal is to help patients maintain community living.
2. *Diagnosis:* The presence or absence of a diagnosis (such as recurring substance dependence) is of interest clinically, but generally it is inappropriate to reflect subtle changes in outcomes for chronic disorders (such as schizophrenia) that will remain with the patient for life. Comorbid conditions associated with a primary disorder (such as depressive symptoms associated with substance use disorders) are sometimes helpful to explain how well patients may be doing under a clinical program. Comorbid conditions can be assessed either as a presence or absence of the disease or, when multiple conditions are considered, summarized by counting the number of conditions reported. Counts of comorbid conditions usually are classified as chronic, treated with medication, diagnosed by a qualified clinician, or patient-reported as causing problems. Using comorbid conditions either as a predictor variable of health outcome or as a secondary measure of health outcomes will pose problems for studies evaluating the impact of neuropsychological services. For example, neuropsychological tests can be useful to clinicians in identifying or delineating certain disorders, and ultimately to inform consumers of the consequences of those disorders. Furthermore, without such tests, some disorders may go undetected and thus would be underreported among control patients who did not benefit from neuropsychological testing.
3. *Symptoms:* Patient symptomatology usually is represented as the presence or absence of specific symptoms, as a count of symptoms, or as a count of symptoms weighted by patient self-reported levels of symptom severity. Data may be obtained from structured lay or clinical interviews. Symptom measures are popular among health professionals because symptom relief frequently is the primary aim of clinical programs.
4. *Functioning outcomes:* These are designed to measure what patients are able to do. Examples include the capacity to work, walk, and rest; conduct home management, communicate, and interact socially with others; perform physical activities of daily living such as eating, dressing, and grooming; and instrumental activities such as taking medication, using the telephone, and getting to places. Measures of functioning can be disease-specific or reflect disability in terms of bed days, days in which the patient restricted activities for health reasons, mortality and life expectancy, or globally as indices of "physical," "mental," or "social" status.
5. *Quality of life:* Quality of life reflects health in terms of its impact on what the patient is able to achieve. Quality of life is represented in terms of the security, privacy, and autonomy of the patient's living environment, including income and ability to live in the community, number and quality of contacts with family and friends, intimate contacts, leisure activities, finances, employment and school participation, legal and safety issues, and contacts with criminal justice system. Assessing the

impact of health services on quality of life is important to patients, families, and the community.

6. *Satisfaction*. Outcomes reflecting patient satisfaction usually are classified into those reflecting patient opinion regarding access to and provision of care, concerns about the health-care system generally, perception of overall health status, and satisfaction with life and circumstances in general. Satisfaction measures are popular with public policymakers looking for votes, third-party payers looking for customers, and health-care administrators looking for paying patients.
7. *Combined measures*. There is a trend in the literature to combine morbidity and mortality data into a single index. The purpose is to find one assessment tool that can be applied to different illnesses, such as those with high mortality rates (heart disease, stroke) and those with high morbidity rates (major depressive disorder, substance use). The Quality Adjusted Life Years (QALY; Torrance & Feeny, 1989) estimate how long a person is likely to live in "life years" that are adjusted to reflect the morbidity patients are expected to experience during those years.

The choice of outcome measures to assess a clinical program should certainly depend on the psychometric properties of the measure (validity, reliability, ease and feasibility of administration, and generalizability). However, far too often investigators evaluate clinical programs by selecting outcome measures that will get attention from the public (quality of life, employment rates, community living, contacts with the criminal justice system) rather than measures that reflect the goals of the program (symptom reduction, compliance with treatment). Measures that are removed from the clinical program goals will be *statistically challenged* to show a detectable change, even though the program may, in fact, accomplish its clinical mission.

When more than one outcome measure is being considered, it is recommended that the *primary* outcome measure should be selected to assess directly whether or not the clinical goals of the program are met. Thus, one should evaluate an addictions treatment program by determining if subjects reduce substance use. Second, select other related outcome measures as *confirmatory*. Confirmatory measures are anticipated to show favorable effects, provided the clinical goals of the program are met. Thus, a confirmatory measure for an addictions program would be reductions in substance use-related symptoms (such as liver dysfunction and dizziness). A third category would be *exploratory* outcomes, enabling researchers to explore how far-reaching program success may be to impact patient life and well-being.

☐ Comparing Costs and Outcomes

In the simple case, the choice as to whether to accept or reject adding neuropsychological evaluations to a clinical program becomes clear if the inclusion is shown to lead to lower (higher) costs and better (worse) outcomes, as in Table 21.2.

Here, neuropsychological services should be included in routine practice if such procedures reduce costs without deteriorating patient outcomes, or if costs remain the same and patient outcomes improve. On the other hand, such an approach would suggest that assessments should not be performed automatically if costs increase without some direct or indirect benefit to the patient, or if costs remain the same but outcomes get worse. Problems arise for decision makers when neuropsychological testing leads

TABLE 21.2. Potential Policy Choices to Include or Exclude Neuropsychological Evaluations with Routine Care

		Costs		
		Increase	no difference	Decrease
Outcome	Improve	*Unclear*	Include	Include
	No change	Exclude	*Equivalent*	Include
	Worsen	Exclude	Exclude	*Unclear*

either to better outcomes but at the expensive of higher costs or to lower costs but with a tradeoff of poorer outcomes.

Whenever the choice is unclear, two cost-outcome statistics are useful. The cost–outcome ratio of differences statistic is based on Jerrell and Hu's (1989) formulation, which that can be used to measure how much additional outcome is produced for each additional health-care dollar expended for neuropsychological examinations. This can be computed by:

$$\text{Ratio of Differences} = \frac{\bar{o}_A - \bar{o}_U}{\bar{c}_A - \bar{c}_U}, \qquad \text{Eq.1A}$$

where $\bar{o}_A$ and $\bar{o}_U$ are average outcomes and $\bar{c}_A$ and $\bar{c}_U$ are average costs for patients with and without neuropsychological examinations, respectively. This statistic is intended to help policymakers balance improvements in health outcomes with increases in care costs. For example, suppose a neuropsychological consultation added $500 to the average cost of care for patients following traumatic brain injury, but the results of the evaluation were shown to be associated with a 50% reduction in the likelihood of multiple doctor and emergency room visits secondary to concerns about postconcussional symptoms. For these health and cost outcomes, one would calculate a cost–outcome ratio of difference of 1%; that is, the services of a neuropsychologist would reduce the likelihood of relapse by 1% for each additional dollar spent on the patient in the practice offering neuropsychological evaluations compared to the practice not offering such services.

It also is possible that the introduction of neuropsychological testing into some clinical settings may lead patients to use more, rather than fewer, health services. Thus, better outcomes may result from more care rather than from more efficacious treatments coming from clinicians who benefit from information obtained from neuropsychological testing. The cost outcome difference in ratios statistic measures the extent to which neuropsychological examinations improve the productivity of the practice for each dollar spent on care.

Mathematically, measuring the *difference in ratios* in cost outcomes between two programs is not straightforward. To understand these calculations, consider the health-care costs a practice spends to provide for the resources (inputs) needed to produce the care that, in turn, leads to changes in health outcomes (outputs). The relationship between costs of services and outcomes of those services can be represented by a function. Here, let o_A (c) and o_U (c) be health outcomes when a practice, with and without neuropsychological examinations, respectively, spends "c" dollars for the average. Then the change in outcome for each additional dollar spent on care, which economists call *marginal productivity,* can be calculated by: $[o(c_0 + \$1) - o(c_0)]/\$1$, where c_0 is the initial "cost" the practice spends on the average patient. Comparing the difference in marginal productivities between patients with and without neuropsychological examinations, one can calculate:

$$\text{Differences in Ratios} = \frac{[o_A(c_0 + \$1) - o_A(c_0)]}{\$1} - \frac{[o_U(c_0 + \$1) - o_U(c_0)]}{\$1} \qquad \text{Eq. 1B}$$

For example, a cognitive therapist in a clinical practice may reduce the risk of relapse for patients with major depressive disorder by 1% for each $100 the clinic spends on behalf of the patient. Suppose another program employing neuropsychological services was able to yield 1.5% for each $100 spent by the clinic? The difference of .5% per $100 represents an increase in the productivity of the second practice over the first. Dollar for dollar, the second clinic employing neuropsychological testing was able to produce an overall "bigger bang" for each dollar expended.

Summary

The constructs of economics and the application of cost–outcome assessment procedures are new to neuropsychology. Research in this area poses a number of challenges to the field (e.g., choice of variables to measure "outcome"), but it is time to begin to understand and address these issues. Clinical algorithms may provide a basis for helping to make sense of managed care by allowing experts and consumers to decide, based on scientific evidence, what should be done clinically that, in the end, will balance outcomes with costs. These endeavors provide rich opportunities to demonstrate the value of neuropsychological services while informing consumers and third-party payers who are interested in getting the most for limited health-care dollars. To play in such an arena, neuropsychologists must begin to systematically address issues of clinical utility and cost effectiveness by designing appropriate studies that would document their cost–outcomes. These studies should (a) take advantage initially of existing databases that contain information relevant to how services are provided in actual clinical settings; (b) include global measures of health-care costs; and (c) include outcome measures that reflect, at minimum, the clinical goals of neuropsychological evaluation and treatment.

References

American Medical Association. (1998). *Current procedural terminology* (4th ed.). Reston, VA: St. Anthony.

Barnett, P. G. (1997). Research without billing data: Econometric estimation of patient-specific costs. *Medical Care, 35,* 553–563.

Battistella, R., & Southby, R. M. (1968). Crisis in American medicine. *The Lancet, 7542,* 581–586.

Burner, S. T., & Waldo, D. R. (1995). National health expenditure projections, 1994–2005. *Health Care Financing Review, 16,* 221–242.

Clark, R. E., Ricketts, S. K., & McHugo, G. J. (1996). Measuring hospital use without claims: a comparison of patient and provider reports. *Health Services Research, 31,* 153–169.

Cullum, C. M. (1999, November). *Cognitive signatures.* Presidential Address for The National Academy of Neuropsychology, San Antonio, TX.

Donabedian, A. (1973). *Aspects of medical care administration*. Cambridge, MA: Harvard University Press.

Dresser, M. V. B., Feingold, L., Rosencranz, S. L., & Coltin, K. L. (1997). Clinical quality measurement: Comparing chart review and automated methodologies. *Medical Care, 35*, 539–552.

Drummond, M. F., O'Brien, B. J., Stoddard, G. L., & Torrance, G. W. (1997) *Methods for the economic evaluation of health care programmes*. Oxford: Oxford University Press.

Elixhauser, A., Halpern, M., Schmier, J., & Luce, B. R. (1998). Health care CBA and CEA from 1991 to 1996: An updated bibliography. *Medical Care, 36*, MS1–MS9.

Feldstein, P. J. (1979). *Health care economics*. New York: John Wiley.

Fowles, J. B., Lawthers, A. G., Weiner, J. P., Garnick, D. W., Petrie, D. S., & Palmer, R. H. (1995). Agreement between physicians' office records and Medicare Part B Claims data. *Health Care Financing Review, 16*,189–199.

Fuchs, V. R. (1974). *Who shall live?* New York: Basic Books.

Gaynor, M., Haas-Wilson, D., & Vogt, W. B. (2000). Are invisible hands good hands? Moral hazard, competition, and the second-best in health care markets. *Journal of Political Economy, 108*, 992–1005.

Gilbert, D. A., Altshuler, K. Z., Rago, W. V., Shon, S. P., Crismon, M. L., Toprac, M. G., & Rush, A. J. (1998). Texas Medication Algorithm Project: Definitions, rationale and methods to develop medication algorithms. *Journal of Clinical Psychiatry, 59*, 345–351.

Gold, M. R., Siegel, J. E., Russell, L. B., & Weinstein, M. C. (Eds.). (1996). *Cost-effectiveness in health and medicine*. New York: Oxford University Press.

Health Professions Education Assistance Acts of 1963 and 1976, PL 94-484.

Hill-Burton Act of 1946, PL 79-725.

Jerrell, J. M., & Hu, T. W. (1989). Cost-effectiveness of intensive clinical and case management compared with an existing system of care. *Inquiry, 26*, 224–234.

Kashner, T. M. (1998). Agreement between administrative files and written medical records: A case of the Department of Veterans Affairs. *Medical Care, 36*,1324–1336.

Kashner, T. M. (1990). Present-future gratification tradeoffs: Does economics validate psychometric studies?." *Journal of Economic Psychology, 11*, 247–268.

Kashner, T. M. (1982). Cost effectiveness of lead screening, comment. *New England Journal of Medicine, 307*, 1260.

Kashner, T. M., & Rush, A. J. (1999). Measuring cost offsets of psychotherapy. In N. E. Miller & K. M. Magruder (Eds.), *The cost effectiveness of psychotherapy: A guide for practitioners, researchers and policymakers* (pp. 109–121). New York: Oxford University Press.

Kashner, T. M., Rush, A. J., & Altshuler, K. Z. (1999). Measuring costs of guideline-driven mental health care: The Texas Medication Algorithm Project. *Journal of Mental Health Policy and Economics, 2*, 111–121.

Kashner, T. M., Rush, A. J., & Altshuler, K. Z. (1997). Managed care and the focus on outcomes research. *Journal of Practical Psychiatry and Behavioral Health, 3*, 135–145.

Kashner, T. M., Suppes, T., Rush, A. J., & Altshuler, K. Z. (1999). Measuring use of outpatient mental health services: A comparison of self reports and provider records. *Evaluation and Program Planning, 22*, 31–39.

Mishan, E. J. (1971). Evaluation of life and limb: A theoretical approach. *Journal of Political Economy, 79*, 687–705.

Naugle, R. I., Cullum, C. M., & Bigler, E. D. (1998). *Introduction to clinical neuropsychology*. Austin, TX: Pro-Ed.

Nurse Training Act of 1964, PL 88-581.

Patrick, D. L., & Erickson, P. (1993). *Health status and health policy: Allocating resources to health care*. New York: Oxford University Press.

Public Health Service Acts (Regional Medical Programs) of 1965, PL 89-239; (Comprehensive Health Planning) of 1966, PL-89-749; (Partnership for Health) of 1967, PL 90-174.

Rice, D. P., Hodgson, T. A., & Kpstein, A. N. (1985). The economic costs of illness: A replication and update. *Health Care Financing Review, 7*, 61–80.

Rush, A. J., & Prien, R. F. (1995). From scientific knowledge to the clinical practice of psychopharmacology: Can the gap be bridged? *Psychopharmacological Bulletin, 31,* 7–20.

Rush, A. J., Rago, W. V., Crismon, M. L., Toprac, M. G., Shon, S. P., Suppes, T., Miller, A. L., Trivedi, M. H., Swann, A. C., Biggs, M. M., Shores-Wilson, K., Kashner, T. M., Pigott, T., Chiles, J. A., Gilbert, D. A., & Altshuler, K. Z. (1999). Medication treatment for the severely and persistently mentally ill: The Texas Medication Algorithm Project. *Journal of Clinical Psychiatry, 60,* 284–291.

Social Security Act Amendments, Section 1122, PL 92-603; and the National Health Planning and Resources Development Act (Health Systems Agencies) of 1974, PL 93-641.

Social Security Act of 1965, PL 89-97; Amendments of 1972, PL 92-603; Tax Equity and Fiscal Responsibility Act of 1982, PL 97-248.

St. Anthony's DRG guidebook (1998). Reston, VA: St. Anthony, Inc.

Starmer, C. (2000). Developments in non-expected utility theory: The hunt for a descriptive theory of choice under risk. *Journal of Economic Literature, 38,* 332–382.

Torrance, G. W., & Feeny, D. (1989). Utilities and quality-adjusted life years. *International Journal of Technology Assessment in Health Care, 5,* 559–575.

Weinstein, M. C., Siegel, J. E., Gold, M. R., Kamlet, M. S., & Russell, L. B. (1996). Recommendations of the panel on cost-effectiveness in health and medicine. *Journal of the American Medical Association, 276,* 1253–1258.

Weinstein, M. C., & Stason, W. B. (1977). Foundations of cost-effectiveness analysis for health and medical practices. *New England Journal of Medicine, 296,* 716–721.

Zakzanis, K. K., Leach L., & Kaplan, E. (1999). *Neuropsychological differential diagnosis.* Lisse, The Netherlands: Swets & Zeitlinger.

POSTSCRIPT

Reflections and Future Directions

George P. Prigatano
Neil H. Pliskin

Reflections

Kashner and Rush (1999) reviewed the health-care costs in the United States and noted that in 1932, "Medical costs amounted to only 4% of the gross domestic product (GDP)" (p. 109). By 1960, the figure was 5.4%. By 1995, the figure increased to 14.2%, with a projected estimate of 17.9% by 2005. In Chapter 1 of this volume, it was noted that the 15% figure was considered unacceptable by many and, in the attempt to curb the tide, managed care was upon us by the mid-1990s. While the battle with managed care organizations continues, the need for clinical neuropsychologists to be fiscally responsible in the conduct of their professional duties should continue indefinitely.

Like other health professionals, clinical neuropsychologists must acquaint themselves with health-care economics and demonstrate the clinical utility and cost–outcome of their work. This book, as noted in the preface, is a beginning step in that direction.

As we reflect on the various chapters in this volume, we are impressed that clinical neuropsychologists have numerous services to provide that have clear value for health care in the United States and abroad. Moreover, those services can impact a wide variety of individuals. These services include careful and systematic documentation of impairments of higher cerebral functioning that aid in treatment planning, differential diagnosis, assessment of treatment efficacy, helping make clinically sensitive decisions about capacity of an individual to return to work, and clarifying the extent of that disturbance for legal matters.

Clinical neuropsychologists also are actively engaged in meaningful education and training programs for family members faced with managing a brain-dysfunctional individual. Clinical neuropsychologists are at the forefront of rehabilitation programs aimed at returning brain-dysfunctional patients back to productive lifestyles or at least independence. They have articulated the need to address both cognitive and affective disturbances in the assessment of various forms of neurological disorders and psychological treatment. They also are actively involved and concerned about how neuropsychological test findings can be translated into more appropriate educational programs.

The impact of neuropsychological assessment in cases involving medical legal issues also has been clearly established.

Clinical neuropsychologists are beginning to talk to health-care economists, as Chapter 21 documents. They also are systematically assessing the economics of private practice (Sweet, Moberg, & Suchy, 2000). We see these as positive signs for the future. It may be worthwhile to also reflect on possible future directions.

Future Directions

As noted in Chapter 2, the value of any neuropsychological service can be measured in both objective and subjective terms. In fact, we encourage this line of thinking, as we feel both dimensions are necessary to determine the degree to which someone (the patient, family, hospital administrator, insurance carrier, managed care representative, physician, attorney, etc.) is willing to pay for such services. This not only determines charges and fees for service, but ultimately affects the salary levels and rates of reimbursement for different services. These are important issues for clinical neuropsychologists throughout the world.

Second, clinical neuropsychologists, like many other health-care professionals, are typically not trained or interested in measuring the direct and indirect costs of their services. Yet, as a profession, if we do not take on this responsibility, someone else will calculate these for us. The end result is that the economic analysis may select variables and methods of comparison and have others' economic interests in mind rather than the interests of our patients, or the profession we work to develop. Thus, we must take on this responsibility to remain professionally strong. We encourage academic departments of psychology to provide graduate courses on health-care economics and the practice of psychology. That course should include specific discussions on how to assess the cost–outcomes of various psychological services including those considered under clinical neuropsychology. We strongly recommend that students be exposed not only to mathematical formulas for doing this type of research but also to theoretical readings in the area. Even more importantly they should have an opportunity to talk directly with health-care economists about their concerns and their views of our discipline. In this regard, it is worthwhile to have insurance companies and representatives from managed care organizations talk with psychologists during their training years regarding what they consider important sources of information necessary to continue to economically support what psychologists do.

Certainly psychologists in general, as well as clinical neuropsychologists in particular, vary in their understanding of the concepts and methods health-care economists use when evaluating their services. Yet, as we have hoped to demonstrate, we are indeed capable of addressing this problem if we put our professional energies to it. We are hopeful that the authors of this volume have examined the topics that are professionally stimulating and helped to provide ideas relevant to conducting future research in this broad area. In order for our profession to go beyond this beginning, many more neuropsychologists are going to have to dedicate themselves to conducting research in this area. This is necessary if neuropsychologists' work is going to impact health-care policy and methods of reimbursement. Neuropsychologists need to take a broad view of what is, in fact, cost–outcome research and how they can demonstrate their value within the context of this model of analyzing both the economic and noneconomic value of their work. Our profession has survived managed care and will continue to survive it. However, the quality of our professional life is highly dependent on our ability to demonstrate the value of what we do and how it truly impacts the health care of the persons we serve. As we can show that our services are not only useful but economically sound, we are in a much better position to make an argument for appropriate reimbursement for services we provide.

Future outcome research by clinical neuropsychologists might consider some of the points that were made in Chapter 1. It was noted in that chapter that health-care economists not only look at the cost of the service, they look at the severity of the health-care problem that service attempts to address. They then consider the scientific evidence for the efficacy of existing services or treatments to substantially reduce the health-care problem that is being addressed.

This type of thinking is important for clinical neuropsychologists. What are, in fact, the biggest problems our patients face? How severe are those problems as they impact the economics of health care in the United States and throughout the world? Finally, how effective are our methods for reducing these problems.

This type of thinking not only makes neuropsychologists better businessmen and women, it makes them better scientists and clinicians. With this type of thinking, we can begin to reformulate what are the relevant questions and, therefore, look for answers that are most useful to our field.

For example, we found it intriguing that neuropsychological test findings may predict mortality better than neuroimaging findings in patients with certain types of brain tumors, particularly those of the metastatic type (see Chapter 8). Neuropsychological test findings may help document when the elderly are, in fact, capable of driving, even when they show early signs of dementia (Chapter 9). This could greatly contribute to their quality of life. Neuropsychological assessment can guide rehabilitation activities (see Chapters 3 and 14) and help in cases of differential diagnosis (Chapters 4 and 9). Furthermore, neuropsychological assessments can help determine when it would be dangerous for someone to return to work (see Chapter 18) as well as when someone is feigning neuropsychological deficits (Chapter 20).

To date, there are no cost-effectiveness studies on neuropsychological services, but there are studies that help demonstrate the economic benefits of neuropsychologically oriented rehabilitation (see Mehblye & Larson, 1994, cited in Chapter 14) and the relative value of training patient caregivers in managing demented patients versus purely providing them with support groups (see Chapter 10).

In the future, neuropsychological test findings undoubtedly will be coupled with neuroimaging findings to aid our diagnostic mission and reveal important facts about brain function. This should greatly improve our ability to use neuropsychological assessment in evaluating patients with epilepsy (Chapter 11) as well as patients showing nonepileptic seizure-like events (Chapter 12). We will refrain from commenting on each chapter, but simply highlight these points as fruitful areas to think about when conducting research on clinical neuropsychology and cost–outcomes.

☐ Cost Outcome Research and the "Evidence-Based Movement" in Medicine: A Final Comment

Undoubtedly, one of the factors contributing to the evidence-based movement in medicine was the avoidance of costly treatments that were ineffective. Friedland (1998), in introducing the topic of evidence-based medicine, nicely summarized the traditional medical paradigm for making decisions regarding patients with the evolving paradigm that uses quantitative analyses, statistically based decision rules, and ultimately cost-effectiveness analysis. He noted,

> Although the new evidence-based medicine paradigm does not always provide a definitive answer, it does provide an explicit framework that helps us evaluate the validity of the relevant literature and, with application of certain key concepts and calculations, better estimate the net benefit of this intervention for our patients. (p. 3)

These are nice words, but in reality, there are both objective and subjective markers of value for each patient that drive consumer spending and the willingness of third-party payers to pay for various clinical services. No one would argue that there should not be "evidence" to justify what we do, and clinical practice should be conducted with the notion that there are finite economic resources. Yet what constitutes evidence is not always clear, and many variables can influence the human experience of satisfaction or lack of satisfaction with a given intervention. In the name of evidence-based medicine, errors can be made. For example, a review of the effectiveness of cognitive rehabilitation for persons with TBI was considered "systematic" because it employed certain experimental and statistical criteria for papers reviewed (Carney et al., 1999). Papers that did not meet inclusionary criteria were excluded for review using evidence-based criteria. The end result was less than a systematic review. Conclusions completely missed the complexity of providing and evaluating cognitive rehabilitation after TBI (Prigatano, 1999). Also, a recent prospective, randomized control study on cognitive rehabilitation (Salazar et al., 2000) came to inaccurate conclusions because the author's research findings were not placed in the proper clinical or scientific context (Prigatano, 2000a). More than 20 years ago, before the evidence-based movement, Yalom (1980) articulately noted the problems of measuring important psychological changes in people following psychotherapy.

These examples are provided not to dismiss the importance of "data" when making decisions. They highlight, however, the point that in some instances it is difficult to define what actually constitutes evidence; more importantly, it is often difficult to properly interpret that evidence. Clinical neuropsychologists must constantly ask what, in fact, is their clinical experience working with patients and not easily dismiss that experience. Moreover, they must better understand what the patient actually experiences when undergoing a given service (Prigatano, 2000b). The question then becomes: How can evidence-based methods and cost-outcome research analyses, including cost-effective analyses, aid our clinical decision making—not replace it. The same point can be found in the writings of Sackett et al. (2000) who has promoted evidence-based movement in Western medicine.

References

Carney, N., Chesnut, R. M., Maynard, H., Mann, N. C., Patterson, P., & Helfand, M. (1999). Effect of cognitive rehabilitation on outcomes for persons with traumatic brain injury: A systematic review. *Journal of Head Trauma Rehabilitation, 14*(3), 277–307.

Friedland, D. J. (1998). Introduction. In D. J. Friedland, A. S. Go, J. B. Davoren et al. (Eds.), *Evidence-based medicine: A framework for clinical practice* (pp. 1–8). Stamford, CT: Appleton & Lange.

Kashner, T. M., & Rush,, A. J. (1999). Measuring medical offsets in psychotherepy. In N. E. Miller & K. M. Magruder (Eds.), *Cost-effectiveness of psychotherapy: A guide for academic research and policymakers* (pp. 109–121). New York: Oxford University Press.

Mehlbye, J., & Larsen, A. ((1994). Social and economic consequences of brain damage in Denmark: A case study. In A. L. Christensen & B. P. Uzzell (Eds.), *Brain injury and neuropsychological rehabilitation: International perspectives* (pp. 257–265). Hillsdale, NJ: Lawrence Erlbaum Associates.

Prigatano, G. P. (1999). Commentary: Beyond statistics and research design. *Journal of Head Trauma Rehabilitation, 14*(3), 308–311.

Prigatano, G. P. (2000a). Rehabilitation for traumatic brain injury (Letter). *Journal of the American Medical Association, 284*(14), 1783.

Prigatano, G P. (2000b). Neuropsychology, the patient's experience, and the political forces within our field. *Archives of Clinical Neuropsychology, 15*(1), 71–82.

Sackettt, D. L., Straus, S. E., Richardson, W. S., Rosenberg, W., & Haynes, R. B. (2000). *Evidence-based medicine: How to practice and teach ERM.* New York: Chruchill Livingstone.

Salazar, A. M., Warden, D. L., Schwab, K., et al. (2000). Cognitive rehabilitation for traumatic brain injury: A randomized trial. *Journal of the American Medical Association, 283,* 3075–301.

Sweet, J. J., Moberg, P. J., & Suchy, Y. (2000). Ten-year follow-up survey of clinical neuropsychologists, Part II: Private practice and economics. *The Clinical Neuropsychologist, 14*(4), 479–495.

Yalom, I. D. (1980). *Existential psychotherapy.* San Francisco: Harper Collins.

Chapter Learning Objectives

Chapter 1

At the completion of this chapter the reader will be able to:

1. Understand the concepts and challenges to neuropsychology involved in conducting cost outcome research.
2. Become acquainted with a new vocabulary, new sources of information and new research questions and methodologies, as it relates to health care economics and cost outcome research.

Chapter 2

At the completion of this chapter the reader will be able to:

1. Understand the concepts of objective and subjective markers of value as it relates to clinical neuropsychological work.
2. Describe different methods of conducting cost outcome research.

Chapter 3

At the completion of this chapter the reader will be able to:

1. Describe the neuropsychological impairments and outcomes following traumatic brain injury.
2. Describe a method for studying cost outcome of neuropsychological assessment after traumatic brain injury.

Chapter 4

At the completion of this chapter the reader will be able to:

1. Describe the clinical features of post-concussion syndrome.
2. Articulate the utility of the neuropsychological assessment for patients with persistent post-concussional disorder.

Chapter 5

At the completion of this chapter the reader will be able to:

1. Cite literature addressing the most common reactions, problems, and needs of families of traumatically brain injured adults and children.
2. Describe a method for demonstrating cost-effectiveness of services provided by neuropsychologists to family members after a traumatic brain injury.

Chanter 6

At the completion of this chapter the reader will be able to:

1. Cite studies supporting the cost effectiveness of neuropsychological services in stroke populations.
2. Describe a method for studying cost outcome in neuropsychological assessment after traumatic brain injury.

Chapter 7

At the completion of this chapter the reader will he able to:

1. Describe the neurobehavioral and neuroanatomical features associated with ACoA aneurysm rupture.
2. Describe potential cost outcome studies for neuropsychological services with ACoA patients.

Charter 8

At the completion of this chapter the reader will be able to:

1. Describe relevant literature supporting the utility of neuropsychological assessment in the evaluation of patients with neoplasms.
2. Describe a method for studying cost outcome of neuropsychological services in patients receiving treatment for neoplasms.

Chapter 9

At the completion of this chapter the reader will be able to:

1. Describe the clinical features of Alzheimer's Disease.
2. Describe several "markers of value" for neuropsychological services in the care of patients with dementia.

Chapter 10

At the completion of this chapter the reader will be able to:

1. Describe the clinical utility of neuropsychological services with the family of dementia patients.
2. Describe a method for analyzing economic value of consultation and treatment of family members with dementia.

Chapter 11

At the completion of this chapter the reader will be able to:

1. Articulate the utility of neuropsychological services commonly provided to patients with epilepsy.
2. Describe several potential ways for evaluating the cost effectiveness of neuropsychological services in the treatment of patients with epilepsy.

Chapter 12

At the completion of this chapter the reader will be able to:

1. Describe the relevant clinical issues in the diagnosis of nonepileptic seizures.
2. Understand the socioeconomic impact of nonepileptic seizures.

Chapter 13

At the completion of this chapter the reader will be able to:

1. Gain an understanding of the advantages and disadvantages between traditional psychoeducational assessment and neuropsychological assessment in determining whether a learning disability exists.
2. Learn about one method of investigating cost effectiveness of neuropsychological assessment in determining whether a learning disability exists.

Chapter 14

At the completion of this chapter the reader will be able to:

1. Define the key features of comprehensive holistic day-treatment programs.
2. Articulate the clinical utility of holistic day-treatment programs.

Chapter 15

At the completion of this chapter the reader will he able to:

1. Articulate the key issues in doing psychotherapy after brain injury.
2. Describe the clinical utility of psychotherapy with brain-dysfunctional patients.

Chapter 16

At the completion of this chapter the reader will he able to:

1. Describe the theoretical bases for cognitive rehabilitation.
2. Articulate relevant studies and research designs documenting the effectiveness of cognitive rehabilitation.

Chapter 17

At the completion of this chapter the reader will be able to:

1. Describe the unique role for neuropsychologists in the assessment of sports-related traumatic brain injury.
2. Articulate relevant cost effectiveness variables in sport neuropsychology.

Chapter 18

At the completion of this chapter the reader will be able to:

1. Describe the major contributions of neuropsychologists in the evaluation of the physician's cognitive capacity to practice medicine.
2. Describe a model for evaluating the cost outcome of neuropsychological services in the assessment of physician competency.

Chapter 19

At the completion of this chapter the reader will be able to:

1. Understand the role for neuropsychology in civil and criminal litigation.
2. Describe relevant "markers of value" for forensic neuropsychological services.

Chapter 20

At the completion of this chapter the reader will be able to:

1. Cite ways in which neuropsychological assessment can be cost effective through the detection of malingering claimants.
2. Describe the characteristics of different neuropsychological measures in the detection of malingering.

Chapter 21

At the completion of this chapter the reader will be able to:

1. Describe changes in health care economics that could influence the practice of neuropsychology.
2. Articulate a method for designing cost effectiveness studies that would emphasize the clinical goals of neuropsychological evaluation and treatment.

CME QUESTIONS

Chapter 1: Health-Care Economics and Clinical Neuropsychology

1. What percent of the gross domestic product (GDP) has been spent on healthcare in the United States in the last several years?
   a. Less than 5%
   b. 10%
   c. 15%
   d. 20%

2. The purpose of this book is to
   a. Help clinical neuropsychologists learn how to demonstrate the economic value of their work.
   b. Show the impact of clinical neuropsychological services on healthcare economy in the United States.
   c. Provide clinical neuropsychologists with a summary of the utility of their work.
   d. Provide an integrated overview of a large literature dealing with cost-effectiveness in clinical neuropsychology.

3. The challenge facing clinical neuropsychologists is to increase the standard of living for people without substantially increasing the proportion of the GDP devoted to healthcare costs in this country.
   a. True
   b. False

4. There are four basic forms of cost outcome measures.
   a. True
   b. False

5. Cost-effectiveness studies measure the dollars saved by the healthcare system given a clinical service.
   a. True
   b. False

6. Cost-effectiveness studies are based solely on randomized controlled studies.
   a. True
   b. False

7. In its simplest form, cost-effective analysis attempts to establish a ratio between the cost of a service divided by its outcome (the so-called cost-effectiveness analysis ratio).
   a. True
   b. False

8. When judging cost-effectiveness outcomes, policymakers often ask "how serious is a certain healthcare problem" as well as "how effective is a given intervention for it?"
   a. True
   b. False

Chapter 2: The Clinical Neuropsychological Examination: Scope, Cost, and Health-Care Value

1. Many factors guide the selection of a test battery for a given patient. Which of the following should not be one of the primary factors in selecting a battery of tests to be administered?
   a. The examiner's skill or knowledge
   b. The patient's clinical presentation
   c. Insurance reimbursement rates
   d. The diagnostic question

2. Typically, comprehensive neuropsychological examination assesses functions across numerous dimensions; this chapter discusses 10 such dimensions. Often, however, brief evaluations or cognitive screening instruments neglect to assess which of the following functions?
   a. New memory and learning
   b. Emotional expression/perception
   c. Attention/concentration
   d. Speech and language skills

3. In the current managed care environment, the cost-benefit of neuropsychological examinations is under scrutiny. Which of the following would be considered a subjective marker of the value of a neuropsychological examination?
   a. Reducing the patient's level of distress
   b. Directing treatment decision
   c. Reducing costs and liabilities
   d. Improving decision making

4. In assessing the cost-effectiveness of neuropsychological evaluations, the costs, charges, fees, and value of the examination must be considered. Which of the following terms refers to the amount of dollars actually paid for services?
   a. Cost
   b. Value

c. Charges
d. Fees

5. The benefit or value of neuropsychological evaluations can be evaluated in terms of both objective and subjective markers. Neuropsychological examinations can help determine which of the following?
   a. A person's ability or readiness to return to work or school
   b. The effectiveness of treatment or surgery
   c. Differentiating neurologic versus psychiatric processes
   d. All of the above

6. In a typical nonprofit hospital or medical center, which of the following statements best describes the economic balance for neuropsychological evaluations and payment for service?
   a. Charges for the neuropsychological examination and fees collected tend to be equivalent.
   b. Neuropsychologists tend to be overpaid for their work and generate high profits.
   c. Revenue generated by neuropsychologists falls below the cost of providing the service.
   d. Participating in forensic evaluations or research activities does not help improve the amount of revenue generated.

7. Drummond (1997) proposed several equations to help study the cost-benefit of health services quantitatively. Which of the following is not included as a component of his equations?
   a. Healthcare costs
   b. Willingness to pay
   c. Patient/family resources
   d. Prognosis

8. Potential topics to further investigate the cost-effectiveness and value of neuropsychological evaluation were presented. Which of the following was not discussed?
   a. Investigating the actual dollar value patients and families would place on the services provided
   b. Training psychometrists to conduct a greater portion of the evaluation
   c. The economic societal costs of working 50 to 60 hours/week to improve revenue
   d. Comparing the cost of a neuropsychological service to an alternative service intended to achieve the same outcome

Chapter 3: Neuropsychological Assessment After Traumatic Brain Injury in Adults

1. Information obtained from a neuropsychological evaluation can be used in which of the following ways?
   a. To assess the impact of new medications
   b. To increase the injured person's awareness of cognitive strengths and weaknesses

c. To provide a means of assessing the effectiveness of cognitive rehabilitation
d. All of the above

2. Neuropsychological evaluation after a severe TBI would be reasonable at what intervals?
   a. When the patient's Glasgow Coma Scale score reaches 12
   b. 3, 6, and 12 months after injury
   c. Monthly after post-traumatic amnesia resolves
   d. At yearly intervals after injury; earlier evaluation is not fruitful

3. Given the importance of cognition to daily functioning, performance on neuropsychological evaluation should be the predominant predictor of return to activities such as competitive employment, living independently, and driving.
   a. True
   b. False

4. In most cases, neuropsychological tests were not intended to address the capacity to return to functional activities. New tests are needed to address issues such as the capacity to make financial decisions, to return to driving, and to resume employment.
   a. True
   b. False

5. Which of the following deficits is least likely to persist after severe TBI due to blunt head trauma?
   a. Memory impairment
   b. Slowed cognitive speed
   c. Aphasia
   d. Decreased attention

6. Which of the following contributes most to family stress after TBI?
   a. Neurobehavioral problems
   b. Physical limitations
   c. Cognitive impairment
   d. Vestibular disturbance

7. Empirical studies have shown positive associations between neuropsychological test findings and all the following except
   a. Return to work
   b. Stability of employment
   c. Return to driving
   d. Need for supervision

8. What percent of inpatient rehabilitation charges is due to neuropsychological services?
   a. 20%
   b. 15%
   c. 10%
   d. <5%

Chapter 4: Neuropsychological Assessment and Management of Patients with Persistent Postconcussional Disorders

1. Which of the following was not proposed as an explanation for prolonged recover/disability after MTBI?
    a. Depression
    b. Post-traumatic stress disorder
    c. Systemic lupus
    d. "Vulnerable" personality styles

2. What was discussed as a cost-effective scenario for the delivery of neuropsychological services, including
    a. Test and treat in the first 3 months *post*-injury.
    b. Test in the emergency room
    c. Test only after 2 years post-injury.
    d. Clinical interview within 3 months of injury followed by comprehensive assessment.

3. What types of information might be helpful to render more conclusive opinions within an assessment context?
    a. Results of past standardized tests e.g. (GRE, SAT).
    b. Completion of significant other rating scale
    c. Records of previous psychiatric treatment
    d. None of the above
    e. All of the above

4. Approximately how many individuals sustain an MTBI each year in the United States?
    a. 1.3 million
    b. 8 million
    c. 130,000
    d. 5 million

5. The research literature seems to suggest which of the following as the most likely explanation for the prolonged recovery from MTBI?
    a. Psychogenic explanations
    b. Neurogenic explanations
    c. The interaction between neurogenic and psychogenic explanations
    d. Malingering

6. Approximately what percentage of individuals who sustain a documented MTBI go on to make a complete or near complete recovery?
    a. 50%
    b. 80%–90%
    c. 10%–20%
    d. 60%

7. Which of the following was discussed in terms of providing a definition of MTBI?
    a. DSM–IV
    b. Glasgow Coma Scale

   c. American Academy of Rehabilitation Medicine criteria
   d. All of the above

8. The need for future research tools with MTBI patients might best be provided by which of these?
   a. Separating at baseline those patients who fall into the "miserable minority" from those who are likely to make a full recovery
   b. Develop, standardize, and norm one nationwide neuropsychology test battery
   c. Develop better malingering measures
   d. Further investigating the assessment potential of the Internet.

Chapter 5: Providing Psychological Services to Families of Brain-Injured Adults and Children in the Present Health-Care Environment

1. Family members report ongoing needs for information and professional support even two or more years after the occurrence of their relative's brain injury.
   a. True
   b. False

2. Which of the following consistently relates to measures of caregiver burden or distress?
   a. caregiver report of physical deficits (for the injured person)
   b. caregiver report of behavioral and emotional problems (for the injured person)
   c. length of time since injury
   d. all of the above

3. When working with families in which a child has sustained a moderate to severe brain injury, clinicians should evaluate:
   a. the child's cognitive and emotional/behavioral status
   b. parental stress/alliance with the child
   c. marital adjustment and family functioning
   d. all of the above

4. Mild head injury in adults and children may only cause transient cognitive or behavioral difficulties so there is little need for family assessment or intervention within this population.
   a. True
   b. False

5. When counseling family members of TBI patients, clinicians should be prepared to help with:
   a. the family member's sense of grief or loss in response to perceived changes in their brain-injured relative
   b. questions about how to best deal with difficult behaviors or cognitive limitations of the injured family member
   c. concerns regarding the well being of all family members, not just the injured person
   d. all of the above

6. Hosack & Rocchio (1995) observed that the effects of managed health care on family services in TBI rehabilitation have:
    a. improved the quality of staff-family relationships during rehabilitation
    b. allowed adequate preparation of family members to serve as caregivers for the injured family member
    c. increased the need for early agreement between staff and families on rehabilitation goals to be addressed
    d. led to the development of more comprehensive family programs

7. A researcher interested in a *cost-benefit analysis* of family services might measure costs of treatment in relation to:
    a. decreased behavioral problems for the TBI family member
    b. extent of improvement in a caregiver's level of depression
    c. expenditures for attendant care for the TBI family member
    d. comparison of amount of staff time required for two different family services

8. Smith & Godfrey (1995) found that family members in their family support program had fewer physician visits compared to comparison group family members. This is an example of:
    a. cost-utility comparison
    b. cost-effectiveness of family services
    c. false-positive findings
    d. medical cost offset changes

Chapter 6: Neuropsychological Assessment of Patients with Cerebrovascular Accidents

1. There are a number of biological and lifestyle factors that contributes to one's risk for ischemic stroke. Which of the following has not consistently been shown to be a risk factor for ischemic stroke?
    a. Hypertension
    b. Modest alcohol consumption
    c. Concurrent cigarette smoking
    d. Obesity

2. The risk of mortality due to stroke varies among individuals. Which of the following effects one's mortality risk?
    a. Age
    b. Gender
    c. Severity of aphasia after stroke
    d. All of the above

3. Which of the following is not included in the most recent estimates of the costs of stroke in Western countries?
    a. Cost of inpatient medical care
    b. Cost of nursing home care
    c. Cost of cognitive and emotional sequelae of stroke
    d. Lost earnings due to premature disability/death due to stroke

4. Neuropsychological deficits are common among stroke patients. Which cognitive domain frequently shows the most prominent impairments?
   a. Attention and information processing speed
   b. Visual-spatial skills
   c. Learning and memory
   d. Language skills

5. Which of the following is the best predictor of poor functional outcome following ischemic stroke?
   a. Aphasia
   b. Memory impairment
   c. Hemi-neglect
   d. Slowed mentation

6. In which area do scientific studies exist that document the efficacy of using neuropsychological testing in stroke patients?
   a. Prediction of functional outcome
   b. Recognition of executive dysfunction and unawareness
   c. Diagnosis of co-morbid dementia
   d. All of the above

7. Which of the following is true regarding post-stroke depression?
   a. It typically develops in the chronic phase of stroke recovery
   b. It is an uncommon occurrence
   c. It differs in presentation from idiopathic clinical depression
   d. It occurs more commonly following cerebral vascular accident in frontal-subcortical regions of the brain

8. All of the following parties can *directly* benefit from neuropsychological services except:
   a. Patient and family
   b. Referral source
   c. Third party payors
   d. All of the above

Chapter 7: Neuropsychological Assessment of Patients Who Have Undergone Surgical Repair of Anterior Communicating Artery Aneurysms

1. The highest incidence of aneurysmal rupture is between the ages of ________ and is occurs more frequently in ____________.
   a. 30–40, males
   b. 30–40, females
   c. 40–70, males
   d. 40–70, females

2. What are the 3 neurobehavioral impairments collectively referred to as "ACoA Syndrome"?
   a. abulia, mutism and confabulation
   b. amnesia, confabulation, personality changes

c. amnesia, language disorders, confabulation
d. confabulation, motor disorders and language disorders

3. The following are neurobehavioral impairments that can be observed following ACoA:
   a. mutism
   b. Alien hand syndrome
   c. abulia
   d. confabulation
   e. all of the above

4. The following, is NOT an example of treatment contributions that neuropsychologist can provide in the treatment of ACoA patients ______.
   a. behavioral monitoring of pharmacological interventions
   b. decision making for surgical interventions
   c. vocational planning
   d. family education
   e. none of the above

5. Depending on the stage of recovery (acute, chronic, etc), the neuropsychologist's main activity with ACoA patients include ______.
   a. cognitive, emotional and behavioral assessment and treatment
   b. primarily testing cognitive functions
   c. making decisions for surgical interventions
   d. deciding if the patient should return to work

6. Neuropsychological services for people with ACoA aneurysm have _____.
   a. been shown to significantly improve cognitive abilities in everyday life
   b. proven effective in only a subset of individuals
   c. not been well documented or studied
   d. not been well integrated into rehabilitation plans

7. The "dual-lesion" hypothesis of confabulation states that _____.
   a. Two different lesions in the brain are required to make a diagnosis of the ACoA syndrome
   b. confabulation is only observed when a lesion of both the basal forebrain and frontal lobes coexist
   c. confabulation has both a psychiatric and an "organic" component
   d. confabulations are due to temporal order displacements and language dysfunction

8. While studies have shown that up to 84% of ACoA survivors are able to return to work and have a "good" recovery, this should be viewed cautiously because _____.
   a. significant psychological, emotional and cognitive problems have been observed even in survivors with little to no neurological impairment.
   b. these patients never return to the same level of work activity as they had premorbidly
   c. return to work is a poor measure of neurological recovery
   d. patients often return to work against the recommendations of the rehabilitation team

Chapter 8: Neuropsychological Assessment and Treatment of Patients with Malignant Brain Tumors

1. Which of the following does not contribute substantially to the neuropsychological functioning of patients with primary brain tumors?
    a. Tumor location
    b. Type of chemotherapy given
    c. Radiation treatment
    d. Tumor growth rate

2. Which of the following are uses of neuropsychological services in brain cancer settings?
    a. Neurosurgical planning
    b. Safety monitoring in clinical trials
    c. Determination of treatment efficacy
    d. All of the above

3. Which of the following are barriers to the practice of neuropsychological services in brain cancer settings?
    a. Patients generally have a poor prognosis and short life span
    b. Patients are unwilling to cooperate with testing
    c. Relatively few brain cancer health care teams have knowledge of or access to neuropsychological services
    d. Neuropsychological services are too expensive

4. In which of the following settings can neuropsychological services be of utility?
    a. End-of-life care
    b. Palliative rehabilitation strategies
    c. Palliative drug strategies
    d. All of the above

5. Which of the following describes the clinical benefit of a new drug according to the FDA?
    a. Survival
    b. Time to tumor recurrence
    c. Improvement of disease-related symptoms
    d. All of the above

6. Which of the following analyses is appropriate to assess which individuals benefit from a given treatment?
    a. Cost-utility analysis
    b. Cost minimization analysis
    c. Regression analysis
    d. Analysis of variance

7. Which of the following are desirable characteristics of a clinical trial battery of tests?
    a. Extremely comprehensive
    b. Able to be completed by most patients, even those who are ill
    c. High rate of false negative results
    d. All of the above

8. Which of the following is not true of brain cancer?
   a. It represents a small number of all newly diagnosed cancers
   b. Age at diagnosis is a major prognostic factor
   c. Patients with metastatic brain cancer do not have cognitive problems
   d. Most patients receive surgery, radiation, and chemotherapy

Chapter 9: The Clinical Utility of Neuropsychological Evaluation of Patients with Known or Suspected Dementia

1. Alzheimer's disease is a diagnosis of exclusion.
   a. True
   b. False

2. Quality adjusted years refers to:
   a. Years of functioning at maximum independence
   b. The number of years remaining before dementia sets in
   c. The number of years estimated before the patient will be institutionalized
   d. The number of years that a patient is taking an anticholinesterase inhibitor

3. Neuropsychological consultation can be especially beneficial in cases of suspected Alzheimer's disease to:
   a. Assist in differential diagnosis
   b. Assess the patient's functional status
   c. Evaluate and assist in patient management
   d. All of the above

4. Level of cognitive impairment is related to utilization of health care services.
   a. True
   b. False

5. The goals of neuropsychological intervention with dementia patients are to:
   a. Assist in adjustment to illness
   b. Provide focused cognitive training related to daily living in order to enhance autonomy
   c. Provide family education and behavioral management strategies
   d. All of the above

6. A cost utility analysis regarding the use of neuropsychological evaluation for differential diagnosis with an ambiguous onset of cognitive decline could result in findings supporting which of the following as a result of testing:
   a. A relative increase in QAY's for the patient
   b. A savings of about $40,000 due to the initiation of proper treatment and the delay in institutional care
   c. A savings of several hundred dollars due to the early implementation of early planning and decreased therapy
   d. None of the above

7. Early diagnosis of Alzheimer's disease with the help of neuropsychological testing can benefit:
    a. The patient and their families in allowing them to plan for their future
    b. The patient so that secondary treatment strategies can be implemented
    c. Society by delaying the progression and thereby the cost of the disease
    d. All of the above

8. Empirical evidence exists for increased diagnostic accuracy and prediction of dementia with neuropsychological evaluation.
    a. True
    b. False

Chapter 10: Neuropsychological Consultation and Training of Family Members of Patients with Dementia

1. Studies on Donepezil have suggested long-term cost savings among patients with mild to moderate Alzheimer's disease.
    a. True
    b. False

2. The leading cause of dementia is:
    a. Alzheimer's disease
    b. Pick's disease
    c. Lewy-Body disease
    d. Toxic exposure

3. Diagnostic accuracy in neuropsychological evaluation can be greatly enhanced in progressive dementias by:
    a. Administering the correct tests
    b. Obtaining collateral information from informants
    c. Adhering to the fixed battery approach
    d. Adhering to the flexible battery approach

4. Behavioral psychotherapy with Alzheimer's disease patients has shown minimal results.
    a. True
    b. False

5. Neuropsychological intervention is usually designed to target
    a. Cognition
    b. Affect
    c. Functional skills
    d. a, b and c

6. A study recently suggested that both individual and small-group intervention with mild dementia patients yielded equivalent results. If the relative costs of each treatment were compared, which type of cost analysis would be conducted?
    a. Efficiency
    b. Effectiveness

c. Benefit
d. Utility

7. Reality Orientation Therapy has been shown to be a potential effective, low-cost therapeutic approach with mild to moderate Alzheimer's disease patients.
   a. True
   b. False

8. Techniques such as spaced retrieval have recently been shown to enhance both subjective memory functioning and emotional well-being.
   a. True
   b. False

Chapter 11: Neuropsychological Evaluation of Patients with Epilepsy

1. How is *epilepsy* best defined?
   a. Repeated, unprovoked seizures
   b. Attacks arising primarily from the temporal lobes (e.g., TLE).
   c. A disorder usually originating in childhood with alterations in consciousness.
   d. A combination of grand mal and petit mal attacks in most people.

2. What are the two basic types of seizures?
   a. Temporal lobe seizures and generalized seizures
   b. Temporal lobe seizures and partial seizures
   c. Partial seizures and generalized seizures
   d. Grand mal seizures and petit mal seizures

3. The annual direct and indirect cost of epilepsy in the United States is approximately
   a. $2,000,000,000
   b. $12,000,000,000
   c. $20,000,000,000
   d. $50,000,000,000

4. Established quality of life correlates of epilepsy include
   a. Markedly increased unemployment rates
   b. Diminished probability of marriage
   c. Increased fears of various types
   d. All of the above

5. Which is true of the medications for epilepsy introduced in recent years?
   a. There are very few of these and they tend to have many side effects.
   b. There are very few of these but they are unusually effective in controlling seizures.
   c. There are a number of these, but their side effects are sufficiently great that they are of limited value.
   d. There are a number of these, but they have been of limited effectiveness in terms of controlling seizures which were previously uncontrolled by the older medications.

6. Neuropsychological evaluations conducted in connection with surgery for epilepsy should emphasize
   a. Functions associated with the temporal lobes
   b. Functions associated with the posterior hippocampus
   c. Emotional and psychosocial factors above cognitive factors
   d. None of the above

7. The Intracarotid Amobarbital Procedure or Wada Test is
   a. Only infrequently accomplished in modern times due to the risks involved.
   b. Of value in preventing adverse cognitive changes after surgery.
   c. Of best established value in predicting seizure relief after surgery.
   d. Accomplished most effectively by a neurologist rather than a neuropsychologist.

8. While the cost-effectiveness of neuropsychological evaluations in epilepsy is difficult to establish due to a number of factors, the existing data indicate that
   a. These evaluations are not cost-effective.
   b. These evaluations may be cost-effective but there is a serious question about this.
   c. These evaluations likely are cost-effective although supporting data are incomplete.
   d. These evaluations are definitely cost-effective as a number of long term definitive studies have already demonstrated conclusively.

Chapter 12: Nonepileptic Seizures and Their Costs: The Role of Neuropsychology

1. Approximately ??? of all Americans will have at least one seizure at some point during their lives requiring medical evaluation and treatment.
   a. 1%
   b. 5%
   c. 10%
   d. 12%

2. From ??? of the two million persons treated yearly for epilepsy in the United States are thought to have nonepileptic seizures (NEPS).
   a. 1 to 10 %
   b. 5 to 15%
   c. 10 to 20%
   d. 5 to 20%

3. Life time costs of treating individuals diagnosed as having NEPS is estimated at ??? per case.
   a. $100,000
   b. $200,000
   c. $300,000
   d. $400,000

4. The rate of primary care physician's visits by patients with diagnosed mental disorders is twice that of other patients, with ??? percent of visits to primary care physicians, primarily for psychologically-based complaints and symptoms.
   a. 10 to 30%
   b. 30 to 50%
   c. 50 to 70%
   d. 70 to 90%

5. It is estimated that ??? of patients with NEPS demonstrate abnormal neuropsychological test findings.
   a. 10%
   b. 20%
   c. 30%
   d. 50%

6. This is about the same for patients with documented epilepsy.
   a. True
   b. False

7. Patients with NEPS are a heterogenous group of individuals and do not present with clearly defined neuropsychological or psychiatric findings.
   a. True
   b. False

8. Clinical neuropsychologists evaluating patients on EMU often are the primary person to help patients understand the potential psychological basis of their symptoms and help them obtain appropriate psychiatric treatment.
   a. True
   b. False

Chapter 13: The Use of Neuropsychological Assessment in Clarifying the Educational Needs of Children with Learning Disabilities

1. The term "phonological processing" refers to
   a. The ability to associate sounds with letter-symbols.
   b. The ability to understand words heard in a song.
   c. The ability to understand what is said to you on a telephone.

2. What skill has the angular gyrus been associated with?
   a. Expressive language
   b. Visual motor integration
   c. Phonemic awareness

3. A concern of the IQ/Achievement discrepancy model is:
   a. Children with higher IQ scores are more often identified than those with lower IQ scores.
   b. Many children with learning disabilities are not identified using this model.
   c. Both of the above

4. The difference in training between a school psychologist and a neuropsychologist is:
    a. School psychologists can have either a masters level or a doctoral level degree whereas neuropsychologists must have a doctoral degree.
    b. Neuropsychologists receive intensive training on brain/behavior relationships whereas school psychologists receive more training on services provided by the school system.
    c. Neuropsychologists determine domains to be assessed using brain research whereas school psychologists' assessments are based on the IQ/Achievement learning disability paradigm.
    d. All of the above

5. A primary symptom associated with a reading disability would be poor phonological awareness, whereas a secondary symptom would be irregular eye movements.
    a. True
    b. False

6. The computer "games" designed by the Tallal group which are designed to drive improvements in temporal processing skills represent a compensatory strategy for auditory processing delays.
    a. True
    b. False

7. A concern that should be addressed in designing a cost efficiency study to compare outcome of the psychoeducational versus a neuropsychological exam would be selection bias given the greater investment (of both time and money) of the neuropsychological assessment.
    a. True
    b. False

8. Most people outgrow all symptoms of a learning disability by the time they are adults.
    a. True
    b. False

Chapter 14: The Clinical Utility and Cost-Effectiveness of Comprehensive (Holistic) Brain Injury Day-Treatment Programs

1. A holistic program may be characterized by which of the following?
    a. Emphasis on cognitive remediation
    b. Emphasis on retraining skills
    c. A primary concern with improvement on neuropsychological tests
    d. None of the above

2. Which of the following must a holistic program have?
    a. Physical therapy
    b. Speech therapy
    c. Milieu therapy
    d. Occupational therapy

3. A treatment time budget refers to which?
    a. How a staff member spends his or her time
    b. How a patient spends his or her time
    c. A way of plotting program expenses
    d. None of the above

4. The evidence for holistic rehabilitation indicates which of these?
    a. It does not work
    b. The benefits are confined to anecdotes and case studies
    c. It cannot be recommended as a standard of care
    d. There are clinical trials demonstrating efficacy

5. Which of the following is true for costs of rehabilitation?
    a. They are uniform for different payers
    b. They are public information
    c. They may involve direct and indirect outlay of funds
    d. They are impossible to calculate

6. For students of cost-effectiveness, which body of data is *most* available at present?
    a. Outcome measures
    b. Indirect costs
    c. Direct costs
    d. Revenue information

7. Which is the best method for demonstrating cost-benefits of holistic neuropsychologic rehabilitation?
    a. Long-term follow up studies
    b. Accumulation of individual case studies
    c. Outcomes of treatments with measured costs
    d. Comparing people who go to work and those who do not following rehabilitation

8. Which are direct costs involved in rehabilitation?
    a. Lost wages
    b. Actual payments to providers of rehabilitation services
    c. Extra household expenses for a family in providing care
    d. Emotional suffering due to the injury

Chapter 15: Psychotherapy After Brain Injury: Costs and Benefits

1. The rationale for individual psychotherapy after brain injury is readily apparent when one looks at:
    a. The nature and extent of acquired brain injury
    b. Preinjury abilities and deficits
    c. Each patient's unique emotional reaction and coping with new problems in function
    d. All of the above

2. Which of the following are indirect financial costs that may be incurred when troubled patients do not receive essential psychotherapy after brain injury? (Circle all that apply)
   a. Increased use of medications by family members
   b. Increased patient visits to primary care physicians occur
   c. Reduced levels of employment and taxes paid by family members staying home to care for patients
   d. Reduced enrollment by brain injured patients at local community colleges

3. What are some of the patient characteristics known to be associated with poor treatment outcome for individual psychotherapy after brain injury?
   a. Profound cognitive impairment
   b. Prior outpatient psychotherapy treatment
   c. High degree of religiosity
   d. Family history of alcoholism

4. What is one important patient characteristic found to be associated with benefit from individual psychotherapy after brain injury?
   a. Patient was "psychological-minded" before the injury
   b. Patient is able to form a therapeutic alliance
   c. Patient is very likable, with good emotional intelligence
   d. Patient is willing to come for two to three sessions a week if needed

5. What is the primary reason way that a good neuropsychological evaluation can contribute to the effectiveness of psychotherapy after brain injury? (Choose one)
   a. The evaluation and report can clearly delineate and prioritize strengths and weaknesses that should guide the focus of treatment.
   b. The testing process gives patients a chance to get comfortable with a psychologist via an all day evaluation and is likely to smooth the course of treatment.
   c. The neuropsychological evaluation provides useful information regarding patient endurance and levels of fatigue that may impact treatment.
   d. The neuropsychological evaluation provides useful information regarding patient commitment and effort that may impact treatment.

Chapter 16: Does Cognitive Rehabilitation Work? Clinical and Economic Considerations and Outcomes

1. Holistic rehabilitation approaches emphasize that:
   a. Emotional and cognitive problems should be treated separately.
   b. Emotional problems should be addressed before attempts are made to reduce cognitive problems.
   c. Cognitive problems should be addressed before attempts are made to reduce emotional problems.
   d. Emotional and cognitive problems should be addressed in parallel.

2. Evaluation of cognitive rehabilitation may be especially evaluated by:
   a. Double blind randomized control trials

b. Single blind randomized control trials
c. Selecting the appropriate design to answer the research question
d. Single case experimental designs

3. The patient/client's response to treatment should be measured primarily by:
   a. Change on questionnaires, checklists, and rating scales
   b. Change on measures of disability and handicap
   c. Change on standardized neuropsychological tests
   d. Change on therapists' observations

4. Single case experimental designs are particularly useful for:
   a. Monitoring an individual's change over time
   b. Monitoring the average change of a group of individuals
   c. Monitoring change of a single point during rehabilitation
   d. Monitoring the influence of motivation on rehabilitation

5. Presently, most cognitive rehabilitation programs work through:
   a. Restoring damaged cognitive functions
   b. Retraining damaged cognitive functions
   c. Developing alternative pathways to take over damaged cognitive functions
   d. Compensating for damaged cognitive functions

6. We can enhance learning in people with severe memory deficits by:
   a. Avoiding trial-and-error learning
   b. Repeating material or information to be learned
   c. Helping people to learn from their mistakes
   d. Teaching the use of mnemonic strategies

7. NeuroPage provides an excellent example of a cost-saving approach in the rehabilitation of brain injured patients:
   a. True
   b. False

8. The major influences on cognitive rehabilitation have been:
   a. Cognitive neuroscience
   b. Cognitive neuropsychology
   c. Cognitive rehabilitation
   d. Cognitive behavioral therapy

Chapter 17: Neuropsychological Assessment of Sport-Related Mild Traumatic Brain Injury

1. Which of the following test **is not** included in the NFL neuropsychological test battery?
   a. The Hopkins Verbal Learning Test
   b. A concussion symptom inventory
   c. The Rey Complex Figure Test
   d. Symbol Search from the WAIS-III.
   e. The Trail Making Test

2. Decisions regarding retirement of the professional athlete is often complicated by the following factor(s)
   a. Financial incentives to play
   b. No current criteria for retirement
   c. A culture of "playing hurt"
   d. A history of multiple concussions
   e. All of the above

3. Which of the following is not true regarding the NHL Neuropsychology program?
   a. It is primarily a research project rather than a clinical program
   b. The program utilizes a network of neuropsychologists throughout Canada and the United States
   c. Implementation of the program was affected by the inclusion of athletes for whom English is a second language
   d. Baseline testing is a primary component of the program
   e. All of the above are true

4. The use of Baseline testing in sports neuropsychology is important because:
   a. It provides pre-injury data against which post-concussion data may be compared.
   b. It helps to account for the marked variability that exists in athletes' neurocognitive functioning.
   c. The athlete can be used as his or her own control.
   d. All of the above.

5. Return to Play following cerebral concussion is:
   a. Based solely on the published guideline for return to play.
   b. Is a complex interaction of many different variables including neuropsychological data.
   c. A decision that should be made based on symptoms alone.
   d. None of the above

6. Neuropsychological testing of athletes is often conducted at which of the following sites?
   a. A bar
   b. A locker room
   c. On the sidelines
   d. In the parking lot

7. Sports Neuropsychology has it's origins in the study of mild TBI focused on the general clinical population.
   a. True
   b. False

8. The Sports as a Laboratory Assessment Model (SLAM) was developed:
   a. to study the acceleration forces in athletics.
   b. to study mild TBI in a controlled setting.
   c. to provide evidence for the equivalence of animal and human models of concussion.
   d. to test helmet protection designs.

9. Concussion in college football follows a five to ten day recovery curve.
    a. True
    b. False

Chapter 18: Neuropsychological Assessment of Physicians Whose Competency to Practice Medicine Is Being Questioned

1. Neuropsychological assessment of cognitive competency to practice medicine relies on which of the following?
    a. Physician-specific norms
    b. Considerations of the age of physician
    c. A unique battery of tests
    d. Good clinical judgement

2. When should physicians whose competency to practice medicine is being questioned be referred for neuropsychological evaluation?
    a. They have had a stroke
    b. They are 75 years or older
    c. They fail a Mental Status Exam
    d. Colleagues comment on memory problems
    e. All of the above

3. Research exploring the relationship between physician residents' cognitive test performances and performance ratings has suggested which of the following?
    a. Cognitive test performance is less strongly related to ratings than medical test scores
    b. Cognitive test performance is more highly related than medical test scores
    c. Neither cognitive performance nor medical test score performance is related to resident ratings.

4. Reasons reported for physicians not seeking early medical treatment for symptoms include which? (Circle all that apply.)
    a. Overconfidence in their own ability
    b. Concerns about confidentiality
    c. Worry about the impact on their practice
    d. Lack of faith in the medical profession

5. Cognitive impairment is perceived to cause poor medical practice in what percentage of cases that come to the attention of legal or regulatory agencies?
    a. Almost all
    b. A majority
    c. About half
    d. A small minority

6. Advantages of comprehensive neuropsychological evaluation in the assessment of physician competency to practice medicine include which?
    a. Low cost
    b. Physician-specific norms
    c. Breadth and depth of coverage
    d. Known sensitivity to subtle physician impairment

7. Advantages of neuropsychological screening in the assessment of physician competency to practice medicine include which?
    a. Low cost
    b. Physician-specific norms
    c. Breadth and depth of coverage
    d. Known sensitivity to subtle physician impairment

8. Interviews with professionals involved in the assessment of physician competency revealed that neuropsychological evaluation is perceived as which?
    a. Worthless
    b. Cheap
    c. Objective
    d. Definitive

Chapter 19: Clinical Neuropsychology in the Forensic Arena

1. All of the following are markers of value of neuropsychological assessment for attorneys EXCEPT:
    a. There is a viable professional making statements about brain functioning based on normative data.
    b. The credibility of a client's testimony can be reinforced by neuropsychological examination findings.
    c. The neuropsychological test data can determine if a client is guilty or innocent.
    d. Determination of the gravity of reported is greatly enhanced by having an objective evaluation conducted by an individual bound by a code of ethics.

2. Neuropsychologists are commonly utilized in which of the following cases:
    a. Disability determination
    b. Education due process within public school systems
    c. Personal injury
    d. Child custody
    e. All of the above

3. Which is true about forensic neuropsychological work?
    a. There are no differences between forensic neuropsychological work and neuropsychological work conducted in a university medical center.
    b. There is a special certification required for forensic neuropsychological work.
    c. Forensic neuropsychological work by it very nature is adversarial and antagonistic.
    d. The neuropsychological work is not recognized as meeting the Frye test.

4. All of the following are potential mitigating factors in the eyes of the court, during criminal proceedings, except:
    a. Mental retardation
    b. Crossed handedness
    c. Learning disability
    d. Psychosis

5. The value of neuropsychology in civil litigation is most often judged in monetary terms
   a. True
   b. False

6. Neuropsychological data can support making a decision about competency to stand trial in all instances except:
   a. Divorce proceedings
   b. Not guilty by reason of insanity
   c. Diminished capacity
   d. Diminished responsibility

7. A man with a history of frontal lobe injury impulsively assaults a stranger. His neuropsychological impairment suggests that he likely has:
   a. Diminished capacity
   b. Diminished responsibility
   c. Insanity
   d. Hysteria

8. The standard that courts recognize to indicate that neuropsychological tests are generally accepted in the field of neuropsychology is the:
   a. Daubert
   b. Frye Test
   c. McNaughten Standard
   d. The American Law Institute Standard

Chapter 20: The Neuropsychological Examination in the Detection of Malingering in the Forensic Arena: Costs and Benefits

1. As used in the chapter, "dissimulators" are individuals who
   a. are healthy but fake a mental illness
   b. are healthy but fake a physical illness
   c. have a mental disorder but fake being healthy
   d. fake either a physical disorder or mental disorder

2. Base rate information influences test effectiveness most when
   a. there is a 50% base rate for the condition being diagnosed
   b. when the base rate is extremely low or high
   c. when the test has a very low combined error rate
   d. none of the above

3. According to the USDOJ, what percentage of civil lawsuits filed go to trial
   a. 1%
   b. 3%
   c. 5%
   d. 15%

4. According to Wetter and Corrigan (1995), what percentage of attorneys believed it was their job to advise clients about validity measures in psychological testing?
   a. 22%
   b. 49%
   c. 63%
   d. 74%

5. One should routinely ask clients what they have learned from their attornies about psychological evaluation procedures and validity testing.
   a. True
   b. False

6. Rank order the following costs of malingering from least costly to most costly:
   a. defense costs, settlement and trial awards, medical expenses
   b. medical expenses, defense costs, settlement and trial awards
   c. defense costs, medical expenses, settlement and trail awards
   d. medical expenses, settlement and trial awards, defense costs

7. High test specificity guards primarily against
   a. Type I false positive errors
   b. Type II false negative errors
   c. Type I and Type II errors equally
   d. none of the above

8. High test sensitivity guards primarily against
   a. Type I false positive errors
   b. Type II false negative errors
   c. Type I and Type II errors equally
   d. none of the above

Chapter 21: Measuring the Economics of Neuropsychology

1. Treatment algorithms can potentially inform service providers, patients and third party payers by:
   a. providing them with a framework regarding available treatment approaches and a means of proceeding through options in sequential steps.
   b. determining the relative costs of various treatments in different geographic regions.
   c. identifying the frequency with which a given provider administers a particular treatment and his/her rate of success with that approach.
   d. Calculating a "treatment valence" by multiplying the cost of a given disease state times its prevalence and dividing by the number of clinicians capable of providing treatment within a specified geographical region.

2. Determining the extent to which health care resources are utilized to treat various disease states is a challenge to researchers. There are several means of establishing "use of care," each of which has its advantages and disadvantages. Which of the

following methods is least likely to produce reliable results if a given health problem was minor, remote, or the patient sustained cognitive impairment?

a. the abstraction of information from patients' medical records that are maintained by health care providers.
b. the patients' self report of his/her health state and treatments received to maintain health.
c. the extraction of health care utilization information from administrative or computerized databases maintained from managed care organizations.
d. Each of the above methods is equally likely to provide accurate information regarding use of care.

3. The healing arts pose additional challenges to the theory of the invisible hand, which refers to the role of competition in balancing the demand of the consumer and the producers' capacity to supply. One of those challenges is described as "moral hazard." "Moral hazard" in this context refers to the fact that:
   a. some health care professionals will offer less than satisfactory or insufficient services in the interest of containing their costs.
   b. consumers of health care reap the benefits of that care but pay for only a portion of its cost due to third party payers, which potentially leads to higher costs than would otherwise be the case.
   c. irresponsible, high-risk behavior places increased demands on health care providers, thereby reducing the potential for those providers to supply health care to treat unavoidable illnesses.
   d. limitations in the supply of health care results in providers treating some affected individuals while denying treatment to others.

4. Cost research takes two forms: "Cost of Illness" and "Cost Outcome" studies. Which of the following is <u>not</u> an example of information that is incorporated in research regarding "Cost of Illness" studies:
   a. the affected individual's lost wages and productivity as a result of his/her illness.
   b. the care giver's lost wages and productivity as a result of caring for the affected individual
   c. the evaluation of an intervention that is implemented to treat a given health problem versus its result in improving the individual's health state.
   d. the total cost of all diagnostic, assessment, and treatment of the given illness or injury.

5. Two approaches used to determine the value of human life are "human capital" and "willingness to pay" measures. The first approach establishes the value of human life in terms of the production potential of the patient in the home and the labor market. The second approach establishes the amount of money that patients are willing and able to spend to avoid the symptoms of a given disease state. The use of such estimates has been criticized because
   a. they implicitly undervalue the very young because they are not currently working and will not be for a long period of time.
   b. they implicitly undervalue the elderly who typically have a shorter remaining productive life.

c. they introduce a "wealth bias" that places greater value on the health values of individuals with more financial resources.
d. all of the above.

6. Establishing the value of clinical services sometimes involves ascertaining the undesirability of the disease state that those services are designed to treat. One means of establishing the undesirability of a given health state is the use of "standard gamble." This refers to:
   a. The risk of death that a patient is willing to accept in pursuing a treatment to end a given health state.
   b. The length of time that an individual is willing to forgo health insurance in order to allocate those financial resources to other purposes and, in essence, "gamble" that illness or injury is unlikely.
   c. The willingness of an individual to accept a less costly treatment alternative that has been determined to be only slightly less effective than a much more expensive intervention.
   d. The amount of money that an individual is willing to pay for health care insurance or membership in a health maintenance organization to avoid incurring other costs of treatment.

7. Receiving neuropsychological services has the potential to result in reduced health care costs. A reason for this outcome is:
   a. "Substitution:" Patients might otherwise attempt to get neuropsychological services from a more costly health service provider.
   b. "Adherence:" Physicians who are better informed regarding the patient's condition may be better able to help the patient comply with a treatment regimen and improve the outcome of that treatment.
   c. "Treatment productivity:" The referring physician may be more efficient in utilizing health care services and achieve the patient's health goals with fewer resources if s/he is informed about the patient's neurocognitive status.
   d. All of the above.

8. The application of neuropsychological services has the potential to result in increased medical costs, because:
   a. The neuropsychologist might identify a health state that would otherwise have gone undetected and, consequently, not received costly treatment.
   b. Patients who receive and benefit from neuropsychological services may begin to place greater importance on their health and consume more medical care to maintain good health.
   c. Patients who benefit from neuropsychological intervention and are able to re-enter the work force may gain the financial resources to consume more health care services, which in turn would help to drive up costs."
   d. All of the above.

AUTHOR INDEX

SUBJECT INDEX

ABOUT THE EDITORS

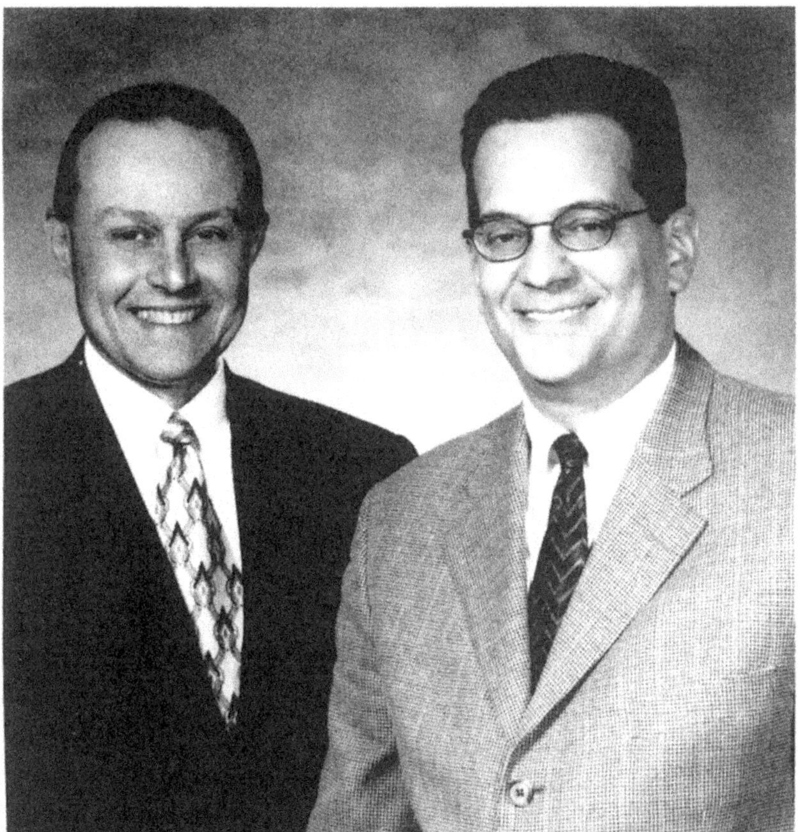

George P. Prigatano is the Newsome Chairman of the Section of Clinical Neuropsychology at the Barrow Neurological Institute and Past President (1998) of the National Academy of Neuropsychology.

Neil H. Pliskin is Professor and Chief of the Neuropsychology Division at the University of Illinois College of Medicine and the Vice-Chair of the Policy and Planning Committee of the National Academy of Neuropsychology.

www.ingramcontent.com/pod-product-compliance
Ingram Content Group UK Ltd.
Pitfield, Milton Keynes, MK11 3LW, UK
UKHW022005180926
475701UK00003B/201
9780415763578